Cardiac Pacing and ICDs

Cardiac Pacing and ICDs

7th Edition

EDITED BY

Kenneth A. Ellenbogen, MD

Kimmerling Professor of Cardiology and Chairman of the Division of Cardiology
VCU / Pauley Heart Center
Director of Clinical Cardiac Electrophysiology and Pacing
Medical College of Virginia / VCU School of Medicine
Richmond, VA, USA

Karoly Kaszala, MD, PhD

Associate Professor of Medicine
VCU / Pauley Heart Center
Medical College of Virginia / VCU School of Medicine
Director of Electrophysiology
Hunter Holmes McGuire VA Medical Center
Richmond, VA, USA

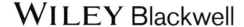

Registered Office(s)
John Wiley & Sons, Inc., 111 River Street, Hoboken, NJ 07030, USA
John Wiley & Sons Ltd, The Atrium, Southern Gate, Chichester, West Sussex, PO19 8SQ, UK

Editorial Office
9600 Garsington Road, Oxford, OX4 2DQ, UK

For details of our global editorial offices, customer services, and more information about Wiley products visit us at www.wiley.com.

Wiley also publishes its books in a variety of electronic formats and by print-on-demand. Some content that appears in standard print versions of this book may not be available in other formats.

Library of Congress Cataloging-in-Publication Data

Names: Ellenbogen, Kenneth A., editor. | Kaszala, Karoly, editor.
Title: Cardiac pacing and ICDs / edited by Kenneth A. Ellenbogen, Karoly Kaszala.
Description: Seventh edition. | Hoboken, NJ : John Wiley & Sons, 2020. | Includes bibliographical references and index.
Identifiers: LCCN 2020005340 (print) | LCCN 2020005341 (ebook) | ISBN 9781119578338 (paperback) | ISBN 9781119578352 (adobe pdf) | ISBN 9781119578284 (epub)
Subjects: MESH: Cardiac Pacing, Artificial | Pacemaker, Artificial | Defibrillators, Implantable
Classification: LCC RC684.P3 (print) | LCC RC684.P3 (ebook) | NLM WG 166.5.C2 | DDC 617.4/120645–dc23
LC record available at https://lccn.loc.gov/2020005340
LC ebook record available at https://lccn.loc.gov/2020005341

Cover Design: Wiley
Cover Images: © toysf400/Shutterstock, © Richman Photo/Shutterstock

Set in 9.5/12pt Minion Pro by SPi Global, Pondicherry, India

Printed in Great Britain by Bell & Bain Ltd, Glasgow

10 9 8 7 6

Contents

List of Contributors

Jeffrey A. Brinker, MD
Professor of Medicine
Johns Hopkins University School of Medicine
Baltimore, MD, USA

T. Jared Bunch, MD
Professor of Medicine
Division of Cardiovascular Medicine
University of Utah School of Medicine
Salt Lake City, UT, USA

Yong-Mei Cha, MD
Consultant and Professor of Medicine
Department of Cardiovascular Diseases
Division of Heart Rhythm Services
Mayo Clinic
Rochester, MN, USA

John D. Day, MD
Intermountain Heart Rhythm Specialists
Intermountain Heart Institute
Intermountain Medical Center
Salt Lake City, UT, USA

Kenneth A. Ellenbogen, MD
Kimmerling Professor of Cardiology and Chairman of
the Division of Cardiology
VCU / Pauley Heart Center
Director of Clinical Cardiac Electrophysiology and Pacing
Medical College of Virginia / VCU School of Medicine
Richmond, VA, USA

Michael E. Field, MD
Cardiac Electrophysiologist, Professor of Medicine
Medical University of South Carolina
Charleston, SC, USA

Michael R. Gold, MD
Michael Assey Chair in Cardiology
Professor of Medicine
Medical University of South Carolina
Charleston, SC, USA

Michael Hoosien, MD
Cardiac Electrophysiologist, Piedmont Heart Institute
Piedmont Atlanta Hospital
Atlanta, GA, USA

Jose F. Huizar, MD
Director, Arrhythmia and Device Clinic
Hunter Holmes McGuire VA Medical Center
Associate Professor of Medicine
VCU School of Medicine
Richmond, VA, USA

Kevin P. Jackson, MD
Associate Professor of Medicine
Duke University, School of Medicine
Durham, NC, USA

Roy M. John, MBBS, PhD, FRCP
Director, Center for Advanced Management
of Ventricular Arrhythmias
Northshore University Hospital
Manhasset, NY, USA

Karoly Kaszala, MD, PhD
Associate Professor of Medicine
VCU / Pauley Heart Center
Medical College of Virginia / VCU School of Medicine
Director of Electrophysiology
Hunter Holmes McGuire VA Medical Center
Richmond, VA, USA

Ammar M. Killu, MBBS
Consultant and Assistant Professor of Medicine
Department of Cardiovascular Diseases, Division of
Heart Rhythm Services
Mayo Clinic
Rochester, MN, USA

Justin Z. Lee, MD
Clinical Cardiac Electrophysiology Fellow
Mayo Clinic
Rochester, MN, USA

Charles J. Love, MD
Professor of Medicine
Johns Hopkins University School of Medicine
Baltimore, MD, USA

Joseph E. Marine, MD
Vice-Director, Division of Cardiology
Associate Professor of Medicine
Johns Hopkins University School of Medicine
Baltimore, MD, USA

Siva K. Mulpuru, MD
Consultant, Division of Cardiovascular Diseases
Associate Professor of Medicine
Mayo Clinic
Rochester, MN, USA

Jeffrey S. Osborn, MD
Intermountain Heart Rhythm Specialists
Intermountain Heart Institute
Intermountain Medical Center
Salt Lake City, UT, USA

Kristen K. Patton, MD
Professor of Medicine
University of Washington
Seattle, WA, USA

Arun R.M. Sridhar, MD, MPH
Assistant Professor of Medicine
University of Washington
Seattle, WA, USA

Bruce S. Stambler, MD
Cardiac Electrophysiologist, Piedmont Heart Institute
Piedmont Atlanta Hospital
Atlanta, GA, USA

Vaibhav Vaidya, MD
Clinical Cardiac Electrophysiology Fellow
Mayo Clinic
Rochester, MN, USA

Niraj Varma, MD, PhD
Staff Physician
Cardiac Electrophysiology and Pacing
Heart and Vascular Institute
Cleveland Clinic
Cleveland, OH, USA

Preface

Management of an aging population with increasing co-morbidities challenges each of us every day and individualizing patient treatment using an evidence-based approach is a common goal of health care providers. Device therapy to treat cardiac arrhythmias remains relevant as device indications expand and survival in chronic disease increases. Our aim with this new edition of the book is to provide an up-to-date source of basic principles and a resource for device technicians, industry representatives, medical students, nurses, residents and fellows and anyone interested in the care of patients with cardiac implantable electronic devices (CIEDs) or interest in cardiac device therapy. Most sections of this book have undergone extensive revision with several key chapters being completely revised. All chapters were updated to include the most relevant clinical progress. Discussions about indications for device therapy now reflects the most current ACC/AHA clinical guidelines. We took a fresh look at different device and lead components and pacing physiology and hemodynamics. Basic pacemaker function and pacing algorithms are extensively discussed along with troubleshooting. The hemodynamic, pacemaker timing cycles, device algorithm and troubleshooting sections all are updated to summarize the most current, clinically relevant scenarios. Since the last edition, several important advances in device therapy became commonplace. Novel technologies, such as leadless pacemakers, His bundle pacing, and subcutaneous ICDs offer alternative therapies to patients and these therapies have reached mainstream application. Beyond discussing the basics of pacing and defibrillation, in the current edition there are step-by-step instructions for the implant procedure. Indications, best uses, and the nuts and bolts of these novel technologies are added and explained. Numerous real-life examples are included to illustrate specific problems and troubleshooting. It is hard to believe that 8 years ago we had only limited availability and acceptance of quadripolar left ventricular pacing leads for cardiac resynchronization therapy and now this is the norm. These chapters have been updated with new information on multi-site pacing. Over the last five years, patient follow-up has been revolutionized with widespread use of remote monitoring and the final chapter provides a thorough review of current evidence and standard practice for patient follow-up.

Of course this book would have never come to fruition without the support of Wiley and the meticulous work of the authors to whom we are greatly indebted. Their outstanding contributions are reflected through each chapter, with excellent summaries of complex topics written in a simplified yet clinically relevant manner and supported by great illustrations. We hope that this new edition will continue to be a helpful resource to all of our colleagues who are interested in learning about cardiac device therapy

Kenneth A. Ellenbogen, MD
Karoly Kaszala, MD, PhD
VCU / Pauley Heart Center
Medical College of Virginia/VCU School of Medicine
Richmond, VA, USA
February 2020

Acknowledgments

To my parents, Roslyn and Leon Ellenbogen, who inspired a lifelong thirst for learning. To my wife, Phyllis, and children, Michael, Amy, and Bethany, whose patience and love made this project successful.

Kenneth A. Ellenbogen, MD

To my parents, the late Karoly and Dr Agnes Kaszala for their guidance, unconditional support and love, to my wife Gabriella, and children Julia, Dalma, and Balazs for their love, patience and understanding.

Karoly Kaszala, MD, PhD

CHAPTER 1

Indications for permanent cardiac pacing

Roy M. John

Center for Advanced Management of Ventricular Arrhythmias, Northshore University Hospital, Manhasset, NY, USA

Introduction

Defects of cardiac impulse generation and conduction can occur at various levels in the cardiac conduction system. In general, intrinsic disease of the conduction system is often diffuse. For example, normal atrioventricular (AV) conduction cannot necessarily be assumed when a pacemaker is implanted for a disorder seemingly localized to the sinus node. Similarly, normal sinus node function cannot be assumed when a pacemaker is implanted in a patient with AV block. Conduction disorders that lead to important bradycardia or asystole may result from reversible or irreversible causes. Recognition of reversible causes is critical to avoid unnecessary commitment to long-term pacemaker therapy. This chapter reviews the common disorders that warrant cardiac pacing and lists the recommended indications set out by published guidelines.

Anatomy and physiology of the conduction system

For a complete understanding of rhythm generation and intracardiac conduction, and of their pathology, a brief review of the anatomy and physiology of the specialized conduction system is warranted.

Sinus node

The sinus node or sinoatrial (SA) node is a crescent-shaped subepicardial structure located at the junction of the right atrium and superior vena cava along the terminal crest. It measures 10–20 mm (with larger extension in some studies) and has abundant autonomic innervation and blood supply, with the sinus node artery commonly coursing through the body of the node. Endocardially, the crista terminalis overlies the nodal tissue, although the inferior aspect of the node has a more subendocardial course. Histologically, the sinus node comprises specialized nodal cells (P cells) packed within a dense matrix of connective tissue. At the periphery, these nodal cells intermingle with transitional cells and the atrial working myocardium, with radiations extending toward the superior vena cava, the crista terminalis, and the intercaval regions [1,2]. The absence of a distinct border and the presence of distal fragmentation explain the lack of a single breakthrough of the sinus node excitatory wavefront. The radiations of the node, although histologically distinct, are not insulated from the atrial myocardium. Hence, a clear anatomical SA junction is absent. The sinus node is protected from the hyperpolarizing effect of the surrounding atria, probably by its unique structure wherein electrical coupling between cells and

Cardiac Pacing and ICDs, Seventh Edition. Edited by Kenneth A. Ellenbogen and Karoly Kaszala.
© 2020 John Wiley & Sons Ltd. Published 2020 by John Wiley & Sons Ltd.

expression of ion channels vary from the center of the node to the periphery. The pacemaker cells at the center of the node are more loosely coupled, while those at the periphery are more tightly coupled with higher density I_f (funny current, a mixed sodium and potassium current carried by the HCN channels) and I_{Na} currents [2].

The SA node has the highest rate of spontaneous depolarization (automaticity) in the specialized conduction system and is responsible for the generation of the cardiac impulse under normal circumstances, although normal human pacemaker activity may be widely distributed in the atrium. The unique location of the sinus node astride the large SA nodal artery provides an ideal milieu for continuous monitoring and instantaneous adjustment of heart rate to meet the body's changing metabolic needs.

Impulse generation in the sinus node remains incompletely understood. Sinus nodal cells have a low resting membrane potential of −50 to −60 mV.

Spontaneous diastolic (phase 4) depolarizations are probably triggered by several currents, including I_f. The predominant inward current in the center of the node is I_{CaL} that generates a "slow" action potential. The action potentials spread peripherally into the musculature of the terminal crest. In the periphery of the node, I_{Na} is operative and necessary for providing sufficient inward current to depolarize the larger mass of atrial tissue. Defects of a number of molecular and biophysical factors that govern the ionic channels of the sinus node can lead to sinus node dysfunction (Figure 1.1).

Differential sensitivity to adrenergic and vagal inputs exists along the nodal pacemaker cells, such that superior sites tend to dominate during adrenergic drive while the inferior sites predominate during vagal stimulation [3]. Interventions including premature stimulation, autonomic stimulation, and drugs have been shown to induce pacemaker shifts (due to multicentric origins) with variable exit locations [4].

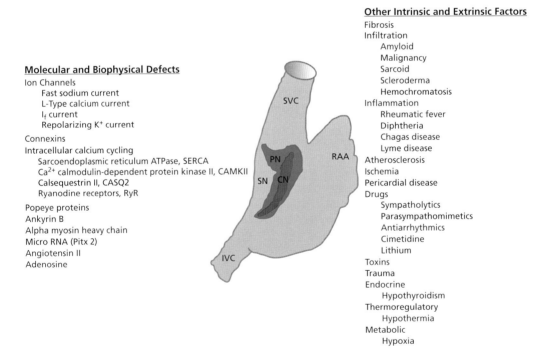

Other Intrinsic and Extrinsic Factors
Fibrosis
Infiltration
    Amyloid
    Malignancy
    Sarcoid
    Scleroderma
    Hemochromatosis
Inflammation
    Rheumatic fever
    Diphtheria
    Chagas disease
    Lyme disease
Atherosclerosis
Ischemia
Pericardial disease
Drugs
    Sympatholytics
    Parasympathomimetics
    Antiarrhythmics
    Cimetidine
    Lithium
Toxins
Trauma
Endocrine
    Hypothyroidism
Thermoregulatory
    Hypothermia
Metabolic
    Hypoxia

Molecular and Biophysical Defects
Ion Channels
    Fast sodium current
    L-Type calcium current
    I_f current
    Repolarizing K^+ current
Connexins
Intracellular calcium cycling
    Sarcoendoplasmic reticulum ATPase, SERCA
    Ca^{2+} calmodulin-dependent protein kinase II, CAMKII
    Calsequestrin II, CASQ2
    Ryanodine receptors, RyR
Popeye proteins
Ankyrin B
Alpha myosin heavy chain
Micro RNA (Pitx 2)
Angiotensin II
Adenosine

Figure 1.1 Summary of factors contributing to sinus node (SN) dysfunction. The central node (CN) shown in red is surrounded by the peripheral nodal (PN) structure in blue. RAA, right atrial appendage; SVC, superior vena cava; IVC, inferior vena cava. Source: modified from Monfredi O, Boyett MR. Sinus sinus syndrome and atrial fibrillation in older persons: a view from the sinoatrial nodal myocyte. *J Mol Cell Cardiol* 2015;83:88–100. Reproduced with permission of Elsevier.

Atrioventricular node

The compact AV node is a subendocardial structure situated within the triangle of Koch and measuring 5–7 mm in length and 2–5 mm in width [5,6]. On the atrial side, the node is an integral part of the atrial musculature, in contrast to the AV bundle which is insulated within the central fibrous body and merges with the His bundle. Based on action potential morphology in rabbit hearts, atrial (A), nodal (N), and His (H) cells have been defined. Intermediate cell types such as AN and NH define areas toward the atrial and His bundle ends of the compact node, respectively. Histologically, the mid nodal part has densely packed cells in a basket-like structure interposed between the His bundle and the loose atrial approaches to the node. The AN cells are composed primarily of transitional cells. Distinct electrical and morphological specialization is seen only in the progressively distal His fibers. Rightward and leftward posterior extensions of the AV node were described by Inoue and Becker [7]. These extensions have clinical implications for defining reentrant circuits that act as a substrate of AV nodal reentrant tachycardia.

The AV node has extensive autonomic innervation and an abundant blood supply from the large AV nodal artery, a branch of the right coronary artery, in 90% of patients, and from the left circumflex artery in 10% (Figure 1.2). AV nodal conduction is mediated via "slow" calcium-mediated action potential and demonstrates decremental conduction due to post-repolarization refractoriness as a result of delayed recovery of the slow inward currents. AV nodal tissue closer to the His bundle (NH and proximal His bundle area) generates junctional escape rhythms (Figure 1.3). Escape rates are dependent on the site of dominant pacemaker activity. Isoproterenol stimulation, for example, accelerates junctional escape and shifts the dominant activity to the transitional cells in the AN region and posterior extensions of the node [8–10].

His–Purkinje system

Purkinje fibers emerging from the area of the distal AV node converge gradually to form the His bundle, a narrow tubular structure that runs through or around the membranous septum to the crest of the muscular septum, where it divides into the bundle branches. The bulk of the His bundle cells contribute to the left bundle branch with a smaller contribution to the right bundle. Longitudinal strands of Purkinje fibers, divided into separate parallel compartments by a collagenous skeleton, can be discerned by histological examination of the His bundle [11]. The collagen sheathing minimizes lateral spread of impulses from the main body of the bundle branches. The rapid conduction of electrical impulses across the His–Purkinje system is responsible for the almost simultaneous activation of the right and left ventricles. The His bundle has relatively sparse autonomic innervation, although its blood supply is quite ample, emanating from both the AV nodal artery and the septal branches of the left anterior descending artery (Figure 1.2).

The bundle branch system is a complex network of interlaced Purkinje fibers that varies greatly among individuals. It generally starts as one or

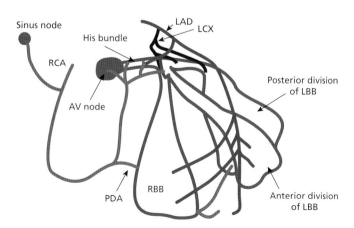

Figure 1.2 Schematic of the conduction system with arterial supply shown. LAD, left anterior descending coronary artery; LBB, left bundle branch; LCX, left circumflex coronary artery; RBB, right bundle branch; RCA, right coronary artery.

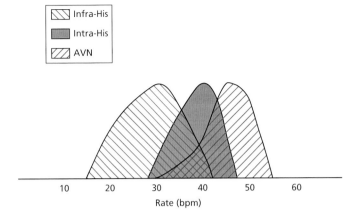

Figure 1.3 Rate of escape rhythm from various areas of the atrioventricular conduction system. AVN, atrioventricular node; infra-His, below the bundle of His; intra-His, within the bundle of His.

more large fiber bands that split and fan out across the ventricles until they finally terminate in a Purkinje network that interfaces with the myocardium (Figure 1.2). In some cases, the bundle branches clearly conform to a tri- or quadri-fascicular system. In other cases, however, detailed dissection of the conduction system has failed to delineate separate fascicles. The right bundle is usually a single discrete structure that extends down the right side of the interventricular septum to the base of the anterior papillary muscle, where it divides into three or more branches. The left bundle more commonly originates as a very broad band of interlaced fibers that spread out over the left ventricle, sometimes in two or three distinct fiber tracts. There is relatively little autonomic innervation of the bundle branch system, but the blood supply is extensive, with most areas receiving branches from both the right and left coronary systems.

His–Purkinje conduction disease may be relatively proximal in some patients and can potentially be overcome by pacing distal to the site of block. His bundle pacing is thus feasible in some patients with left bundle branch in order to normalize QRS complexes and synchronize ventricular contraction [12].

Indications for permanent pacemakers

Permanent pacing is considered in a number of clinical situations, some of which are unambiguous whereas others require a higher level of expertise for determination of potential benefit. The main factors that determine the need for cardiac pacing

are (i) symptoms associated with a bradyarrhythmia, (ii) the site of conduction abnormality in the conduction system, and (iii) the presence of conditions associated with progressive AV conduction abnormalities (e.g. genetic cardiomyopathies). In addition, the determination will depend on whether the conduction disease is likely to be permanent or reversible, such as due to a drug effect or acute inflammatory or ischemic process. A permanent pacemaker is generally a lifelong commitment for a patient; the need for generator changes and surgical revisions for malfunction become important considerations in younger patients. Hence, the decision to implant a pacemaker is not to be taken lightly.

A joint committee of the American College of Cardiology (ACC) and the American Heart Association (AHA) was formed in the 1980s to provide uniform criteria for pacemaker implantation. A recent update in conjunction with the Heart Rhythm Society was published in 2018 [13]. It is recognized that there will be cases that cannot be categorized based on these guidelines. Nevertheless, these guidelines have wide endorsement.

All guideline recommendations are subdivided into three classes to reflect the magnitude of treatment effect (Table 1.1). A class I indication pertains to a condition in which the procedure or intervention confers definite benefits. A class III indication is one where the intervention is not helpful and potentially harmful, and hence not recommended.

Additionally, the evidence supporting recommendations is ranked by the following criteria for level of evidence.

- *Level A*: Data derived from multiple randomized controlled trials (RCTs) involving a large number

Table 1.1 Classes of guideline recommendations

Class I	Conditions for which there is evidence and/or general agreement that a pacemaker implantation is beneficial, useful, and effective
Class II	Conditions for which there is conflicting evidence and/or a divergence of opinion about the usefulness/efficacy of pacemaker implantation
Class IIa	Weight of evidence/opinion in favor of efficacy
Class IIb	Usefulness/efficacy less well established by evidence/opinion
Class III	Conditions for which there is evidence and/or general agreement that a pacemaker is not useful/effective and in some cases may be harmful

of patients; meta-analysis of high-quality RCTs; one or more RCTs corroborated by high-quality registry studies.

- *Level B-R* (randomized): Moderate-quality evidence from one or more RCTs or from meta-analyses of moderate-quality RCTs.
- *Level B-NR* (non-randomized): Moderate-quality evidence from one or more non-randomized studies, observational studies or registry studies; meta-analyses of such studies.
- *Level C-LD* (limited data): Randomized or non-randomized observational or registry studies with limitations of design or execution; meta-analyses of such studies; physiological or mechanistic studies in human subjects.
- *Level C-EO* (expert opinion): Consensus based on clinical experience.

Some class I indications will necessarily lack support from level A evidence due to early non-randomized studies documenting clear benefits such that randomized trials become unethical.

Sinus node dysfunction

Disorders of the sinus node can be divided into those primarily due to intrinsic pathology of the node and surrounding atrium, or extrinsic factors such as autonomic stimulation or drug effects (Figure 1.1). The terms sinus node disease (SND), sick sinus

syndrome, and SA disease are often used interchangeably. All refer to a broad range of abnormalities in the sinus node and atrial impulse formation and propagation (Table 1.2). They include persistent sinus bradycardia and/or chronotropic incompetence without identified cause, intermittent or persistent sinus arrest, and SA exit block. Frequently, atrial arrhythmias and sinus nodal dysfunction coexist and cause symptomatic sinus pauses at cessation of an atrial arrhythmia (Figure 1.4). The term tachy–brady syndrome is applied because of the frequent need for bradycardia support with pacing to allow antiarrhythmic therapy for the tachycardia.

Pathology intrinsic to the sinus node is quite common, and its incidence increases with advancing age. Several patterns have been identified: a diffuse or localized atriopathy has been suggested. Electrophysiological studies have shown structural remodeling, particularly along the long axis of the crista terminalis, and associated with a more caudal migration of the atrial pacemaker activity [8]. Progressive downregulation of the I_{CaL} channel and loss of connexin-43 expression are features in the guinea pig model [14]. In humans, such atriopathy is also associated with atrial arrhythmias, particularly atrial fibrillation that develops in 50% of patients with SND. Atrial arrhythmias further aggravate SND, and catheter ablation of fibrillation and flutter has been shown to reverse some of the adverse electrical remodeling of the sinus node [15]. Atrophic or hypoplastic sinus node has been described in association with congenital anomalies. A familial form of SND is also recognized. Finally, idiopathic SND without any detectable morphological abnormality can occur and may be related to abnormal neural innervation.

In patients with sinus node dysfunction, the correlation of symptoms with bradyarrhythmias is *critically* important. This is because there is a great deal of disagreement about the absolute heart rate or length of pause required before pacing is indicated. If the symptoms of SND are dramatic (e.g. syncope, recurrent dizzy spells, seizures, or severe heart failure), then the diagnosis may be relatively easy. However, symptoms are often non-specific (e.g. easy fatigability, depression, listlessness, early signs of dementia) and may be easily misinterpreted in the elderly. Electrophysiological studies have a low sensitivity for detection of SND and

Table 1.2 Manifestations of sinus node dysfunction and their diagnosis

Sinus bradycardia	Sinus rates persistently <50 bpm and associated with symptoms. Prolonged sinus node recovery time (following atrial pacing) is helpful in diagnosing sinus node disease but has low sensitivity
Chronotropic incompetence	Inadequate sinus rate response to exercise, defined as failure to achieve 80% of expected heart rate during exercise. Diagnosis made with exercise test or ambulatory ECG monitoring
Sinoatrial (SA) block	Sinus beats are "dropped" in a regular pattern (e.g. 2 : 1 SA block, 3 : 2 SA Wenckebach, etc.) due to blocking of impulses in the perinodal area between the sinus node and atrial muscle (by disease, medications, etc.). Diagnosis is by ECG or ambulatory monitoring
Sinus pause >3.0 s	Failure of impulse formation in the sinus node due to pathology, medications, etc. The diagnosis is made electrocardiographically by an absence of sinus P waves that occurs without any discernible pattern
Tachy–brady syndrome	The diagnosis is made electrocardiographically by alternating periods of bradycardia and tachycardia. It may be due to (i) overdrive suppression of sinus node by atrial fibrillation, flutter or tachycardia with sinus pauses that occur at the termination of tachycardia; (ii) periods of paroxysmal atrial arrhythmia with rapid rates superimposed on underlying sinus bradycardia; or (iii) persistent atrial fibrillation with periods of fast and slow AV conduction. Note that the tachy–brady syndrome associated with persistent atrial fibrillation is related to disease in the AV node and not sinus node

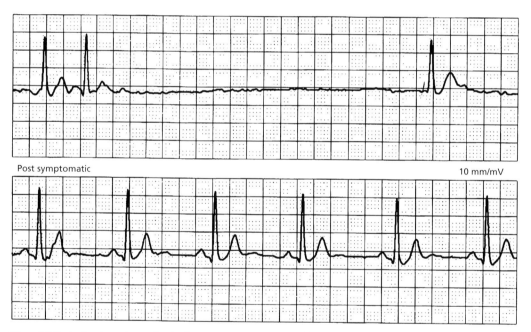

Post symptomatic   10 mm/mV

Figure 1.4 Tachy–brady syndrome due to sinus arrest at termination of atrial fibrillation. Patient-triggered event recording during presyncope in a 56-year-old male with paroxysmal atrial fibrillation shows an asystolic pause in excess of 4 s at termination of fibrillation. The sinus offset pause is intercepted by a junctional escape beat before resumption of normal sinus rhythm.

ambulatory monitoring with symptom correlation has the best diagnostic yield.

Essential drugs used for coexisting conditions can accentuate SND (Figure 1.5). If cessation of a drug is anticipated to cause deterioration of the primary condition, permanent pacing may be needed to allow continuation of medical therapy in some patients. Chronotropic incompetence is an underdiagnosed condition where patients fail to augment their heart rate with exercise, with marked

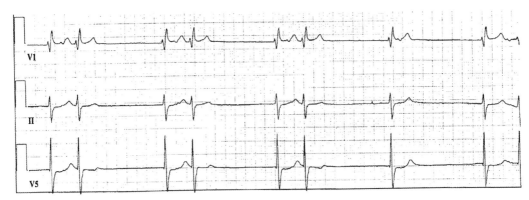

Figure 1.5 A 69-year-old male had been started on atenolol 75 mg/day for treatment of hypertension approximately 2 weeks earlier. He was seen in the emergency room complaining of feeling weak and lightheaded. The ECG shows a slow junctional escape rhythm followed by a sinus beat in a pattern termed "escape–capture bigeminy." Discontinuation of atenolol resulted in return of normal sinus rhythm within 36 hours. Patients with sinus node dysfunction may be dependent on sympathetic stimulation, and beta-blockers, even in low doses, may result in profound bradycardia.

exercise intolerance in some patients. Although no specific parameter has been established as a diagnostic standard, the most commonly used definition for chronotropic incompetence is the inability to achieve 80% of expected heart rate reserve for age; expected heart rate reserve is defined as the difference between age-predicted maximal heart rate (220 – age) and the resting heart rate.

Patients with SND may have associated disease in the AV node and His–Purkinje conduction system. However, the rate of lone SND progressing to AV block is low. The mean annual incidence of complete AV block developing in patients implanted with AAI pacemakers for SND is 0.4–1.7% [16,17]. The natural history of untreated SND is highly variable. Syncope resulting from sinus arrest tends to be recurrent and may result in falls and significant orthopedic injuries, especially in the elderly. The incidence of sudden death is low and SND very rarely affects survival regardless of whether or not it is treated with a pacemaker.

Indications for permanent pacing in sinus node dysfunction
Class I indications
1 Sinus node dysfunction with symptoms directly attributable to SND. (Level of evidence: C-LD)
2 Sinus node dysfunction as a result of essential long-term drug therapy of a type and dose for which there are no acceptable alternatives. (Level of evidence: C-EO)

Class IIa indications
1 Tachy–brady syndrome and symptoms attributable to bradycardia. (Level of evidence C-EO)
2 Symptomatic chronotropic incompetence. (Level of evidence: C-EO)

Class III (permanent pacing not indicated)
1 Permanent pacing is not indicated in asymptomatic patients with SND. (Level of evidence: C)

Acquired atrioventricular block

In the majority, sclerodegenerative changes account for progressive conduction system disease. However, in a significant proportion, AV block is secondary to other causes that are potentially reversible or associated with progressive heart disease with added risk of ventricular arrhythmias such that an implantable cardioverter–defibrillator (ICD) should be considered as a means of providing pacing therapy. In a recent review of unexplained heart block in patients under 55 years of age, cardiac sarcoidosis or giant cell myocarditis accounted for 25% of cases and these patients had a high incidence of sudden death, ventricular tachycardia (VT), or need for cardiac transplantation [18]. In younger patients presenting with advanced conduction system disease, further evaluation with cardiac magnetic resonance (CMR) imaging or positron emission tomography (PET) is useful for detection of

pathology that merits the use of an ICD as opposed to provision of cardiac pacing alone.

Based on electrocardiography (ECG) characteristics, AV block is classified as first, second, and third degree. Anatomically, block can occur at various levels in the AV conduction system: above the His bundle (supra-His), within the His bundle (intra-His), and below the His bundle (infra-His). First-degree AV block is defined as abnormal prolongation of the PR interval to greater than 200 ms and is commonly due to delay in the AV node irrespective of QRS width. Type I second-degree heart block refers to progressive PR prolongation before a non-conducted beat and a shorter PR interval after the first blocked beat. This is the classical Wenckebach type AV block usually seen in conjunction with narrow QRS complexes, implying a more proximal level of block, usually in the AV node (Figure 1.6). Type II second-degree heart block is characterized by fixed PR intervals before and after blocked beats, and is usually associated with a wider QRS complex, indicating distal levels of block in the conduction system. Type II second-degree AV block is usually below the level of the AV node (within or below the His bundle); symptoms and progression to complete AV block are common. AV conduction in a 2 : 1 pattern can be due to proximal or distal block, although the width of the QRS can help differentiate these based on the above principle. Advanced second-degree block or "high-grade" AV block refers to two or more non-conducted sinus P waves, but with resumption of conducted beats suggesting preservation of some AV conduction (Figure 1.7). In the setting of atrial fibrillation or flutter, a prolonged pause (e.g. >5 s) is often due to advanced second-degree AV block. Third-degree AV block is defined as the absence of AV conduction. In the case of atrial fibrillation, complete AV block often manifests as a regularized slow ventricular rate (Figure 1.8).

The site of AV block will to a great extent determine the adequacy and reliability of the underlying escape rhythm (Figures 1.9 and 1.10). While ECG characteristics are helpful in defining levels of block, they are not always reliable and occasionally an electrophysiological study is required. Type I second-degree block, for example, can occasionally be infranodal, even with a narrow QRS, and may warrant the consideration of pacing [19]. Certain clinical maneuvers may be helpful in determining the level of block. Increased AV conduction with exercise and atropine generally indicate block at the AV nodal level, while maneuvers that slow the atrial rate, such as carotid massage, improve His–Purkinje conduction by allowing for recovery from refractoriness (Table 1.3).

There is considerable variation in the symptomatic manifestation of AV block, ranging from an asymptomatic status to syncope and sudden death. First-degree AV block and asymptomatic type I second-degree AV block are in general benign and not an indication for cardiac pacing. However,

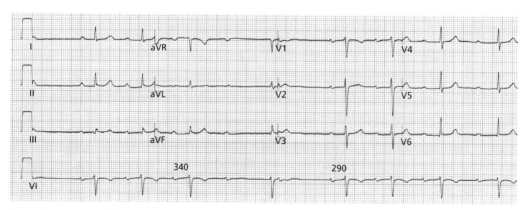

Figure 1.6 Type I second-degree AV block associated with Lyme disease. This 32-year-old male presented with complaints of palpitation due to heart beat irregularity. He had features of Lyme disease several weeks previously. There is progressive PR prolongation before the fourth P wave fails to conduct. The fourth QRS complex is a junctional escape beat. The sixth P wave that conducts has a shorter PR interval (290 ms) compared to the last conducted beat before block occurred (340 ms).

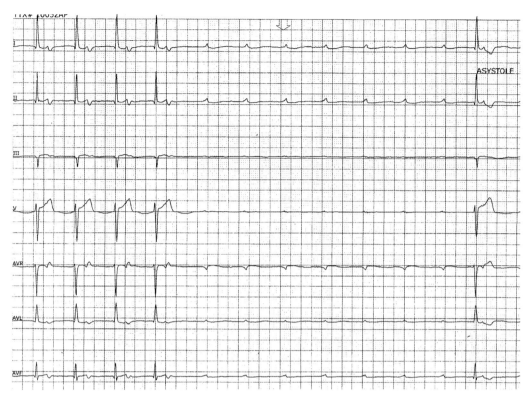

Figure 1.7 High-grade AV block. This 60-year-old female with hypertension and coronary artery disease presented with syncope. Baseline ECG showed marked first-degree AV block and voltage changes of left ventricular hypertrophy. Telemetry recorded abrupt interruption of AV conduction with multiple non-conducted P waves with spontaneous recovery. Her β-adrenergic blockers were continued as essential treatment for coronary artery disease and a permanent pacemaker was implanted.

rarely, first-degree block with marked PR prolongation can potentially cause atrial systole to occur in close proximity to the preceding ventricular systole and give rise to symptoms similar to those of a pacemaker syndrome [20]. Prolongation of the PR interval is particularly important in patients with left ventricular (LV) dysfunction as marked PR prolongation in excess of 250–300 ms can lead to impaired LV filling, increased pulmonary capillary wedge pressure, and decreased cardiac output [21]. Similar consequences can ensue in patients with type I second-degree AV block even in the absence of bradycardia-related symptoms.

Type II second-degree AV block is important as it has a high rate of progression to third-degree AV block. It usually reflects diffuse conduction system disease and often warrants permanent pacing even in the absence of symptoms. Third-degree AV block with a wide QRS escape rhythm often presents with fatigue,

dyspnea, presyncope or frank unheralded syncope. Rarely, ventricular fibrillation and torsades de pointes VT can result from marked bradycardia and prolonged pauses. Permanent cardiac pacing should be strongly considered even if the escape rate is greater than 40 bpm, because it is not necessarily the escape rate that determines a safe and reliable heart rhythm but the site of origin of the escape rhythm. Infra-His escape rhythms are more likely associated with prolonged asystole, syncope, and death (Figure 1.10).

AV block, usually with 2 : 1 AV conduction, can be provoked by exercise (Figure 1.11). Patients typically complain of exertional dyspnea and dizziness. The abnormality is often reproducible by exercise testing. Once ischemia is excluded as a cause, permanent pacing is remarkably effective for symptom relief. Without pacing, these patients have a poor prognosis because the site of conduction block is below the AV nodal level [22].

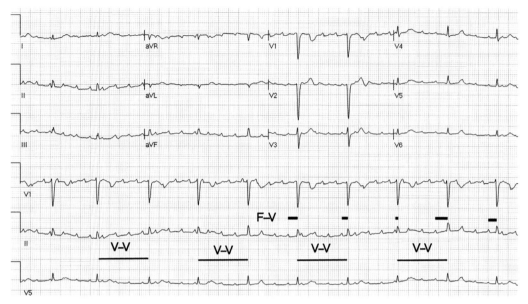

Figure 1.8 Third-degree AV block and junctional escape during atrial flutter. Identification of complete AV block during atrial flutter or atrial tachycardia may be challenging as high-level conduction block has to be considered as well. In this tracing the second QRS is likely conducted but the rest of the recording shows a regular atrial rhythm dissociated from a regular ventricular rhythm. Note that F wave to QRS duration (F–V) is variable while the ventricular rate (V–V) is stable, ruling out AV conduction. Source: courtesy of Karoly Kaszala, MD.

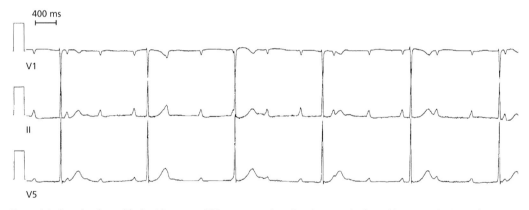

Figure 1.9 Complete heart block with narrow QRS escape rhythm. This 70-year-old male presented with fatigue. Rhythm strips reveal complete AV block and a slow junctional escape rhythm with narrow QRS complexes. A permanent dual-chamber pacemaker completely relieved his symptoms.

In general, the presence of symptoms documented to be due to AV block is an indication for permanent pacing regardless of the site of the block (e.g. above as well as below the His bundle). However, it is important to recognize potentially reversible causes of AV block despite their presentation with symptoms. Important examples include acute myocarditis (particularly that associated with Lyme carditis), AV block related to drug toxicity, transient vagotonia, and hypoxic events. Many of these conditions tend to resolve with disease-specific treatment and although temporary pacing may be required, permanent pacing is seldom necessary. One exception is drug-related AV block that may not always resolve completely on cessation of the medication and may need permanent pacing (see discussion of temporary pacing indications in subsequent sections).

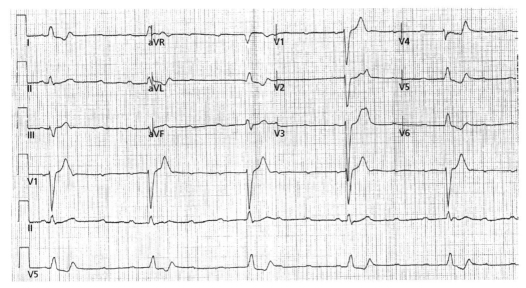

Figure 1.10 Complete AV block with wide QRS escape rhythm. This 77-year-old male presented with syncope without warning and sustained facial injuries. The slow ventricular escape rhythm at 30 bpm likely originates from the right bundle branch. Intermittent asystole due to unstable escape rhythm was the most likely cause of syncope.

Table 1.3 Responses to maneuvers to identify level of block in patients with 2 : 1 atrioventricular (AV) block

	Block above AV node	Block below AV node
Exercise	+	± or −
Atropine	+	± or −
Carotid sinus massage	−	+ or ±
Isoproterenol	+	− or ±

+, improved AV conduction; −, worsened AV conduction.

The indications for permanent pacing for heart block due to increased vagal tone (reflex syncope), acute myocardial infarction (MI), and congenital AV block are discussed separately.

Indications for permanent pacing in acquired AV block
Class I indications
1 In acquired second-degree Mobitz type II AV block, high-grade AV block or complete AV block not attributable to reversible or physiological causes, permanent pacing is recommended regardless of symptoms. (Level of evidence: B-NR)
2 Patients with neuromuscular disease, such as muscular dystrophy or Kearns–Sayre syndrome, who have second- or third-degree AV block or His–ventricular (HV) interval ≥70 ms should be considered for permanent pacing with a defibrillator regardless of symptoms.[1] (Level of evidence: B-NR)
3 Permanent atrial fibrillation with symptomatic bradycardia. (Level of evidence: C-LD)
4 Symptomatic AV block during clinically indicated guideline-directed medical therapy for which there is no reasonable alternative. (Level of evidence: C-LD)

Class IIa indications
1 Second-degree Mobitz type II AV block, high-grade AV block or complete heart block in patients with inflammatory or infiltrative cardiomyopathies (e.g. sarcoidosis): permanent pacing with additional defibrillator is reasonable.[1] (Level of evidence: B-NR)
2 PR interval >240 ms and left bundle branch block (LBBB) in patients with lamin A/C gene mutations, including limb girdle and Emery–Dreifuss muscular dystrophies: permanent pacing with defibrillation capability should be considered. (Level of evidence: B-NR)

---

[1] Defibrillator implants are for patients with an expected meaningful survival of more than 1 year.

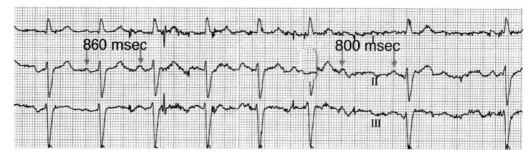

Figure 1.11 Exercise-induced AV block. This 68-year-old male presented with exertional dyspnea. His baseline ECG showed sinus rhythm with first-degree AV block and left anterior hemiblock. With gentle leg elevation exercise in the examination room while connected to the ECG, 2 : 1 AV block developed as the PP intervals shortened from 860 to 800 ms. This finding is typical of block below the AV node. Permanent dual-chamber cardiac pacing relieved his symptoms.

3 Permanent pacing is reasonable in patients with marked first-degree or second-degree Mobitz type I AV block if symptoms can be attributed to the AV block. (Level of evidence: C-LD)

Class IIb indications

1 In patients with neuromuscular diseases, such as myotonic dystrophy type 1, with PR >240 ms, QRS duration >120 ms or fascicular block, permanent pacing with defibrillation is reasonable.

Conduction system disease in the presence of 1 : 1 AV conduction

Conduction disease may involve the bundle branches or the individual fascicles of the left bundle. In bifascicular block, the ECG shows evidence of conduction delay or block in both bundles such as complete right bundle branch block (RBBB) with anterior or posterior hemiblock or complete LBBB alone. The term "alternating bundle branch block" (or bilateral bundle branch block) refers to evidence for impaired conduction in the right bundle and both fascicles of the left bundle on successive ECGs. In strict terms, evidence for disease in all three fascicles should justify the term "trifascicular block." However, the term trifascicular block has also been loosely applied to bifascicular block with first-degree AV block where the block may actually be due to a combination of AV nodal and infra-His conduction disease (Figure 1.12).

The prevalence of bundle branch block increases with age (approximately 1% in middle age, rising to 17% at age 80) [23]. LBBB is less common but its presence is associated with a higher incidence of structural heart disease. In bifascicular block, the risk of progression to advanced heart block is related to the presence of symptoms. Syncope is the sole predictor. In the absence of syncope, the annual incidence is 0.6–0.8%, whereas syncopal patients have a 5–11% annual risk of progression to AV block [24,25]. The finding of an HV interval of greater than 100 ms or the demonstration of intra- or infra-His block during incremental atrial pacing at a rate of less than 150 bpm is highly predictive for the development of high-grade AV block (Figure 1.13), but their prevalence is low and hence sensitivity is low [26,27]. Care has to be exercised during atrial pacing so as not to misinterpret the physiological AV block that is often seen with long–short intervals. The majority of patients with bifascicular block who undergo electrophysiological studies will have normal or mildly prolonged HV intervals. However, in patients with bundle branch block and a normal electrophysiological study, implantable loop monitors have shown that recurrent syncope is often due to a bradyarrhythmia, most commonly sudden-onset paroxysmal AV block [28]. The current guidelines recommend permanent pacing for syncope, bundle branch block, and HV interval >70 ms.

Because chronic bifascicular block is associated with other forms of heart disease, pacing alone, although successful for symptom relief, has not been shown to improve mortality. Echocardiography is indicated for assessment of LV function. In the presence of ventricular dysfunction, VT is an alternative mechanism for syncope and sudden death. Programmed stimulation of the ventricle may demonstrate inducibility for ventricular arrhythmia, necessitating consideration of an ICD.

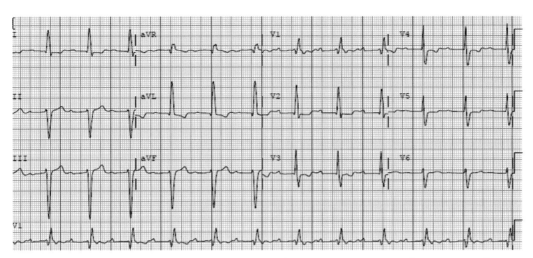

Figure 1.12 Bifascicular block due to right bundle branch block and left anterior hemiblock (note that left anterior fascicular block is diagnosed by left-axis deviation, qR in aVL, R peak time in aVL >45 ms, and rS pattern in leads II, III and aVF). There is PR prolongation to 320 ms. First-degree AV block in such patients is not always predictive of HV interval. When PR interval >300 ms, AH prolongation is present in more than 90% of patients. HV prolongation is present in 50% of patients but not predictive of progression to complete heart block, Thus, in the absence of symptoms, there is no indication for invasive study or cardiac pacing.

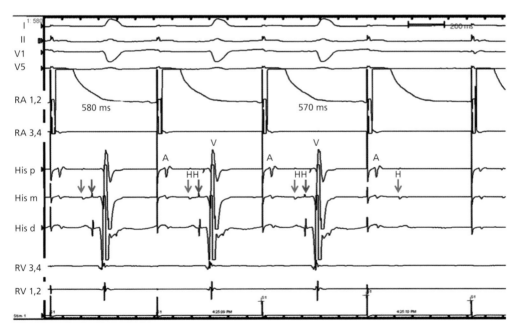

Figure 1.13 Intra- and infra-His AV block induced with atrial pacing. A 68-year-old male was admitted complaining of recurrent dizziness and syncope. His baseline 12-lead ECG showed a PR interval of 0.25 s and a left bundle branch block QRS morphology. The His bundle is split and denoted by H and H′ (blue and red arrows). With decremental atrial pacing, intra-His block (blue arrow) is demonstrated at a cycle length of 570 ms (105 bpm). These findings are indicative of severe diffuse conduction system disease. A permanent dual-chamber pacemaker was implanted, and the patient's symptoms resolved. From top to bottom: I, II, V1 and V5 are standard ECG leads; intracardiac recording from the right atrial appendage (RA 1, 2 and RA 3, 4); and His bundle (His-p, His-m, and His-d are proximal, mid and distal His recordings respectively). A, atrial depolarization; H, proximal His bundle depolarization; H′, distal His bundle depolarization; V, ventricular depolarization.

Indications for pacing in conduction system disease with 1 : 1 AV conduction
Class I indications
1   Patients with syncope and bundle branch block who are found to have an HV interval ≥70 ms at electrophysiological study. (Level of evidence: C-LD)
2   Patients with alternating bundle branch block. (Level of evidence: C-LD)

Class III (not indicated)
1   Bifascicular block with or without first-degree AV block and no symptoms.

Reflex syncope

Reflex syncope includes a group of conditions that are neurally mediated and result in a common cardiovascular response of vasodilation and/or bradycardia. Cerebral hypoperfusion results in loss of consciousness. Any one of the two components of the reflex may predominate. The cardioinhibitory response with predominant bradycardia results from increased parasympathetic tone and is characterized by sinus slowing, sinus arrest (Figure 1.14), prolongation of the PR interval and, less commonly, AV block that occurs alone or in combination. The vasodepressor response is secondary to a reduction in sympathetic activity and marked by loss of vascular tone and hypotension. This effect is independent of heart rate changes.

The two most common types of reflex syncope are neurocardiogenic (vasovagal) and carotid sinus hypersensitivity syndrome. The other types are generally referred to as situational syncope because they are generally associated with a particular stimulus (Table 1.4). Several forms are recognized based on the triggering mechanism, although the triggers may vary considerably in and between individual patients. Classical vasovagal syncope is most common in young patients and occurs as isolated episodes. Generally, patients experience a distinct prodrome of dizziness, nausea, diaphoresis, and visual changes, followed by loss of consciousness. Recovery is gradual but occurs within minutes and it is unusual to experience post-ictal states. However, one-third of patients (commonly older adults) may have minimal or no prodromal symptoms and syncope can be sudden with bodily injuries. When vasovagal syncopal spells begin at

an older age, they may be an expression of a pathological process heralding early autonomic failure.

Reflex syncope becomes important when frequent syncope alters quality of life, occurs with a very short prodrome exposing patients to risk of trauma, or occurs during high-risk activity such as driving, flying, or heavy machine operation. Non-pharmacological therapy, such as avoidance measures, physical counter-pressure maneuvers, and tilt training, are useful initial interventions for control of vasovagal syncope [30]. Pharmacological interventions such as fludrocortisone and midodrine predominantly address the vasodepressor component and may occasionally be effective for individual patients, but randomized trials have not proven clear benefit from any particular drug. Although beta-blockers can lessen the degree of mechanoreceptor activation in neurocardiogenic syncope, randomized trials have not shown benefit [31]. In carotid sinus syncope, beta-blockers may, in fact, worsen symptoms.

The role of cardiac pacing in vasovagal syncope has been evaluated in multiple clinical trials with varying results. Meta-analysis of these studies suggested a 17% non-significant reduction in syncope in double-blind studies when both the paced and unpaced groups received pacemaker implants (thereby eliminating a placebo effect). More recent trials using implantable loop recorders (ILRs) to document asystole during vasovagal syncope have been more favorable to permanent cardiac pacing for symptom relief. The ISSUE 3 study randomized patients aged 40 years or older, with three or more syncope episodes and documentation of syncope with greater than 3-s asystole or 6-s asystole without syncope, to pacing-activated or -inactivated modes after implantation. The study showed a significant reduction in recurrent syncope at 2 years, from 57% in the pacing-inactivated group to 25% in the paced group [32]. However, it should be noted that 511 patients with highly symptomatic vasovagal syncope underwent implantation of an ILR in order to identify 89 (17%) patients with important asystole.

In the presence of predominantly cardioinhibitory responses, cardiac pacing tends to be effective for attenuation of symptoms and is a reasonable consideration in older patients. Dual-chamber pacing is generally preferred as VVI pacing can potentially worsen symptoms. Pacemakers that

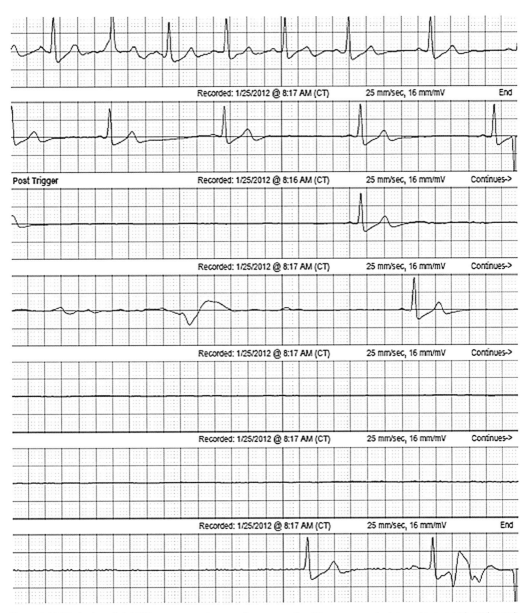

Figure 1.14 Marked cardioinhibitory response to neurally mediated syncope. This 45-year-old female presented with syncope preceded by nausea while wearing an event monitor. There was gradual sinus slowing with prolonged sinus arrest resulting in syncope. Intense vagal stimulation can suppress junctional escape rhythms.

offer closed-loop stimulation, a form of rate-adaptive pacing in response to myocardial contraction dynamics derived from right ventricular (RV) impedance changes, has shown benefit over conventional dual-chamber pacing [33]. Because the cardioinhibitory and vasodepressor components can variably manifest in the same patient during different episodes, patients should be warned of the possibility of recurrence relating to hypotension. In younger patients, however, simple measures should be exhausted before considering commitment to lifelong pacemaker therapy. In the ISSUE 3 study, pacemaker implantation was associated with complications in 6%. Longer-term complications of pacemaker generator changes and lead malfunction are more pertinent to younger patients.

Table 1.4 Types of neurally mediated syncope

Vasovagal	Mediated by emotional stress, such as fear, pain, sight of blood, instrumentation Mediated by orthostatic stress
Carotid sinus syncope	Mediated by pressure to the carotid sinus area, e.g. shaving, turning of the head, tight neck collar
Situational	Cough, sneeze Gastrointestinal stimulation: swallow, defecation, visceral pain Micturition syncope Post exercise Postprandial
Other	Triggered by increased intrathoracic pressure, e.g. laughing, playing brass instruments, weightlifting
Atypical forms	No identified precipitant Adenosine-sensitive syncope

Source: adapted from Shen et al. [29].

One variant of neurally mediated syncope is the hypersensitive carotid sinus syndrome. A mildly abnormal response to vigorous carotid sinus massage may occur in up to 25% of patients, especially if coexisting vascular disease is present. Some patients with an abnormal response to carotid sinus massage may have no symptoms suggestive of carotid sinus syncope. On the other hand, the typical history of syncope such as blurred vision and lightheadedness or confusion in the standing or sitting position, especially during movement of the head or neck, should suggest the diagnosis. Classical triggers of carotid sinus syncope are head turning, tight neckwear, shaving, and neck hyperextension. Syncopal episodes are generally reproducible in a given patient. Because of the predominantly bradycardic (cardioinhibitory) response to carotid hypersensitivity, permanent pacing has a high success rate for alleviating symptoms (Figure 1.15).

Paroxysmal AV block
A distinct form of paroxysmal AV block associated with syncope has been described in patients with no structural heart disease or evidence for conduction disturbance on ECG [34]. Patients present with abrupt syncope associated with abrupt onset

of high-grade AV block and prolonged asystole, with recovery of normal AV conduction soon afterward. The classical sinus slowing prior to onset of AV block that is typical of vagally mediated AV block is usually absent. Electrophysiological studies show normal His–Purkinje conduction and tilt table testing is usually negative. Patients have an adenosine profile opposite to that of vasovagal syncope and characterized by low plasma adenosine levels, low expression of adenosine A_{2A} receptors, and high induction rate for transient AV block with exogenous adenosine. Cardiac pacing in these patients prevents recurrence of syncope. The entity may be similar to the one termed "low adenosine syncope" that tends to respond to theophylline and cardiac pacing [35]. Further studies are needed to define this syndrome more clearly.

Indications for pacing in neurally mediated syncope and hypersensitive carotid sinus syndrome (2018 European Society of Cardiology guidelines)
Class IIa indications
1 In patients aged >40 years, permanent pacing should be considered to reduce syncopal recurrence with documented symptomatic asystolic pauses >3.0 s or asymptomatic pauses >6 s due to sinus arrest, AV block, or the combination of both. (Level of evidence: B-R)
2 Pacing should be considered for reducing syncope recurrence in patients with cardioinhibitory carotid sinus syndrome who are aged >40 years with recurrent frequent unpredictable syncope. (Level of evidence: B)

Class IIb indications
1 Cardiac pacing may be considered for reducing syncope recurrence in patients with tilt-induced asystolic response who are aged >40 years with recurrent frequent unpredictable syncope. (Level of evidence: B)
2 Cardiac pacing may be considered for reducing syncope recurrence in patients with clinical features of adenosine-sensitive syncope. (Level of evidence: B)

Class III (not indicated)
1 Pacing is not indicated in the absence of cardioinhibitory response.

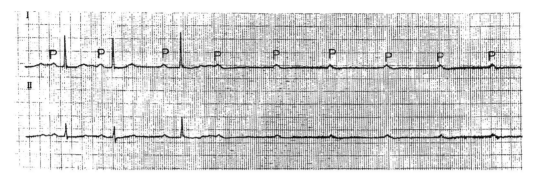

Figure 1.15 Response to gentle carotid massage in carotid hypersensitivity syndrome. A 69-year-old male complained of near-syncope, which typically occurred while shaving or turning his neck. Carotid sinus massage was performed shortly before the second QRS complex. Note that the sinus rate slows prior to the third QRS complex, followed by complete heart block with ventricular asystole.

Spinal cord injury

Based on the level and severity of spinal cord injury, bradycardia may accompany the acute phase of recovery due to a marked reduction in sympathetic tone. Cervical cord injuries are most likely to cause sinus arrest and asystole in the initial 2–4 weeks and may require temporary pacing if atropine and sympathetic stimulation are ineffective. The bradyarrhythmia is the result of unopposed parasympathetic stimulation. Hence, the use of theophylline as an adenosine receptor blocker can be effective and its use is supported by small case series [36]. Permanent pacing is best reserved for intractable cases as recurrent infections and bacteremia are common in these patients, increasing the risk of lead-related endocarditis in the longer term.

Ictal bradycardia

Rarely (<0.5%), profound bradycardia due to sinus arrest or AV block at the nodal level can complicate seizures, mostly temporal lobe epilepsy. Prolonged ictal asystole (>6.0 s) is more common with left temporal lobe epilepsy than right, and can worsen and extend the duration of syncope associated with such seizures. Pacing has been shown to reduce syncopal events and is a consideration if antiepileptic measures such as drugs and surgery fail to control epilepsy. In the 2018 guidelines for bradycardia, permanent pacing is considered a class IIa indication based on limited data [37,38].

Specific conditions associated with cardiac conduction disease

Chronic neuromuscular disorders

A number of neuromuscular disorders are associated with cardiomyopathy and a high incidence of sudden death. In general, the direct consequence of the neuromuscular defects, such as respiratory failure, limits lifespan. However, in some of these conditions, cardiac disease may be responsible for greater morbidity and mortality. Most often, bradyarrhythmias in neuromuscular disorders are due to direct involvement of the specialized AV conduction system. The relatively small numbers of patients involved and the absence of randomized placebo-controlled clinical trials make it difficult to provide definitive guidelines for pacemaker implantation. Since mortality and the incidence of sudden cardiac death are high in this group of disorders, and because conduction system disease tends to be unpredictable, the development of second- or third-degree AV block, even in the absence of symptoms, is considered a class I indication for permanent pacing. In addition, suggestive symptoms such as syncope should be promptly and aggressively investigated. Some authorities recommend yearly ECGs and 24-hour ambulatory recordings for patients with one of these disorders to facilitate early recognition of AV block. It should also be realized, however, that life-threatening ventricular arrhythmias are also fairly common in this population, especially when LV function is impaired or complicated by hypertrophic cardiomyopathy (HCM), so use of a permanent pacemaker will not necessarily prevent sudden cardiac death.

The neuromuscular disorders most frequently associated with symptomatic conduction system disease are as follows.

Myotonic muscular dystrophy

The type 1 form (Steinert disease) is the most common adult form of neuromuscular disease and is inherited as an autosomal dominant disorder that usually becomes clinically manifest in the third decade. One-third of deaths are sudden and related to heart block or ventricular tachyarrhythmias [39,40]. Permanent pacemakers are warranted for second- or third-degree AV block, even in the absence of symptoms. A recent large non-randomized study of type 1 myotonic dystrophy patients compared an invasive electrophysiological evaluation when PR interval exceeded 200 ms and/or QRS was prolonged in excess of 100 ms with a non-invasive clinical approach. The invasive group, which underwent pacemaker implantation based on the finding of an HV interval greater than 70 ms, had a significant reduction in sudden death [41].

Duchenne muscular dystrophy

This progressive X-linked disease usually becomes clinically apparent in the mid-teens and is fatal by the end of the third decade. The ECG typically shows prominent R waves in V1 with deep narrow Q waves in the lateral precordial leads. Although cardiac involvement is almost universal, the incidence of arrhythmias is variable, with many patients dying from heart failure. In the absence of definitive data, it seems prudent to recommend permanent pacemaker implantation in patients who develop second-degree or higher degrees of AV block, especially in the setting of a wide QRS complex.

Becker muscular dystrophy

This is an X-linked condition closely related to Duchenne muscular dystrophy. It has similar electrocardiographic abnormalities, but progresses more slowly. The severity of cardiac involvement does not parallel the severity of neuromuscular disease. Although there is less experience with this disorder, the indications for permanent pacing are similar to those for patients with Duchenne muscular dystrophy.

Emery–Dreifuss muscular dystrophy

This is a slowly progressive X-linked muscular dystrophy with a high incidence of conduction system disease and arrhythmias. Sudden cardiac death due to bradyarrhythmias has been well documented, and permanent pacemakers are often necessary.

Limb girdle muscular dystrophy

This is a heterogeneous group of disorders that usually begin with weakness in the upper legs and pelvic musculature. Cardiac involvement is variable, although there is a familial form with a high incidence of conduction system disease. Patients with a family history of heart block or sudden death should be considered for permanent pacing relatively early in the course of their disease.

Kearns–Sayre syndrome

This is a multisystem mitochondrial disorder characterized by progressive external ophthalmoplegia, pigmentary retinal degeneration, and AV block. Involvement of the distal conduction system is the rule and high-degree AV block is common. Although definitive data are lacking, it seems prudent to implant a permanent pacemaker prophylactically when marked first-degree AV block becomes manifest.

Infiltrative and inflammatory disorders

The infiltrative cardiomyopathies are characterized by deposition of abnormal substances that commonly lead to stiffening of the ventricular myocardium, causing diastolic dysfunction. Many of these diseases increase wall thickness, and may present with small ventricular volume and occasional LV outflow tract (LVOT) obstruction so as to mimic HCM. Some may have minimal structural abnormalities by echocardiography but involve the conduction system early such that initial presentation may be with heart block or ventricular arrhythmias. Infiltrative and inflammatory cardiomyopathies particularly prone to manifest cardiac conduction disease include sarcoidosis, giant cell myocarditis, amyloidosis, Wegener granulomatosis, metabolic diseases such as hemochromatosis, primary oxaluria, and hematological malignancies and cardiac tumors. Some metabolic diseases such as Fabry disease and the glycogen storage diseases (e.g. Danon disease) demonstrate frequent cardiac involvement. AV block, although rare, is well recognized in these conditions. In South American countries, Chagas disease is a common cause of bradyarrhythmias requiring cardiac pacing.

The prognosis of many of these disorders is usually more closely related to the underlying disease, although the actual cause of death may be cardiac. For example, malignancies involving the heart, especially "solid" tumors, tend to have a uniformly poor prognosis. Nonetheless, infiltrative disorders may directly affect the conduction system and cause life-threatening bradyarrhythmias and tachyarrhythmias. In these situations, permanent pacemakers or defibrillators can be life-saving.

Sarcoidosis

This is a relatively common disorder of unknown etiology and is characterized by formation of non-caseating granulomas in various organs, including the myocardium. After an early stage of granulomatous inflammation, sarcoidosis may resolve completely or progress with end-organ fibrosis. Cardiac involvement is common in autopsy studies but infrequently recognized clinically, and is a common cause of death. Approximately 5% of patients will have cardiac-predominant disease without evidence for other organ involvement [42]. Granulomas typically involve the basal septum and posterior wall, resulting in conduction system disease, localized LV aneurysms, and VT. Definitive diagnosis requires demonstration of cardiac granulomas, but patchy myocardial involvement reduces yield from cardiac biopsy to a low 25–30%. Imaging with fluorodeoxyglucose (^{18}F-FDG) and PET or CMR can identify inflammation and has better diagnostic accuracy compared with older techniques [43].

Although conduction abnormalities are the most common cardiac presentation, the risk of sudden death from ventricular arrhythmias is high in the presence of significant cardiac involvement. Hence, once a diagnosis of cardiac sarcoidosis is established, it is common to consider an ICD [44]. Treatment with corticosteroids has been shown in retrospective studies to stabilize LV function, but has no significant impact on conduction disease or ventricular arrhythmias [45].

Amyloidosis

The amyloidoses are a group of multisystem diseases characterized by deposition of the extracellular proteinaceous material amyloid. These deposits occur as a result of misfolding of a precursor protein [46]. The most common clinical amyloidoses that involve the heart are those due to deposition of light chains (AL amyloid), and a hepatically expressed protein, transthyretin (TTR). A form of wild-type TTR infiltration is seen in men aged older than 70 years and is termed senile amyloidosis. Cardiac involvement is the most common cause of death in amyloidosis and manifests as marked wall thickening due to infiltration in all anatomical distributions, including the atria, ventricles, and perivascular space. Because the infiltration is extracellular, despite the appearance of increased wall thickness on echocardiography, the voltage on surface ECG will be low and is a clue to the diagnosis. Perivascular fibrosis can affect the specialized conduction system, causing SND, intraventricular conduction defects, or AV block. Conduction system disease is common to all forms of cardiac amyloidosis but patients with senile cardiac amyloidosis most commonly progress to heart block. Permanent pacing is helpful in alleviating symptoms, but has not been demonstrated to provide a survival benefit [47,48].

Collagen vascular diseases

Several systemic inflammatory diseases can involve the heart and vascular structures, resulting in pericarditis, myocarditis, and vasculitis, including coronary artery disease. Arrhythmias are not common, but fibrosis of the conduction system has been reported to cause AV block, particularly in Wegener granulomatosis and polymyositis. An acute inflammatory AV block that reverses with treatment has been reported with Wegener granulomatosis. Congenital heart block associated with the transmission of anti-SSA/Ro antibodies from the mother occurs in systemic lupus erythematosus and to a lesser extent in primary Sjögren syndrome (see section Pacing for children and adolescents) [49].

Chagas disease

This chronic inflammatory disease, caused by the protozoan *Trypanosoma cruzi*, is largely restricted to endemic areas in Central and South America.

The acute phase of the infection usually goes unrecognized and is rarely life-threatening. Approximately 20% of patients will develop chronic Chagas disease several (10–20) years after the initial infection. Conduction system disease precedes other manifestations, such as localized cardiac aneurysms, thromboembolism, and a diffuse cardiomyopathy with marked cardiomegaly. Sinus bradycardia, atrial fibrillation, AV block, and ventricular arrhythmias are common. Even the early phases of conduction abnormalities, such as RBBB and fascicular block, are associated with an increased risk of sudden death [50].

Genetic cardiomyopathies

Familial or genetic cardiomyopathies account for 20–30% of disease originally diagnosed as idiopathic dilated cardiomyopathy. The work-up of these cardiomyopathies shares common management strategies. Once the proband is recognized, evaluation of family members can identify clinically silent cardiomyopathy and allow for early interventions. Genetic testing can be helpful in some diseases, especially if the pathogenic mutation is identified [51].

Dilated cardiomyopathy

Cardiomyopathies resulting from mutations in the gene coding for the nuclear envelope protein lamin A and C (*LMNA*) and mutations in the *SCN5A* gene are particularly associated with conduction system disease and ventricular arrhythmias [51]. Mutations in *LMNA* associated with cardiomyopathy are highly penetrant, with most carriers demonstrating some evidence of cardiac involvement by 65 years of age. Initial manifestations may be first-degree AV block with gradual progression to complete heart block. Associated atrial arrhythmias are common. Cardiomyopathy usually follows the development of conduction system disease by several years and risk of ventricular arrhythmias is highest when significant systolic dysfunction is present [51]. The diagnostic possibility of an inherited cardiomyopathy has two implications for the relatively young patient presenting with complete heart block: (i) a cardiac evaluation is warranted prior to permanent pacemaker implantation and (ii) periodic assessment of LV function is essential after cardiac pacing for early detection of LV dysfunction. Indications for pacing in dilated cardiomyopathy are discussed in the section Pacing for systolic heart failure.

Hypertrophic cardiomyopathy

This is a common disease entity caused by autosomal dominant mutations in genes encoding protein components of the sarcomere and its constituent myofilament elements. It is characterized by excessive myocardial hypertrophy without cavity dilatation, but varying degrees of phenotypic expression exist. The disease may manifest with LVOT obstruction, diastolic dysfunction, mitral regurgitation, myocardial ischemia, arrhythmias including atrial fibrillation, and sudden death. The distinction between the obstructive and non-obstructive varieties is important because management strategies are largely dependent on symptoms of obstruction. LVOT obstruction is well recognized to be dynamic. Although initially attributed to systolic contraction of the hypertrophied basal ventricle encroaching on the outflow tract, recent studies emphasize the importance of drag forces on an abnormally positioned mitral apparatus that push the leaflets into the outflow tract during systole [52].

In HCM with significant LVOT obstruction, atrial synchronized RV apical pacing results in decrease in outflow gradient and symptomatic improvement in a subset of patients. The exact mechanism of improvement is unclear, but may be related to paradoxical septal movement during systole, although alternate or additional mechanisms such as ventricular dilatation and chronic remodeling may play a part.

Initial enthusiasm for dual-chamber pacing in obstructive HCM was tempered by randomized trials that eliminated a placebo effect. In three randomized crossover trials of continuous DDD pacing compared with AAI pacing, the overall reduction in outflow tract gradient with DDD pacing was modest (20–40%), with substantial variation among individual patients, and symptomatic improvement was no different from that in AAI-paced patients [52]. Acute hemodynamic studies and echocardiographic LV morphology do not predict long-term benefit from dual-chamber pacing. One subgroup that appears to derive most benefit is patients over the age of 65 years [53]. When pacing is performed to relieve outflow tract obstruction in HCM, it is important to optimize AV delay to allow ventricular preexcitation, but not to compromise ventricular filling with too short a delay. In addition, rate-adaptive AV delay is necessary to maintain ventricular preexcitation during exercise. The position of the ventricular lead should be such that it provides distal apical capture.

Permanent pacing is currently not considered an early mode of intervention for symptomatic obstructive HCM. Surgical myomectomy or alcohol septal ablation has been shown to provide more reliable and consistent clinical improvement. Pacing is therefore considered only for patients who are not candidates for these interventions or for those with preexisting dual-chamber pacing devices. Approximately 10–20% of patients will develop persistent complete heart block following alcohol septal ablation and will require permanent cardiac pacing. The risk of ventricular arrhythmias following septal ablation ranges in various reports from 2 to 5% per year. The choice of pacemaker versus ICD should be based on current guideline recommendations [52].

Indications for permanent pacing for HCM (adapted from ACC/AHA guidelines published in 2011 [53] and ESC guidelines in 2014 [54])

Class I indications
1 Class I indications for sinus node dysfunction or AV block as previously described. (Level of evidence: C)

Class IIa indications
1 In patients with HCM who have had a dual-chamber device implanted for non-HCM indications, it is reasonable to consider a trial of dual-chamber AV pacing from the RV apex for the relief of symptoms attributable to LVOT obstruction. (Level of evidence: B)

Class IIb indications
1 AV sequential pacing may be considered in medically refractory symptomatic patients with obstructive HCM in sinus rhythm, with resting or revocable gradient >50 mmHg and who are not candidates for septal reduction therapy. (Level of evidence: C)

Pacing for systolic heart failure

Early studies suggested that dual-chamber pacing, especially with a short AV delay, improved hemodynamics by optimizing ventricular filling or reducing diastolic mitral regurgitation. However, randomized studies failed to confirm these beneficial effects. In contrast, there is considerable evidence that the use of biventricular pacing, by providing cardiac resynchronization therapy (CRT), reduces heart failure symptoms and lowers heart failure mortality with or without an ICD [55]. CRT has been well studied in randomized trials involving over 6000 patients and has demonstrated favorable structural remodeling with improved LV function and reduced mitral regurgitation in 70% of patients. Recent trials of less symptomatic patients (NYHA class I and II) show a reduction in composite end points of heart failure hospitalization and death, but mortality reduction is limited to class II patients [56,57]. All but one trial of CRT involved the use of an ICD as opposed to a CRT pacemaker. Consequently, it is common practice to incorporate defibrillator therapy when CRT pacing is indicated. However, CRT pacing alone has a significant impact on improving quality of life and functional status, and is a reasonable choice in older patients when prolongation of life is not the primary consideration. In addition, for patients who demonstrate a cardiomyopathy as a result of dyssynchrony induced by RV pacing, addition of a LV pacing lead to provide biventricular pacing alone may result in adequate reversal of cardiomyopathy and avoid the need for an ICD.

CRT device implantation is more difficult than placement of a non-CRT pacemaker or ICD and complication rates are greater, usually related to the additional manipulations required for the lead and its delivery systems. Lead dislodgement requiring revision is particularly more common [58]. Appropriate patient selection for this therapy is therefore crucial for ensuring benefit. In post-hoc subgroup analyses of clinical trials, factors associated with the most benefit from CRT include non-ischemic dilated cardiomyopathy, the presence of LBBB, and QRS duration of 150 ms or longer [59]. The recent 2012 focused update guideline of the ACC, AHA and Heart Rhythm Society (HRS) limits the class I indication for CRT to patients with

LBBB and QRS duration of 150 ms or longer [55]. Between 2011 and 2016, several national societies published guidelines for CRT in heart failure creating some inconsistencies, especially with respect to QRS duration and non-LBBB QRS. For example, earlier recommendations suggested QRS duration greater than 120 ms as an indication for CRT. The ECHO CRT study, published in 2013, showed increased cardiovascular mortality with CRT in patients with QRS duration less than 130 ms [60]. Hence, more recent guidelines have set the cutoff at 130 msec below which CRT is not a recommendation.

The role of biventricular pacing in atrial fibrillation is less well established. As the purpose of pacing is to correct LV dyssynchrony, adequate heart rate control in atrial fibrillation is essential to allow for consistent biventricular pacing. Often this requires AV nodal ablation [61].

Indications for pacing in heart failure and impaired LV systolic function (based on the 2013 ACC/AHA guideline [62] and the 2016 ESC Heart Failure Society guideline [63])

Class I indications

1 Class I indications for sinus node dysfunction or AV block as previously described. (Level of evidence: C)

2 CRT pacing in patients with an LV ejection fraction (LVEF) of 35% or less, sinus rhythm, LBBB, and QRS duration of 150 ms or longer, and heart failure with reduced ejection fraction on guideline-directed medical therapy (GDMT). (Level of evidence: A for NYHA III/IV and B for NYHA class II)

Note that the ESC Heart Failure Society guideline extends the class I indication to patients with the above characteristics and LBBB with QRS >130 ms. (Level of evidence: B)

3 CRT rather than RV pacing is recommended for patients with heart failure and reduced ejection fraction regardless of NYHA class for patient with an indication for ventricular pacing in order to reduce morbidity (Level of evidence: A)

Class IIa indications

1 CRT pacing can be useful in patients with an LVEF of 35% or less, sinus rhythm, LBBB with a QRS duration of 130–149 ms, and NYHA class II, III

or ambulatory IV symptoms on GDMT. (Level of evidence: B). Note that this is a class I indication according to ESC Heart Failure Society 2016 guideline.

2 CRT can be useful in patients with an LVEF of 35% or less, sinus rhythm, non-LBBB pattern with a QRS duration of 150 ms or longer, and heart failure with reduced ejection fraction on GDMT. (Level of evidence: B)

3 CRT can be useful in patients with atrial fibrillation and an LVEF of 35% or less on GDMT if:

  a the patient requires ventricular pacing or otherwise meets CRT criteria; and

  b AV nodal ablation or pharmacological rate control will allow near 100% ventricular pacing with CRT. (Level of evidence: B)

4 CRT can be useful in patients on GDMT who have an LVEF of 35% or less and are undergoing device placement or replacement with anticipated requirement for significant (>40%) ventricular pacing. (Level of evidence: B)

Class IIb indications

1 CRT may be considered for patients who have an LVEF of 35% or less, sinus rhythm, non-LBBB pattern with a QRS duration 130–149 ms, and NYHA class III/ambulatory class IV symptoms on GDMT. (Level of evidence: B)

Class III (not indicated)

1 CRT pacing is not recommended for patients with a QRS duration <130 ms. (Level of evidence: A)

Pacing to prevent or terminate tachycardias

Pacing techniques may terminate arrhythmias that depend on a reentrant mechanism. For supraventricular tachycardias (SVTs) and atrial arrhythmias, antiarrhythmic drugs or catheter-based ablation is often effective in preventing recurrence and hence, in contemporary practice, the use of cardiac pacing is limited to patients who have associated bradyarrhythmias. Rarely, a patient who fails one or is unsuitable for drugs or ablation may benefit from antitachycardia pacing if reliable and repetitive termination of the arrhythmia can be demonstrated without proarrhythmic effects (Figure 1.16). Such devices for pacing without defibrillation capability

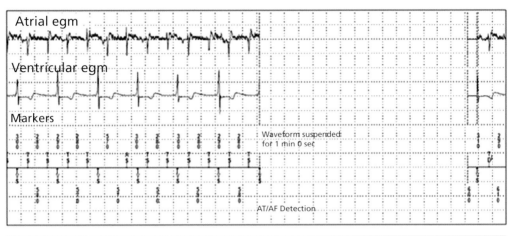

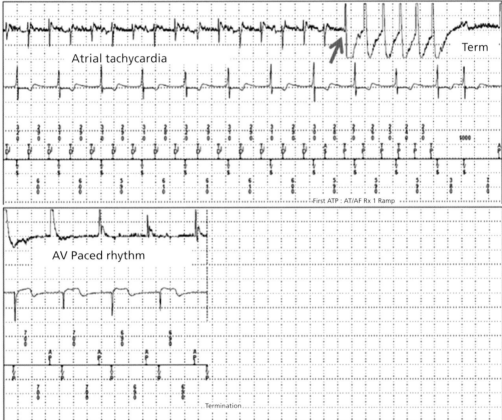

Figure 1.16 Atrial overdrive pacing to terminate atrial tachycardia. This 75-year-old female with pulmonary hypertension and recurrent atrial tachycardia had a dual-chamber pacemaker for tachy–brady syndrome. Her atrial arrhythmia was reproducibly terminated with atrial overdrive pacing. (*Top to bottom*) Atrial bipolar electrograms, ventricular electrograms, and marker channels. At baseline, an atrial tachycardia at a cycle length of 250 ms (240 bpm) was present. A burst of atrial overdrive pacing was delivered (blue arrow) and resulted in termination of tachycardia (term) with resumption of AV synchronized pacing.

are limited to the atrium. Ventricular antitachycardia pacing is currently only available with ICDs.

Ventricular arrhythmias may be pause dependent and pacing prevents prolonged pauses and can prevent the arrhythmia in some patients. Typically, the onset of torsades de pointes VT in patients with a prolonged QT interval is preceded by long RR intervals (Figure 1.17). Pacing combined with β-adrenergic blockers has been shown to reduce the occurrence of sudden cardiac death in patients with the congenital long-QT syndrome [64]. In patients with long-QT syndrome at high risk for sudden death, however, such pacing is usually provided via an ICD.

Several modes of permanent pacing therapy have been tested for prevention of atrial fibrillation. However, none of the special pacing techniques, such as dual-site atrial pacing, biatrial pacing, alternative sites for atrial pacing in the region of the Bachmann bundle or low septum, or atrial overdrive pacing algorithms, has shown significant benefit [65]. In patients with SND, the use of atrial-based pacing is superior to VVI pacing in reducing atrial fibrillation and stroke. Benefit is maximal when ventricular pacing is minimized.

Indications for permanent pacing to prevent or terminate tachycardias

Class I indications
1 Permanent pacing is indicated for sustained pause-dependent VT, with or without QT prolongation. (Level of evidence: C)

Class IIa indications
1 Permanent pacing is reasonable for high-risk patients with congenital long-QT syndrome. (Level of evidence: C). Note that most of these patients will qualify for an ICD.
2 Symptomatic recurrent SVT that is reproducibly terminated by pacing in the unlikely event that catheter ablation and/or drugs fail to control the arrhythmia or produce intolerable side effects. (Level of evidence: C)

Class IIb indications
1 Prevention of symptomatic, drug-refractory recurrent atrial fibrillation in patients with coexisting sinus node dysfunction. (Level of evidence: B)

Class III (not indicated or recommended)
1 The presence of accessory pathways with the capacity for rapid anterograde conduction whether

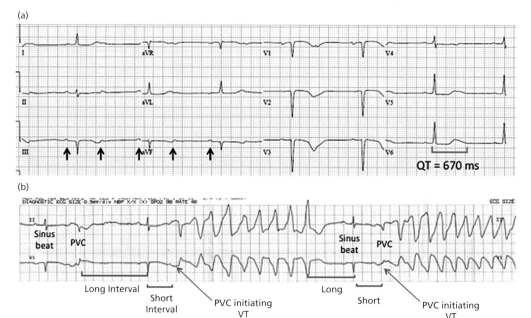

Figure 1.17 Bradycardia-related torsades de pointes ventricular tachycardia (VT). (a) Marked QT prolongation related to 2 : 1 AV block in an 80-year-old woman hospitalized with syncope and facial injuries. The black arrows denote P waves. (b) A premature ventricular contraction (PVC) that arises on the T wave causes a post-PVC pause, further lengthening QT interval. Self-limiting torsade de pointes VT is initiated by a long–short RR interval and is repeated.

or not the pathway(s) participate in the mechanism of the tachycardia.

2 Frequent or complex ventricular ectopic activity without sustained VT in the absence of the long-QT syndrome.

3 Torsades de pointes VT due to reversible causes.

Pacing for children and adolescents (including all patients with congenital heart block)

There are no randomized clinical trials of permanent pacing in pediatric patients and those with congenital heart disease. Hence, the level of evidence for most recommendations is consensus based. The general indications for pacing in children and adolescents are similar to those for adults but with several additional considerations. The diagnosis of important bradycardia in children is age dependent. Whereas a heart rate of 45 bpm would be considered normal for an adult, the same rate would indicate profound bradycardia in a newborn or infant with marked hemodynamic consequences. In addition, the abnormal cardiovascular physiology resulting from palliative surgery for congenital heart diseases can place postsurgical patients at risk for decompensation from bradycardia or loss of AV synchrony that may have been well tolerated by patients with normal physiology. Further, the risk of paradoxical embolism from thrombus on endocardial leads is a consideration in patients with significant intracardiac shunts. Finally, the technical challenges of vascular access and long-term consequences of endovascular leads in children often prompt the consideration of epicardial systems at early ages. While this may be appropriate for children weighing less than 10–15 kg, in larger children the risks of thoracotomy and the higher rate of epicardial lead failures have to be balanced against vascular occlusions from endovascular lead placement. Long-term RV pacing can lead to ventricular dysfunction and periodic assessment by echocardiography is helpful in the detection of early LV dysfunction, especially in patients with congenital heart disease and genetic cardiomyopathies.

The common indications for pacing in children, adolescents, and patients with congenital heart disease can be broadly divided into (i) sinus bradycardia, (ii) tachy–brady syndrome, and (iii) congenital or postsurgical advanced second- or third-degree AV block. SND is rare in pediatric patients but, when present, may be associated with mutations in the *SCN5A* gene [66]. Pacing is usually reserved for situations where symptoms such as syncope can be correlated with bradyarrhythmias (<40 bpm or >3-s pause). It should be recognized that apnea, seizures, and neurocardiogenic mechanisms might cause concurrent bradycardia. Correction of the primary abnormality is more effective than long-term pacing for these conditions.

The common form of tachy–brady syndrome seen in children follows surgery for congenital heart disease. Intra-atrial reentrant tachycardia with loss of sinus node function can manifest as recurrent palpitation, hemodynamic compromise, and prolonged sinus pauses at termination of the atrial tachycardia. Although permanent atrial-based pacing, including antitachycardia pacing to terminate intra-atrial reentry, is a potential treatment option, catheter-based ablation of these arrhythmias is optimal if it can be achieved successfully.

Congenital complete AV block is a rare anomaly that results from abnormal embryonic development of the AV node and is not associated with structural heart disease in 50% of cases. Patients can be broadly divided into groups that are antibody (maternal anti-SS/Ro and/or anti-SSb/La antibodies) positive and antibody negative. When anti-SSA/Ro antibodies are present in the sera of mothers with connective tissue disease, the incidence of congenital heart block in live births has been reported to be 1–2% [67]. The antibodies cross the placenta and damage the conduction system; heart block develops *in utero* and in the early neonatal stage. Less commonly, late postnatal development of heart block has been described. The antibody-negative group tends to present at a later stage and heart block is progressive.

Most children with isolated congenital complete AV block have a stable escape rhythm with a narrow complex. The indications for pacing continue to evolve. Pacing is generally indicated in symptomatic children with complete heart block or if the heart rate in the neonate is less than 55 bpm. In the asymptomatic child or adolescent with complete congenital AV block, several criteria, including average heart rate, pauses in intrinsic rate, associated structural heart disease, QT interval, and exercise tolerance, have been suggested as indications for pacing [68,69].

Congenital heart diseases such as corrected transposition of the great arteries, ostium primum atrial septal defects, and ventricular septal defects may be associated with complete heart block. Patients who develop permanent postsurgical complete AV block have a poor prognosis without cardiac pacing. Hence, advanced AV block that persists for longer than 7–10 days postoperatively is considered a class I indication for pacing.

Indications for permanent pacing in children and adolescents (based on 2018 ACC/AHA/HRS guidelines [13])
Class I indications
1 In adults with congenital heart disease (CHD) and symptomatic SND or chronotropic incompetence, atrial-based permanent pacing is recommended. (Level of evidence: B-NR)
2 In adults with CHD and symptomatic bradycardia due to AV block, permanent pacing is recommended. (Level of evidence: B-NR)
3 In adults with congenital complete AV block with any symptomatic bradycardia, a wide QRS escape rhythm, mean daytime heart rate below 50 bpm, complex ventricular ectopy or ventricular dysfunction, permanent pacing is recommended. (Level of evidence: B-NR)
4 In adults with CHD and postoperative second-degree Mobitz-type II AV block, high-grade AV block or complete AV block that is not expected to resolve, permanent pacing is recommended. (Level of evidence: B-NR)
5 Congenital third-degree AV block in an infant with a ventricular rate of less than 55 bpm or with congenital heart disease and a ventricular rate of less than 70 bpm. (Level of evidence: C-EO)

Class IIa indications
1 In asymptomatic adults with congenital complete AV block, permanent pacing is reasonable. (Level of evidence: B-NR)
2 In adults with repaired CHD who require permanent pacing for bradycardia indications, a bradycardia device with atrial antitachycardia pacing capabilities is reasonable. (Level of evidence: B-NR)
3 In adults with CHD with preexisting sinus and/or AV conduction disease who are undergoing

cardiac surgery, intraoperative placement of epicardial permanent pacing is reasonable. (Level of evidence: C-EO)

Class IIb indications
1 In adults with CHD and pacemakers, atrial-based permanent pacemakers for the prevention of atrial arrhythmias maybe considered. (Level of evidence: B-NR)

Class III (not indicated or harm)
1 In selected patients with adult CHD and venous-to-systemic intracardiac shunts, placement of endocardial leads is potentially harmful. (Level of evidence: B-NR)

Permanent pacing after the acute phase of myocardial infarction

Bradyarrhythmias and conduction defects are relatively common after acute myocardial infarction (MI). They are the result of both autonomic stimulation and ischemia or necrosis of the conduction system. In a large randomized trial of thrombolysis in acute MI, AV block occurred in approximately 7% [70]. The location of the infarction influences the type of conduction defect. AV block associated with inferior wall MI is often at the AV nodal level with narrow QRS escape rhythms, is usually transient, and has a good prognosis. Permanent pacing is rarely required. AV block in association with an anterior MI is most often due to extensive myocardial necrosis that includes the conduction tissue, tends to be infranodal with unstable wide QRS escape, and carries a high mortality, although acute revascularization strategies have improved outcomes in these patients (Figures 1.18 and 1.19). Intraventricular conduction defects (IVCDs) after acute MI occur transiently in up to 18.4% of patients and in a permanent form in 5.3% [71]. The incidence of AV block is higher in post-MI patients who develop transient AV block associated with a persisting peri-infarct IVCD other than isolated left anterior fascicular block.

Although temporary pacing is often necessary in the acute phase of infarction, the need for permanent pacing is less common and mostly dictated by the presence of IVCDs and not necessarily by the presence of symptoms. The long-term

(a)

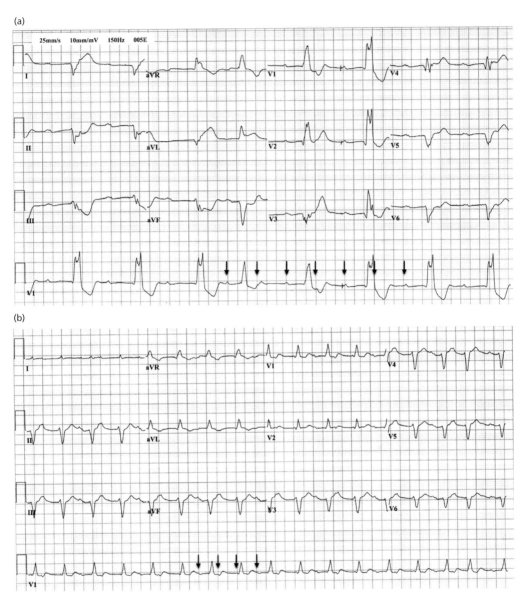

(b)

Figure 1.18 Acute anterior myocardial infarction complicated by complete AV block. This 82-year-old male presented with acute left main coronary artery occlusion in cardiogenic shock. (a) The initial ECG shows complete AV block with wide complex escape and evidence of ST-elevation myocardial infarction. The fourth and probably also the fifth complexes are conducted beats. P waves are indicated by arrows. He underwent temporary pacing, percutaneous intervention for acute revascularization, and hemodynamic support with a percutaneous left ventricular assist device. (b) ECG on the following day shows persistent complete AV block and an accelerated junctional rhythm with right bundle branch block and left anterior hemiblock. Although the conduction abnormalities are indications for pacing, the associated myocardial damage and hemodynamic compromise limit prognosis. This patient succumbed to progressive multiorgan failure.

prognosis for patients who develop AV block and an IVCD is strongly influenced by the extent of myocardial injury and hemodynamic status (Figure 1.18). The need for temporary pacing in the acute stages of infarction is not by itself an indication for permanent pacing. Patients who have an indication for permanent pacing after ST-elevation MI and severe LV dysfunction should be

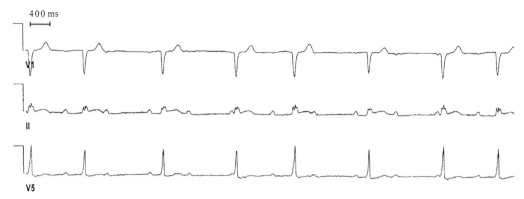

Figure 1.19 AV block associated with acute inferior myocardial infarction. Rhythm strips recorded from a 63-year-old female with an acute inferior wall myocardial infarction showing high-grade AV block with junctional escape beats. Some of the P waves are conducted with a prolonged PR interval (e.g. second QRS is captured by atrial conducted beat). The presence of junctional escape beats precludes typical Wenckebach conduction. Because the patient was asymptomatic, no therapy was administered. Normal AV conduction resumed the following morning.

evaluated for an ICD indication if recovery of ventricular function is not anticipated.

Indications for permanent pacing following acute myocardial infarction
Class I indications

1   Patients who present with sinus node dysfunction or AV block in the setting of an acute MI should undergo a waiting period before determining the need for permanent pacing. (Level of evidence: B-NR)
2   In patients presenting with an acute MI with second-degree Mobitz type II AV block, high-grade AV block, alternating bundle branch block or complete AV block (persistent or infranodal), permanent pacing is indicated after a waiting period. (Level of evidence: B-NR)

Class III (not indicated or harm)

1   In patients with an acute MI and transient AV block that resolves, permanent pacing should not be performed. (Level of evidence: B-NR)
2   In patients with an acute MI and a new bundle-branch block or isolated fascicular block in the absence of second- or third-degree AV block, permanent pacing should not be performed. (Level of evidence: B-NR)

Pacing after cardiac surgery and transcatheter aortic valve implantation

Approximately 3–5% of patients will develop persistent bradyarrhythmias after open heart surgery, with a higher incidence following repeat surgery. Sinus node dysfunction may result from right atrial cannulation for cardiopulmonary bypass, but mostly resolves within a week. The development of paroxysmal atrial arrhythmia in conjunction with SND can be particularly troublesome to treat without temporary pacing support. However, once sinus node function recovers, antiarrhythmic drugs can often be employed safely for postoperative atrial arrhythmias.

In adults, persistent AV block is most common after valvular surgery, particularly tricuspid valve replacement (12%). Risk is higher with multivalvular surgery, up to 25% for triple valve replacement [72]. In one large retrospective study, preexisting RBBB was more predictive than LBBB, but preoperative PR prolongation, repeat surgery, and age over 70 years were all predictors for the need for permanent pacing [72]. The aortic valve is closely related to the His bundle and surgical valve replacement carries a higher risk for persistent AV block. Hence, the threshold for pacing for heart block complicating aortic valve surgery is lower. Mitral valve surgery more commonly affects the AV node partly due to injury to the AV nodal artery. As the block is at the nodal level, threshold for pacing is higher. The majority of patients who develop postoperative bradyarrhythmias recover conduction and hence it is customary to wait 5–7 days before consideration of permanent pacing. If there is evidence for continued improvement in sinus node function or AV block at the nodal level, longer waiting times may be justified. Patients who ultimately undergo permanent cardiac pacing tend to have a good prognosis and only about 40% remain dependent on pacing in the longer term [73]. Septal myomectomy or alcohol septal ablation for hypertrophic obstructive cardiomyopathy is associated with AV block requiring pacing in 10–14% of patients [74]. The risk of sudden death is estimated to be approximately 1% per year and does not warrant the routine use of defibrillators. However, in the presence of other risk factors such as marked LV thickening, family history, or syncope, a defibrillator rather than a pacemaker is indicated.

Transcatheter aortic valve replacement (TAVR) is rapidly evolving as an effective alternative to valve surgery for patients with aortic stenosis. Unlike in the surgical procedure where the valve is excised prior to replacement, the calcified valve remains *in situ* in TAVR. Transcatheter placement of a valve prosthesis and balloon dilatation within this calcified valve produce a mass effect in the region of the membranous septum and adjoining conduction system. This potential mechanism leads to persistent heart block requiring cardiac pacing in 2–20% of patients, with the more recent studies documenting a lower incidence of persistent conduction defects [75,76]. New LBBB occurs in 20–50% of patients, and high-grade AV block in approximately 10% of patients but half of these resolve before discharge [75]. QRS duration of less than 120 ms was predictive of recovery [77]. Patients with new LBBB that persists after TAVR are also at risk of late heart block after discharge. In one study, an HV interval of more than 65 ms after TAVR had an 80% sensitivity and specificity for subsequent risk for heart block [78].

Earlier studies had shown a higher propensity for AV block based on type of prosthesis used but newer valves and better positioning have reduced the incidence. However, the risk of AV block in patients who develop new LBBB and timing of pacemaker implant remain ill-defined. Current guidelines recommend that a pacemaker may be considered for persisting LBBB after TAVR (class IIb indication) [13]. As more patients undergo non-surgical aortic valve replacement, larger studies will be needed to define risk of persistent AV block.

Drug-induced bradycardia

A number of medications may produce transient bradycardia that may require temporary pacing until the effect of the drug dissipates. These drugs may cause sinus node dysfunction and/or AV block; if drugs are used in combination, their effects may become more potent and exacerbate mild or latent conduction system disease. If long-term therapy with these agents is necessary for an underlying disorder and a substitute cannot be found, permanent pacing may be required (Figure 1.5). Drug-induced AV block might not always resolve after discontinuation of the potentially offending drug. In one series, approximately half of patients who developed heart block in the context of therapy with an AV nodal blocking agent required permanent pacing for persistent or recurrent AV block [75]. Cessation of digoxin therapy has the best chance of recovery of AV nodal conduction, but β-adrenergic blocker therapy often unmasks underlying conduction disease [79,80].

Sleep-disordered breathing and bradycardia

Nocturnal bradycardia is common in the young and conditioned athletes. Sinus bradycardia, sinus arrest, and varying degrees of AV block at the nodal level are observed and, in most circumstances, is physiological and vagally mediated. No intervention is required in the asymptomatic patient [81]. The prevalence of nocturnal bradyarrhythmia is lower in middle-aged and older healthy individuals.

A higher prevalence of sleep-related bradycardia is seen in patients with sleep apnea syndrome; the bradyarrhythmia tends to correlate with hypopneic events. Sinus node dysfunction is most common (7–40%) but second- or third-degree AV block is observed in 1–13% of patients [82]. Prevalence of bradyarrhythmias correlates with severity of sleep apnea. These patients have normal rhythm during wakeful hours. Continuous positive airway pressure reduces sleep-related bradyarrhythmia by 70–80% and eliminates the need for cardiac pacing in the majority. Symptomatic bradycardia is rare during long-term follow-up.

Summary

In patients with symptomatic and potentially life-threatening bradyarrhythmias, cardiac pacing is a cost-effective intervention to relieve symptoms and prevent death. However, the possible complications and the potentially complex longer-term management of permanent pacemaker systems require that careful consideration be given to the indications before implantation.

Acknowledgment

The author would like to acknowledge Robert W. Peters, Pugazhendhi Vijayaraman and Kenneth A. Ellenbogen for use of figures from the fifth edition.

References

1 Sanchez-Quintana D, Cabrera JA, Farre J, *et al.* Sinus node revisited in the era of electroanatomical mapping and catheter ablation. *Heart* 2005;91(2):189–194.

2 Boyett M, Honjo H, Kodama I. The sinoatrial node, a heterogeneous pacemaker structure. *Cardiovasc Res* 2000;47(4):658–687.

3 Boyett MR, Honjo H, Yamamoto M, *et al.* Regional differences in effects of 4-aminopyridine within the sinoatrial node. *Am J Physiol* 1998;275(4):H1158–H1168.

4 Opthof T. The mammalian sinoatrial node. *Cardiovasc Drugs Ther* 1988;1(6):573–597.

5 Mazgalev TN, Ho SY, Anderson RH. Anatomic–electrophysiological correlations concerning the pathways for atrioventricular conduction. *Circulation* 2001;103(22): 2660–2667.

6 Lee P-C, Chen S-A, Hwang B. Atrioventricular node anatomy and physiology: implications for ablation of atrioventricular nodal reentrant tachycardia. *Curr Opin Cardiol* 2009;24(2):105–112.

7 Inoue S, Becker AE. Posterior extensions of the human compact atrioventricular node. *Circulation* 1998;97(2): 188–193.

8 Sanders P, Morton JB, Kistler PM, *et al.* Electrophysiological and electroanatomic characterization of the atria in sinus node disease. *Circulation* 2004; 109(12):1514–1522.

9 Fedorov VV, Ambrosi CM, Kostecki G, *et al.* Anatomic localization and autonomic modulation of atrioventricular junctional rhythm in failing human hearts. *Circ Arrhythm Electrophysiol* 2011;4(4):515–525.

10 Dobrzynski H, Nikolski VP, Sambelashvili AT, *et al.* Site of origin and molecular substrate of atrioventricular junctional rhythm in the rabbit heart. *Circ Res* 2003; 93(11):1102–1110.

11 James TN, Sherf L. Fine structure of the His bundle. *Circulation* 1971;44(1):9–28.

12 Vijayaraman P, Chung MK, Dandamudi G, *et al.* His bundle pacing. *J Am Coll Cardiol* 2018;72(8):927–947.

13 Kusumoto FM, Schoenfeld MH, Barrett C, *et al.* 2018 ACC/AHA/HRS Guideline on the evaluation and management of patients with bradycardia and cardiac conduction delay: A Report of the American College of Cardiology/American Heart Association Task Force on Clinical Practice Guidelines and the Heart Rhythm Society. *Heart Rhythm* 2019;16(9):e128–e226.

14 Jones SA, Boyett MR, Lancaster MK. Declining into failure: the age-dependent loss of the L-type calcium channel within the sinoatrial node. *Circulation* 2007;115(10): 1183–1190.

15 Hocini Mlz, Sanders P, Deisenhofer I, *et al.* Reverse remodeling of sinus node function after catheter ablation of atrial fibrillation in patients with prolonged sinus pauses. *Circulation* 2003;108(10):1172–1175.

16 Adachi M, Igawa O, Yano A, *et al.* Long-term reliability of AAI mode pacing in patients with sinus node dysfunction and low Wenckebach block rate. *Europace* 2008; 10(2):134–137.

17 Kristensen L, Nielsen JC, Pedersen AK, *et al.* AV block and changes in pacing mode during long-term follow-up of 399 consecutive patients with sick sinus syndrome treated with an AAI/AAIR pacemaker. *Pacing Clin Electrophysiol* 2001;24(3):358–365.

18 Kandolin R, Lehtonen J, Kupari M. Cardiac sarcoidosis and giant cell myocarditis as causes of atrioventricular block in young and middle-aged adults. *Circ Arrhythm Electrophysiol* 2011;4(3):303–309.

19 Zipes DP. Second-degree atrioventricular block. *Circulation* 1979;60(3):465–472.

20 Kim YH, O'Nunain S, Trouton T, *et al.* Pseudo-pacemaker syndrome following inadvertent fast pathway ablation for atrioventricular nodal reentrant tachycardia. *J Cardiovasc Electrophysiol* 1993;4(2):178–182.

21 Brecker SJD, Xiao HB, Sparrow J, Gibson DG. Effects of dual-chamber pacing with short atrioventricular delay in dilated cardiomyopathy. *Lancet* 1992;340(8831):1308–1312.

22 Chokshi SK, Sarmiento J, Nazari J, *et al.* Exercise-provoked distal atrioventricular block. *Am J Cardiol* 1990;66(1):114–116.

23 Eriksson P, Hansson P-O, Eriksson H, Dellborg M. Bundle-branch block in a general male population. *Circulation* 1998;98(22):2494–2500.

24 McAnulty JH, Rahimtoola SH, Murphy E, *et al.* Natural history of high-risk bundle-branch block. *N Engl J Med* 1982;307(3):137–143.

25 Scheinman MM, Peters RW, Morady F, *et al.* Electrophysiologic studies in patients with bundle branch block. *Pacing Clin Electrophysiol* 1983;6(5):1157–1165.

26 Dhingra RC, Palileo E, Strasberg B, *et al.* Significance of the HV interval in 517 patients with chronic bifascicular block. *Circulation* 1981;64(6):1265–1271.

27 Petrac D, Radic B, Birtic K, Giurovic J. Prospective evaluation of infrahisal second-degree AV block induced by atrial pacing in the presence of chronic bundle branch block and syncope. *Pacing Clin Electrophysiol* 1996; 19(5):784–792.

28 Brignole M, Menozzi C, Moya A, *et al.* Mechanism of syncope in patients with bundle branch block and negative electrophysiological test. *Circulation* 2001;104(17):2045–2050.

29 Shen WK, Sheldon RS, Benditt DG, *et al.* 2017 ACC/AHA/HRS guideline for the evaluation and management of patients with syncope: executive summary. A Report of the American College of Cardiology/American Heart Association Task Force on Clinical Practice Guidelines and the Heart Rhythm Society. *J Am Coll Cardiol* 2017;70(5):620–663.

30 Krediet CT, van Dijk N, Linzer M, *et al.* Management of vasovagal syncope: controlling or aborting faints by leg crossing and muscle tensing. *Circulation* 2002;106(13):1684–1689.

31 Sheldon R, Connolly S, Rose S, *et al.* Prevention of Syncope Trial (POST): a randomized, placebo-controlled study of metoprolol in the prevention of vasovagal syncope. *Circulation* 2006;113(9):1164–1170.

32 Brignole M, Menozzi C, Moya A, *et al.* Pacemaker therapy in patients with neurally mediated syncope and documented asystole. Third International Study on Syncope of Uncertain Etiology (ISSUE-3): a randomized trial. *Circulation* 2012;125(21):2566–2571.

33 Palmisano P, Dell'Era G, Russo V, *et al.* Effects of closed-loop stimulation vs. DDD pacing on haemodynamic variations and occurrence of syncope induced by head-up tilt test in older patients with refractory cardioinhibitory vasovagal syncope: the Tilt test-Induced REsponse in Closed-loop Stimulation multicentre, prospective, single blind, randomized study. *Europace* 2017;20(5):859–866.

34 Brignole M, Deharo J-C, De Roy L, *et al.* Syncope due to idiopathic paroxysmal atrioventricular block. *J Am Coll Cardiol* 2011;58(2):167–173.

35 Brignole M, Guieu R, Tomaino M, *et al.* Mechanism of syncope without prodromes with normal heart and normal electrocardiogram. *Heart Rhythm* 2017;14(2):234–239.

36 Hurley KF, Magee K, Green R. Aminophylline for bradyasystolic cardiac arrest in adults. *Cochrane Database Syst Rev* 2015;(11):CD006781.

37 Bestawros M, Darbar D, Arain A, *et al.* Ictal asystole and ictal syncope: insights into clinical management. *Circ Arrhythm Electrophysiol* 2015;8(1):159–164.

38 Tenyi D, Gyimesi C, Kupo P, *et al.* Ictal asystole: a systematic review. *Epilepsia* 2017;58(3):356–362.

39 Groh WJ, Groh MR, Saha C, *et al.* Electrocardiographic abnormalities and sudden death in myotonic dystrophy type 1. *N Engl J Med* 2008;358(25):2688–2697.

40 Lazarus A, Varin J, Babuty D, *et al.* Long-term follow-up of arrhythmias in patients with myotonic dystrophy treated by pacing. *J Am Coll Cardiol* 2002;40(9):1645–1652.

41 Wahbi K, Meune C, Porcher R, *et al.* Electrophysiological study with prophylactic pacing and survival in adults with myotonic dystrophy and conduction system disease. *JAMA* 2012;307(12):1292–1301.

42 Doughan AR. Cardiac sarcoidosis. *Heart* 2006;92(2):282–288.

43 Buckley O, Doyle L, Padera R, *et al.* Cardiomyopathy of uncertain etiology: complementary role of multimodality imaging with cardiac MRI and ^{18}FDG PET. *J Nucl Cardiol* 2009;17(2):328–332.

44 Al-Khatib SM, Stevenson WG, Ackerman MJ, *et al.* 2017 AHA/ACC/HRS guideline for management of patients with ventricular arrhythmias and the prevention of sudden cardiac death: A Report of the American College of Cardiology/American Heart Association Task Force on Clinical Practice Guidelines and the Heart Rhythm Society. *J Am Coll Cardiol* 2018;72(14):e91–e220.

45 Lakdawala NK, Givertz MM. Dilated cardiomyopathy with conduction disease and arrhythmia. *Circulation* 2010;122(5):527–534.

46 Merlini G, Bellotti V. Molecular mechanisms of amyloidosis. *N Engl J Med* 2003;349(6):583–596.

47 Falk RH. Cardiac amyloidosis: a treatable disease, often overlooked. *Circulation* 2011;124(9):1079–1085.

48 Barbhaiya CR, Kumar S, Baldinger SH, *et al.* Electrophysiologic assessment of conduction abnormalities and atrial arrhythmias associated with amyloid cardiomyopathy. *Heart Rhythm* 2016;13(2):383–390.

49 Knockaert DC. Cardiac involvement in systemic inflammatory diseases. *Eur Heart J* 2007;28(15):1797–1804.

50 Bern C, Montgomery SP, Herwaldt BL, *et al.* Evaluation and treatment of Chagas disease in the United States. *JAMA* 2007;298(18):2171.

51 Ackerman MJ, Priori SG, Willems S, *et al.* HRS/EHRA expert consensus statement on the state of genetic testing for the channelopathies and cardiopathies. *Heart Rhythm* 2011;8(8):1308–1339.

52 Gersh BJ, Maron BJ, Bonow RO, *et al.* 2011 ACCF/AHA guideline for the diagnosis and treatment of hypertrophic cardiomyopathy. *J Am Coll Cardiol* 2011;58(25):e212–e260.

53 Maron BJ, Nishimura RA, McKenna WJ, *et al.* Assessment of permanent dual-chamber pacing as a treatment for drug-refractory symptomatic patients with obstructive hypertrophic cardiomyopathy. *Circulation* 1999;99(22):2927–2933.

54 Elliott PM, Anastasakis A, Borger MA, *et al.* 2014 ESC guidelines on diagnosis and management of hypertrophic cardiomyopathy: The Task Force for the Diagnosis and Management of Hypertrophic Cardiomyopathy of the European Society of Cardiology (ESC). *Eur Hevart J* 2014;35(39):2733–2779.

55 Epstein AE, DiMarco JP, Ellenbogen KA, *et al.* 2012 ACCF/AHA/HRS focused update incorporated into the ACCF/AHA/HRS 2008 guidelines for device-based therapy of cardiac rhythm abnormalities: a report of the American College of Cardiology Foundation/American

Heart Association Task Force on Practice Guidelines and the Heart Rhythm Society. *J Am Coll Cardiol* 2013;61(3): e6–e75.

56 Tang ASL, Wells GA, Talajic M, *et al*. Cardiac-resynchronization therapy for mild-to-moderate heart failure. *N Engl J Med* 2010;363(25):2385–2395.

57 Moss AJ, Hall WJ, Cannom DS, *et al*. Cardiac-resynchronization therapy for the prevention of heart-failure events. *N Engl J Med* 2009;361(14):1329–1338.

58 van Rees JB, de Bie MK, Thijssen J, *et al*. Implantation-related complications of implantable cardioverter-defibrillators and cardiac resynchronization therapy devices. *J Am Coll Cardiol* 2011;58(10):995–1000.

59 Zareba W, Klein H, Cygankiewicz I, *et al*. Effectiveness of cardiac resynchronization therapy by QRS morphology in the Multicenter Automatic Defibrillator Implantation Trial–Cardiac Resynchronization Therapy (MADIT-CRT). *Circulation* 2011;123(10):1061–1072.

60 Ruschitzka F, Abraham WT, Singh JP, *et al*. Cardiac-resynchronization therapy in heart failure with a narrow QRS complex. *N Engl J Med* 2013;369(15):1395–1405.

61 Gasparini M, Auricchio A, Regoli F, *et al*. Four-year efficacy of cardiac resynchronization therapy on exercise tolerance and disease progression: the importance of performing atrioventricular junction ablation in patients with atrial fibrillation. *J Am Coll Cardiol* 2006;48(4):734–743.

62 Yancy CW, Jessup M, Bozkurt B, *et al*. 2013 ACCF/AHA guideline for the management of heart failure: a report of the American College of Cardiology Foundation/American Heart Association Task Force on practice guidelines. *Circulation* 2013;128(16):e240–e327.

63 Ponikowski P, Voors AA, Anker SD, *et al*. 2016 ESC Guidelines for the diagnosis and treatment of acute and chronic heart failure: the Task Force for the diagnosis and treatment of acute and chronic heart failure of the European Society of Cardiology (ESC). Developed with the special contribution of the Heart Failure Association (HFA) of the ESC. *Eur J Heart Fail* 2016;18(8):891–975.

64 Eldar M, Griffin JC, Van Hare GF, *et al*. Combined use of beta-adrenergic blocking agents and long-term cardiac pacing for patients with the long QT syndrome. *J Am Coll Cardiol* 1992;20(4):830–837.

65 Ellenbogen KA. Pacing therapy for prevention of atrial fibrillation. *Heart Rhythm* 2007;4(3):S84–S87.

66 Lei M, Zhang H, Grace A, Huang C. SCN5A and sinoatrial node pacemaker function. *Cardiovasc Res* 2007;74(3):356–365.

67 Costedoat-Chalumeau N, Amoura Z, Villain E, *et al*. Anti-SSA/Ro antibodies and the heart: more than complete congenital heart block? A review of electrocardiographic and myocardial abnormalities and of treatment options. *Arthritis Res Ther* 2005;7(2):69–73.

68 Michaëlsson M, Jonzon A, Riesenfeld T. Isolated congenital complete atrioventricular block in adult life. *Circulation* 1995;92(3):442–449.

69 Villain E, Coastedoat-Chalumeau N, Marijon E, *et al*. Presentation and prognosis of complete atrioventricular block in childhood, according to maternal antibody status. *J Am Coll Cardiol* 2006;48(8):1682–1687.

70 Meine TJ, Al-Khatib SM, Alexander JH, *et al*. Incidence, predictors, and outcomes of high-degree atrioventricular block complicating acute myocardial infarction treated with thrombolytic therapy. *Am Heart J* 2005;149(4):670–674.

71 Newby KH, Pisano E, Krucoff MW, *et al*. Incidence and clinical relevance of the occurrence of bundle-branch block in patients treated with thrombolytic therapy. *Circulation* 1996;94(10):2424–2428.

72 Koplan BA, Stevenson WG, Epstein LM, *et al*. Development and validation of a simple risk score to predict the need for permanent pacing after cardiac valve surgery. *J Am Coll Cardiol* 2003;41(5):795–801.

73 Raza SS, Li J-M, John R, *et al*. Long-term mortality and pacing outcomes of patients with permanent pacemaker implantation after cardiac surgery. *Pacing Clin Electrophysiol* 2011;34(3):331–338.

74 Fitzgerald P, Kusumoto F. The effects of septal myectomy and alcohol septal ablation for hypertrophic cardiomyopathy on the cardiac conduction system. *J Interv Card Electrophysiol* 2018;52(3):403–408.

75 Nazif TM, Dizon JM, Hahn RT, *et al*. Predictors and clinical outcomes of permanent pacemaker implantation after transcatheter aortic valve replacement: the PARTNER (Placement of AoRtic TraNscathetER Valves) trial and registry. *JACC Cardiovasc Interv* 2015;8:60–69.

76 Toggweiler S, Stortecky S, Holy E, *et al*. The electrocardiogram after transcatheter aortic valve replacement determines the risk for post-procedural high-degree AV block and the need for telemetry monitoring. *JACC Cardiovasc Interv* 2016;9:1269–1276.

77 Schroeter T, Linke A, Haensig M, *et al*. Predictors of permanent pacemaker implantation after Medtronic CoreValve bioprosthetic implantation. *Europace* 2012;14:1759–1763.

78 Rivard L, Schram G, Asgar A, *et al*. Electrocardiographic and electrophysiological predictors of atrioventricular block after transcatheter aortic valve replacement. *Heart Rhythm* 2015;12:321–329.

79 Osmonov D, Erdinler I, Ozcan KS, *et al*. Management of patients with drug-induced atrioventricular block. *Pacing Clin Electrophysiol* 2012;35(7):804–810.

80 Zeltser D, Justo D, Halkin A, *et al*. Drug-induced atrioventricular block: prognosis after discontinuation of the culprit drug. *J Am Coll Cardiol* 2004;44(1):105–108.

81 Viitasalo MT, Kala R, Eisalo A. Ambulatory electrocardiographic recording in endurance athletes. *Br Heart J* 1982;47(3):213–220.

82 Mehra R, Benjamin EJ, Shahar E, *et al*. Association of nocturnal arrhythmias with sleep-disordered breathing: The Sleep Heart Health Study. *Am J Respir Crit Care Med* 2006;173(8):910–916.

CHAPTER 2

Basics of cardiac pacing: components of pacing, defibrillation, and resynchronization therapy systems

Justin Z. Lee, Vaibhav Vaidya, and Siva K. Mulpuru
Heart Rhythm Services, Mayo Clinic, Rochester, MN, USA

Introduction

Significant strides in our understanding of human cardiac physiology and the manipulation of pathological states with technology have been made since the first implantation of a pacemaker by Åke Senning in 1958. In this chapter we attempt to explain the underlying physiology of cardiac rhythm and the fundamentals of cardiac stimulation and discuss various devices currently in practice. We also explore various components of the devices with particular relevance to the clinical manifestations of malfunction and component failure.

Basics of pacing

Myocardial potential

Transmembrane potential

The presence of a transmembrane potential difference forms the basis for the electrical activation of the myocardium The myocyte cell membrane is composed of a phospholipid bilayer, arranged such that the hydrophobic phospholipid domains face one another and the hydrophilic ends are exposed to the extracellular and intracellular fluid (Figure 2.1a). The phospholipid bilayer forms a barrier to the free passage of charged ions across the cell membrane, except through specialized ion channels. An actively maintained difference in the concentrations of positively and negatively charged ions (known as cations and anions, respectively) across the cell membrane results in a potential difference across the cell membrane, and is known as the transmembrane potential [1]. During cellular diastole, the transmembrane potential across myocyte cell membranes is negative, with the intracellular space having a greater net negative charge compared to the extracellular space. This net negative potential during cellular diastole is also known as the resting membrane potential (RMP), with differences in the absolute value of the RMP in pacemaker, specialized conduction, atrial and ventricular cells. The Na^+/K^+-ATPase ion channel is integral to the maintenance of the negative transmembrane potential. This channel uses ATP to transport $3Na^+$ ions to the extracellular space while exchanging $2K^+$ ions to the intracellular space, resulting in fewer positively charged ions in the intracellular space and a negative resting membrane potential.

Action potential

When stimulated by electric current, myocytes can undergo a change in the transmembrane potential to less negative values (depolarization), followed by a return of the transmembrane potential to baseline values (repolarization). This sequence of

Cardiac Pacing and ICDs, Seventh Edition. Edited by Kenneth A. Ellenbogen and Karoly Kaszala.
© 2020 John Wiley & Sons Ltd. Published 2020 by John Wiley & Sons Ltd.

(a)

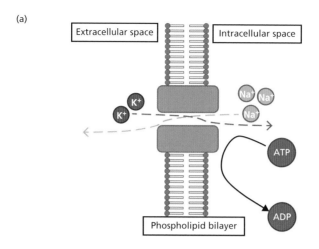

(b)

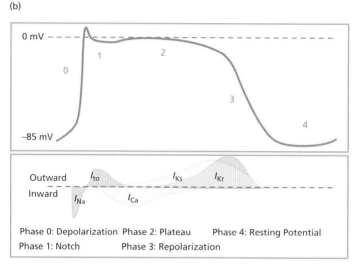

Figure 2.1 (a) Transmembrane potential. The cell membrane is composed of a phospholipid bilayer (blue) that forms a barrier to the passage of charged ions across the membrane. Ion channels, such as the Na$^+$/K$^+$-ATPase ion channel shown here (orange), are responsible for generation of a negative transmembrane potential. This channel uses ATP to transport 3Na$^+$ ions from the intracellular to the extracellular space and 2K$^+$ ions from the extracellular to the intracellular space, resulting in a net negative intracellular charge. (b) Schematic of the ventricular myocardial action potential with five phases: 4, resting; 0, rapid depolarization; 1, early repolarization; 2, plateau; 3, late repolarization.

changes in the transmembrane potential is known as the action potential and forms the basis for electrical activation of all excitable tissues [2]. The cardiac action potential has been extensively studied through patch clamp and microelectrode techniques and the ionic basis for action potential has been well elucidated.

The cardiac action potential in ventricular myocytes consists of five phases (Figure 2.1b). Phase 4 is the resting state, where a negative intracellular potential is maintained by the sodium/potassium channels and the sodium/calcium exchangers. Phase 0 is the depolarization phase, where conformational changes in the voltage-gated sodium channels (I_{Na}) allow the influx of positively charged sodium ions into the myocytes, resulting in depolarization of the cell membrane. Phase 1 is the rapid repolarization phase, mediated by the I_{to} channels,

(b)

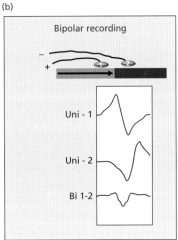

(a)

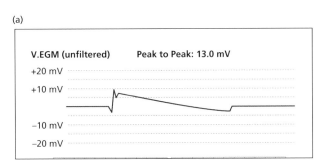

Figure 2.2 (a) Current of injury recorded during placement of a ventricular active fixation lead. Current of injury approximates the monophasic action potential of cardiac myocytes. (b) Spread of depolarization across a myocardial sheet recorded by two electrodes. The unipolar electrograms are recorded between the electrodes and a distant electrode (electrode not pictured). The resultant electrograms encompass both "near field" and "far field" myocardial activation due to the large antenna. The bipolar electrogram is derived from the unipolar electrograms of two electrodes and is more representative of near-field activation and less likely to detect non-cardiac far-field signals.

resulting in early repolarization. Differences in distribution of the I_{to} channels across the myocardial layers are one determinant of cardiac repolarization. Compared to these phases, phase 2 is a prolonged phase where depolarization is maintained by the influx of calcium through the L-type calcium channels, resulting in calcium-induced calcium release from the sarcolemmal membrane. There is also an efflux of potassium from the cell through the rapid (I_{Kr}) and slow (I_{Ks}) inward delayed rectifier potassium channels, such that the myocyte remains depolarized in phase 2. Contraction of the myocyte occurs during this phase of the action potential. In phase 3, the closure of calcium channels, while the potassium channels remain open, results in an efflux of potassium ions and repolarization of the cell membrane toward the resting membrane potential (see Online Video 2.1).

Sensing

A fundamental function of pacemakers and defibrillators is the detection of the presence and timing of cardiac electrical activity, commonly known as sensing. Accurate sensing is critical to the normal pacing performance, so that pacing stimuli can be delivered in the absence of intrinsic cardiac activity, and withheld in the presence of intrinsic cardiac activity. Accurate sensing is also critical for defibrillation, where detection of tachyarrhythmias requires sensing of these rhythms. While the action potential occurs on a cellular level, it cannot be measured in a sheet of myocardial cells without the use of intracellular electrodes. Damage to the cell membranes by mechanical pressure or active fixation of a pacemaker lead results in recording of a monophasic action potential, which closely parallels the cellular action potential (Figure 2.2a) [3]. However, these recordings are only transiently present at the time of device implantation, and cannot serve as the basis for long-term sensing of myocardial cellular activity.

Instead, sensing in clinical cardiac electrophysiology involves the measurement of the wavefront of depolarization as it spreads from cell to cell (Figure 2.2b). The spread of depolarization across the myocardial muscle sheet inscribes a waveform measured between two electrodes. Bipolar sensing constitutes the detection of the electrical wavefront between two closely spaced recording electrodes present within the pacing lead (such as the tip and ring electrodes), while unipolar sensing involves recording between the lead tip and a remote electrode such as the pacing generator. In implantable cardioverter–defibrillator (ICD) leads, it is possible to sense from the tip of the ICD lead to the defibrillation coil, known as integrated bipolar sensing (Figure 2.3). Bipolar sensing constitutes a far smaller "antenna" and mainly records the activation wavefront as it passes between the two closely spaced recording electrodes. Meanwhile, unipolar sensing has a wider antenna and records not only the local myocardial activation wavefront but also the wavefront of activation across the entire heart. Hence, unipolar sensing is more susceptible to the detection of unwanted biologic signals (such as electrical activity from the opposite cardiac chamber, repolarization signals, myopotentials) and extrinsic signals (electromagnetic interference). Satisfactory sensing amplitudes for P waves are around 1.5–5 mV and for R waves are around 5–25 mV [4].

The analog signals acquired through the leads are digitized, filtered, amplified, and rectified before application of threshold values for declaration of an event by the device (Figure 2.4). The sensing threshold values are fixed in pacemakers while the values are dynamic in defibrillators to account for varying amplitudes during fibrillation.

Stimulation physics

Sensing, pacing threshold and impedance comprise three fundamental parameters in the evaluation of pacemakers and defibrillators.

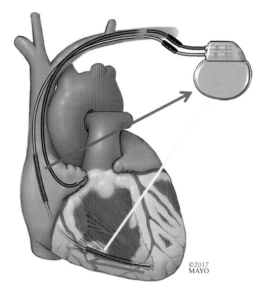

Figure 2.3 Various manufacturer-specific sensing vectors are available with implantable cardioverter–defibrillators. These include tip to ring (bipolar sensing, not shown) and tip to right ventricular (RV) defibrillation coil (integrated bipolar sensing, blue arrow). Additional vectors that can be used for telemetry or to record and discriminate arrhythmias include the shock electrogram (RV coil to generator, yellow arrow) and the leadless electrogram (SVC coil to generator, green arrow). Source: used with permission of Mayo Foundation for Medical Education and Research, all rights reserved.

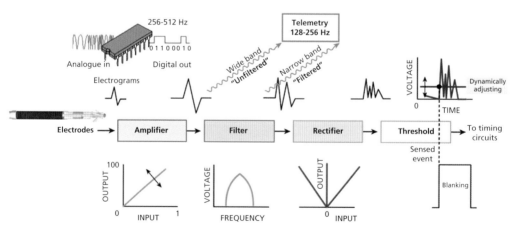

Figure 2.4 Signal processing in implantable cardioverter–defibrillators. The analog signal recorded between two electrodes is sampled at a rate of 256–512 Hz, followed by amplification, bandpass filtering to remove high- and low-frequency noise, rectification of negative signals to positive, and finally sensing based on the programmed sensitivity. Source: Swerdlow CD, Asirvatham SJ, Ellenbogen KA, Friedman PA. Troubleshooting implanted cardioverter defibrillator sensing problems I. *Circ Arrhythm Electrophysiol* 2014;7(6):1237–1261. Reproduced with permission of Wolters Kluwer Health, Inc.

Threshold

Delivery of energy to the myocardium via external methods can raise the transmembrane potential, resulting in depolarization of the local myocardium. The minimum amount of energy required to depolarize the myocardium is known as the pacing threshold [4]. The threshold is determined by the strength or magnitude or amplitude of the delivered impulse (measured in volts or milliamperes) and the duration for which the impulse is delivered (in milliseconds). It is imperative to appraise the relative contribution of both components of the pacing threshold in order to understand energy-efficient programming of pacemakers and defibrillators.

Strength–duration curve

The strength–duration curve is a graphical plot of the strength or magnitude of the impulse required to depolarize the myocardium at any given pulse duration or pulse width (Figure 2.5). In general, at a lower pulse duration or pulse width, the strength or magnitude of the pulse delivered needs to be greater for myocardial capture, and vice versa. The strength–duration curve can be constructed for any pacemaker and finds important applications in programming energy-efficient output parameters. Two points of critical importance on the strength–duration curve are the chronaxie and rheobase.

The current required to depolarize the myocardium at an infinite pulse width is known as the rheobase. As the pulse duration is increased, the current required for myocardial depolarization decreases, such that beyond a pulse width of 2 ms there is very little decrease in the threshold current magnitude, resulting in a "flat portion" of the strength–duration curve. For practical purposes, a pulse width greater than 2 ms does not result in lower pulse amplitude for myocardial capture. The chronaxie is the pulse width required to depolarize the myocardium at a current that is twice the rheobase. If one plots the aggregate energy required to depolarize the myocardium, the pulse width and amplitude at the chronaxie approximates the minimum required energy for pacing. The pulse width at chronaxie has been measured in a large number of pacing leads and is approximately 0.3 ms for atrial and ventricular leads [5].

The energy required for myocardial depolarization can be estimated from the formula:

$$E = VIt$$

where E represents energy, I current, V voltage, and t pulse duration.

Since $V = IR$ by Ohms law (where R is resistance), this equation can also be expressed as:

$$E = I^2 R t$$

or

$$E = V^2 t / R$$

Thus, the energy expended during myocardial capture is directly proportional to the pulse duration and directly proportional to the square of the applied voltage and current.

The current generations of device generators have non-rechargeable batteries with a finite amount of charge, and programming minimal required outputs that result in consistent myocardial capture is paramount to optimizing the battery life. In modern pacemakers, it is estimated that about half of estimated battery life is used for

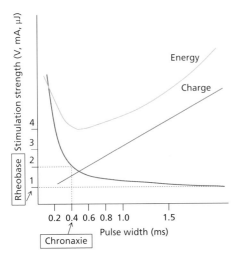

Figure 2.5 The strength–duration relationship (red curve) is a plot of the strength of impulse required for myocardial depolarization versus the pulse duration. The rheobase is the strength of impulse (current/voltage) required for myocardial depolarization at infinite pulse duration. The chronaxie is the pulse duration at twice the rheobase current/voltage. The chronaxie and rheobase approximate the minimum required energy for myocardial capture (green curve).

pacing function and the other half for housekeeping functions. Understanding the strength–duration curve is critical to the goal of programming energy-efficient outputs. For instance, programming outputs with a pulse duration above 2 ms is rarely justified. This would result in greater pulse duration and increased depletion of battery life, while output at below 2 ms would have a similar likelihood of capturing the myocardium. Furthermore, testing the threshold voltage at a pulse width between 0.3 and 0.4 ms can find the pulse amplitude required for myocardial capture that requires the minimal amount of energy to be expended by the device battery.

The programmed output for pacemakers is programmed at 2–2.5 times the measured threshold. This is because the capture threshold can vary based on autonomic tone, medication use, electrolyte imbalances, and changes occurring at the lead–myocardial interface (Table 2.1). A safety margin of 2–2.5 times the threshold allows for uninterrupted capture of the myocardium while avoiding the adverse effects of loss of capture.

Impedance

The third critical parameter to evaluate while interrogating the status of a pacemaker or defibrillator is the pacing impedance. Impedance is the cumulative resistance to the passage of electrical current in the circuit. The entire path that current must traverse between the battery terminals contributes to the pacing impedance: the generator (in the case of unipolar stimulation), leads, and the lead–myocardial interface. Practically, the impedance offered by the leads is designed to be minimal, such that the major source of impedance occurs at the lead–myocardial interface. Normal bipolar pacing impedance is variably characterized as 400–1200 Ω, and can be lower for unipolar pacing.

Absolute values and trends in the pacing impedance can both be indicative of a malfunction. For example, low impedance values suggest an insulation breach, while high impedance values may indicate a lead fracture or air in the header (Table 2.2) [6]. Diagnosis of malfunctions based on impedance is discussed in detail in Chapters 7 and 10. Another important concept is the relationship between impedance and battery life. Voltage bears a constant relationship with the impedance and current flowing in a circuit (Ohm's law: voltage = current × impedance). Thus, for a constant voltage energy source such as a pacing generator, the greater the impedance, the lower the magnitude of current required to create a potential difference to depolarize the myocardium. Thus, higher pacing impedance can result in reduced current drain from the generator and increase battery life [4].

Table 2.1 Factors affecting pacing threshold

	Increased threshold	Decreased threshold
Antiarrhythmic medications	Quinidine Procainamide Flecainide Propafenone Amiodarone Ibutilide	Sotalol Dofetilide
Other medications	Beta-blockers Mineralocorticoids	Glucocorticoids Catecholamines Atropine
Metabolic factors	Acidosis Hypoxemia Hyperkalemia	Hypokalemia
Physiological variables	Eating Sleeping	Exercise Increased sympathetic tone
Device-related variables	Large electrode size Smaller output capacitance	Small electrode size Larger output capacitance

Table 2.2 Diagnostic considerations with changes in pacing, defibrillation or battery impedance

	Increased impedance	Decreased impedance
Pacing impedance	Pace-sense conductor fracture Loose set-screw Air in the header	Pace-sense insulation breach (can be intermittent)
Defibrillation impedance	Pneumothorax High-voltage conductor/coil fracture	High-voltage insulation breach Short-circuiting due to inside-out or outside-in lead abrasion (additional details in lead design section)
Battery impedance	Battery depletion	Design factors such as anode corrugation to increase surface area

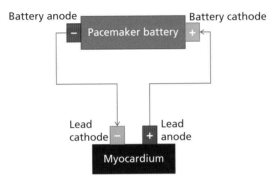

Figure 2.6 Typical bipolar pacing circuit composed of a galvanic cell/battery and bipolar pacing between the lead tip and ring. The battery anode (red) donates electrons and has a negative polarity. The electrons are accepted by the lead tip, which is the lead cathode (green) and also has a negative polarity. The lead ring or lead anode (red) donates electrons and has a positive polarity. Electrons are accepted by the battery cathode (green), which has a negative polarity.

Anodal versus cathodal stimulation

A clear understanding of the anode and cathode, the distinction between battery and lead anode and cathode, and the polarities of these terminals facilitates further discussion of pacing biophysics and the important concept of anodal versus cathodal stimulation. An electric circuit constitutes a flow of electrons through a conductive medium that is driven by a potential difference supplied by a battery. Battery terminals either electrons donors or electron recipients. Donation of electrons is defined as oxidation, and the terminal undergoing oxidation is always known as the anode. The terminal receiving electrons undergoes reduction, and is always known as the cathode. The polarity of the anode and cathode as "positive" and "negative" can be confusing, but can be deduced by recalling the principles of oxidation and reduction, and distinguishing between the battery and lead anode and cathode (Figure 2.6).

Cells can convert chemical energy into electrical energy (galvanic/voltaic cells) or can convert electrical energy into chemical energy (electrolytic cells). In a galvanic cell, such as a pacemaker generator, spontaneous chemical reactions drive electron loss/oxidation from one terminal (anode), resulting in the battery anode having a negative charge, and electron gain/reduction at the other terminal (cathode), resulting in a positive charge at the battery cathode. In a conventional bipolar pacing lead, the electrons travel from the battery anode to the lead tip. As the lead tip receives electrons, it is the lead cathode and it has a negative polarity. Electrons travel back to the battery cathode from the lead ring. Since the electrons are donated by the lead ring, this is the lead anode and it has a positive charge since it is connected to the positive terminal of the battery. In modern pacemaker systems, the lead cathode is almost always the lead tip, as mentioned in the present discussion, while the anode is

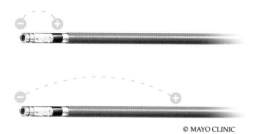

Figure 2.7 Multiple pacing vectors in an ICD lead. (*Top*) Bipolar pacing between the ICD lead tip (cathode) and ring (anode). (*Bottom*) Integrated bipolar pacing between the ICD lead tip (cathode) and right ventricular defibrillation coil (anode). Source: used with permission of Mayo Foundation for Medical Education and Research, all rights reserved.

programmable and can be the ring electrode, defibrillation coil, or the generator itself (Figure 2.7).

Modern devices, especially cardiac resynchronization therapy (CRT) devices, allow for the programming of multiple different pacing vectors. CRT leads are routinely constructed with four electrodes, allowing any of the four electrodes to be programmed as the cathode. Furthermore, depending on the device manufacturer, the anode can be programmed to the right ventricular (RV) lead ring electrode, RV defibrillation coil or the generator, in addition to these four electrodes. These multiple programmable pacing vectors allow greater flexibility of device programming and permit selection of pacing vectors that have the minimum threshold.

Figure 2.8a depicts the typical pacing stimulus applied to the myocardium by cardiac devices. The typical pacing pulse is direct current with a constant voltage and fixed pulse duration, applied from the cathode (depolarizing stimulus), with sudden changes in voltage at the initiation ("make") and termination ("break") of the pulse. Pacing pulses can also be applied from the anode and result in hyperpolarization. Most clinical stimulation of tissue is during the cathodal "make." Both "make" and "break" can result in stimulation of tissue at the cathode or anode. Other than certain special circumstances such as pacing in the relative refractory period, the cathodal "make" stimulation requires the lowest energy for myocardial capture [7]. Regular pacemaker leads are designed so the anode has a larger surface area, resulting in lower charge density and thereby reducing the probability of anodal capture.

However, in cases where the anode has a small surface area, and the output voltage is programmed high, anodal capture can occur and result in undesirable consequences. This situation can be encountered in CRT programming with a left ventricular (LV) lead [8]. When programmed to pace between the LV lead tip cathode and the RV ring anode at high outputs due to elevated LV tip thresholds, there can be capture of the RV myocardium at the anode, while failing to capture at the LV lead tip, resulting in RV-only pacing and loss of CRT (Figure 2.8b). Understanding the principle of anodal stimulation can help clinicians be cognizant of this and observe for loss of LV pacing due to anodal stimulation. Programming the anode to an electrode with a large surface area (such as a defibrillation coil) can reduce the charge density at the anode and avoid anodal stimulation.

Polarization

Application of a potential difference across a conductive medium results in the flow of electrons from the negative to positive terminals, which constitutes an electric current (conventional notation is the flow of positive charges). The direct flow of electrons across a conductive medium constitutes Faradic current. However, current can still conduct when the circuit comprises charged ions instead of conductive media with free electrons. For instance, at the lead–myocardial interface within the human body, there cannot be a direct transfer of electrons from the lead to the myocardium, but electric current can still pass from the pacing lead to the myocardium. A potential difference applied to metallic electrodes in contact with a medium containing charged ions results in migration of positively charged ions to the negative terminal and negatively charged ions to the positive terminal, resulting in passage of electric current. This process of the passage of electric current without the actual exchange of electrons is known as non-Faradic current. Myocardial pacing at conventional pacing outputs occurs via non-Faradic current, but at high pacing outputs, electrolysis at the lead–myocardial interface can result in Faradic current. The byproducts of electrolysis, such as hydroxide (OH^-) ions, can corrode the leads.

The sequence of events underlying non-Faradic current is more complex than previously described.

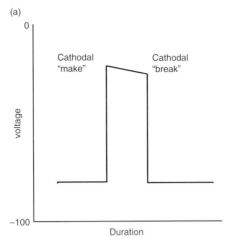

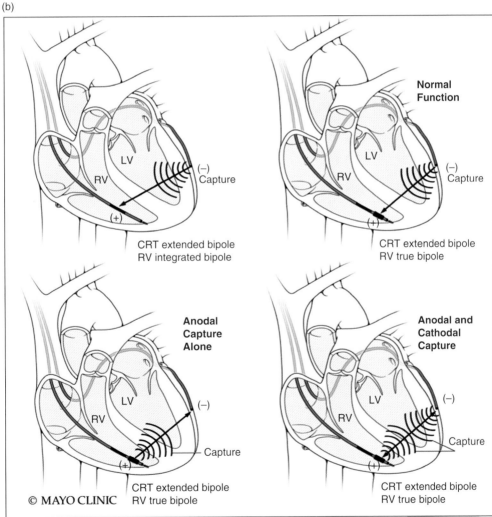

Figure 2.8 (a) Typical cathodal pacing pulse with constant voltage and fixed pulse duration. Myocardial capture occurs usually during the cathodal "make" rather than cathodal "break". (b) Concept of anodal stimulation. High-output stimulation between the left ventricular (LV) lead tip cathode and a right ventricular (RV) ring anode can result in anodal RV capture. Increasing the anodal surface area by programming the RV coil as anode can reduce the charge density and prevent anodal capture. CRT, cardiac resynchronization therapy. Source: used with permission of Mayo Foundation for Medical Education and Research, all rights reserved.

Application of a charge to the lead–myocardial interface results in attraction of a layer of ions of the opposite charge. Ions of the opposite polarity to the first layer can then be attracted to the first layer, which can culminate in multiple layers of charged ions. The presence of two charged surfaces separated by a non-conductive or dielectric medium constitutes a capacitor, and myocardial pacing involves the formation of a temporary capacitor with each pacing pulse (Figure 2.9a). This concept was first described by Helmholtz in 1879 and is termed Helmholtz capacitance or as double-layer or bilayer capacitance [3]. After the pacing pulse has terminated, the temporary double layer capacitor discharges, and this discharge is recorded on the pacing leads and is known as the polarization artifact (Figure 2.9b). The presence of this artifact can interfere with accurate functioning of auto-capture algorithms, as discussed subsequently.

A solution to the problem of polarization artifact is the development of fractal leads. Fractal leads involve deposition of conductive material on the

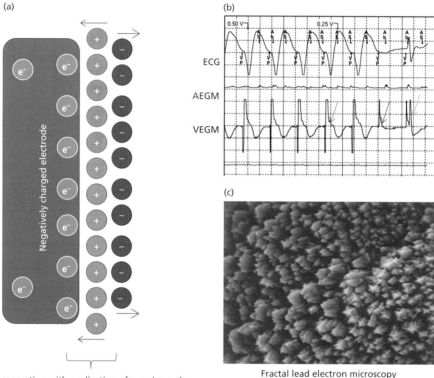

(a)

Negatively charged electrode

Charge separation with application of a pacing pulse – development of a temporary bilayered capacitor

(b)

ECG

AEGM

VEGM

(c)

Fractal lead electron microscopy

Reproduced with Permission from Abbott

Figure 2.9 (a) Non-Faradic current and formation for a double layer or bilayer capacitance (Helmholtz capacitance). Application of current to an electrode results in electron build-up and a negatively charge electrode. At the electrode–myocardial interface, there is not direct transfer of electrons (Faradic current). Instead, charge transmission occurs due to attraction (violet arrows) of positively charged ions (cations) in the interstitial fluid (non-Faradic current). A thin layer of cations is attracted to the negatively charged electrode. A layer of negatively charged ions (anions) is then attracted to the cations and multiple such layers can be formed. These separated charged layers constitute a temporary capacitor and form with each pacing pulse, and are responsible for the polarization artifact. (b) Ventricular threshold testing in a patient with atrial fibrillation. The first five pacing pulses result in right ventricular (RV) capture, followed by loss of capture on the sixth beat, and loss of capture with intrinsic conduction to the right ventricle on the seventh beat. The polarization artifact is visible on the sixth beat (red arrow). During RV capture, the polarization artifact occurs along with the electrogram (EGM) created by RV depolarization (evoked potential, blue arrow). In the seventh beat the polarization artifact is again visible, with EGM from intrinsic RV conduction following soon after. (c) Electron micrograph of a fractal lead.

lead tip in an irregular manner at a microscopic scale (Figure 2.9c). This greatly increases the electrochemically active surface area of the lead. As capacitance is proportional to the surface area of the capacitor, fractal leads result in formation of double-layer capacitors with increased capacitance compared to conventional leads. While it might seem counterintuitive to increase the capacitance of pacing electrodes, a greater capacitance reduces the charge held per unit area, resulting in reduced amplitude of the polarization artifact.

Changes with lead fixation

Active fixation leads are implanted by advancing a tiny screw at the tip of the lead into the myocardium, while passive fixation leads bear tines that are embedded into trabeculated regions of the myocardium. Pressure on the local myocardium by active or passive leads results in ST elevation on the local electrogram (EGM), known as the current of injury. The injury current is representative of the local multicellular action potential and is a form of monophasic action potential recording, as discussed previously [3].

Active fixation results in a more prominent current of injury and is a marker of sufficient acute fixation of the leads (see Figure 2.2a). The current of injury has the greatest magnitude a few minutes after implantation, followed by a reduction in magnitude over the next few minutes to hours. A positive current of injury indicates an endocardial position of the lead tip, while a negative current of injury should alert the implanter to the possibility of myocardial perforation and an epicardial lead tip position [9].

Evoked potentials

Pacing outputs are a critical determinant of battery life, and there is a constant push towards lowering pacing outputs while retaining reliable capture of the myocardium. Conventionally, pacing outputs were programmed at a safety margin of 2–2.5 times the measured capture threshold. One approach to lowering the pacing outputs safely involves automated measurement of the pacing threshold and adjustment of pacing outputs slightly above the measured threshold. Each device manufacturer has a different algorithm for automated threshold measurement, but the concept of evoked potentials or an evoked response is central to all approaches.

Output of the pacing pulse results in multiple recorded deflections on bipolar EGM recordings, including a saturation artifact, polarization artifact and, when myocardial capture occurs, the local EGM, also known as the evoked response in pacing parlance (see Figure 2.9b). The challenge in the detection of the evoked response is the exclusion of the saturation and polarization artifacts. The saturation artifact occurs a few milliseconds after the pacing pulse as a result of direct saturation of the sensing amplifiers. The saturation artifact can be separated from the evoked response by opening the sensing window for evoked responses a few milliseconds after pulse delivery. However, separation of the polarization artifact from the evoked response is technically far more complex and sometimes not possible. Engineering advances such as fractal leads can minimize the polarization artifact and aid in the detection of the evoked response.

Types of cardiac implantable electronic devices

Many cardiac implantable electronic devices (CIEDs) have been developed over the years and many of them improve patient outcomes by pacing or defibrillation.

Pacemaker

The basic function of the pacemaker is to maintain a desired heart rate or synchrony between cardiac chambers (atrioventricular or interventricular synchrony). Modern devices have many additional functions, such as diagnostic capabilities, activity sensors, and fluid retention monitoring.

A pacemaker system generally comprises a pulse generator connected to the myocardium by leads (Figure 2.10). The pulse generator is made of a header block and a device enclosure. These components are hermetically sealed together at production. The header block contains the set-screws for lead connection and, in some cases, an embedded radiofrequency antenna. Within the enclosure can be found the power source and integrated circuit boards containing the sensing circuit, timing circuit, output circuit, memory, logic circuits, physiological sensors, and inductive telemetry coil. The leads are securely connected to the pulse generator with the use of set-screws. Leads traverse from the

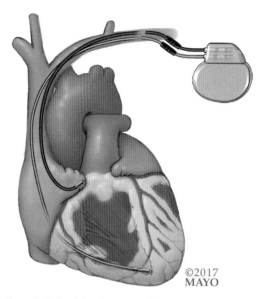

Figure 2.10 Dual-chamber pacemaker with a right atrial lead (blue) and a right ventricular lead (green). The pulse generator is in the prepectoral area and is connected by leads to the myocardium by active fixation leads. Source: used with permission of Mayo Foundation for Medical Education and Research, all rights reserved.

pocket through the veins (transvenous leads) or are implanted directly on the surface of the heart by surgery (surgical leads). The leads can be fixed to the heart by active fixation or passive fixation. Connection failure between the components of a pacemaker system may result in an "open circuit" leading to absence of electrical continuity. Intermittent contact between the components of the pacemaker system may also inhibit pulse generator output due to detection of potentials mistaken as intrinsic electrical activity. In the past few years, there is a growing interest in conduction system pacing where the goal is to pace the conduction system to reproduce a narrow QRS morphology. The His bundle has emerged as an alluring target of pacing to achieve a more physiological activation of the ventricles via the native conduction system (Figure. 2.11).

Implantable cardiac defibrillator

An implantable cardioverter–defibrillator (ICD) system includes a pulse generator connected to the heart with one or two coils in addition to the components that are used for sensing and pacing

(a)

(b)

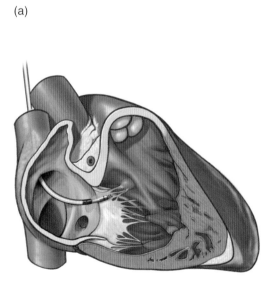

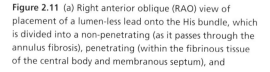

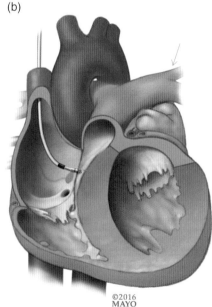

Figure 2.11 (a) Right anterior oblique (RAO) view of placement of a lumen-less lead onto the His bundle, which is divided into a non-penetrating (as it passes through the annulus fibrosis), penetrating (within the fibrinous tissue of the central body and membranous septum), and branching portion (at the crest of the muscular ventricular septum). (b) Left anterior oblique (LAO) view of conduction system pacing demonstrating its septal location. Source: used with permission of Mayo Foundation for Medical Education and Research, all rights reserved.

(a)

(b)

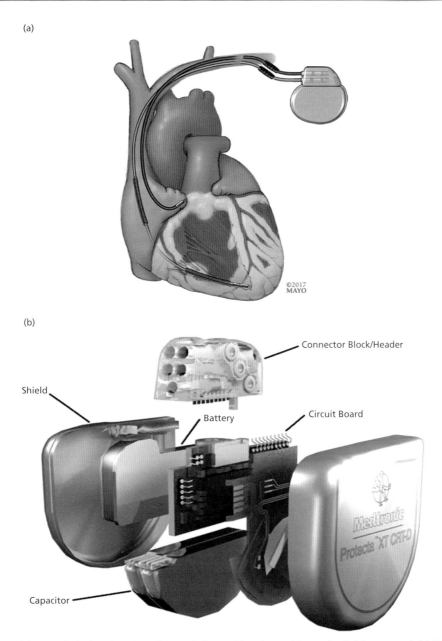

Connector Block/Header

Shield

Battery

Circuit Board

Capacitor

Figure 2.12 (a) ICD with shock coils in the right ventricular and the superior vena cava. The right ventricular lead is connected to the myocardium by passive fixation. Source: used with permission of Mayo Foundation for Medical Education and Research, all rights reserved. (b) ICD components: the sealed titanium can contains circuits, high-voltage capacitor, and battery. Source: Medtronic, Inc. Reproduced with permission of Medtronic, Inc.

(Figure 2.12). The ICD pulse generator includes the battery, hybrid integrated circuit board, telemetry communication coil, and high-voltage components including the transformer, capacitor, and output circuitry. The high-voltage capacitor consists of two conductors separated by an insulator.

The basic function of a capacitor is to store electrical charge and release this energy to the circuit. The high-voltage charging circuit (Figure 2.13) converts the low-voltage output of the battery to the high-voltage output that charges the output capacitor for delivery of the shock.

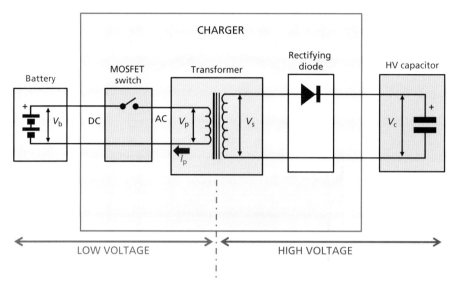

Figure 2.13 High-voltage (HV) charging circuit converts the low-voltage output of the battery to the high-voltage output that charges the output capacitor for delivery of the shock. V_b, V_p, V_s, and V_c represent voltages across the battery, primary winding of the transformer, secondary winding of the transformer, and the capacitor. I_p denotes current in the primary circuit. DC, direct current; AC, alternating current.

Cardiac resynchronization therapy devices

The goal of CRT is to restore electrical synchrony. The most common CRT component configuration includes a three-lead pulse generator, and right atrial, RV, and LV leads (Figures 2.14 and 2.15). The right atrial lead permits sensing or tracking of atrial rhythm to synchronize ventricular activation to atrial activity. The RV lead is used to sense intrinsic ventricular activity, and to pace alongside the LV pacing stimulus. Current CRT devices use separate RV and LV output and sensing circuits with multiple options for programming the stimulation vector. The LV pacing lead may have one (unipolar), two (bipolar), or four (quadripolar) electrodes with independent programmability of the stimulation configuration. Therefore, the left ventricle can be stimulated in a unipolar configuration from a single electrode in the coronary vein with the pulse generator casing being the electrode of opposite polarity. It can also be stimulated in a bipolar configuration using two electrodes in the coronary vein. Stimulation can also be performed with any of up to four electrodes in a quadripolar LV lead as the cathode and either the RV ring electrode or the pulse generator as the anode. The advantages of multiple stimulation configuration options are (i) minimizing LV capture threshold, (ii) reducing the chances of left phrenic nerve stimulation, (iii) independent timing of LV and RV stimulation, and (iv) the option of using automatic capture algorithms in both ventricular chambers. Modern CRT devices also have capabilities to pace simultaneously in multiple vectors (multipoint pacing, Abbott Laboratories, Abbott Park, IL) and to pace from LV lead alone synchronized to native RV conduction (Adaptive CRT, Medtronic, Minneapolis, MN).

Subcutaneous ICD

The subcutaneous ICD (S-ICD) was developed to avoid endocardial lead placement. The components of a subcutaneous ICD include a pulse generator and subcutaneous lead. The pulse generator is placed laterally in the midaxillary–anterior axillary line and is connected to the subcutaneous lead tunneled next to the sternum (Figure 2.16) [10]. The current second-generation S-ICD, the EMBLEM™ MRI (Boston Scientific, Marlborough, MA), contains a pulse generator that has a volume of 60 cm^3 (83 × 69 × 12 mm), weighs 130 g, and utilizes an LiMnO$_2$ battery with a projected longevity of 7.3 years [11]. The subcutaneous lead has an 8-cm shocking coil that separates the distal and

(a)

(b)

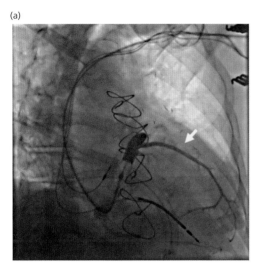

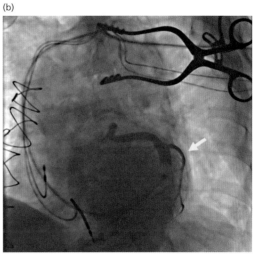

Figure 2.14 (a) Right and (b) left anterior oblique views of balloon occlusion venography during cardiac resynchronization therapy device implant. A good target vein is identified along the lateral border of the heart (yellow arrow).

(a)

(b)

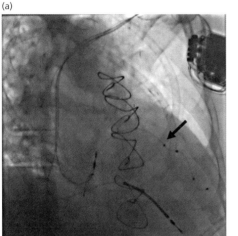

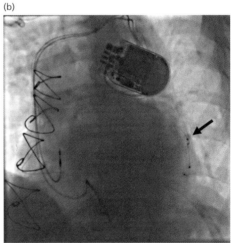

Figure 2.15 Placement of a quadripolar lead in (a) right and (b) left anterior oblique views in the identified coronary sinus branch. The four electrodes on the quadripolar lead provide several options for programming the left ventricular pacing vector.

proximal sensing electrodes with respect to the pulse generator.

In comparison with closely spaced endocardial electrodes, the S-ICD recording has a lower amplitude and frequency, and the device software must process the waveform to distinguish QRS from T wave and P wave. The vector that provides the optimal waveform that allows this distinction in various body postures will be selected (Figure 2.17). The two methods of screening patients are manual screening and automated screening. With manual screening, ECG strips are recorded in both the supine and standing position. The manual screening tool is then used to evaluate if all the QRS complexes and T waves in at least one sensing vector are suitable in both the supine and standing position (Figure 2.18). Automated screening utilizes an automated screening tool which may be more objective [12].

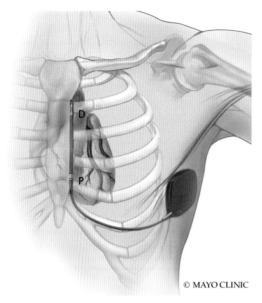

© MAYO CLINIC

Figure 2.16 Components of the subcutaneous ICD system. The pulse generator is implanted in the left lateral axillary area and is connected to a subcutaneous lead with an 8-cm shocking coil, which separates the distal (D) and proximal (P) electrodes. This coil is tunneled adjacent to the sternum. Source: used with permission of Mayo Foundation for Medical Education and Research, all rights reserved.

Leadless pacemaker

The single-component leadless pacemaker refers to a device in which all the components of the pacemaker (battery, electronics, stimulating electrodes, rate-adaptive sensors) are contained within a single system. The two main single-component system are the Micra transcatheter pacing system (TPS) (Medtronic, Minneapolis, MN) and the Nanostim leadless cardiac pacemaker (LCP) (Abbott Laboratories, Abbott Park, IL) (Figure 2.19). However, the Nanostim LCP is currently not clinically available due to issues with malfunctioning batteries and problems with the docking button during device retrieval. Nevertheless, clinicians may see patients with devices implanted during clinical trials. Leadless pacemakers may be suitable for patients that meet indications for permanent single-chamber RV pacing (VVIR) [13]. This may include patients with chronic atrial fibrillation with atrioventricular (AV) block or sinus bradycardia with infrequent pauses.

The Micra TPS has a shorter, smaller, and lighter profile compared to the Nanostim LCP (Table 2.3). The rate-modulating mechanism in the Micra TPS is based on the three-axis accelerometer, whereas the Nanostim LCP utilizes blood temperature.

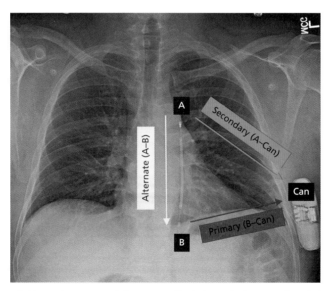

Figure 2.17 The three available sensing vectors of the subcutaneous ICD. There is a primary vector (from proximal electrode ring to can), secondary vector (from distal electrode ring to can), and alternate vector (from distal to proximal electrode).

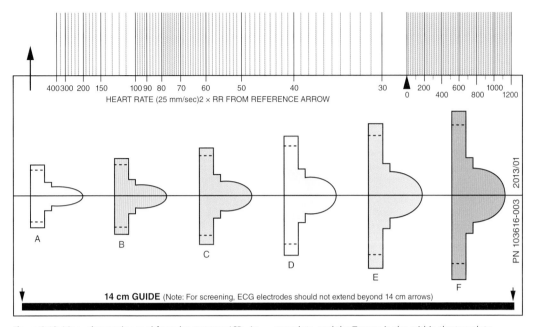

HEART RATE (25 mm/sec)2 × RR FROM REFERENCE ARROW

14 cm GUIDE (Note: For screening, ECG electrodes should not extend beyond 14 cm arrows)

Figure 2.18 Manual screening tool for subcutaneous ICD. An acceptable waveform is when the tip of the QRS complex is within the dashed line and the top or bottom part of the template, and the T wave is also within the template. Source: courtesy of Boston Scientific. © 2017 Boston Scientific Corporation or its affiliates. All rights reserved.

(a)

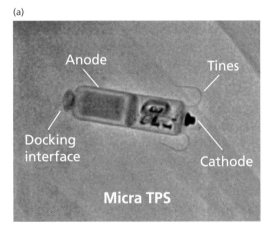

(b)

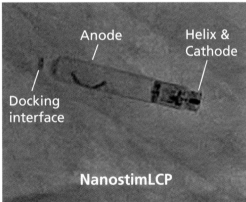

Figure 2.19 (a) Micra TPS has a centrally located cathode between the passive fixation tines, while the ring electrode is on the body. (b) The Nanostim LCP has a longer profile with an active fixation mechanism. The active helix is also the cathode, while the body acts as the anode.

For pacemaker communication, the Micra TPS utilizes radiofrequency telemetry, whereas the Nanostim LCP uses conductive telemetry. The Micra TPS also has an autocapture threshold algorithm to potentially prolong battery life.

Both devices are implanted via a sheath (23 Fr for Micra and 18 Fr for Nanostim) inserted in the femoral vein and delivered to the right ventricle. The positioning of the device is typically facilitated by fluoroscopic guidance and contrast injections. The fixation mechanism of the Micra TPS is via passive fixation with four integrated self-expanding electrically inert nitinol tines. On the other hand, Nanostim LCP utilizes an active fixation helix that is secured into the RV apical septum via rotation of the delivery catheter handle control knob.

Table 2.3 Comparison of components of the Micra and Nanostim leadless pacemakers

	Micra (TPS)	Nanostim (LCP)
Indications	VVI(R)	VVI(R)
Size (height × width in mm)	26 × 6.7	42 × 6
Volume (cm³)	0.8	1.0
Weight (g)	2.0	2.0
Delivery sheath diameter	23-F inner diameter and 27-F outer diameter	18-F inner diameter and 21-F outer diameter
Battery technology	Lithium–silver–vanadium oxide/carbon monofluoride	Lithium–carbon monofluoride
Estimated longevity (years)[a]	4.7 (2.5 V @ 0.4 ms)	9.8 (2.5 V @ 0.4 ms)
Longevity based on nominal settings (years)	9.6 (1.5 V @ 0.24 ms)	14.7 (1.5 V @ 0.24 ms)
Autocapture threshold algorithm	Available, optimizes pacing output to 0.5 V above pacing threshold	Not available
Fixation mechanism	Passive fixation with electrically inert nitinol tines	Active fixation with screw-in helix
Rate modulation mechanism	Three-axis accelerometer	Blood temperature
Pacemaker communication	Radiofrequency telemetry	Conductive telemetry: requires placement of skin patches for pacemaker communication

[a] Longevity based on ISO (International Organization for Standardization) for reporting battery longevity: 2.5 V, 0.4 ms, 600 Ω, 60 bpm, and 100% pacing.

For Micra, the conventional Medtronic programmer is used for communication with the device via radiofrequency telemetry. For Nanostim, a dedicated programmer is required. Signal transmission would require application of skin electrodes for communication via conductive telemetry.

At end of service, proposed options include (i) programming the device off, which permanently deactivates pacing and sensing, and implanting a new pacemaker; or (ii) retrieving the device and implanting a new pacemaker. Both devices have a docking interface for percutaneous retrieval provided the device is not encapsulated; although this may complicate device retrieval, it does lead to a theoretically reduced risk of infection.

Wireless cardiac resynchronization system

The wireless cardiac resynchronization system (WiSE-CRT, EBR Systems, Sunnyvale, CA) utilizes a multicomponent strategy for leadless cardiac resynchronization (Figure 2.20). A receiver titanium electrode covered by polyester is delivered into the left ventricle utilizing a percutaneous aortic retrograde approach and implanted endocardially in the left ventricle via three self-expanding nitinol tines. A separate device, which consists of a battery and an ultrasound transmitter, is implanted subcutaneously in the left thorax. The transmitter generates ultrasound pulses directed to the implanted receiver-electrode. The receiver-electrode converts the acoustic energy to an electrical pacing pulse. There is no battery in the endocardial receiver-electrode. This can be co-implanted with any device capable of performing RV pacing to achieve synchronous biventricular capture by sensing the RV signal.

Components of the CIED system

Battery

The power source for most pacemakers today is a solid chemical battery. At implant, the battery's electrochemical potential represents the total

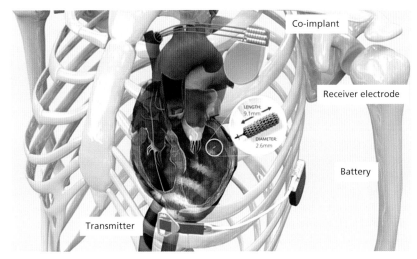

Figure 2.20 Components of the wireless cardiac resynchronization system. Source: EBR Systems, Inc. Reproduced with permission of EBR Systems, Inc.

energy available to the device over its service life for all monitoring, processing, and therapeutic functions. The lithium–iodine battery has been used in the vast majority of cardiac pacemakers as it has an unsurpassed record of reliability. However, as pacemakers have become more complicated, their power needs have grown. As a result, the demands on the power source have increased exponentially. Lithium–carbon monofluoride (LiCFx), lithium–manganese dioxide ($LiMnO_2$), and hybrid batteries are increasingly being used in pacemakers (Table 2.4).

Lithium (Li) is located in the anode of the battery (electrically negative) and provides electrons to the external load. An oxide or halogen-rich compound (PI_2) is located in the cathode (electrically positive) and receives electrons. The electrolyte separates the anodal and cathodal reactions and is capable of conducting ions but not electrons. A dissolved lithium salt (a complex of iodine and poly-2-vinylpyridine) is the electrolyte used in lithium–iodine batteries. As the battery is drained, the mass of electrolyte increases, as does the internal battery impedance. The internal impedance of a cell determines its current carrying capability. Low internal resistance allows high currents.

An important consideration for device functionality is the peak power requirement. For the treatment of bradycardia, microampere-level currents are sufficient to stimulate the heart (peak current drains <100 μA). Batteries with a low rate of self-discharge, such as most lithium–iodine batteries,

Table 2.4 Summary of battery chemistries

Battery chemistries	Characteristics
Lithium–iodine (Li/I)	Reliable, good longevity, small size Low power capability and not suitable if higher power is needed
Lithium–carbon monofluoride (LiCFx)	Medium power capability Less predictable end-of-service properties due to abrupt voltage decline near end of battery life
Lithium–silver–vanadium oxide (Li/SVO)	High power capability Most ICD batteries Voltage as an indicator of battery life
Lithium–manganese dioxide ($LiMnO_2$)	Good power capability Stable charge times up to end of service without battery pulsing Cell voltage remains nearly constant until elective replacement indicator (ERI). Therefore, charge time and battery energy consumed is used to monitor battery status
Lithium/hybrid (Li/SVO and CFx)	High power capability More predictable end-of-service properties

are typically adequate. This is in contrast to the treatment of tachycardia requiring shock therapy, where ampere-level pulse currents are required. ICD batteries must be able to deliver high current (up to 3 A) and high power (up to 10 W) for several seconds to charge the high-voltage capacitors. Therefore, high-rate batteries, such as lithium–silver–vanadium oxide, are needed. However, there is a growing complexity of pacemakers and the need for more power delivery for a variety of uses, such as inductive and radiofrequency telemetry, EGM storage, rate modulation, and sensors. Therefore, medium-rate batteries have been developed to treat bradycardia and meet these other demands. The lithium–carbon monofluoride (Li/CFx) battery is an example of a medium-rate primary cell capable of milliampere-level (up to 300 mA) pulse currents. Although Li/CFx cells have high current density and are capable of higher power delivery than lithium–iodine batteries, they exhibit an abrupt decline in voltage near the end of their life, making it difficult to design adequate replacement-time indicators. Nevertheless, this battery chemistry is increasingly being used in today's devices in combination with other battery chemistries to yield the desired properties. For example, silver–vanadium oxide (SVO) may be combined with CFx in the cathode to produce a hybrid cathode. This battery is capable of supporting high power needs and also has more predictable end-of-service properties. The composition (ratio) of the two chemistries can be varied to suit the needs of the device.

The importance of battery chemistry is not in the nuances of chemical reaction, but rather in the clinical implications. Battery chemistry determines initial voltage, voltage decay, and discharge rate characteristics. The rate of unwanted chemical reactions that cause internal current leakage between the positive and negative electrodes of the cell, like all chemical reactions, increases with temperature, thus increasing battery decay. Though not clinically relevant after implant, this may be a factor that impacts storage conditions of devices on the shelf.

Longevity of the battery is defined as the interval between device implantation and detection of the end-of-service indicator. The longevity of the battery is dependent on the usage conditions, but also the number and efficiency of the associated components of the integrated circuit boards. Clinically, once a system is implanted, it is important to maximize the longevity of the device by careful programming of outputs and selection of options. The use of capture management features, reducing the frequency of capacitor reformations

(ICDs), and programming outputs to clinically safe margins is the first step. Second, disabling unused features, such as pre-detection EGM storage, can help preserve battery longevity. All modern devices have an end-of-service indicator that alerts the clinician to impending battery depletion and allows adequate time for replacement of the device. These indicators include monitored battery voltage, battery impedance, and capacitor reformation times (ICDs only).

Circuitry: complementary metal-oxide semiconductor

Complementary metal-oxide semiconductor (CMOS) is a technology used to produce integrated circuits. Within a pacemaker, the integrated circuit board contains the sensing circuit, timing circuit, output circuit, and telemetry circuit (Figure 2.21).

Sensing circuit

The intracardiac EGM is conducted from the electrodes to the sensing circuit of the pulse generator, where it is amplified and filtered (see Figure 2.4). The intracardiac EGM is filtered to remove unwanted frequencies, a process that markedly affects the amplitude of the processed signal. A bandpass filter attenuates components of the EGM on either side of the center frequency. The bandpass filters of different manufacturers vary significantly with regard to center frequency (from approximately 20 to 40 Hz), so intracardiac EGMs measured with a pacing system analyzer from one manufacturer may produce considerably different EGM amplitudes from those produced by the pulse generator sensing amplifier of another manufacturer. Following filtering of the intracardiac signal, the processed signal is compared with a reference voltage to determine if the signal exceeds a threshold detection level (programmed sensitivity). Signals with amplitudes greater than the sensitivity threshold level are sensed as intracardiac events, whereas signals of lower amplitude are discarded as noise. Signals that exceed the threshold level are sent to the timing circuit and logic circuits.

Most permanent pacemakers also contain noise reversion circuits that change the pulse generator to an asynchronous pacing mode when the sensing threshold level is exceeded at a rate faster than the noise reversion rate. The noise reversion mode

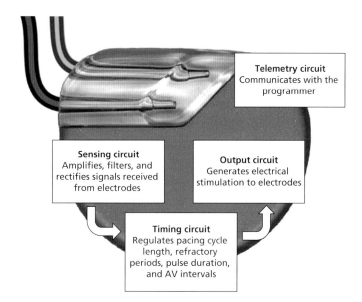

Telemetry circuit
Communicates with the
programmer

Sensing circuit
Amplifies, filters, and
rectifies signals received
from electrodes

Output circuit
Generates electrical
stimulation to electrodes

Timing circuit
Regulates pacing cycle
length, refractory
periods, pulse duration,
and AV intervals

Figure 2.21 Basic pacemaker circuits
and function.

prevents inhibition of pacing in the presence of electromagnetic interference.

Timing circuit

The pacing cycle length, sensing refractory and alert periods, pulse duration and AV interval are precisely regulated by the timing circuit of the pulse generator. The timing circuit of a pulse generator is a crystal oscillator that generates a very accurate signal with a frequency in the kilohertz range. The output of the crystal oscillator is sent to a digital timing and logic control circuit that operates internally generated clocks at divisions of the oscillator frequency. The output of the logic control circuit is a logic pulse that triggers the output pacing pulse, the blanking and refractory intervals, and the AV delay. The timing circuit also receives input from the sense amplifier to reset the escape intervals of an inhibited pacing system or trigger initiation of an AV delay for triggered pacing modes. The pulse generator also contains a rate-limiting circuit that prevents the pacing rate from exceeding an upper limit in the case of a random component failure. This runaway protection rate is typically in the range of 180–200 pulses per minute.

Output circuit

The output circuit contains the output section and voltage multipliers. Pacing outputs of greater than the specified voltage of a cell are achieved by a variety of methods. One approach is to use capacitors located on the output circuits. These capacitors are charged by the battery in parallel, but then discharged in series to minimize battery drain and to have desired output. Multiple capacitors can be used to achieve the desired output voltages. The use of these voltage multipliers has a significant impact on battery longevity. For example, a programmed output of 5.6 V requires two capacitors but results in a fourfold increase in the current drain from the lithium–iodine battery. When a capacitor-based output circuit is used to deliver a specified voltage for a programmed pulse width, the actual waveform shows a drop from the leading edge to the trailing edge. The magnitude of the voltage drop is a function of the pacing impedance but is not clinically important.

An alternative approach to capacitor-based voltage multipliers is to use the electromagnetic principle of inductance. An inductor, also known as a reactor, is simply a coil of wire that has specific electrical properties when subjected to a magnetic field. When an electrical current is passed through it, a magnetic field is created. This magnetic field helps to store the electrical current for a short time, even if the input is removed. When the magnetic field around the coil collapses, the electrical current is discharged. This method allows for a more efficient current draw from the battery. However, the choice of method used is related to the overall design of the pacemaker and their relative efficiencies can only be viewed in this context.

Zener diode

The electronic circuitry of the pulse generator must also be protected from damage caused by overwhelming electrical energy generated in the clinical environment. The Zener diode is designed to protect the integrated circuit from high external voltages such as may occur during defibrillation shocks or electrocautery. Zener diode is a semiconductor that behaves as a short circuit by allowing current to flow away from the device if the detected voltage exceeds a certain value above the output voltage of the pulse generator.

Telemetry systems

Current-generation implanted devices have the capability to establish a two-way communication with a programmer. This communication is typically accomplished with radiofrequency (inductive) telemetry or conductive telemetry.

Radiofrequency (inductive) telemetry

Inductive telemetry is based on the principle of inductive coupling, where two conductors are inductively coupled so that a change in current through one (e.g. wand) induces a voltage across the other (e.g. device) by electromagnetic induction. Near-field (wand) and far-field (wandless) communication utilizes radiofrequency for transmission. Most pulse generators require the radiofrequency signal to be pulsed with a specific frequency in a sequence that is typically 16 pulses in duration. Thus, the radiofrequency signal is quite precise, decreasing the likelihood of inappropriate alteration of the program by environmental sources of radiofrequency energy or magnetic fields. This characteristic also prevents the programmers of one manufacturer from programming the pulse generator of another. The detected telemetry bursts from the programmer are sent as digital information from the radiofrequency demodulator to the telemetry control logic circuit of the pulse generator. This logic circuit also provides for properly timed pulses to be sent from the antenna of the pulse generator to the programmer. "Real-time telemetry" is the term used to describe the capability of a pulse generator to transmit information to the programmer regarding measurements of pulse amplitude and duration, lead impedance, battery impedance, and delivered current, charge, and energy.

Recently, Bluetooth® technology has also been incorporated into pacemakers to enable communication between pacemakers and smartphones and tablets. Bluetooth is a wireless technology that uses a radiofrequency of 2.4 GHz for communication.

Conductive telemetry

Conductive telemetry is based on exchange of signals from electrodes on the skin and the implanted device. This allows the pacemaker to be smaller as it removes the need for a coil for electromagnetic coupling such as that in inductive telemetry. It is also more energy efficient as compared to radiofrequency telemetry, which requires larger amounts of power [14]. With these properties, its use is seen in the Nanostim LCP. The programmer transmits signals to the implanted Nanostim LCP with 250-kHz pulses applied to skin electrodes. This communication is visible on the surface EGM (Figure 2.22).

Sensors

Beyond prevention of symptomatic or potentially life-threatening bradyarrhythmias, the more nuanced role of a pacemaker is in the maintenance of adequate heart rate in response to specific physiological stressors. Under normal physiological situations, patients do not maintain a fixed heart rate. Rather, heart rate may vary depending on the clinical situation – whether the patient is at rest, exercising, or under conditions of emotional or physical stress, such as a febrile illness that may require a higher heart rate to maintain adequate cardiac output. In the absence of a sufficient heart rate response to physiological stress, patients may develop symptoms ranging from shortness of breath to frank syncope.

One common condition under which inadequate heart rate responses to physiological stress may be seen is sinus node dysfunction, which may be due to older age, medication use, prior sinus node ablation, prior heart transplant, or other cause. In addition, in patients with atrial fibrillation with either a slow ventricular response or prior AV node ablation, pacemakers may be required to augment the ventricular rate to similarly maintain adequate cardiac output.

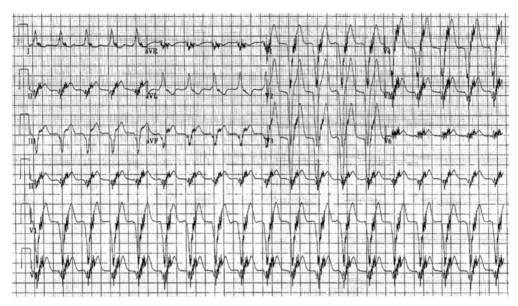

Figure 2.22 Surface electrocardiography obtained during active conductive telemetry communication between the leadless cardiac pacemaker and programmer shows high-frequency pulses. Source: tracing courtesy of Paul Friedman, MD.

Means of using a pacemaker to allow for adaptation of the pacing rate to the physiological need may range from the decision to implant a dual- versus a single-chamber pacemaker so that the ventricular rate can be coupled to the atrial rate, to more advanced use of sensors and programmable algorithms that offer a mechanism by which conditions of increased physiological stress are identified and the pacing rate altered. In the former case, some patients may have adequate sinus response to physiological stress but the ventricular response may not similarly augment due to AV node dysfunction. In such cases, the pacemaker, in the absence of a means of sensing the atrial rhythm, may not augment the ventricular rate and thus will not maintain AV synchrony. Special types of single-chamber leads that sense in both the atrium and ventricles but only pace the ventricle are available, and may be of utility in patients with normal sinus node function and impaired AV node function. However, most commonly, patients receive a true dual-chamber system, in which dedicated separate atrial and ventricular leads are used.

Regardless of the decision to use a single- or dual-chamber system there are many patients in whom the heart is unable to intrinsically respond to metabolic demands. In such cases, several different types of sensing technologies and programming algorithms have been developed that work to identify when there is a condition of increased metabolic demand requiring a change in the pacing rate. We focus here on the different types of sensors clinically available, considerations related to their programming, and special conditions of sensor-based pacing adaptations that extend beyond changing the heart rate alone.

Accelerometers (body motion)

An accelerometer measures rate of change in velocity. It consists of an arm mounted on a circuit board that flexes in response to body movements. Movement and flexion of the arm of the accelerometer results in deformation of an attached piezoelectric or piezoresistive material. The arm does not respond to pressure on the device per se as it is mechanically insulated from the can, but rather to changes in velocity. These changes in velocity are detected by the device and, based on a variety of programmable and non-programmable set points, will result in a change in heart rate. With triaxially mounted accelerometers, acceleration signals in the x-axis, y-axis, and z-axis can be detected. The frequency of typical body motion, such as during walking or stair climbing, is 1–8 Hz.

Table 2.5 Mechanism, advantages, and disadvantages of accelerometer and minute-ventilation sensors

	Accelerometer	*Minute-ventilation sensor*
Mechanism	Deformation of an attached piezoelectric or piezoresistive material	Changes in transthoracic impedance
Advantages	Good speed of response	Good proportionality to exercise
Disadvantages	Affected by environmental vibration Limited proportionality to exercises with prolonged activity but with constant velocity Non-movement-based exertion like febrile illness not detected by accelerometer	Affected by electromagnetic interference Inappropriate activation with coughing or upper extremity movement Affected by voluntary hyperventilation

Various studies have demonstrated that accelerometers are quite consistent in response between patients and under different physiological conditions, regardless of the degree and type of activity. When compared with vibration sensors, they offer better rate modulation that is proportional to exercise workload. Other advantages include the ability to respond rapidly to the onset of activity, as well as filter out environmental noise more effectively compared with vibration sensors.

However, accelerometers have several limitations. For example, prolonged activity may be associated with a constant velocity and thus no further acceleration will be seen even though metabolic demand will continue to increase concomitantly with the duration of exercise. In turn, rates of acceleration may not directly correlate with the physiological need, as when comparing moving uphill versus downhill. Finally, non-movement-based exertion, such as emotional stress or febrile illness, will not be detected by an accelerometer, limiting its ability to offer rate adaptation under all conditions.

The Micra (Medtronic, Minneapolis, MN) leadless pacemaker has an accelerometer-based sensor and the rate response sensing vector can be programmed along three axes. The same sensor is used to identify passive ventricular filling and atrial contraction so that the ventricular pacing pulse can be adequately timed to the atrial electrical event.

Minute-ventilation sensors

Under conditions of isometric exercise or where a constant velocity is maintained over a prolonged period of time, vibration or acceleration sensors may inadequately identify the level of metabolic demand. In turn, in some patients, such as those with heart failure or the elderly, the degree of metabolic demand may far outstrip the degree of physical motion (i.e. small degrees of physical activity may result in large increases in metabolic demand). Thus, sensors that depend on evaluating changes in minute ventilation have been developed (Table 2.5). Minute-ventilation sensors rely on the changes in transthoracic impedance that occur during inspiration and expiration as a surrogate for the change in minute ventilation (equal to respiratory rate × tidal volume). Minute ventilation, in turn, correlates with oxygen consumption (Vo_2), as both respiratory rate and tidal volume increase in proportion to Vo_2 [15]. Thus, minute-ventilation sensors may detect situations of increased metabolic demand in the absence of physical activity.

When the lungs are inflated during inspiration, there is more insulating air between the tip of the pacing lead and the pulse generator, increasing impedance in the circuit. In turn, when the lungs are deflated during expiration, the transthoracic impedance decreases. Low-energy subthreshold 320-mA pulses are delivered at high frequency allowing for frequent impedance measurements. This continuous measurement of impedance allows the sensor to detect fluctuations in transthoracic impedance on the basis of the frequency of changes in impedance (which correlates with the respiratory rate), as well as changes in impedance amplitude (which correlates with tidal volume). Using these parameters, minute ventilation can be calculated.

At the onset of activity, minute ventilation tends to increase more slowly than heart rate in the setting of an intact sinus node, whereas during sustained exercise at high workloads minute ventilation increases out of proportion to heart rate and oxygen consumption, particularly if the anaerobic threshold is crossed. Because of this changing relationship between minute ventilation, oxygen consumption, and heart rate throughout exercise, the minute-ventilation sensor will typically use a steeper slope at the onset of exercise and a flatter slope at high levels of exercise when calculating the target pacing rate.

Limitations of minute-ventilation sensors include inappropriate activation with coughing, abnormal breathing patterns, or even upper extremity movement, which can result in changes in transthoracic impedance. They may also interfere with the respiratory rate monitors that are typically used in the hospital setting. As with all impedance-sensing devices, it will also be affected by electromagnetic interference.

Peak endocardial acceleration sensor

Peak endocardial acceleration (PEA) sensors use a specially designed lead with a microaccelerometer located in the lead tip [16]. This accelerometer measures mechanical vibrations generated by the heart during isovolumetric contraction. This signal directly correlates with contractility and variations in the peak-to-peak value are compared against a reference value. The purpose of this is to identify early changes in contractility that correlate with input from autonomic nervous system feedback to the heart. Even in the absence of appropriate sinus or AV nodal function, the autonomic nervous system will still have a direct impact on myocardial contractility that can be used as a surrogate marker for demonstrating the need for change in heart rate. Thus, increased contractility indicates a need for increased heart rate and cardiac output. However, the PEA sensor is no longer used for rate-adaptive pacing because of concern for long-term stability with special lead sensors. It is now primarily used to monitor hemodynamic function and adjust AV and VV intervals in CRT devices [(17]. Guided by an algorithm, PEA data can be used to adjust VV and AV intervals to achieve optimal intervals to improve long-term outcomes [18].

Closed-loop stimulation: right ventricle impedance sensor

Contractility of the ventricles increases with catecholamine stimulation during physiological stress. Contractility can be measured using intracardiac impedance from the RV impedance sensor. One such sensor that is clinically available in Biotronik (Berlin, Germany) devices is termed "closed loop stimulation" (CLS). This system works by analyzing contractility based on impedance changes on a beat-to-beat basis to determine the pacing rate required to match hemodynamic needs. This system works on the same principle as minute-ventilation sensors, but instead of looking for ventilation-related impedance changes, the algorithm is optimized to measure impedance changes in response to cardiac contraction. The system works by triggering rate increases in response to prespecified impedance triggers. In diastole, when the right ventricle is filled, there will be a smaller fraction of myocardium interfacing with the lead tip, and the impedance will be lower. In systole, the impedance will be higher. During exercise, when there is inadequate rate response, exercise will induce a higher contractility. When contractility increases, the right ventricle will be less filled and thus the impedance will be higher. This, in turn, is used to trigger the device to pace faster. Once rate response is adequate, the augmentation in contractility is less, thus establishing a negative feedback loop. This negative feedback loop establishes a closed-loop system as opposed to an open-loop system (Figure 2.23).

Trials have suggested the superiority of this algorithm when compared with standard accelerometer-based sensors, and utility in conditions such as neurocardiogenic syncope [19]. As this sensor also responds to contractility changes from other, non-exertional, neurocardiogenic triggers, it may provide heart rate support during emotional or mental stress.

The limitation of CLS is that ventricular ischemia and cardioactive medications will likely affect CLS-determined rate response. Furthermore, patients with severely impaired RV function may not be suitable for the CLS sensor.

Blended-sensor devices

While activity sensors respond rapidly, they are not proportional at higher levels of workload. They overpace at low activity levels but underpace at higher activity levels. However, proportional sensors are typically slow to response. With a dual-sensor combination, such as combining minute-ventilation sensors with an activity sensor, measured data from both sensors can be combined to form a "blended sensor" that may provide an even better rate-adaptive response to exercise than either sensor

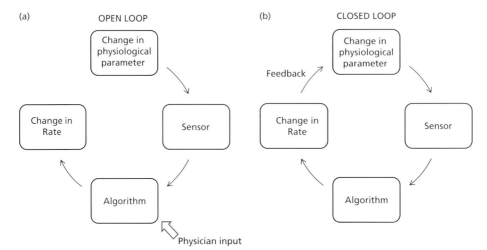

Figure 2.23 (a) Open loop sensor, where induced rate change does not procedure negative feedback in the physiological parameter. Physician input on adjustment of the algorithm is also needed to optimize rate response. (b) Closed loop sensor, where change in rate (increased pacing rate) leads to change in the physiological parameter (decreased augmented contractility when rate response is adequate) in the opposite direction, establishing a negative feedback loop.

alone [20]. Information from the activity sensor is typically weighted more heavily at the onset of exercise, when physical motion is more prominent than increased respiration, and the minute-ventilation sensor is more prominent after more sustained activity and in recovery, when metabolic needs remain elevated after physical motion has slowed or stopped. With this sensor combination, the rapid increase in pacing rate with the onset of activity and the more gradual decline of heart rate in recovery can closely approximate the physiological heart rate response pattern of the intact sinus node. Several studies have demonstrated the utility of such blended sensors [21]. Furthermore, sensor cross-checking in dual-sensor devices also enhances the specificity of each sensor. For example, if one sensor registers "no physiologic stress," changes in the other sensor can be ignored or have its response attenuated.

Lead design

Pacing and defibrillation leads are designed to carry electric current from the pulse generator to the electrodes in the heart. To effectively perform this task all leads have two components: a metallic conductor with low internal resistance separated from surrounding structures with an insulation material. All leads have a connector pin that connects in the header, and a main body that contains the insulation material and conductor cables that are connected to the electrodes at their respective locations (tip, ring, RV coil, superior vena cava coil, etc.). The leads placed in a human body are subject to stress from body movements, heart chamber movements, interactions with other physical objects (e.g. other leads), and growth of connective tissue. The essential property of any lead is to be malleable but at the same time withstand stress to prevent degradation. The materials should also withstand oxidative stress from contact with electrolytic currents. The conductor elements are often woven helically along the long axis of the cable and are referred to as filars. The number of filars in each conductor cable is also variable. The properties of these materials are summarized in Table 2.6.

Depending on the arrangement of the conductor elements in the lead body, they can be classified broadly into three types (Figure 2.24).

1 *Coaxial design*: In this lead design the conductor elements are arranged one outside of the other rotationally around the longitudinal axis. The conductor to the ring electrode is often arranged on the outside while the conductor to the tip electrode is on the inside of the lead. If there is a breach in insulation around the outer conductor cable, the device has diagnostic capabilities to sense change in impedance and to switch the lead from bipolar to unipolar, thereby eliminating the outer conductor cable.

Table 2.6 Components used in modern pacing and defibrillation leads

Component	Material used	Advantages	Disadvantages
Conductor	MP35N alloy made of cobalt, nickel, chromium, and molybdenum. It can be combined with silver to form drawn brazen strand and drawn filled tubes	Low resistance	
Electrodes	Platinum–iridium alloy. Some of the pace-sense electrodes incorporate titanium	Low resistance	
Defibrillation coils	• Platinum-coated titanium • Platinum-clad tantalum • Platinum–iridium • Platinum–iridium-clad tantalum	Low resistance Minimal oxidation with shocks	
Insulation	• Silicone	Inert, biostable and resistant to metal ion oxidation	Breaks down easily and is subject to cold flow
	• Polyurethane	Excellent tensile strength and abrasion resistance	Environmental stress cracking and metal ion oxidation
	• Fibropolymers: PTFE, ETFE • Copolymer hybrids: Elast-Eon	Good biocompatibility	Stiffness

PTFE, polytetrafluoroethylene; ETFE, ethyltetrafluoroethylene.

2 *Coradial design*: The metal conductor elements are arranged side by side, each with its own insulation covering, rotationally around a central long axis. The lumen can be hollow to facilitate insertion of a stylet. An external breach is likely to affect both the tip and ring conductor cables, resulting in short-circuiting and loss of effective current delivery to the electrodes. The coradial design facilitates leads with smaller diameter.

3 *Multilumen design*: Defibrillation and multielectrode leads (quadripolar LV leads) have a complex design as the number of conductor cables increases dramatically. A coaxial design with all the conductor cables would increase the diameter of the lead. A multilumen design is an advance in lead design whereby the diameter is kept to a minimum and additional empty spaces are left in the lead to accommodate stress from other cables in the lead. Because of the multilumen design, breakdown in insulation can occur from outside to inside (outside in) in between the conductors (inside out) in the individual lumens. Figure 2.25 shows the cross-sectional details of various ICD leads currently available in clinical practice.

The header connection component of the lead has been standardized for pacing and defibrillation circuits. Pacing cables and defibrillation cables are connected by IS1 and DF1 pins, respectively, to their corresponding cavity-receiving port in the header. Although IS1 and DF1 pins cannot be mistakenly inserted into other corresponding cavity-receiving ports, there is potential for reversal of superior vena cava (SVC) and RV coil DF1 pins (Figure 2.26). When the DF1 pins are reversed, the defibrillation shock vector is suboptimal and the shock therapy may not be successful. The reversal can also lead to inappropriate detection as the sensing antenna is enlarged from RV tip to coil in SVC position instead of desired RV tip to RV coil (integrated bipolar configuration). A new standard DF4 connector was introduced to standardize and minimize operator-related errors in securing the pins in the header. With the advent of quadripolar LV leads, IS4 pins are increasingly used in clinical practice. While the IS4 and DF4 pins look alike, the dimeter of the DF4 pin is narrower and meticulous attention should be paid to prevent inadvertent placement of the pins in the header.

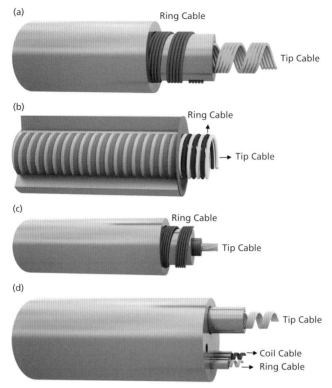

Figure 2.24 (a) Coaxial lead design. In this lead design the conductor cable to the tip electrode (green) is inside the conductor cable to the ring electrode (blue). The number of filars, and their arrangements, turns and spacing between each turn vary greatly between leads. A central lumen still exists in a coaxial lead design for a stylet to be inserted. (b) Coradial lead design. In this lead design the conductor cables are beside one another (conductor cable to the ring electrode is blue and the conductor cable to the tip electrode is green). (c) Lumen-less pacing lead (Medtronic Select Secure). In this lead design the cable to the tip electrode is in the middle of the lead (green), while the cable to the ring electrode is on the outside (blue). (d) Multilumen lead design. In this lead design the cable to the tip electrode (yellow) is usually separated from rest of the other conductor cables. A compression lumen is normally present to allow for movement of individual cables inside the lead.

The conductor cables are attached to the electrodes or coils using spot welding, crimp joints, or stake joints [22]. The defibrillation shock electrodes have spaces between the coil turns and are prone to issue ingrowth, making extraction difficult. Various strategies have been adopted to reduce ingrowth of fibrous tissue, including backfilling with silicone, flat cable coil design with gentler curve, and use of porous expanded polytetrafluoroethylene (ePTFE or GoreTex).

Surgically implanted leads
These leads can be sutured directly on the epicardial surface of the heart. Each electrode is individually sutured and then connected to the device based on unipolar or bipolar lead configuration. Bipolar screw leads with steroid elution are also currently available in the market (Figure 2.27). These leads can be placed under direct visualization or via a minimally invasive thoracotomy procedure. Defibrillation coils can be placed in the pericardial space and secured with sutures or in the transverse sinus.

Additional components for pacing for defibrillation circuit
Pacing lead extenders are available when a pacing lead has to be tunneled and extended to the contralateral side. Additional defibrillation coils and subcutaneous coils can be added to the defibrillation circuit to optimize the defibrillation vector (Figure 2.28). The additional coil is added to a

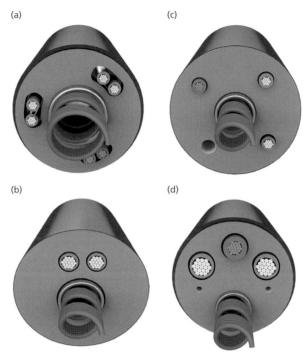

Figure 2.25 (a) Durata (Abbott Laboratories, Abbott Park, IL) lead. The central lumen is surrounded by a conductor cable to the tip electrode (blue). There are three pairs of cables surrounding the cable to the tip electrode. Two pairs of cables supply the superior vena cava (SVC) and right ventricular (RV) coils (yellow) and the remaining pair supplies the RV ring electrode (gray). Each individual cable is covered by it is own insulation. On top of it the whole lead may be covered by an additional layer of insulation (Optim). (b) Reliance (Boston Scientific, Natick, MA) defibrillator lead. The conductor cable to the tip electrode (blue) is in the center of the lead. The cables to RV coil and SVC coil are depicted as yellow. (c) Linox (Biotronik, Germany) defibrillator lead. The conductor cable to the tip electrode (blue) is in the center of the lead. The cables to the SVC coil and RV coil are depicted as yellow. The conductor cable to the ring electrode is depicted as gray. Each of the conductor cables has its own insulation covering. A compression lumen (green) accommodates movements of individual cables inside the lead. (d) Quattro (Medtronic, Minneapolis, MN) defibrillator lead. The conductor cable to the tip electrode (blue) is in the center of the lead. The cables to the SVC and RV coils are depicted as yellow. The cable to the ring electrode is depicted as gray. Compression lumens (green) can be seen in the lead.

DF1 splitter. DF4 connectors act as replacers but can be configured to additional coils (Figure 2.29).

Special situations

Magnetic resonance imaging with modern devices

The three main electromagnetic fields used to create a magnetic resonance imaging (MRI) scan include a static magnetic field to align the protons, a pulsed radiofrequency field to excite the nuclear spin of the proton, and a gradient magnetic field to localize in space the signal emitted after the radiofrequency signal is turned off. These use a variety of different magnetic field strengths, ranging from 0.2 to 9 T.

The adverse effects of MRI on CIEDs can be divided into six main components (Table 2.7) [23].

1 The magnetic field can induce force and torque due to ferromagnetic materials.
2 Electrical current in conductive wires can be induced by the gradient magnetic field.
3 Radiofrequency fields can lead to CIED component heating and thermal tissue damage.
4 Radiofrequency energy pulses or changing magnetic field gradients can lead to electromagnetic interference. This may lead to oversensing and inappropriate inhibition of demand pacing or inappropriate shocks in ICDs.

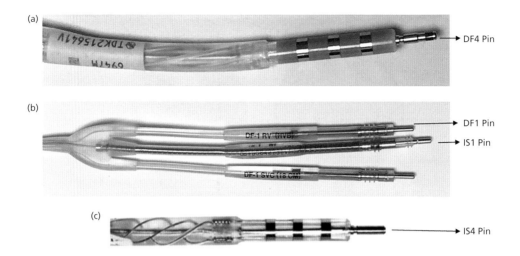

(a) ··············▶ DF4 Pin

(b) ··············▶ DF1 Pin
··············▶ IS1 Pin

(c) ··············▶ IS4 Pin

Figure 2.26 (a) DF4 connector pin. The tip of the pin is narrower in diameter compared to the IS4 connector pin. (b) DF1/IS1 connector pins connecting to the yolk of a defibrillator lead. (c) IS4 connector pin from a quadripolar left ventricular lead.

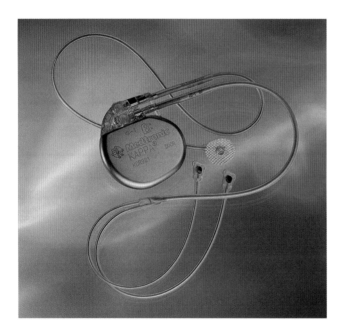

Figure 2.27 Two types of surgical epicardial leads available for pacing. Bipolar leads can be screwed down to the myocardium or each electrode can be individually sutured to the myocardium. Source: Medtronic, Inc. Reproduced with permission of Medtronic, Inc.

5 The high electromagnetic interference can lead to power-on reset, where the device reverts to default factory settings.
6 The static magnetic field can activate the reed switch, leading to asynchronous pacing and inhibition of tachycardia therapies.

With the increasing use of MRI, magnetic resonance-conditional pacemakers were subsequently developed (Figure 2.30). These are defined as devices for which there are no known hazards under a specific MRI environment and conditions of use [23]. Leads have been designed to minimize heating at the tip and to reduce the antenna effect in order to reduce risk of current induction. These are achieved by altering the number of filars or winding turns, coating the tip with a substance resistant to polarization, and applying a heat-dissipating filter at the near-distal end of the lead [23].

(a)

(b)

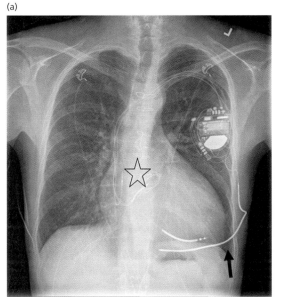
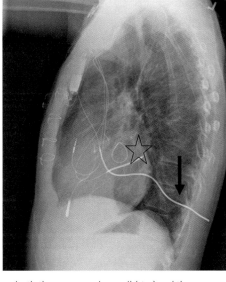

Figure 2.28 (a) Anteroposterior chest X-ray of a patient with high defibrillation threshold showing coronary sinus (star) and subcutaneous coil (arrow). (b) Lateral chest X-ray shows both the coronary sinus coil (star) and the subcutaneous coil (arrow) extending posteriorly.

(a)

(b)

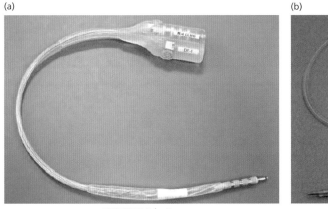
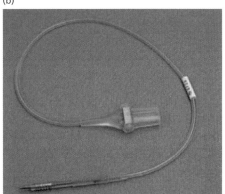

DF4 5019 Adapter

DF 1 6726 Splitter

Figure 2.29 (a) DF4 adapter available on the market. Additional coils are added to the system to enhance or replace an SVC coil with a subcutaneous array or other high-voltage lead. (b) DF1 adapter, used for the same purpose.

Generators have been designed to have reduced ferromagnetic content, replacement of reed switches with Hall sensors, shielding with filters to reduce risk of damage to circuitry and internal power supply, and dedicated MRI programming pathway to be turned on and off before and after a scan [23].

Scanning should also meet the prerequisites specified for the device, with the goal of limiting energy deposition on CIEDs. Most systems have been approved for 1.5 T scanning, maximum gradient slew rate of 200 T/m per second, maximum specific absorption rate of 2 W/kg, and limited number and length of imaging sequences.

Other requirements include active reprogramming before and after scanning. Continuous monitoring of ECG and pulse oximetry during scanning by a provider with advanced cardiac life support training is also required. It is important to have a standardized institutional workflow that includes assessment of the benefits of MRI compared with

Table 2.7 Potential adverse effects of MRI in patients with a pacemaker

Potential interactions	Incidence and risk factors	Prevention
Mechanical forces on ferromagnetic components	Movement of device is very rare Torsional force from 1.5-T scanner is typically not significant	MRI-conditional devices and leads minimize ferromagnetic material Delay MRI in fresh implants to allow for lead stabilization
Induced electrical current resulting in myocardial electrical stimulation and arrhythmia	Current generated clinically is too low to capture myocardium	Continuous monitoring during scan Limit lead length and looped leads
Heating and tissue damage	Risk of tissue heating depends on lead length and lead configuration Epicardial, fractured, and abandoned leads are more likely to cause local heating Risk higher with thoracic CMR Changes in lead impedance, sensing, and threshold that warrant device reprogramming or revision are rare Temporary changes in battery voltage often recover over time	Minimize SAR while still ensuring adequate image quality Avoid MRI in patients with epicardial, fractured, or abandoned leads Appropriate selection of MRI landmark Assessment of lead immediately after MRI
Electromagnetic interference causing oversensing	Rare reports of magnet mode and pauses in dependent patients	Program-asynchronous pacing in pacemaker-dependent patients Program demand pacing in non-dependent patients Continuous monitoring during scan Newer devices are better shielded from EMI
Power-on reset to default factory settings	Incidence ranges from 0.7 to 3.5% More likely in devices released before 2002	Discontinue scan if noted during monitoring Avoid MRI in dependent patients with devices released before 2002
Change in reed switch behavior	Incidence ranges from 0 to 38%	Some MRI-conditional devices use Hall sensor

CMR, cardiac magnetic resonance; EMI, electromagnetic interference; SAR, specific absorption rate.

alternative imaging or diagnostic methods, evaluation of CIED before and after the scan, and appropriate magnetic resonance-conditional programming during the scan. Table 2.8 summarizes the pre- and post-scan steps (note that some steps and requirements may be manufacturer specific).

A CIED system is only MRI-conditional if both the generator and the leads are MRI-conditional, and there are no abandoned, fractured, or epicardial leads. For MRI non-conditional CIEDs, there are increasing data on successful MRI scanning without clinically significant

changes in CIED function or patient harm. It is important to maintain a standardized collaborative institutional protocol to guide decisions on performing MRI in these patients.

Perioperative programming

The primary issue during a surgical procedure pertaining to CIEDs is electromagnetic interference (EMI). This can originate from an electrosurgery unit or other equipment in the operating room, such as nerve stimulators or radiofrequency ablation devices. The main risks of EMI in

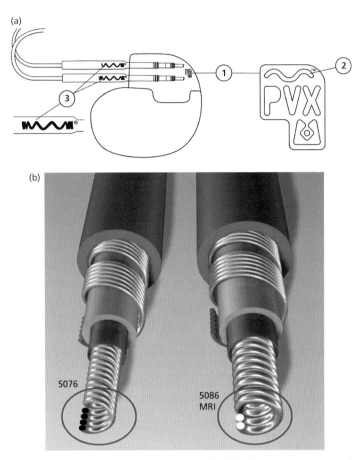

Figure 2.30 Select features of an MRI-conditional pacemaker system. (a) The fluoroscopic markers found on the header block (1, 2) of the MRI-conditional pacemakers Revo™ and Advisa™ (Medtronic, Inc.). The fluoroscopic marker found on the proximal portion of the lead (3) identifies it as MRI-conditional. (b) The two-filar inner conductor of the 5086® lead and the four-filar inner conductor of the 5076® lead. Source: Medtronic, Inc. Reproduced with permission of Medtronic, Inc.

Table 2.8 Confirmation of MRI safety with MRI-conditional devices

Cardiologist-verified scan conditions
Confirm implanted system is MRI-conditional
Implant >6 weeks
Stable pacing, sensing, and impedance parameters
No other devices, abandoned leads, adaptors or extenders
Programming changes recommended by manufacturer ("MRI mode")

Radiologist-verified scan conditions
1.5-T closed-bore MRI
Maximum gradient slew rate per axis ≤200 T/m per s
SAR <2 W/kg
Monitoring of patient vital signs
Available external defibrillator

SAR, specific absorption rate.

a patient with a CIED are inhibition of pacing due to oversensing and delivery of inappropriate shock from misinterpretation of EMI as a tachyarrhythmia [24].

A number of methods are available to minimize the risk of EMI, such as use of bipolar electrosurgery as it does not cause EMI unless it is directly applied to the CIED. If monopolar electrosurgery is used, the CIED should not be located in the current path of the grounding pad and the electrosurgery site. Electrosurgery applied above the umbilicus is more likely to cause device interference than when applied below the umbilicus (Figure 2.31). Therefore, in monopolar electrosurgery above the umbilicus, the general recommendation is for inactivation of ICD detection and rendering a pacemaker asynchronous in a pacemaker-dependent

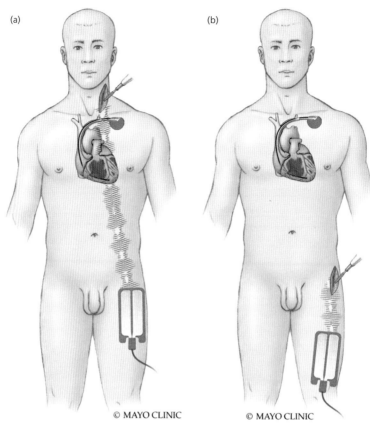

© MAYO CLINIC   © MAYO CLINIC

Figure 2.31 (a) Monopolar electrosurgery above the umbilicus where the current path crosses the device may lead to device interference. (b) Current path is distant from the device in monopolar electrosurgery below the umbilicus. Therefore in monopolar electrosurgery above the umbilicus the general recommendation is for inactivation of ICD detection and rendering a pacemaker asynchronous in a pacemaker-dependent patient. Source: used with permission of Mayo Foundation for Medical Education and Research, all rights reserved.

patient [24]. The length of the monopolar electro-surgery burst should also be less than 5 s. It is important to know that, typically, magnets deacti-vate therapies in ICDs and cause asynchronous pacing in pacemakers. Magnet response is pro-grammable and an example where reprogramming would be needed is in a patient with an ICD who is pacemaker dependent. Some devices have an audi-ble tone with correct magnet application over the device. The optimal magnet positioning for ade-quate response is also different for different devices.

Radiation therapy guidance

Current-generation CIEDs use CMOS, which can be impaired by radiation therapy due to damage to the silicon and silicon oxide insulators within sem-iconductors [25]. The susceptibility of CIEDs to radiation therapy may occur from either direct irradiation or scatter radiation. The damage from radiation therapy is a dose-dependent effect, with increasing malfunction with greater cumulative dose [26]. Radiation therapy-induced damage can present as transient safety mode pacing, changes in pacing rate, rapid runaway pacing, or sudden device failure [25,27]. In patients with CIEDs undergoing ionizing radiation, there should be a discussion between the CIED team, medical physi-cist, and radiation oncologist on how to minimize the risk of device damage while providing the best treatment for the patient. Significant risk of dam-age occurs when the dose is above 10 Gy, which is a measure of energy deposited. If the amount of pro-posed ionizing radiation is above a safe level, either the treatment plan must change or the device

Table 2.9 Summary of management before, during, and after radiation therapy

Before radiation therapy
Treatment team should be informed of type of device, pacemaker-dependency, minimum and maximum pacemaker rates
CIED relocation if its current location will interfere with adequate tumor treatment
During radiation therapy
Continuous visual and voice contact
Weekly CIED evaluation for patients who are pacing dependent or those undergoing neutron-producing radiotherapy
After radiation therapy
Complete CIED evaluation at the conclusion of radiation therapy

CIED, cardiac implantable electronic device.

should be relocated to a position farther from the treatment field. Relocation is not recommended for devices receiving a maximum cumulative incident dose of less than 5 Gy [23]. Prior to initiation of radiation treatment, the treatment team should be aware of the type of device, whether the patient is pacemaker dependent, the minimum programmed pacing rate, and the maximum programmed tracking and sensor rates [23]. Weekly CIED evaluations should also be performed in patients undergoing radiation therapy (Table 2.9).

References

1 Wright SH. Generation of resting membrane potential. *Adv Physiol Educ* 2004;28(1–4):139–142.

2 Grant AO. Cardiac ion channels. *Circ Arrhythm Electrophysiol* 2009;2(2):185–194.

3 Iravanian S, Langberg JJ. A review of bioelectrodes for clinical electrophysiologists. *Heart Rhythm* 2019;16(3):460–469.

4 Mulpuru SK, Madhavan M, McLeod CJ, *et al.* Cardiac pacemakers: function, troubleshooting, and management: Part 1 of a 2-part series. *J Am Coll Cardiol* 2017;69(2):189–210.

5 Coates S, Thwaites B. The strength–duration curve and its importance in pacing efficiency: a study of 325 pacing leads in 229 patients. *Pacing Clin Electrophysiol* 2000;23(8):1273–1277.

6 Swerdlow CD, Ellenbogen KA. Implantable cardioverter–defibrillator leads: design, diagnostics, and management. *Circulation* 2013;128(18):2062–2071.

7 Dekker E. Direct current make and break thresholds for pacemaker electrodes on the canine ventricle. *Circ Res* 1970;27(5):811–823.

8 Thibault B, Roy D, Guerra PG, *et al.* Anodal right ventricular capture during left ventricular stimulation in CRT-implantable cardioverter defibrillators. *Pacing Clin Electrophysiol* 2005;28(7):613–619.

9 van Gelder BM, Bracke FA. Current of injury (COI) pattern recorded from catheter delivered active fixation pacing leads. *Pacing Clin Electrophysiol* 2008;31(6):786–787; author reply 787.

10 McLeod CJ, Boersma L, Okamura H, Friedman PA. The subcutaneous implantable cardioverter defibrillator: state-of-the-art review. *Eur Heart J* 2017;38(4):247–257.

11 Ali H, Lupo P, Cappato R. The entirely subcutaneous defibrillator: a new generation and future expectations. *Arrhythm Electrophysiol Rev* 2015;4(2):116–121.

12 Bogeholz N, Pauls P, Guner F, *et al.* Direct comparison of the novel automated screening tool (AST) versus the manual screening tool (MST) in patients with already implanted subcutaneous ICD. *Int J Cardiol* 2018;265:90–96.

13 Tjong FV, Reddy VY. Permanent leadless cardiac pacemaker therapy: a comprehensive review. *Circulation* 2017;135(15):1458–1470.

14 Ferguson JE, Redish AD. Wireless communication with implanted medical devices using the conductive properties of the body. *Expert Rev Med Devices* 2011;8(4):427–433.

15 Kay GN, Bubien RS, Epstein AE, Plumb VJ. Rate-modulated cardiac pacing based on transthoracic impedance measurements of minute ventilation: correlation with exercise gas exchange. *J Am Coll Cardiol* 1989;14(5):1283–1289.

16 Greco EM, Ferrario M, Romano S. Clinical evaluation of peak endocardial acceleration as a sensor for rate responsive pacing. *Pacing Clin Electrophysiol* 2003;26(4 Pt 1):812–818.

17 Bordachar P, Garrigue S, Reuter S, *et al.* Hemodynamic assessment of right, left, and biventricular pacing by peak endocardial acceleration and echocardiography in patients with end-stage heart failure. *Pacing Clin Electrophysiol* 2000;23(11 Pt 2):1726–1730.

18 Delnoy PP, Ritter P, Naegele H, *et al.* Association between frequent cardiac resynchronization therapy optimization and long-term clinical response: a post hoc analysis of the Clinical Evaluation on Advanced Resynchronization (CLEAR) pilot study. *Europace* 2013;15(8):1174–1181.

19 Lindovska M, Kamenik L, Pollock B, *et al.* Clinical observations with closed loop stimulation pacemakers in a large patient cohort: the CYLOS routine documentation registry (RECORD). *Europace* 2012;14(11):1587–1595.

20 Coman J, Freedman R, Koplan BA, *et al.* A blended sensor restores chronotropic response more favorably than an accelerometer alone in pacemaker patients: the LIFE study results. *Pacing Clin Electrophysiol* 2008;31(11):1433–1442.

21 Shukla HH, Flaker GC, Hellkamp AS, *et al.* Clinical and quality of life comparison of accelerometer, piezoelectric crystal, and blended sensors in DDDR-paced patients with sinus node dysfunction in the mode selection trial (MOST). *Pacing Clin Electrophysiol* 2005;28(8):762–770.

22 Kalahasty G, Ellenbogen KA. ICD lead design and the management of patients with lead failure. *Card Electrophysiol Clin* 2009;1(1):173–191.

23 Indik JH, Gimbel JR, Abe H, *et al.* 2017 HRS expert consensus statement on magnetic resonance imaging and radiation exposure in patients with cardiovascular implantable electronic devices. *Heart Rhythm* 2017;14(7):e97–e153.

24 Crossley GH, Poole JE, Rozner MA, *et al.* The Heart Rhythm Society (HRS)/American Society of Anesthesiologists (ASA) Expert Consensus Statement on the perioperative management of patients with implantable defibrillators, pacemakers and arrhythmia monitors: facilities and patient management. *Heart Rhythm* 2011;8(7):1114–1154.

25 Last A. Radiotherapy in patients with cardiac pacemakers. *Br J Radiol* 1998;71(841):4–10.

26 Maxted KJ. The effect of therapeutic X-radiation on a sample of pacemaker generators. *Phys Med Biol* 1984; 29(9):1143–1146.

27 Katzenberg CA, Marcus FI, Heusinkveld RS, Mammana RB. Pacemaker failure due to radiation therapy. *Pacing Clin Electrophysiol* 1982;5(2):156–159.

CHAPTER 3

Hemodynamics of cardiac pacing and pacing mode selection

Bruce S. Stambler[1], Niraj Varma[2], and Michael Hoosien[1]

[1] Piedmont Heart Institute, Piedmont Atlanta Hospital, Atlanta, GA, USA
[2] Cardiac Electrophysiology and Pacing Heart and Vascular Institute, Cleveland Clinic, Cleveland, OH, USA

Introduction

Cardiac pacing in an individual patient can have either beneficial or detrimental effects on hemodynamic function and clinical outcomes. Appropriate selection of a cardiac rhythm management device for a given patient and optimal management of a patient with a permanent pacing device require proper understanding of the major factors that influence hemodynamic function. While early generations of cardiac pacemakers were sufficient technologically to prevent symptomatic bradycardia, the goal of cardiac pacing over the last few decades has been the attainment of "physiological" pacing. Many variables in pacing systems can affect cardiac hemodynamic function. The ideal pacemaker should maintain and optimize heart rate, atrioventricular (AV) synchrony, and ventricular activation to enable cardiac output to meet the metabolic needs of the patient, whether at rest or during exercise. The concept and definition of physiological pacing have evolved over time in concert with our understanding of pacing-related cardiovascular hemodynamics, as well as with technological sophistication.

In the current era, the goals of physiological pacing include maintaining heart rate, optimizing AV synchrony, minimizing right ventricular (RV) pacing to avoid ventricular desynchronization, using alternative RV pacing sites for improved hemodynamic performance, and selecting appropriate patients for cardiac resynchronization therapy (CRT). Optimization of hemodynamic function in the pacemaker patient is determined to a large extent by a complex interaction between device-related variables (e.g. pacing mode, pacing lead position, pacing rate, rate responsiveness, AV relationships, atrial and ventricular activation sequences, and frequency of RV pacing) and the underlying patient substrate (e.g. atrial rhythm, chronotropic competence, AV and ventricular conduction, ventricular function, history of heart failure and/or myocardial infarction).

Correction of bradycardia

When a patient with AV block or sinus node disease experiences sudden bradycardia, blood pressure and cardiac output fall, leading to reduced cerebral perfusion. The primary therapeutic goal of cardiac pacing in such situations is to correct symptomatic bradycardia. It is currently the only effective treatment that can prevent death or syncope caused by ventricular asystole. Simply increasing the heart rate will result in improvement of the hemodynamic abnormalities, including normalization of systolic blood pressure.

Cardiac Pacing and ICDs, Seventh Edition. Edited by Kenneth A. Ellenbogen and Karoly Kaszala.
© 2020 John Wiley & Sons Ltd. Published 2020 by John Wiley & Sons Ltd.

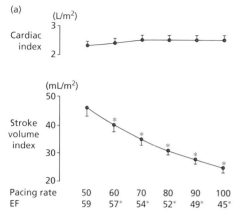
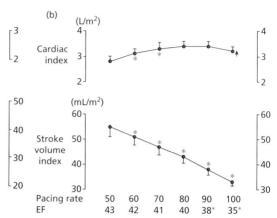

Figure 3.1 Effects of ventricular pacing rate on cardiac index, stroke volume index, and left ventricular ejection fraction (EF) in patients with a normal heart size and ejection fraction (a) and in patients with cardiomegaly and depressed ejection fraction (b). In patients with normal hearts, cardiac index did not change significantly as ventricular pacing rate was increased from 50 to 100 bpm. In contrast, in patients with cardiomyopathy, mean cardiac index was highest at ventricular pacing rates of 70–90 bpm. In both groups, increases in pacing rates resulted in significant linear decreases in stroke volume index. In patients with normal hearts, ejection fraction decreased at pacing rates from 60 to 100 bpm compared to 50 bpm. In patients with cardiomyopathy, ejection fraction was significantly reduced only at pacing rates of 90–100 bpm. Asterisk indicates significantly different ($P <0.05$) from values at lower pacing rates. Source: Narahara and Blettel [1]. Reproduced with permission of Wolters Kluwer Health.

Early work on the ideal pacing rate suggested that a rate between 70 and 90 bpm results in maximal increase in cardiac output during ventricular pacing at rest (Figure 3.1) [1]. Further augmentation of heart rate via ventricular pacing resulted in either no additional increase or a decrease in cardiac output accompanied by an increase in peripheral vascular resistance and decrease in left ventricular ejection fraction (LVEF). Historically, when earliest generation single-chamber ventricular pacemakers were manufactured with only one rate, 70 bpm was the rate usually chosen. However, it should be kept in mind that in an individual patient it is likely that different resting ventricular rates (either higher or lower) may be required to optimize hemodynamics at rest. In patients with systolic and/or diastolic dysfunction or hypertensive hypertrophic heart disease, higher heart rates may limit maximal cardiac output by shortening diastolic filling time, reducing left ventricular (LV) compliance, and increasing systemic vascular resistance (Figure 3.1). Increasing heart rate also augments cardiac oxygen consumption and if this occurs without an enhancement of cardiac output, then a lower pumping efficiency will occur at the higher rate.

Chronotropic incompetence and rate modulation

In addition to maintaining resting heart rate in the physiological range, pacemaker therapy can allow the heart rate to rise during exercise. A variety of terms have been used to describe the capacity of a pacing system to respond to physiological need by increasing or decreasing pacing rate. The earliest term used to describe this physiological property of pacing systems was "rate responsiveness." Significant objection to this term (for grammatical reasons) has led to the more acceptable use of the terms "rate adaptive" and "rate modulating." However, all these terms are used interchangeably.

When the chronotropic function of the sinus node is impaired, the ability of a pacing system to provide rate adaptation depends on the presence of physiological sensors that monitor the need for heart rate modulation. Rate-adaptive pacing is available in almost all modern pulse generators. Rate-adaptive pacing sensors detect physical or physiological indices to mimic the rate response of the normal sinus node. A variety of sensors have been developed to modulate pacing rate according to metabolic demands and to correct chronotropic incompetence. Activity, accelerometer, and minute-ventilation sensors are commercially available. There is no single sensor that ideally mimics normal cardiac physiology and perfectly modulates heart rate according to metabolic demands. A detailed review of the technology of physiological sensors is provided in Chapter 2.

Exercise physiology

The importance of rate modulation in pacing systems is related directly and specifically to the importance of matching cardiac output with physiological need. The predominant need for rate modulation derives from physical activity or exertion. A rise in heart rate with greater workload improves exercise capacity. However, there are other physiological situations in which, normally, there are modulations of heart rate (e.g. during fever and emotional stress). These situations, however, have received less attention, especially in the context of pacing systems.

During exercise – or "work" – the body tissues increase their demand for oxygen. In addition, there is increased need for removal of metabolic by-products, such as CO_2, from tissues. The body has a number of physiological mechanisms in place to provide for increased metabolic demands during exercise. Redistribution of blood flow to working tissues, increased ability of working tissues to extract oxygen from blood, and, most important, increased cardiac output are these mechanisms. Here we focus on the last of these, the body's ability to increase cardiac output with exercise, as this is what rate modulation provides.

The importance of cardiac output during work must be appreciated. A direct, relatively linear relationship exists between the amount of work accomplished and oxygen consumption. Maximal work capacity is therefore specifically related to maximum oxygen consumption. Further, consistent with the Fick principle:

$$\text{Cardiac output} = O_2 \text{ consumption/Arterial} \\ - \text{venous } O_2 \text{ difference}$$

Also:

$$\text{Cardiac output} = \text{Stroke volume} \times \text{Heart rate}$$

By substituting in these equations:

$$O_2 \text{ consumption} = \text{Stroke volume} \times \text{Heart rate} \\ \times \text{Arterial} - \text{venous } O_2 \text{ difference}$$

Because oxygen consumption is directly linearly proportional to work (Figure 3.2):

$$\text{Work} = \text{Stroke volume} \times \text{Heart rate} \\ \times \text{Arterial} - \text{venous } O_2 \text{ difference}$$

Increasing any of these variables will support an increased ability to do work, but the increase in heart rate is the most important determinant. Maximum work, in normal individuals, is accomplished by an increase in stroke volume to approximately 150% of the resting value, an increase in heart rate to approximately 300% of the resting value, and an increase in arterial–venous O_2 difference to approximately 250% of the resting value.

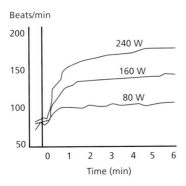
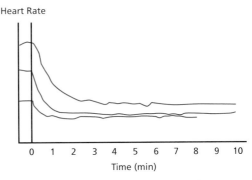
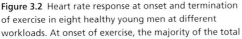

Figure 3.2 Heart rate response at onset and termination of exercise in eight healthy young men at different workloads. At onset of exercise, the majority of the total increment in heart rate occurs in the first minute of effort. Source: Linnarsson [2]. Reproduced with permission of John Wiley & Sons Ltd.

These changes allow an increase in work to over 10 times resting levels. In normal individuals, peak cardiac output can be increased to 300% of resting values simply by an increase in heart rate. During peak exercise, the stroke volume is increased to approximately 150% of the resting value. This increase in stroke volume is not linear and is achieved at approximately the halfway point between the rest and maximal exercise levels. The increased stroke volume is accomplished by an increase in venous return, ventricular filling, and contractility. It is ideal to optimize stroke volume, because this is a more energy efficient way of accomplishing cardiac output (milliliters of cardiac output/milliliters of O_2 consumption) than by an increase in heart rate.

The normal heart rate response to exercise follows a triphasic response (Figure 3.2) [2]. Heart rate increases most rapidly within the first 10–15 s of maximum-effort exercise and reaches 70% of total heart rate increase in this phase. A slower exponential rise in rate follows during the next 60–90 s. Finally, a slow linear increase or plateau phase results from sustained activity. Heart rate deceleration with cessation of exercise is generally slower than acceleration and follows a biphasic or triphasic response.

Chronotropic incompetence

The inability to increase and maintain heart rate appropriately with exercise is called chronotropic incompetence. A number of criteria have been proposed to diagnose chronotropic incompetence, including the inability to increase heart rate with exercise to at least 70–85% of the maximum predicted heart rate (maximum predicted heart rate = 220 – age in years). This is a useful criterion for diagnosing chronotropic incompetence, but it cannot be used in individuals with limitations on their exercise function unrelated to cardiopulmonary status. Thus, the diagnosis of chronotropic incompetence is difficult if the patient cannot undergo formal exercise testing or perform a simple hall walk test. Further, there are patients with delayed chronotropic responses who could benefit from rate-adaptive pacing systems but might be missed by this criterion. More complicated formulas have been developed to allow determination of the presence of chronotropic incompetence by exercise

testing with assessments made by stage. The Wilkoff chronotropic assessment exercise protocol (CAEP) is performed via treadmill testing and is often used for chronotropic competency evaluation [3]. It uses gradual increases in both elevation and speed, and can be used for the evaluation of devices with a variety of sensor types.

Chronotropic incompetence is common among pacemaker patients. However, the frequency of chronotropic incompetence in part depends on the definition used and method of assessment. Among a cohort of pacemaker patients [42% AV block, 56% sinus node disease, and 59% atrial fibrillation (AF)], 51% were diagnosed as having chronotropic incompetence based on the Wilkoff chronotropic index [4]. Among patients in whom sinoatrial disease is the primary indication for pacing, not all will manifest chronotropic incompetence during formal exercise testing. Some individuals with sinus node dysfunction may demonstrate normal chronotropic response to exercise, whereas others may have little or no ability to increase heart rate during exercise. Thus, the need for rate-adaptive pacing is unpredictable in sinoatrial disease. The overall pattern of chronotropic response in an individual is variable and may evolve over time. Some patients are able to achieve the appropriate heart rate for the level of exercise but do so more slowly than is normal. Patients with any form of chronotropic incompetence are candidates for pacing systems with rate-modulation capabilities. It is also noted that making predictions regarding the future need for rate-adaptive pacing is unreliable at the time of implantation. This is usually not a clinical issue, because rate-adaptive pacing is available in almost all modern pacemaker generators and can be programmed "on" if needed after implantation.

Chronotropic incompetence may be provoked by disease, most commonly ischemic heart disease, valvular heart disease, and heart failure, or induced by drugs. In a study of pacemaker patients, significant predictors of chronotropic incompetence included the existence of coronary artery disease, presence of an acquired valvular heart disease, former cardiac surgery, and therapy with digitalis, beta-blockers or amiodarone [4]. Chronotropic incompetence has important prognostic implications in patients with coronary artery disease. It predicts all-cause mortality independent of angiographic severity of coronary artery disease [5]. The prevalence of chronotropic impairment in heart failure patients also is variably reported (25–70%), possibly due to lack of a standardized definition and/or differing assessment methodologies. Chronotropic impairment impacts the physical function and quality of life of heart failure patients.

Advantages and clinical benefits of rate modulation

The ability to increase heart rate is the most important determinant of cardiac output and exercise capacity, especially at higher levels of exertion. Accordingly, an inappropriate chronotropic response to exercise can decrease peak exercise oxygen uptake by as much as 15–20%.

Quantification of the improvement in work capacity in pacemaker populations comparing non-rate-modulated with rate-modulated modes has shown the advantages of the rate-modulated systems. Rate-modulated pacing systems have been shown not only to improve the heart rate response with exercise, but also to increase work capacity. For every 40% increase in paced rate during rate-modulated pacing compared with non-rate-modulated pacing, there is a 10% increase in work capacity. Compared with VVI pacing, VVIR mode improves exercise duration and cardiac index in patients undergoing paired

stress testing. These improvements are independent of patient age and ejection fraction. Even greater improvements in exercise hemodynamics are documented with DDDR pacing compared with either VVIR or DDD modes. Compared with VVIR, DDDR pacing has demonstrated improved exercise capacity, cardiac output, and cardiac metabolic indices, suggesting more efficient cardiac work. In patients with sick sinus syndrome, DDDR pacing provides greater maximal heart rates, longer exercise times, higher maximal oxygen uptake, and higher oxygen uptake at anaerobic threshold than DDD pacing (Figure 3.3). These benefits are attributed largely to the increased heart rate in the rate-adaptive mode.

Despite recognized theoretical benefits of rate modulation on exercise performance, it is realized that many pacemaker recipients are elderly and function at submaximal levels of exertion during virtually all their daily activities. Rarely does the typical pacemaker patient require improvement in maximal work capacity and few are expected to stress to their maximal heart rate, except for the young or extremely vigorous. References are available that provide normal ranges of heart rates in response to moderate exercise according to age, sex, and body surface area, which have relevance to rate-adaptive pacemaker programming. However, such rates are often inappropriate in some patients,

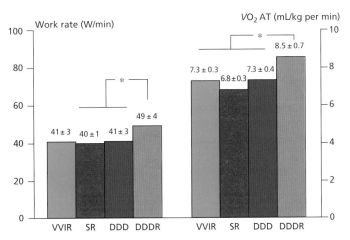

Figure 3.3 Work rate versus oxygen uptake at anaerobic threshold in nine patients with sinus node dysfunction. Each patient underwent testing in sinus rhythm (SR) and VVIR, DDD and DDDR pacing modes using a respiratory sensor pacemaker. Oxygen uptake was greater in DDDR mode compared with all others at anaerobic threshold (AT). Source: Lemke B, Dryander SV, Jäger D, et al. Aerobic capacity in rate modulated pacing. Pacing Clin Electrophysiol 1992;15:1914–1918. Reproduced with permission of John Wiley & Sons Ltd.

such as those with coronary artery disease, valvular disease, or diastolic dysfunction. Optimization of heart rate by providing rate modulation at submaximal levels of exertion during activities of daily living is most often the therapeutic aim. This may require individualized pacemaker programming to suit the unique needs of each patient.

From an evidence-based perspective, it is notable that despite the physiological basis for rate-adaptive pacing and acute improvements in exercise hemodynamics with the use of this technology, it has not been clearly and consistently established that rate-adaptive pacing provides clinically relevant improvements in symptoms, quality of life, or other relevant cardiovascular outcomes. The Advanced Elements of Pacing Trial (ADEPT) studied 872 patients with at least mild chronotropic incompetence and found no significant improvements in quality of life in patients assigned to rate-modulated compared with fixed-rate pacemakers (DDDR vs. DDD) [6]. Furthermore, there were no differences in the composite end point of death, non-fatal myocardial infarction, stroke, hospitalization for heart failure, or AF between the two groups. Interestingly, the DDDR group was significantly more likely to experience hospitalization for heart failure compared with the DDD group (7.3% vs. 3.5%). Thus, it should be concluded that the addition of rate modulation in conventional dual-chamber devices, despite attempting to replicate the normal response to exercise, does not have a positive impact on quality of life or cardiovascular outcomes. It may be speculated that the increased frequency of RV pacing at higher heart rates during rate-modulated pacing, with the resultant forced ventricular dyssynchrony, may increase the risk of heart failure and negate the potential benefits of restoring chronotropic competence. The clinical utility and importance of rate modulation during biventricular pacing has not been well investigated, though small studies are suggestive of improved exercise capacity when rate modulation is utilized during CRT in patients with heart failure and chronotropic incompetence [7].

Although there are a variety of sensors that can be used for rate modulation in currently available pacemakers, there is little evidence to support a major clinical difference in outcomes between sensors and their combinations. Interestingly, when three of the most commonly utilized rate-adaptive sensors (accelerometer, piezoelectric, and blended sensors; see Chapter 2) were compared in DDDR-paced patients with sinus node dysfunction in the Mode Selection Trial (MOST), quality-of-life analyses demonstrated that patients with blended sensors had significantly worse physical function than did patients with the other two sensor systems [8]. There were no significant differences, after adjustment for baseline differences, among the three sensors in clinical end points after long-term follow-up, including no significant differences in the risk of death, heart failure hospitalization, AF, and the combined end point of mortality and stroke.

Atrioventricular synchrony

The introduction of dual-chamber (AV sequential) pacing in 1962 was designed to avoid the AV desynchronization imposed during ventricular-only pacing and to improve hemodynamics. Enthusiasm for AV sequential (DDD) pacing and the importance of maintaining AV synchrony was so high in the 1980s that at that time many in the field believed that these pacemakers could permit the restoration of normal cardiac physiology. Furthermore, at one time, dual-chamber [right atrial (RA) and RV] cardiac pacing was proposed as a possible therapy for heart failure. However, subsequent studies and randomized clinical trials of pacemaker therapy have provided important new insights into the hemodynamics of AV synchrony and pacing mode selection. The widespread recognition of the potential deleterious effects of frequent RV pacing along with the introduction of LV-based pacing and CRT have further complicated consideration of the hemodynamics of AV synchrony, optimal pacemaker mode selection, and dual-chamber pacemaker programming.

The hemodynamic benefits of AV synchrony accrue from its ability to (i) maximize ventricular preload and therefore contractility; (ii) close AV valves before ventricular systole, limiting AV valvular regurgitation; (iii) maintain low mean atrial pressures, thus facilitating venous return; and (iv) regulate autonomic and neurohumoral reflexes involving atrial pressure and volume.

Advantages

The loss of AV synchrony during ventricular pacing in the presence of sinus rhythm is associated most consistently with increases in atrial pressures, alterations in pulmonary and systemic venous flow patterns, and AV valvular regurgitation. Effects of AV desynchronization on systemic blood pressure and cardiac output are more variable between patients. Autonomic activation of the vagal inhibitory reflexes associated with atrial distension can result in an inappropriate decrease in peripheral vascular resistance. Rarely, VVI pacing with loss of appropriate AV synchrony can produce dramatic responses and disabling symptomatology with severe symptomatic hypotension, decreased cardiac output, and syncope.

Atrial pressures

An increase in atrial pressures during ventricular pacing is probably the major mechanism by which symptoms are produced when AV synchrony is not maintained. Increases in atrial pressure during ventricular pacing (VVI) are related primarily to atrial contraction against closed AV valves during ventricular systole. During AV synchrony, atrial contraction augments ventricular end-diastolic filling pressure while maintaining a low mean atrial pressure throughout diastole. In the absence of AV synchrony, a higher mean atrial pressure is required to achieve the same degree of ventricular filling. By this mechanism, AV synchrony is associated with lower venous and left atrial (LA) pressures (Figure 3.4).

In Figure 3.4, the left panel shows recordings of pulmonary capillary wedge pressure in one patient during AV-synchronous pacing [80 pulses per minute (ppm), AV interval 150 ms]. The right panel shows the pulmonary capillary wedge pressure during ventricular pacing (80 ppm) with intact ventriculoatrial (VA) conduction. A relatively normal pulmonary capillary wedge pressure tracing is produced during AV pacing with mean pressures between 4 and 8 mmHg and without significant phasic aberration. In contrast, during ventricular pacing, the mean pressures are elevated to between 8 and 12 mmHg with large A waves (or VA waves) that, at times, exceed 16 mmHg. This elevation in atrial pressures, and specifically the production of giant or "cannon" A waves, occurs because of LA contraction against a closed mitral valve; the increased pressure wave is present not only in the left atrium, but also in the pulmonary veins and pulmonary capillary wedge position. The same phenomenon occurs on the right side of the heart.

Figures 3.5 and 3.6 display simultaneous RA and pulmonary capillary wedge pressure recordings during ventricular pacing (80 ppm) in which VA conduction is intact. In Figure 3.5, 1 : 1 VA conduction is present, while in Figure 3.6 there is 2 : 1 VA conduction. Intact VA conduction produces consistent elevations in pressure in the left atrium and right atrium due to contraction of the atria against closed AV valves. Even when VA conduction is not intact, because of unequal atrial and ventricular rates, there will be frequent periods when atrial contraction occurs during ventricular systole, during which the AV valves are closed; hence, the problems of elevated pressures in the atria and pulmonary veins occur. Some patients are actually more symptomatic when VA conduction is not intact, due to intermittency of these elevated pressures,

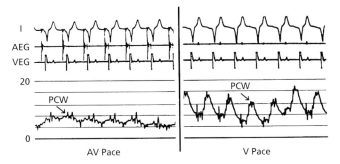

Figure 3.4 Pulmonary capillary wedge (PCW) pressure recordings from a single patient during (*left*) atrioventricular (AV) pacing (AV Pace) with AV interval of 150 ms and (*right*) ventricular pacing (V Pace) at 80 ppm. Scale in mmHg. I, ECG lead I; AEG, atrial electrogram; VEG, ventricular electrogram.

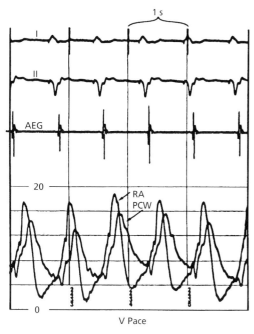

Figure 3.5 Right atrial (RA) and pulmonary capillary wedge (PCW) pressure recordings during ventricular pacing (V Pace) at 80 ppm with 1 : 1 ventriculoatrial conduction. Scale in mmHg. I, II standard ECG leads; AEG, atrial electrogram.

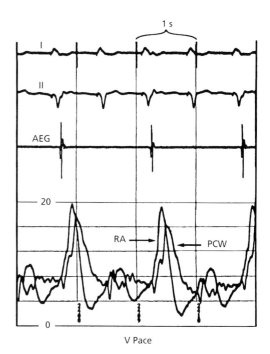

Figure 3.6 Right atrial (RA) and pulmonary capillary wedge (PCW) pressure recordings during ventricular pacing (V Pace) at 80 ppm with 2 : 1 ventriculoatrial conduction. Scale in mmHg. I and II, standard ECG leads; AEG, atrial electrogram.

thus preventing patients from establishing tolerance to this phenomenon.

The relationship of the phasic changes in the pulmonary capillary wedge (and LA) pressures to LV pressures can be seen in Figures 3.7–3.9. Figure 3.7 is a display of normal LV and pulmonary capillary wedge pressure recordings during AV pacing (80 ppm, AV interval 150 ms). The appropriately timed A wave can be seen in both the LV and pulmonary capillary wedge pressure recordings. In contrast, as Figure 3.8 shows, during ventricular pacing (80 ppm) with a consistent 1 : 1 VA relationship, the loss of the A-wave contribution to the upstroke of the LV pressure recording and the giant A wave, late in ventricular systole, can be seen consistently in the pulmonary capillary wedge pressure recording. Figure 3.9 displays this relationship when the atrial contraction is random in relation to ventricular contraction.

Pulmonary venous flow patterns

Doppler echocardiography can provide non-invasive insight into physiological pacemaker-related changes in paced patients, including alterations in pulmonary vein flow and LA mechanical function (Figures 3.10 and 3.11). VA (retrograde) conduction produces a contraction of the atria against closed AV valves, which induces a reversal of blood flow from the left atrium toward the pulmonary veins. This can be recognized by retrograde flow into the pulmonary vein (z wave) on the pulsed-Doppler echocardiographic recording (Figure 3.10). Even when retrograde conduction during ventricular pacing is absent, atrial contraction may still occur shortly after ventricular activation by chance, resulting in intermittent regurgitation into the pulmonary veins (Figure 3.11). Inappropriately timed atrial reverse flow at the time of ventricular systole markedly decreases the systolic flow velocities of pulmonary veins and reverses flow into the pulmonary veins. A study using transesophageal Doppler echocardiography has demonstrated that atrial reverse flow into the pulmonary veins is a consistent finding in patients during VVI pacing when VA conduction is present. Furthermore, during ventricular pacing (VVI) with VA conduction, patients with clinical signs and symptoms of pacemaker

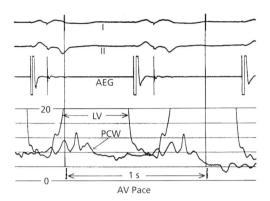

Figure 3.7 Left ventricular (LV) and pulmonary capillary wedge (PCW) pressure recordings during atrioventricular (AV) pacing at 80 ppm with AV interval of 150 ms. Scale in mmHg. I and II, standard ECG leads; AEG, atrial electrogram.

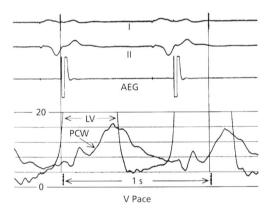

Figure 3.8 Left ventricular (LV) and pulmonary capillary wedge (PCW) pressure recordings during ventricular pacing at 80 ppm with a 1 : 1 ventriculoatrial (VA) relationship (VA interval 150 ms). Scale in mmHg. I and II, standard ECG leads; AEG, atrial electrogram.

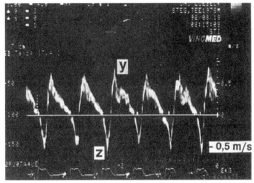

Figure 3.10 Ventricular pacing with 1 : 1 retrograde conduction. In this transesophageal pulsed-Doppler echocardiographic recording, positive values depict antegrade flow in a pulmonary vein, whereas negative values depict retrograde flow. After each ventricular stimulus (see ECG at the bottom of the tracing), a retrograde P wave appears, resulting in regurgitation into the pulmonary vein (z wave). Source: Stierle U, Krüger D, Mitusch R, et al. Adverse pacemaker hemodynamics evaluated by pulmonary venous flow monitoring. *Pacing Clin Electrophysiol* 1995;18:2028–2034. Reproduced with permission of John Wiley & Sons Ltd.

syndrome (i.e. hypotension with dizziness, dyspnea, fatigue) have significantly higher atrial reverse flow velocities into their pulmonary veins than patients without pacemaker syndrome (Figures 3.12 and 3.13).

Atrioventricular valvular regurgitation
Effective and properly timed atrial and ventricular contraction is functionally important for complete mitral valve leaflet closure. Thus, it is not surprising that RV pacing (VVI) is associated with substantial worsening or production of significant

Figure 3.9 Left ventricular (LV) and pulmonary capillary wedge (PCW) pressure recordings during ventricular pacing at 80 ppm with ventriculoatrial dissociation. Scale in mmHg. I and II, standard ECG leads; AEG, atrial electrogram.

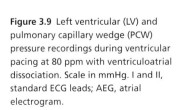
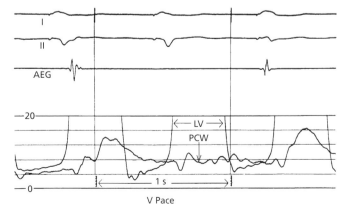

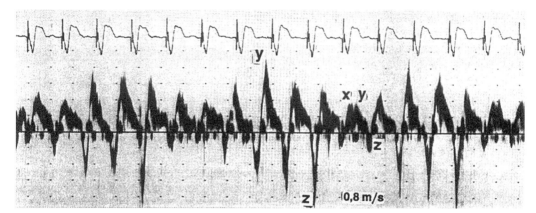

Figure 3.11 Ventricular pacing without retrograde conduction. Transesophageal pulsed-Doppler echocardiographic recording as in Figure 3.10. With a VVI pacing rate (75 bpm) different from the sinus rate, P waves appear shortly after the ventricular stimulus in three of the five cycles, resulting in regurgitation into the pulmonary vein (z wave as in Figure 3.10). Source: Stierle U, Krüger D, Mitusch R, *et al*. Adverse pacemaker hemodynamics evaluated by pulmonary venous flow monitoring. *Pacing Clin Electrophysiol* 1995;18:2028–2034. Reproduced with permission of John Wiley & Sons Ltd.

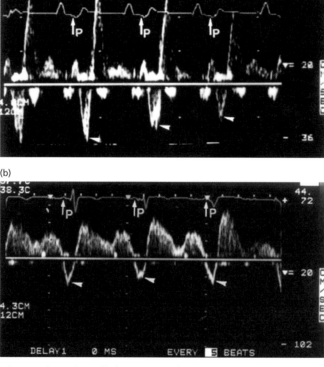

Figure 3.12 Representative Doppler tracings of left pulmonary vein flow in a patient with clinical pacemaker syndrome before (a) and after (b) reprogramming to DDD mode. (a) Atrial reverse flow (arrowheads) of the pulmonary vein regularly occurs after the electrocardiographically retrograde P wave (P). (b) Atrial reverse flow (arrowheads) of the pulmonary vein is noted after the electrocardiographically antegrade P wave (P). Systolic flow velocities of the pulmonary vein are increased compared with those in (a). Source: Lee TM, Su SF, Lin YJ, *et al*. Role of transesophageal echocardiography in the evaluation of patients with clinical pacemaker syndrome. *Am Heart J* 1998;135:634–640. Reproduced with permission of Elsevier.

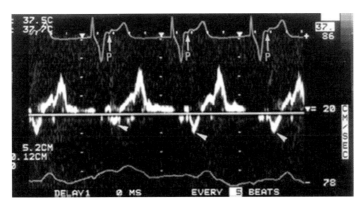

Figure 3.13 Representative Doppler tracings of left pulmonary vein flow together with respiration in an asymptomatic patient during VVI pacing. Atrial reverse flow (arrowheads) of the pulmonary vein is noted after the electrocardiographically retrograde P wave (P), similar to Figure 3.12a. The magnitude of atrial reverse flow is significantly lower than that in Figure 3.12a. Source: Lee TM, Su SF, Lin YJ, *et al*. Role of transesophageal echocardiography in the evaluation of patients with clinical pacemaker syndrome. *Am Heart J* 1998; 135:634–640. Reproduced with permission of Elsevier.

mitral and/or tricuspid regurgitation in some patients due to the loss of AV synchrony or an inappropriately timed AV interval.

A number of case reports have described dramatic reductions in the severity of mitral regurgitation (MR) in patients with severe MR during ventricular pacing after upgrading to a dual-chamber device (Figure 3.14). In one study, the majority of patients (67%) with signs and symptoms of pacemaker syndrome during ventricular pacing (VVI) with retrograde conduction had significant MR (moderate or above) documented. Strikingly, MR disappeared in these patients after reprogramming to DDD mode. Other investigators likewise have demonstrated that the extent of valve regurgitation may be an important factor in the genesis of subclinical pacemaker syndrome. Thus, RV pacing can cause AV valve regurgitation in some patients that may resolve with the resumption of AV synchrony using AAI pacing or AV pacing programming to DDD mode.

When atrial contraction is not followed by an adequately synchronized ventricular contraction, the AV pressure gradient reverses during atrial relaxation and diastolic ventricular pressures exceed those in the atria (VA pressure gradient). This results in diastolic AV valve regurgitation because the mitral and tricuspid valves are incompletely closed. The presence of diastolic MR highlights the importance of adequately timed AV synchrony for optimal diastolic filling of the ventricle. Diastolic mitral and tricuspid

regurgitation is a common finding when AV synchrony is lost, such as during ventricular-only pacing (e.g. VVI) or in the presence of AV conduction abnormalities (Figure 3.15). Significant elevation of LV end-diastolic filling pressures will contribute to worsening of diastolic MR during AV dyssynchrony.

In most pacemaker patients, however, worsening of AV regurgitation appears to play a lesser role in elevating atrial pressure than does the contraction of the atria against closed AV valves during ventricular pacing. Furthermore, in the absence of ventricular dysfunction or structural heart disease, diastolic MR during AV desynchronization is usually a benign phenomenon without significant therapeutic clinical implications. Using transesophageal Doppler echocardiography, significant MR was found during VVI pacing with VA conduction in only 8% of a group of patients without clinical pacemaker syndrome.

Blood pressure

For grouped patient data, AV synchrony generally provides similar or slightly greater systolic and mean blood pressures than ventricular pacing. A typical example of the blood pressure comparison among atrial, AV, and ventricular pacing is shown in Figure 3.16. In this case, essentially no differences exist between the blood pressures when comparing atrial with AV pacing. The blood pressure during ventricular pacing is slightly lower than during either atrial or AV pacing.

(a)

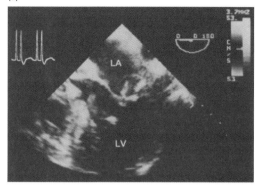

(b)

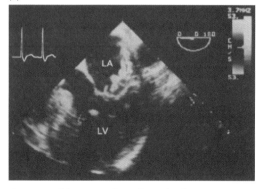

Figure 3.14 (a) Transesophageal Doppler flow image showing mitral regurgitant jet. There was mild mitral regurgitation during atrioventricular sequential pacing. (b) Transesophageal Doppler flow image showing a mitral regurgitation jet during ventricular pacing [10 s after image shown in (a)]. With ventricular pacing, mitral regurgitation is severe. LA, left atrium; LV, left ventricle. Source: Berglund H, Nishioka T, Hackner E, *et al*. Ventricular pacing: a cause of reversible severe mitral regurgitation. *Am Heart J* 1996;131:1035–1037. Reproduced with permission of Elsevier.

Although not the typical response, some individuals do have dramatic and symptomatic decreases in systemic blood pressure when ventricular pacing is instituted (Figure 3.17). Several mechanisms may be responsible for this phenomenon. Loss of LV preload volume from mistimed atrial contraction (loss of atrial "kick") and activation of inhibitory cardiac reflexes (due also to inappropriately timed atrial contraction) have been the mechanisms most commonly implicated. This marked hypotension can produce dramatic symptoms, including syncope. In a clinical setting, if this problem is suspected but hypotension with symptoms cannot be reproduced

in a supine position, an upright or semi-upright posture may unmask the problem, especially if it is related to a LV preload deficiency caused by loss of atrial contribution to ventricular filling. An important consideration in the hemodynamic response to ventricular pacing is VA conduction. VA conduction, the ability to conduct electrical impulses retrograde from the ventricles through the AV junction to the atria, can lead to atrial contraction during ventricular systole or, in cases of long VA conduction, early diastole. This can cause loss of the atrial contribution to ventricular filling as well as other hemodynamic problems. VA conduction has been found in as many as 90% of patients with sick sinus syndrome and in 15–35% of individuals with a variety of degrees of AV block. During ventricular pacing, even when VA conduction is not intact, if the ventricular pacing rate is unequal to the atrial rate, there will be periods when atrial contraction occurs during ventricular systole with the resulting disadvantageous hemodynamics.

Cardiac output

Properly timed atrial contraction provides a significant increase in ventricular end-diastolic volume and is responsible for the so-called atrial kick (Figure 3.18). Studies have shown a wide range in the actual importance of the atrial contribution to ventricular filling depending on the patient population and study conditions. By increasing the end-diastolic volumes (right and left ventricles), the cardiac output is, in turn, increased. The average increase in cardiac output in a pacing population, if AV synchrony is maintained, is between 15 and 25% in comparison with non-AV-synchronized ventricular pacing. In a study in pediatric patients with congenital complete AV block and normal ventricular function, cardiac output was measured using a non-invasive method involving inert gas rebreathing and was shown to be 18% higher in synchronous AV pacing with optimized AV intervals than during VVIR pacing [9].

The hemodynamic benefits of AV-synchronized versus ventricular pacing have also been demonstrated for patients after myocardial infarction and cardiac surgery. Patients with reduced cardiac output – especially if such reduced function is due to relative volume depletion or only mild-to-moderately depressed LV

(a)

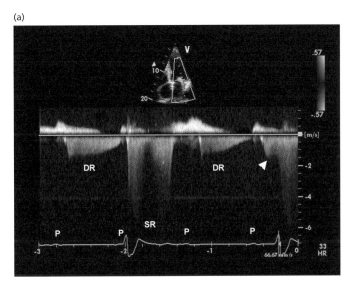

(b)

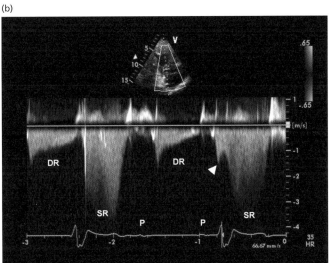

Figure 3.15 Mitral valve (a) and tricuspid valve (b) continuous-wave Doppler recordings from an apical transducer position obtained in an 80-year-old male with complete atrioventricular (AV) block. There is a ventricular escape rhythm at 33–35 bpm (QRS complexes). Note the diastolic AV valve regurgitation that occurs when the P wave is not followed by an appropriately timed ventricular contraction. Also note that diastolic AV regurgitation is reduced (arrowhead) when the ventricular contraction (QRS complex at the right side of each image) happens by chance to fall at an appropriate interval after the P wave (simulating a more synchronized AV relationship). DR, diastolic regurgitation; P, P wave; SR, systolic regurgitation.

function – frequently benefit significantly from maintenance of AV synchrony. In a group of patients with severe LV systolic dysfunction (mean LV ejection fraction 0.21 ± 0.07) and New York Heart Association (NYHA) class II–IV heart failure, there were significant reductions in cardiac index (~12%) with single-chamber VVI pacing compared with pacing modes that maintained AV synchrony (AAI or DDD with ventricular pacing from the RV apex or outflow tract) [10] (Figure 3.19).

There is a general perception that patients with abnormal cardiac function benefit most from maintenance of AV synchrony. This may be true,

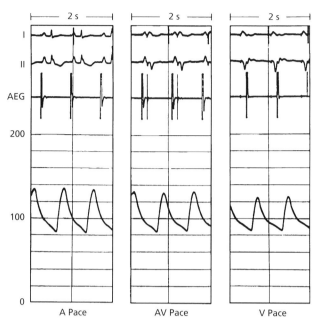

Figure 3.16 Femoral artery pressure recordings from one patient. (*Left to right*) During atrial pacing (A Pace); during atrioventricular (AV) sequential pacing (AV Pace); and during ventricular pacing (V Pace). All tracings are at 80 ppm with an AV interval of 150 ms during AV pacing. Scale in mmHg. I, II, and III, standard ECG leads; AEG, atrial electrogram.

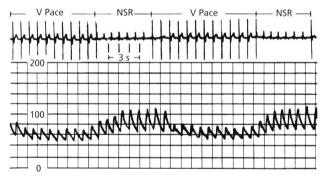

Figure 3.17 Radial artery pressure recording from a patient during right ventricular pacing (V Pace) at 80 ppm and normal sinus rhythm (NSR) (scale in mmHg). This patient's blood pressure, measured by radial artery line, drops from approximately 110/70 mmHg during sinus rhythm to approximately 75/55 mmHg during ventricular pacing.

but the reasons are frequently not due to better cardiac output. In fact, if cardiac output were the only hemodynamic consideration, it is patients with very poor ventricular function (markedly increased end-diastolic volume and depressed ejection fraction) that benefit least from AV synchrony. This can be best understood by using the concept of ventricular function curves that compare stroke volume or cardiac output with LV end-diastolic volume or preload.

Figure 3.20 shows hypothetical ventricular function curves for a patient with normal ventricular function (curve 1), one with moderate LV dysfunction (curve 2), one with very poor LV function and a markedly dilated ventricle (curve 3), and one with hypertrophic cardiomyopathy (curve 4). These curves describe the performance of the left ventricle in generating stroke volume (or cardiac output) in relation to the end-diastolic volume (or preload). In patients with normal LV function

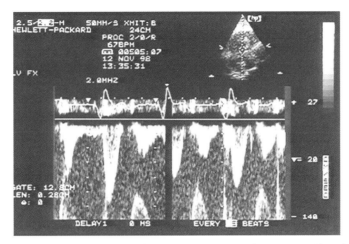

Figure 3.18 Doppler echocardiographic evaluation of the velocity time integral in the left ventricular outflow tract obtained from a patient with a VVI pacemaker originally implanted for complete heart block. The sinus mechanism was intact, and the patient had palpitations and symptoms consistent with a low cardiac output. There is marked beat-to-beat fluctuation in the stroke volume in accord with waxing and waning coincidental atrioventricular (AV) synchrony, clearly demonstrating a benefit of restoring AV synchrony and providing justification for replacement of an otherwise normally functioning VVI pacemaker with a more appropriate dual-chamber system. Source: courtesy of Paul A. Levine, MD.

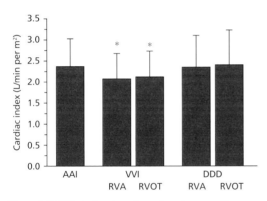

Figure 3.19 Effect of pacing site and mode on cardiac index. Measurements during pacing at a fixed rate were compared in each patient. Pacing was performed in AAI, VVI, and DDD modes from the right ventricular apex (RVA) or outflow tract (RVOT). Means ± SD are shown. Asterisk indicates *P* <0.05 vs. AAI. Source: Gold *et al.* [10]. Reproduced with permission of Elsevier.

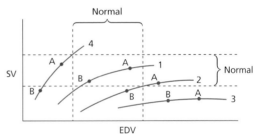

Figure 3.20 Hypothetical ventricular function curves comparing (1) stroke volume (SV) and left ventricular end-diastolic volume (EDV) in patients with normal ventricular function; (2) moderately depressed ventricular function; (3) severely depressed ventricular function; and (4) hyperdynamic ventricular function. Point A, with normal atrioventricular (AV) sequence; point B, without normal AV sequence.

(curve 1), as end-diastolic volume increases, stroke volume (and cardiac output) increases until the flat or descending portion of the curve is reached. In patients with depressed LV function (curves 2 and 3), there is a lesser increase in stroke volume that depends on end-diastolic volume to the point that, in patients with poor LV function (curve 3), there is negligible improvement in stroke volume with further increases in end-diastolic volume. On the other hand, patients with hypertrophic or hypertensive cardiomyopathy tend to have small ventricles that are normal (i.e. normal systolic function) or hyperdynamic in function (curve 4). Small increases in end-diastolic volume can significantly increase stroke volume in this situation. As has been discussed, AV synchrony provides the atrial kick that increases end-diastolic volume. Point A on these curves represents the hypothetical stroke volume and end-diastolic volume during AV pacing. Point B represents stroke volume and end-diastolic volume during ventricular pacing (with associated loss of atrial kick). In the normal situation (curve 1), although end-diastolic volume is greater and hence stroke volume is greater during AV-synchronized pacing, the loss of AV synchrony during ventricular pacing does not drop the end-diastolic volume and the stroke volume significantly. However, this might not be the case if the filling volume were otherwise reduced by volume depletion due to blood loss, diuresis, and so on. In these situations, even with normal LV function, the higher end-diastolic volumes and stroke volumes provided by properly timed atrial contraction might be important. With depressed LV function of a moderate degree (curve 2), although maintenance of AV synchrony provides for a greater end-diastolic volume, the stroke volume advantage is diminished. It is possible that, due to overall reduction in stroke volume (and cardiac output), even this modest increment in stroke volume would be of important benefit. In patients with more severely depressed LV function and extremely flat LV function curves (curve 3), end-diastolic volume can be augmented with maintenance of AV synchrony, but there is little advantage in stroke volume.

With regard to patients with hypertrophic cardiomyopathy or highly non-compliant ventricles (curve 4), maintenance of AV synchrony may be very important in enhancing stroke volume and cardiac output because of the relatively small end-diastolic volumes. This is because small increments in end-diastolic volume may substantially increase the stroke volume due to the steep slope of the curve. This relatively steep-sloped ventricular function curve is also characteristic of patients with ventricular diastolic dysfunction, a group for whom maintenance of AV synchrony also is very important. Figure 3.21 displays this concept in a group of patients studied using quantitative nuclear techniques [11]. Although only data from the supine position at 80 bpm are shown (AV interval 150 ms during AV-synchronized pacing), the same situation hemodynamically was found to be present at a faster pacing rate (100 bpm) and in an upright posture.

The conceptual approach of ventricular function curves is useful for practical understanding of the

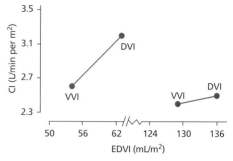

Figure 3.21 Ventricular function curves comparing cardiac index (CI) and left ventricular end-diastolic volume index (EDVI) from (*left*) a group of nine patients with relatively normal ventricular function and (*right*) a group of four patients with markedly depressed ventricular function. The patients were studied in the supine position at a pacing rate of 80 ppm and atrioventricular (AV) interval during DVI pacing of 150 ms. Points are group mean. DVI, AV sequential pacing (AV synchrony); VVI, ventricular pacing (no AV synchrony).

benefits of AV synchrony. However, movement along single ventricular function curves is overly simplistic. A number of variables that can affect hemodynamic function, such as afterload, can be modulated by other factors that might cause shifting from one curve to another, as well as movement along a given curve. In this regard, systemic vascular resistance may be significantly higher during ventricular pacing. The increase in systemic vascular resistance is related mechanistically to an increase in neural reflexes. These autonomic responses to ventricular pacing include increased peripheral sympathetic nerve tone and circulating catecholamine levels supportive of blood pressure when cardiac output is diminished.

A hemodynamic variable that is usually not significantly affected in most individuals during AV versus ventricular pacing is ejection fraction. Although the components of ejection fraction, both end-diastolic volume and stroke volume, are significantly lower during ventricular pacing, ejection fraction is unaffected because both the numerator (stroke volume) and the denominator (end-diastolic volume) of the ejection fraction vary in the same proportion. Ejection fraction is a crude measurement of contractile performance, so it is not surprising that the presence or absence of AV synchrony, which primarily affects preload and cardiac output, has no effect on ejection fraction.

Autonomic neural and neurohormone level alterations

Single-chamber RV pacing is associated with higher levels of sympathetic nerve activity, cardiac norepinephrine spillover, and plasma epinephrine and norepinephrine concentrations than AV synchronous pacing [12]. Catecholamine levels increase most during VVI pacing with retrograde conduction. The enhanced sympathetic outflow appears to be mediated by the arterial and cardiopulmonary baroreflexes.

Plasma levels of natriuretic peptides, including atrial and brain natriuretic peptides (ANP and BNP, respectively), appear to reflect the presence of appropriate AV synchrony and the hemodynamic changes produced by different cardiac pacing modes. RV pacing without AV synchrony (VVI) increases plasma ANP and BNP levels when compared with pacing modes with AV synchrony (AAI or DDD). Increased natriuretic peptide levels develop within several minutes after AV synchrony is lost, both at rest and during exercise. These hormonal alterations persist over the long term but return toward normal after AV synchrony is restored. The release of these hormones occurs in response to worsened cardiac hemodynamics, reflecting atrial distension, higher atrial pressures, and increased LV filling pressures with AV desynchronization. Low levels of natriuretic peptides might be used as a cardiac biomarker reflective of the presence of a physiological pacing mode.

Mortality and cardiovascular outcomes

A meta-analysis summarizing several prospective randomized trials comparing AV synchronous pacing modes (AAI or DDD with or without rate response) with the ventricular-only pacing mode (VVI) has provided insight into the impact of pacing mode selection on mortality and important cardiovascular outcomes in 7000 patients with bradycardia indications for permanent pacemaker implantation [13]. The major conclusions of this systematic review were that (i) atrial-based pacing does not reduce all-cause mortality, cardiovascular death, or heart failure; (ii) atrial-based pacing does reduce the incidence of AF [hazard ratio (HR) 0.80, 95% confidence interval (CI) 0.72–0.89; $P = 0.00003$]; (iii) atrial-based pacing is associated with a reduction of borderline significance in stroke

(HR 0.81, 95% CI 0.67–0.99; $P = 0.035$); and (iv) no patient subgroups derived a special benefit from atrial-based pacing. Aside from these conclusions, there is evidence suggesting that dual-chamber devices modestly improve quality of life and are less likely to be associated with pacemaker syndrome [14]. Thus, most clinicians believe that the clinical evidence is sufficient to justify routine use of pacing modes that provide AV synchrony. Consistent with this clinical practice, the 2012 Heart Rhythm Society (HRS)/American College of Cardiology Foundation (ACCF) Expert Consensus Statement on Pacemaker Device and Mode Selection gives AV synchronous pacing modes a class I recommendation in patients with sinus node dysfunction (DDD or AAI) or AV conduction block (DDD) [15].

Effects of optimal atrioventricular interval timing

The mere presence of a consistent AV relationship may not ensure the best possible hemodynamics or clinical outcomes in a patient with a cardiac pacemaker. An excessively short AV delay may limit active filling of the ventricle and promote systolic AV valvular regurgitation as ventricular contraction begins while the AV valves are open. An excessively long AV delay may result in loss of the booster pump function of the atria related to two factors: (i) inadequate diastolic filling of the ventricle because atrial contraction does not occur near the onset of LV systolic contraction but rather is superimposed on early passive filling; and (ii) diastolic AV valvular regurgitation due to reopening of the valve before ventricular systole.

An optimally timed AV interval maximizes LV filling and stroke volume by the Frank–Starling mechanism. Atrial contraction should occur optimally just before the isovolumic contraction phase. This was well demonstrated in an acute experimental model in canines with complete AV block in which net LV chamber filling was measured with a mitral annular flow probe while the AV timing delay was varied [16]. Increasing the AV delay from 0 (simultaneous AV contraction) to a more physiological range (e.g. around 80–120 ms) enhanced net chamber filling. In the physiological range of AV intervals, atrial systole is completed and the mitral valve closes as LV pressure begins to rise.

At long AV delays (e.g. >275 ms), net filling declines, and at very long delays (e.g. 320 ms) net filling actually falls below that observed at no AV delay. At long AV delays, atrial systole is superimposed on early rapid filling, mitral valve closure is dependent on LV pressure rise, which generates presystolic regurgitation, and net LV filling declines.

In patients at rest with normal ventricular function, the optimal range for the AV interval when the right atrium and ventricle are paced is on average between 150 and 200 ms (Figure 3.22). However, this interval may vary considerably from patient to patient and from time to time in a specific patient (i.e. as short as 100 ms and up to 250 ms). For the reasons noted below, the optimal AV interval when the atrium is sensed will be 20–50 ms shorter than when the right atrium is paced.

Interindividual variation in the optimal AV interval depends on the degree of interatrial and interventricular conduction delays that occur in response to DDD pacing. In conventional right heart pacing systems, the activation sequence of the left-sided chambers may be quite different from the pacemaker-programmed values in situations where marked interatrial and interventricular conduction delays develop in response to pacing or are present intrinsically. Optimal LV contraction should start immediately at the end of LA transport. However,

delays introduced by sensing and pacing of right heart chambers may cause misalignment between electrical and mechanical events, especially of the left heart chambers. Optimal AV pacing may need to account for and correct for these delays introduced by pacing with an appropriately timed AV pacing interval. Such a "physiological" AV interval compensates for pacing- and sensing-induced delays, and assures that LA transport is completed just before LV contraction starts.

For example, RA pacing (especially from the RA appendage or lateral RA wall) prolongs the duration of the P wave and consequently the time from P-wave onset to the end of LA transport, or the atrial transport delay (ATD) (Figure 3.23). Likewise, RV pacing, especially when performed from the RV apex, alters the onset of LV systole and prolongs the interventricular delay (Figure 3.24). In addition to artificial pacing and sensing delays, in patients with underlying, high-grade, interatrial conduction delay in the presence of atrial disease, long AV intervals (250–350 ms) sometimes may be required to provide effective LA systole. Programming a short or "physiological" AV delay in such patients may result in a left atrium that is activated late, producing LA contraction against a closed mitral valve. In patients with interatrial delay or block, consideration may also be given to

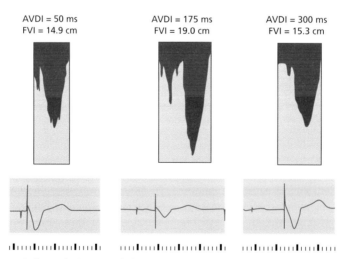

AVDI = 50 ms
FVI = 14.9 cm

AVDI = 175 ms
FVI = 19.0 cm

AVDI = 300 ms
FVI = 15.3 cm

Figure 3.22 Doppler aortic flow velocity integrals (FVI) recorded at varying atrioventricular (AV) pacing intervals. Note the maximal aortic flow velocity at an AV delay interval (AVDI) of 175 ms. Source: Janosik DL, Pearson AC, Buckingham TA *et al*. The hemodynamic benefit of differential atrioventricular delay intervals for sensed and paced atrial events during physiologic pacing. *J Am Coll Cardiol* 1989;14:499–507. Reproduced with permission of Elsevier.

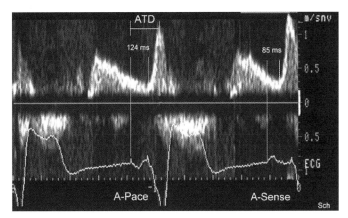

Figure 3.23 Atrial transport delay (ATD) is prolonged during atrial pacing compared with atrial sensing. Atrial-paced and -sensed ATD are shown. ATD is the time from the onset of P wave to the peak of the mitral Doppler A wave, a surrogate for the end of active atrial transport. On the first beat (atrial-paced beat) the time from the pacing pulse to the peak of the mitral Doppler A wave is the paced ATD. On the second beat (atrial-sensed beat) the time from the onset of the P wave to the peak of the A wave is the sensed ATD. Source: Chirife et al. [19]. Reproduced with permission of John Wiley & Sons Ltd.

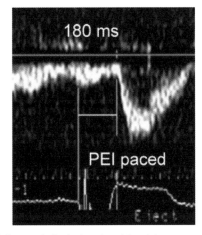
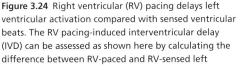
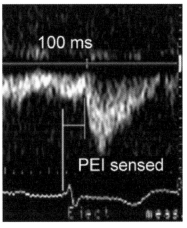

Figure 3.24 Right ventricular (RV) pacing delays left ventricular activation compared with sensed ventricular beats. The RV pacing-induced interventricular delay (IVD) can be assessed as shown here by calculating the difference between RV-paced and RV-sensed left pre-ejection intervals (PEIs). The extent of lengthening of PEI by RV pacing is proportional to IVD. In this example, IVD = 180 − 100 = 80 ms. Source: Chirife et al. [19]. Reproduced with permission of John Wiley & Sons Ltd.

pacing from the RA septum (Bachmann's bundle), coronary sinus, or biatrially to advance LA electrical activation.

The approach of shortening the AV interval during RV pacing in patients with heart failure remains controversial and cannot be advocated. The major benefit of this approach may be confined to the subset of individuals with prolonged PR intervals and diastolic MR. Appropriate patients for dual-chamber pacing with short AV intervals may be those with symptomatic heart failure in sinus rhythm with a long PR interval, prolonged functional diastolic MR (≥450 ms in duration), and a short ventricular filling time (<200 ms at rest). Furthermore, in the setting of marked first-degree AV block (PR interval >300 ms), a pacemaker-like syndrome can occur in the absence of a pacemaker (sometimes referred to as "pseudopacemaker syndrome") (Figure 3.25) [17]. In these cases, atrial systole effectively occurs during or immediately

(a)

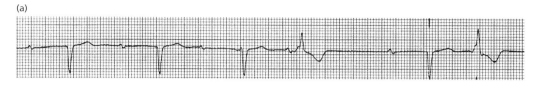

(b)

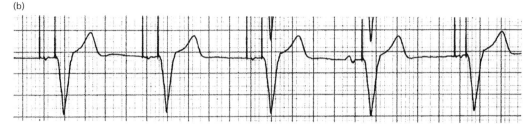

Figure 3.25 ECG tracings from a 74-year-old male with complaints of fatigue and exercise intolerance without syncope or dizziness. (a) Marked first-degree atrioventricular (AV) block is present (PR interval >500 ms) with a normal QRS duration and premature ventricular contractions (PVCs). The Holter monitor from this patient demonstrated first-degree, second-degree (type I), and 2 : 1 AV block with heart rates from 36 to 150 bpm. The longest pause was 2.7 s. There were also frequent PVCs (>9000 in 24 hours). (b) DDD rhythm with appropriate AV intervals (150/120 ms). Following dual-chamber pacemaker implantation, the patient noted a marked improvement in his symptoms and functional capacity, with more energy and overall improved quality of life.

after ventricular systole, resulting in loss of effective AV synchrony. In patients with marked first-degree AV block, dual-chamber (RA and RV) pacing at a short AV interval may improve hemodynamics by optimization of atrial and ventricular synchrony and elimination of diastolic MR. Elimination or reduction of diastolic regurgitation can result in lengthening of the diastolic LV filling time and augmentation of stroke volume and cardiac output (Figure 3.26).

Determination of optimal atrioventricular interval

A variety of invasive and non-invasive techniques have been used to determine the optimal AV interval in pacemaker patients. Doppler echocardiography is often used in clinical trials and has become an accepted method that can be beneficial in determining the optimal AV delay for an individual patient. This approach can analyze diastolic transmitral Doppler flow velocity (E and A waves), stroke volume assessed by aortic velocity time integral (VTI), and AV valve regurgitation for optimization of AV intervals. The Ritter method of AV interval optimization, which uses the mitral valve inflow Doppler profile, is the most widely applied technique. This technique is based on the assumption that the AV delay that maximizes cardiac output is the one that provides the longest LV filling time without interruption of the A wave (atrial contraction wave) and allows ventricular systole to begin immediately subsequent to maximum diastolic ventricular filling, thus avoiding cannon A waves and diastolic MR (Figure 3.27). The goal of AV optimization is to align the end of LA transport with the onset of LV contraction. In the Ritter method, a short AV interval (AV_{short}) is programmed in which there is clear A-wave truncation on the Doppler mitral inflow assessment. The interval from the QRS onset to the completion of the A wave (QA_{short}) is then measured. Next, a long AV delay (AV_{long}) without A-wave truncation is programmed and the interval from QRS onset to the completion of the A wave (QA_{long}) is again measured. The optimal AV delay is defined as: $AV_{opt} = AV_{long} - (QA_{short} - QA_{long})$. An alternative to the Ritter method that uses Doppler echocardiography is the iterative method, which is designed to maximize diastolic filling time by measuring the shortest AV interval that does not result in A-wave attenuation.

Due to the cost, inconvenience, and time required to perform a Doppler echocardiography study, simpler alternatives that use surface electrocardiography (ECG) alone to optimize the AV interval in an individual patient have been proposed and investigated.

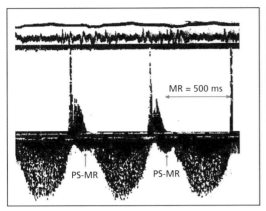

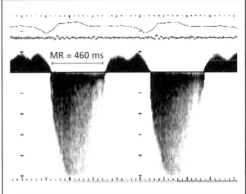

Figure 3.26 Continuous-wave Doppler recordings show mitral regurgitation (MR) in a patient with dilated cardiomyopathy and prolonged PR interval, before and after DDD pacing with AV delay optimization. (*Left*) MR is of long duration (500 ms) during native conduction with a distinct presystolic component (PS-MR) impinging into and abbreviating the left ventricular (LV) filling time. (*Right*)

Shortening the AV delay to 100 ms with DDD pacing eliminates PS-MR, shortens the total MR duration, and increases LV filling time. Source: Salukhe TV, Henein MY, Sutton R. Pacing in heart failure: patient and pacing mode selection. *Eur Heart J* 2003;24:977–986. Reproduced with permission of Oxford University Press.

While ECG-based approaches for AV optimization are of interest, they have not been widely adopted.

One of the surface ECG approaches defines the optimal AV delay based on an arbitrary delay of 100 ms from the end of the surface P wave to the peak/nadir of the paced ventricular complex (Figure 3.28) [18]. The end of the surface P wave represents the end of LA activation, whereas the peak/nadir of the paced ventricular complex coincides with the onset of the isovolumetric contraction period. The AV delay is considered optimal when the end of LA contraction (A wave) coincides with complete mitral valve closure and the onset of the isovolumetric contraction period.

Another ECG-based AV optimization approach uses measurements of P-wave and QRS durations to predict interatrial and interventricular electro-mechanical delays, and calculates the optimal AV interval based on validated regression equations that derive electromechanical timing delays obtained by Doppler echocardiography [19]. This approach is based on the premise that the optimal AV interval is defined by the LA transport delay (ATD), the interventricular delay (IVD) and the P-sense offset (in the case of atrial sensing). The ATD is predicted from measurement of sensed or paced P-wave duration, the IVD from paced QRS duration, and the P-sense offset is 30 ms by default or the time from P onset to P detection using the

surface ECG and pacemaker marker channels. Estimates of ATD and IVD obtained from Doppler echocardiography can then be calculated from validated regression equations using the ECG measurements of P-wave and QRS durations or from tables provided by these investigators and plugged into the proposed optimal AV interval formula (Table 3.1). For example, if measured atrial-paced P-wave duration is 140 ms, the investigators indicate that the expected ATD is 190 ms, and if paced QRS duration is 180 ms, expected IVD is 62 ms. Thus, for RA pacing/RV pacing, optimal AV delay = 190 − 62 = 128 ms.

A highly simplified ECG approach for AV optimization that only uses the surface P wave (a measure of interatrial conduction time) has also been proposed [20]. In this small study, the P-wave duration correlated to the optimal AV delay as calculated by the Ritter method by a factor of 1.26. Based on these data, the authors suggested that by adding one-fourth of the P-wave duration to its baseline measurement, the optimal AV delay during AV pacing can be approximately determined.

Although leaving a device at the nominal AV interval settings may not ensure optimal cardiac hemodynamics, clinical outcomes data on the role of AV optimization have not been definitive. A strategy of AV optimization programming is yet to be implemented or accepted on a wide-scale basis.

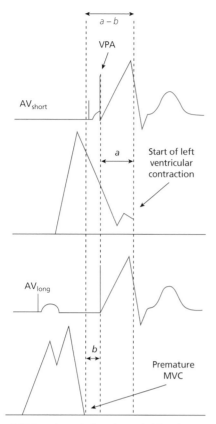

Figure 3.27 Doppler technique for optimizing the atrioventricular (AV) interval. The surface ECG and Doppler mitral inflow pattern are depicted schematically for a very short AV interval (e.g. 50 ms, *top*) and a very long AV interval (e.g. 250 ms, *bottom*). Interval *a* represents the longest time between the ventricular pacing artifact (VPA) and mitral valve closure (MVC) for the short AV interval. Interval *b* represents the time between ventricular pacing and mitral valve closure during the long AV interval, and may be a negative value due to diastolic regurgitation. The optimal AV delay is calculated as the long AV delay minus the difference between intervals *a* and *b*. Source: adapted from Kinderman M, Fröhlig G, Doerr T, Schieffer H. Optimizing the AV delay in DDD pacemaker patients with high degree AV block: mitral valve Doppler versus impedance cardiography. *Pacing Clin Electrophysiol* 1997;20:2453–2462. Reproduced with permission of John Wiley & Sons Ltd.

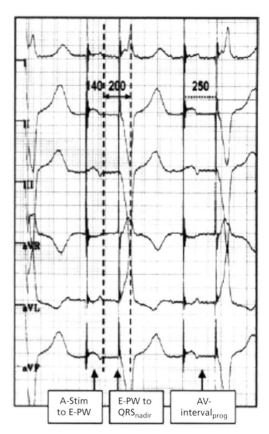

Figure 3.28 Determination of optimal paced atrioventricular (AV) delay (AVD_{opt}) by surface ECG. First, a long AV delay of 250 ms was programmed (AVD_{prog}, programmed interval from atrial to ventricular stimulus). The interval from the end of the P wave to the peak/nadir of the paced ventricular complex (T) was 200 ms. The interval from the atrial stimulus to the end of the P wave (the global atrial conduction time) was 140 ms. According to the algorithm, $AVD_{opt} = AVD_{prog} + 100 - T$, the optimized AV delay was 150 ms. A-Stim to E-PW, interval between the pacing stimulus and the end of P-wave deflection; AV-interval$_{prog}$, long AV delay programmed for testing; E-PW to QRS$_{nadir}$, end of P wave (E-PW) to peak/nadir of paced QRS. Source: Strohmer *et al.* [18]. Reproduced with permission of John Wiley & Sons Ltd.

No consensus exists regarding which patients should undergo AV optimization or when this process should be performed. Much of the evidence regarding AV optimization for pacing derives from small, single-center, acute, non-randomized trials, many of which lack a control group. The echocardiography for CRT guidelines published by the American Society of Echocardiography in 2008 recommended the use of the Ritter or iterative method for calculation of the optimal AV delay [21].

Large-scale randomized controlled trials validating that AV interval optimization results in long-term improvement in clinical outcomes do not exist. Among patients receiving CRT, the SMART-AV (SmartDelay Determined AV Optimization: A Comparison to Other AV Delay Methods Used in Cardiac Resynchronization Therapy) trial prospectively randomized patients

Table 3.1 Determination of optimal atrioventricular (AV) delays using the atrial transport delay (ATD) and interventricular delay (IVD) derived from the P-wave and QRS duration ECG measurements

P or QRS duration (ms)	ATD (ms)	IVD (ms)
80	132	23
90	142	27
100	152	31
110	161	35
120	171	39
130	181	43
140	190	47
150	200	51
160	210	55
170	219	59
180	229	62
190	238	66
200	248	70
210	258	74
220	267	78
230	277	82
240	287	86
250	296	90

Using this table, it is possible to estimate the duration of right atrial (RA)-paced ATD and right ventricular (RV)-paced IVD from the corresponding P or QRS duration column. Once ATD and IVD are found, calculation of the optimal AV follows from ATD – IVD. For example, as shown in this table, if measured RA-paced P-wave duration is 140 ms, expected ATD is 190 ms. If RV-paced QRS duration is 140 ms, expected IVD is 47 ms. Thus, during RA and RV pacing, optimal AV delay is 190 – 47 = 143 ms. In the case of atrial-sensed pacemaker timing cycles with RV pacing, optimal AV delay can be determined by subtracting the P-sensed offset (PSO, i.e. the time from surface P onset to P detection). The value of PSO can be either default (30 ms) or measured from the ECG and pacemaker marker channels. So, in this example, the optimal AV delay during RA sensing and RV pacing is 143 – 30 = 113 ms.
Source: Chirife et al. [19]. Reproduced with permission of John Wiley & Sons Ltd.

to a fixed empirical AV delay (120 ms), an echocardiographically optimized AV delay, or an AV delay optimized with SmartDelay™ (an empirically derived electrogram-based algorithm) [22]. At the end of follow-up, the trial found no differences in LV end-systolic volume or any of the secondary end points: LV end-diastolic volume, ejection fraction, NYHA class, quality of life, and 6-min walk distance. This study indicates that routine use of echocardiographic optimization or algorithm-based AV interval optimization cannot be recommended as being clinically warranted in patients undergoing CRT. Most individuals will exhibit satisfactory hemodynamics using standard "out-of-the-box" settings and do not need to undergo echocardiographically guided AV optimization. Interestingly, in the SMART-AV delay trial, women optimized via echocardiography or with SMART-AV delay responded more favorably than women randomized to the fixed AV interval [22]. Thus, AV optimization in selected patients who do not respond to CRT may be warranted. Also, it is still reasonable to consider individualized AV optimization in patients who are hospitalized with acute heart failure or pacemaker syndrome.

Atrial-sensed versus atrial-paced atrioventricular intervals

Appropriate programming of the AV interval also may depend on whether the atrium is sensed or paced. Programming differential AV intervals for sensing and pacing may give rise to small but significant increases in cardiac output in patients with LV dysfunction, due to differences in atrial-paced versus -sensed conduction times. If atrial activity is sensed, this marks the initiation of the pacemaker AV interval. Because some atrial activation has already occurred at the time that the sensing amplifier detects the presence of a P wave, the AV interval based on sensed atrial activity should be shorter (by about 30 ms on average) than when the atrium is paced to begin both the AV interval and atrial electrical activation (Figure 3.29). Generally, an atrial-sensed AV interval of 20–50 ms less than the atrial-paced AV interval is programmed, but the most appropriate difference is probably variable in different patients.

Atrial versus atrioventricular pacing

Both atrial and AV pacing have the advantage of providing AV synchrony. Aside from differing AV intervals, the major difference between atrial and AV sequential pacing is the ectopic ventricular

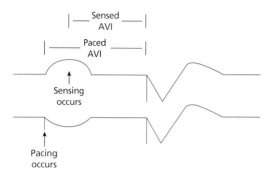

Figure 3.29 Hypothetical relationship of appropriate atrioventricular intervals (AVIs) during atrial sensing versus atrial pacing at initiation of the AVI.

activation with RV pacing in the dual-chamber mode versus intrinsic AV conduction during atrial-only pacing. Over the years, there has been recognition of the potential detrimental effects of RV pacing on hemodynamic function. Studies have shown acute improvements in cardiac output, ejection fraction, and pulmonary capillary wedge pressure with AAI compared with DDD pacing. RV pacing compared with intrinsic ventricular activation produces increases in LV filling pressures and end-systolic volume, as well as reductions in regional septal ejection fraction, ventricular dP/dt, stroke volume, and indices of diastolic function. Chronic RV pacing is associated with an increased risk of AF, heart failure, and mortality in patients with impaired LV systolic function [23]. As a result of the concern over the long-term consequences of chronic RV pacing, interest developed in utilizing pacemaker algorithms that allow for maintenance of AV synchrony and atrial emptying but minimize RV pacing.

However, a meta-analysis summarizing seven separate randomized trials showed no meaningful difference in all-cause mortality, all-cause hospitalization, or incidence of AF with the use of algorithms designed to minimize RV pacing in patients with preserved LV function [24]. These findings likely reflect the fact that ventricular pacing reduction algorithms often excessively prolong the AV delay. Prolonged AV (and PQ) delays, even when followed by intrinsic ventricular conduction or fusion, may compromise atrial transport function, reduce ventricular preload, and promote diastolic MR and AF [25]. As noted earlier, at long AV delays

net LV filling is reduced because atrial systole is superimposed on early rapid filling, and mitral valve closure is dependent on the LV pressure rise, which generates presystolic regurgitation. Thus, a low percent of ventricular pacing may not be desirable when it is associated with very prolonged AV intervals (i.e. AV >275–300 ms or PQ >180–200 ms), especially at higher heart rates.

Rate-adaptive atrioventricular delay

In dual-chamber devices programmed in the DDDR mode, rate-adaptive pacing might be sensor driven (atrial or AV sequential pacing) or result from ventricular tracking of the atrial rhythm. When rate adaptation is activated, a sensor-driven rate is recorded. If the sensor-driven rate exceeds both the intrinsic atrial rate and the lower rate limit, rate-adaptive pacing occurs. A programmed maximum sensor rate determines the fastest rate at which pacing can occur.

Dual-chamber devices allow rate-adaptive AV delays to be programmed that can shorten the AV delay up to the maximum tracking or sensor-driven rate. This feature is designed to simulate normal shortening of the PR interval during exercise and allows AV synchrony to be maintained at higher heart rates. At higher heart rates, optimal hemodynamics may require shorter AV delays than are best at lower rates. With exercise, there is a relatively linear decrease in the normal PR interval as exercise increases from the resting state to near maximal exertion. The total reduction in spontaneous PR interval in normal individuals is about 20–50 ms or approximately 4 ms for each 10-beat increment in heart rate. Rate-adaptive AV interval shortening is a programmable feature in DDD pacemakers, and is designed to mimic the normal physiological response of the PR interval to increasing heart rates. Cardiac output can be more effectively increased and pulmonary capillary wedge pressures (and presumably atrial pressures) can be effectively maintained at lower levels using rate-variable AV intervals rather than fixed AV intervals.

Maintaining optimal AV synchrony may be less important during exercise than at rest in providing ventricular filling. The importance of AV synchrony diminishes at higher heart rates as the early and late diastolic filling phases converge. However, the loss of AV synchrony can compromise stroke volume even during exercise. In Figures 3.30 and 3.31, the relative hemodynamic benefits of rate modulation and stroke volume, and rate modulation and AV synchrony, respectively, scaled from rest to maximum exertion can be seen for a general population. At rest, AV synchrony is of pre-eminent benefit, whereas this benefit diminishes as maximal exercise is approached, especially in relation to rate modulation. Rate modulation is of very little value at rest, but becomes quite important early in exercise and increases in relative benefit as maximal exercise is approached. Rate modulation and AV synchrony are complementary, not competitive, physiological concepts.

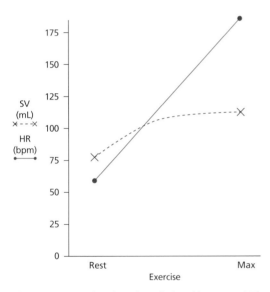

Figure 3.30 Normal stroke volume (SV) and heart rate (HR) response to exercise.

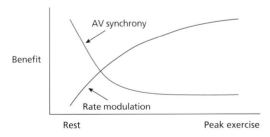

Figure 3.31 Hypothetical general relationship between atrioventricular (AV) synchrony and rate modulation with respect to hemodynamic benefit, both at rest and during exercise.

Pacemaker syndrome

Pacemaker syndrome describes a condition comprising a variety of symptoms and signs produced by ventricular pacing that are relieved by restoration of AV synchrony [26]. Although it is most often the result of VVI pacing, pacemaker syndrome can result from any pacing mode that results in adverse hemodynamic profile, even AAI pacing with long PR intervals.

Two difficulties in ascribing symptoms and signs specifically to pacemaker syndrome are commonly encountered. First, patients who have pacemakers implanted are frequently those with other cardiovascular problems that produce the symptoms and signs described. Second, many pacemaker patients unfortunately have the belief that having the pacemaker, de facto forces them to accept a less than normal sense of well-being. An extreme symptom frequently associated with pacemaker syndrome is syncope. Syncope is very uncommon and is most likely related to profound hypotension – and, in some, a decrease in cardiac output – associated with loss of AV synchrony. Additional symptoms related to blood pressure and cardiac output include malaise, easy fatigability, a sense of weakness, lightheadedness, and dizziness. Symptoms related to higher atrial and venous pressures include dyspnea (frequently at rest), orthopnea, paroxysmal nocturnal dyspnea, a sensation of fullness and/or pulsations in the neck and chest, as well as palpitations, chest pain, nausea, and peripheral edema. Experience has shown that careful questioning is frequently necessary to elucidate these symptoms. It is not uncommon for patients who have had a pacemaker implanted for some time to deny symptoms but, on specific questioning, to admit to having experienced symptoms that can be directly related to ventricular pacing with loss of AV synchrony. Careful examination is necessary to find physical signs related to ventricular pacing. Some of these signs include relative or absolute hypotension that can be continuous or fluctuating, neck vein distension with prominent cannon A waves, pulmonary rales, and rarely peripheral edema.

The incidence of pacemaker syndrome during ventricular pacing is quite variable in the literature, ranging from 2 to 83% depending in part on the definition used to diagnose this clinical entity. Pacemaker syndrome was defined in the Mode Selection Trial (MOST) in patients with sick sinus syndrome as either new or worsened dyspnea, orthopnea, elevated jugular pressure, rales, and edema with VA conduction during ventricular pacing, or symptoms of dizziness, weakness, presyncope, or syncope, and a 20-mmHg reduction in systolic blood pressure when the patient was ventricularly paced compared with atrial pacing or sinus rhythm [27]. Based on this definition, pacemaker syndrome occurred in 18.3% of those in sinus rhythm treated with VVIR pacing ($n = 996$) in MOST. This incidence is similar to the 26% found in the Pacemaker Selection in the Elderly (PASE) trial [28]. The strongest predictor of pacemaker syndrome in MOST was a higher percent of ventricular-paced beats. Pacemaker syndrome caused a marked decrease in quality of life, which improved significantly after reprogramming to the DDDR pacing mode.

In a substudy of the PASE trial, development of pacemaker syndrome in patients programmed to VVIR pacing was diagnosed within the first week after implantation and was associated with elevated plasma ANP levels (>90 pg/mL). After crossover from VVIR to DDDR pacing mode in these patients, there was prompt resolution of the symptoms that led to the diagnosis and a decline in plasma ANP levels (<90 pg/mL). Physiologically, increased release of ANP during VVI pacing may reduce arterial pressure because of its potent vasodilator effects and reflexly result in enhanced sympathetic nervous outflow. This may account for or worsen the signs and symptoms of pacemaker syndrome. ANP release may serve as a clinical marker of pacemaker syndrome in VVIR-paced patients and may be involved in its pathogenesis.

Pacemaker syndrome results from a complex interaction of hemodynamic, neurohumoral, and vascular changes induced by the loss of AV synchrony (Figure 3.32). It is speculated that patients who develop pacemaker syndrome during ventricular pacing may have a failure to increase systemic vascular resistance adequately despite elevated peripheral sympathetic nerve traffic and circulating catecholamines (Figure 3.33). Sympathetic neural activation is a normal physiological response during ventricular pacing. In addition to reduced stroke volume and cardiac output resulting from loss of atrial kick during ventricular pacing, pacemaker syndrome may result in some patients from an inadequate sympathetic response to ventricular pacing, with a failure to compensate for upright posture with augmentation in sympathetic tone. In others, the elevated venous pressures resulting from atrial contraction against closed AV valves may activate inhibitory atrial and cardiopulmonary vagal afferent nerves that can counteract the protective vasoconstrictive reflex, resulting in peripheral vasodilation and hypotension.

Based on this understanding, it has been speculated that pacemaker syndrome might be predicted by a simple hemodynamic evaluation at the time of pacemaker implant. Pacemaker syndrome may be more likely to result from VVI pacing if systolic blood pressure drops by more than 20 mmHg during ventricular pacing (see Figure 3.17). In the PASE trial, need for future crossover to dual-chamber mode was predicted by a decrease in supine systolic blood pressure during VVI pacing at the pacemaker implantation to less than 110 mmHg (relative risk 2.6; 95% CI 1.5–4.5; $P \leq 0.001$) [28]. The sensitivity of a decrease in paced systolic blood pressure to less than 110 mmHg at implantation for predicting intolerance to VVIR pacing was 36%, specificity was 86%, positive predictive power 48%, and negative predictive power 79%. In contrast, in MOST, systolic blood pressure drop with VVIR pacing at implantation was not associated with the development of pacemaker syndrome [27].

It is often thought that pacemaker syndrome is more likely to occur and be more severe when retrograde VA conduction is present. In this regard, although retrograde conduction is common, even in patients with complete heart block, it may be intermittent and not consistently present at implant. Thus, absence of retrograde conduction at implant during sedation may not preclude subsequent development of signs and symptoms of pacemaker syndrome. In the PASE trial, VA conduction or cannon A waves were present in almost 50% of patients who required crossover from VVIR to DDDR pacing. However, in both the MOST and PASE trials, presence of VA conduction at implant was not a significant predictor of development of intolerance to VVIR pacing [27,28].

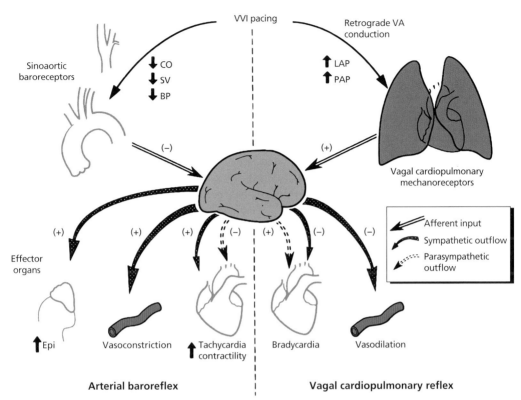

Figure 3.32 Schematic of the multiple reflex pathways involved in pacemaker syndrome. The arterial baroreflexes detect a decrease in stroke volume when atrioventricular (AV) dyssynchrony occurs, leading to sympathetic activation and vasoconstriction. Conversely, AV dyssynchrony leads to increased atrial wall tension and activation of reflex pathways, leading to vagally mediated vasodilation as well as release of humoral substances, such as atrial natriuretic peptide (ANP), which further facilitate baroreflex-mediated vasoconstriction. BP, blood pressure; CO, cardiac output; Epi, epinephrine; LAP, left atrial pressure; PAP, pulmonary artery pressure; SV, stroke volume. Source: Ellenbogen KA, Stambler BS. Pacemaker syndrome. In: Ellenbogen KA, Kay GN, Wilkoff BL, eds. *Clinical Cardiac Pacing*. Philadelphia: WB Saunders, 1995: 419–431. Reproduced with permission of Elsevier.

Despite attempts to identify clinical variables that predict intolerance to ventricular pacing, multiple studies have failed to detect any that consistently predict the development of pacemaker syndrome. Therefore, the vast majority of pacemaker implanters have concluded that because prediction of pacemaker syndrome on clinical criteria alone is imprecise, the most effective way to prevent this problem is to implant atrial-based pacemakers in most patients. Undoubtedly, as a consequence of this shift away from the use of VVI/VVIR pacing in clinical practice, there has been a reduced prevalence of pacemaker syndrome.

Management of patients with VVI pacing-induced pacemaker syndrome includes reprogramming or upgrading to DDD pacing, reducing the lower pacing rate to encourage AV conduction or the native rhythm, use of hysteresis, or withdrawal of medications that impair sinus node function. For the rare patient with pacemaker syndrome present with a dual-chamber system, appropriate programming to ensure atrial capture and avoidance of atrial non-pacing modes (VDD) or atrial non-tracking modes (DDI or DVI) may be useful.

Detrimental effects of right ventricular pacing

Right ventricular pacing can have detrimental effects on myocardial function and result in progression of heart failure, particularly in patients with preexisting LV dysfunction, and can also result

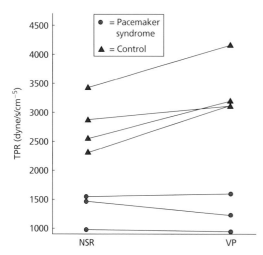

Figure 3.33 Changes in total peripheral vascular resistance (TPR) during normal sinus rhythm (NSR) and ventricular pacing (VP) in four control subjects and three patients with pacemaker syndrome. In the control subjects, there was an approximately 20% increase in peripheral resistance, whereas peripheral resistance failed to increase in the patients with pacemaker syndrome. Source: Ellenbogen *et al*. [26]. Reproduced with permission of John Wiley & Sons Ltd.

in a modest detrimental effect on LV function in patients who have normal systolic function.

RV pacing produces an asynchronous pattern of activation, contraction, and relaxation within and between the left and right ventricles. RV pacing impairs systolic and diastolic function. These hemodynamic derangements occur whether or not normal AV synchrony is present and may be most pronounced when the ventricular pacing site is the RV apex [29]. Ventricular pacing may compromise effective forward stroke volume further by inducing functional MR. RV pacing results in significant regional differences in perfusion and oxygen consumption, and reduced myocardial mechanical efficiency [30].

Asynchronous activation during chronic RV apical pacing leads to long-term adaptations of the myocardium, referred to as remodeling. Chronic RV pacing induces ventricular dilation, asymmetric LV hypertrophy and thinning, altered perfusion distribution, increased myocardial catecholamine concentrations, abnormal histological changes including myofiber disarray, and impairment of LV function. These alterations are due to the LV dyssynchronous contraction present during chronic

RV apical pacing. Thus, when normal AV conduction remains intact, preservation of a physiological ventricular activation sequence during permanent cardiac pacing is of importance for optimization of hemodynamic function.

Several studies have observed a high prevalence of asymptomatic LV dysfunction in pacemaker patients undergoing stimulation from the right ventricle [31–33]. In a single-center study, a history of having a permanent pacemaker with a RV pacing lead was the strongest predictor (HR 6.6; P = 0.002) of a decrease in LVEF (of >7 points) over 18 months' follow-up [32]. In patients with complete AV block and normal ventricular function at permanent lead implantation, chronic RV pacing induced regional myocardial perfusion defects and wall motion abnormalities, and impaired LV systolic and diastolic function [33].

In the MOST trial among a pacemaker population with sinus node disease, there was an association between percent of ventricular pacing (in either single- or dual-chamber modes) and development of heart failure [31,34]. Chronic RV pacing also was associated with an increased risk of AF. Ventricular pacing in the VVIR mode of greater than 80% of the time was associated with increased heart failure risk, and RV pacing in the DDDR mode of greater than 40% conferred a 2.6-fold increased risk of heart failure. In absolute terms, the average risk of heart failure in those receiving RV pacing was approximately 10%; however, the risk was approximately 2% if RV pacing was minimal (<10% of the time). The risk of AF increased linearly with cumulative RV pacing in both groups. From these data, it was concluded that both heart failure progression and AF can be reduced by implementing strategies that minimize ventricular pacing and preserve normal ventricular activation. Consistent with this notion, the SAVE PACe (Search AV Extension and Managed Ventricular Pacing for Promoting Atrioventricular Conduction) trial evaluated a pacing algorithm that minimizes RV pacing in patients with sinus node disease and reported a 40% reduction in persistent AF in those randomized to dual-chamber minimal ventricular pacing (median percent ventricular pacing, 9.1%) compared with those with conventional dual-chamber pacing (median percent ventricular pacing, 99.0%) [35]. However, there were no differences in rates of heart failure or mortality.

Notably, most patients with sinus node dysfunction have normal LV function and tolerate even frequent RV pacing without an increased risk of developing heart failure during long-term follow-up [36,37]. Although RV pacing may result in about a 6–7% absolute decline in LVEF, the risk for clinical heart failure due to RV pacing among patients with pacemakers who have sinus node disease is quite low (approximately 1.2% at 2 years after pacemaker implantation). Furthermore, whether there is a percent of RV pacing that may result in a higher risk of heart failure or AF in patients with sinus node disease is also controversial. Although the aforementioned data from MOST suggest that risk may be increased when RV pacing is greater than 40–50%, in contrast the DANPACE (Danish Multicenter Randomized Trial on Single Lead Atrial Pacing versus Dual-Chamber Pacing in Sick Sinus Syndrome) trial detected no significant association between percent ventricular pacing and the risk of AF or heart failure [25,36,37]. A meta-analysis supports prior findings suggesting that measures to minimize RV pacing fail to positively impact important clinical outcomes (including rates of persistent or permanent AF, all-cause hospitalization, and all-cause mortality) [24].

In patients with structural heart disease and compromised LV function, the deleterious effects of RV pacing appear to have greater clinical consequences. Clinical evidence of the deleterious effects of chronic and frequent RV pacing in this population was demonstrated in the Dual Chamber and VVI Implantable Defibrillator (DAVID) trial [38]. DAVID tested the hypothesis that dual-chamber pacing for rate support would be more efficacious than back-up pacing in patients with impaired ventricular systolic function receiving a dual-chamber implantable cardioverter–defibrillator (ICD). The trial was a multicenter study of patients with standard indications for ICD implantation (ventricular tachycardia/ventricular fibrillation, LVEF <40%), but without indications for bradycardia pacing. All patients had a dual-chamber, rate-adaptive pacing ICD implanted and were randomized to ventricular back-up pacing (VVI 40 bpm) or dual-chamber rate-adaptive pacing (DDDR 70 bpm, average AV delay 180 ms). The study was prematurely discontinued because of increased mortality and hospitalization in patients treated with dual-chamber pacing (73.3% 1-year survival and 22.6% requiring hospitalization) compared with back-up ventricular pacing (83.9% survival and 13.3% hospitalization). A subsequent analysis of the DAVID trial and confirmatory observations from other studies demonstrated that percent RV pacing predicted the primary clinical outcomes (composite end point of death or hospitalization for congestive heart failure) in patients with LV dysfunction receiving ICDs [39]. Patients with DDDR RV pacing of less than 40% had similar or better outcomes compared with the VVI back-up group (mean RV pacing <4%), whereas outcomes were worse among patients with DDDR RV pacing of greater than 40% [40]. The DAVID II trial, which compared AAI pacing at 70 bpm with VVI pacing at 40 bpm in a second group of patients who required ICD but not pacemaker therapy, found no difference between the two groups, effectively excluding the higher base rate pacing as the cause of the worsened outcomes in the DDDR 70-bpm group in the original DAVID trial.

Strategies to minimize right ventricular pacing

Because of evidence that a high proportion of RV pacing, particularly in patients with some degree of LV systolic dysfunction, may be detrimental, there is a growing trend to minimize RV pacing as much as possible. The risks of frequent or continuous RV stimulation may be reduced by using "minimal ventricular pacing" strategies that use back-up ventricular pacing (VVI or VVIR) modes when AV synchrony is not required, or extended AV intervals during dual-chamber pacing, to allow for intrinsic ventricular activation (Figure 3.34).

Simple measures often employed to reduce ventricular pacing include lengthening programmed AV intervals, programming a lower pacing rate below the sinus rate, adding rate hysteresis for periods of inactivity, and adjusting drugs that affect AV nodal conduction. Rate-adaptive AV delay programming can allow long AV delays to be programmed at lower heart rates, but more appropriate AV intervals at higher rates. To further minimize potentially unnecessary ventricular pacing, rate-adaptive AV interval pacing can be reserved for

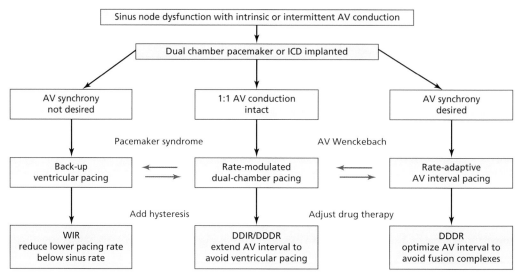

Figure 3.34 Minimal ventricular pacing strategy to promote intrinsic atrioventricular (AV) conduction after implant of a dual-chamber pacemaker or ICD for treatment of sinus node dysfunction with impaired AV conduction (present or anticipated). (*Left*) Back-up VVIR pacing is used if AV synchrony is not required. The lower pacing rate is programmed below sinus rate and rest hysteresis is added when appropriate. Change to dual-chamber pacing if pacemaker syndrome develops (due to retrograde VA conduction). (*Middle*) Rate-modulated dual-chamber pacing is preferred for patients with intrinsic AV conduction. The programmed AV interval is extended to promote normal ventricular activation in patients capable of maintaining 1 : 1 AV conduction. Discontinue or adjust drugs that affect AV conduction when appropriate. Add rate-adaptive pacing if the patient is symptomatic with extended AV delays. (*Right*) Rate-adaptive AV interval pacing is used for patients requiring physiological AV intervals. During programming, sensed and paced AV intervals should be optimized to avoid ventricular fusion complexes.

patients who are symptomatic with long AV delays or high-grade AV block.

These suggested strategies may be the only means available in older device technology to reduce unnecessary RV pacing, but may have limitations. Many dual-chamber pacemakers impose limitations on maximum allowable AV intervals in order to maintain atrial tracking at elevated rates and adequate sensing windows for atrial tachyarrhythmia mode switch algorithms. In ICDs, allowable AV intervals are more restricted to prevent VT underdetection due to cross-chamber blanking periods. Furthermore, long AV delays increase the risk of pacemaker-mediated tachycardias. Finally, if RV pacing continues to occur at long programmed AV delays (>300 ms), this imposes both AV and ventricular desynchronization.

To deal with issues and limitations related to DDD/R pacing with long AV delays, minimal ventricular pacing algorithms have become available that essentially provide atrial [AAI(R)] pacing with ventricular monitoring and back-up ventricular support [DDD(R)] pacing should high-grade AV block develop. These algorithms can extend AV delays beyond 300 ms to avoid ventricular pacing unless high-grade AV block is present. These algorithms are effective in promoting intrinsic AV conduction and reducing ventricular pacing frequency to very low levels (<5–10%) [41]. The results of the SAVE PACe study indicated that use of one of these advanced algorithms in patients with sinus node disease reduced the risk of AF without an increase in heart failure events or mortality [35].

Another approach to minimize RV pacing has been the use of paced and sensed AV delay hysteresis algorithms that enable prolongation of the AV delay after a predetermined number of atrial beats to look for spontaneous AV conduction. The INTRINSIC RV trial among ICD recipients with LV systolic dysfunction included use of AV search hysteresis during DDD programming to reduce RV pacing percent [42]. This trial found that lowest rates of adverse clinical events occurred with RV pacing between 10 and 19% [43]. The event rates (death or heart failure hospitalization) in this group were lower than in those with increasing levels of RV pacing, but interestingly were also lower than in the group with the least amount of RV pacing (0–9%). Thus, some degree of RV pacing is permissible and may even be beneficial in patients with ICDs.

As noted previously, patients with normal hearts usually tolerate some degree of RV pacing without developing heart failure and may benefit from optimized AV synchrony. Notably in contrast to the conclusions of MOST, the DANPACE study in patients with sinus node disease found no difference in mortality, and incidence of chronic AF, stroke, and heart failure between the single-lead atrial and dual-chamber pacing groups, even though ventricular pacing percent in the latter group was 65 ± 33%. In addition, paroxysmal AF occurred more frequently in the AAIR group. In DANPACE, the AV interval was 140–160 ms if no intrinsic conduction was present at an AV interval of greater than 220 ms, but an AV delay hysteresis algorithm was enabled to allow automatic search for intrinsic AV conduction. This algorithm minimized unnecessary ventricular pacing, but reduced it to a percent that was substantially higher than that in the managed ventricular pacing (MVP) group in the SAVE PACe trial (RV pacing percent, 9%) but lower than that in the DDD(R) groups with fixed, short AV delays in SAVE PACe (RV pacing percent, 99%) and MOST (RV pacing percent, 90%). Thus, it seems that strategies to reduce unnecessary RV pacing are appropriate, but it may be best to have optimized AV synchrony by avoiding either very short or long AV conduction intervals.

Alternative site right ventricular pacing

In patients with AV conduction disease in whom reducing the percent of ventricular pacing is not feasible because of the requirement for frequent or continuous ventricular pacing support, more physiological alternatives to RV apical pacing should be considered. Pacing from the para-Hisian region, RV outflow tract (RVOT), or RV septum may offer theoretical advantages over the RV apex that could result in a more synchronous ventricular activation sequence. Despite these potential theoretical

advantages and a meta-analysis suggesting improved long-term LV systolic function during non-apical RV pacing, the clinical benefits of alternative site RV pacing have not been demonstrated convincingly as of yet [44,45].

His bundle pacing

The bundle of His, a rapid conduction path for both ventricles, is an obvious target for alternative site pacing. Criteria for selective His bundle pacing (HBP) include 12-lead ECG equivalence between native and paced QRS, and His–ventricular (HV) interval of spontaneous rhythm equal to the paced ventricular interval.

Though the idea was conceived decades ago, HBP has more recently garnered widespread interest due to availability of new tools that greatly improve acute procedural success. Several small proof of concept studies have assessed the feasibility of permanent Hisian pacing to produce a narrow-paced QRS complex identical to that in intrinsic rhythm [46–48]. Successful HBP results in better hemodynamic performance and more uniform distribution of perfusion when compared with RV pacing. In a small study in patients who underwent AV nodal ablation for permanent AF, Deshmukh et al. [49] compared hemodynamic changes during direct His pacing, RV apical pacing, and high and low septal pacing and showed that His pacing provided the best acute chronotropic and lusinotropic response (Figure 3.35). As all patients had underlying AF and complete AV block, the confounding effect of atrial filling and RV fusion was eliminated in this study.

A less obvious role of His pacing is for correction of underlying left bundle branch block (LBBB) to resynchronize LV contraction. The theory of longitudinal dissociation of the His explains how His pacing may correct some LBBBs [50]. Direct and exclusive stimulation of predestined fibers to the LBB within the Hisian trunk, below a lesion within the Hisian bundle responsible for the conduction deficit, causes QRS normalization, with resumption of electrical and mechanical LV synchrony. In one study, patients meeting CRT implant indications but treated with His pacing sustained significant improvement in LV function [51]. However, little is known of the proportion of heart failure patients with LBBB in whom LBBB is

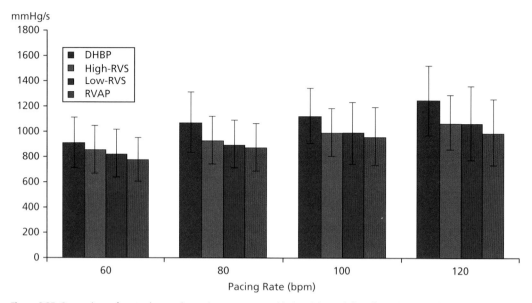

mmHg/s

Figure 3.35 Comparison of acute changes in maximum positive rate of rise of left ventricular systolic pressure (d*P*/dt$_{max}$, a measure of contractility; mmHg/s) in patients with atrial fibrillation who underwent atrioventricular (AV) node ablation. Direct His bundle pacing provided the most advantageous hemodynamic profile. DHBP, direct His bundle pacing; RVS, right ventricular septum; RVAP, right ventricular apex. Source: adapted from Deshmukh *et al.* [49].

a His bundle-based ("central") lesion rather than a reflection of peripheral myocardial conduction deficits that may not be corrected in this manner. In one study comparing permanent HBP with RV pacing, HBP was successfully performed in 304 of 332 patients (92%) requiring permanent pacing. In addition to demonstrating that HBP was both safe and feasible, this pacing modality was found to be associated with a reduction in the primary end point of death, hospitalization for heart failure, and need for upgrade to biventricular pacing [52]. Similar implant success rates were demonstrated in a meta-analysis that included 26 studies of HBP involving more than 1400 patients (84% success rate using stylet-driven leads and 92% using a dedicated delivery sheath and lumenless lead), with an overall 10% improvement in LVEF in those patients with underlying LV systolic dysfunction [53]. Furthermore, as can be seen in Figure 3.36, HBP results in a lower incidence of pacing-induced cardiomyopathy versus RV pacing, in addition to higher LVEF during long-term follow-up. While these initial studies are positive and encouraging, additional randomized controlled trials are needed to more completely understand the role of HBP in clinical practice.

Non-apical right ventricular pacing

Most studies of alternative site RV pacing have focused on the RVOT, and in particular on the septal portion of the outflow tract. It is speculated that RVOT or mid-septal pacing will not be associated with the deleterious effects on hemodynamic function seen with RV apical pacing. However, most of the data comparing alternative pacing sites to RV apical pacing have been equivocal. Some studies have found significant acute hemodynamic advantages, but several randomized controlled chronic studies have demonstrated either modest or negligible benefit of RVOT compared with RV apical pacing [55,56]. It should be noted that among numerous acute and chronic clinical studies, only in one study was RVOT pacing hemodynamically worse than RV apical pacing.

One of the challenges in evaluating the potential benefits of RVOT pacing is that this region, at least up until recently, has been difficult to identify using fluoroscopy and therefore is not standardized anatomically with respect to pacing sites. Thus, confirmation of anatomical lead location remains challenging and not well validated. In addition, many studies of alternative site RV pacing are difficult to interpret because of the small number of

Long-Term Lead Performance and clinical Outcomes

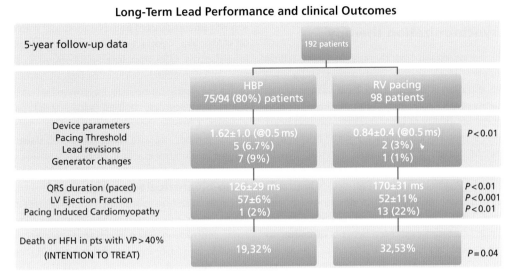

5-year follow-up data			
	192 patients		
	HBP 75/94 (80%) patients	**RV pacing** 98 patients	
Device parameters Pacing Threshold Lead revisions Generator changes	1.62±1.0 (@0.5 ms) 5 (6.7%) 7 (9%)	0.84±0.4 (@0.5 ms) 2 (3%) 1 (1%)	P<0.01
QRS duration (paced) LV Ejection Fraction Pacing Induced Cardiomyopathy	126±29 ms 57±6% 1 (2%)	170±31 ms 52±11% 13 (22%)	P<0.01 P<0.001 P<0.01
Death or HFH in pts with VP>40% (INTENTION TO TREAT)	19,32%	32,53%	P=0.04

Figure 3.36 In this long-term follow-up study of 192 patients undergoing either His bundle pacing (HBP) or right ventricular (RV) pacing there was a statistically significant reduction in the incidence of pacing-induced cardiomyopathy in the HBP group (2% vs. 22%). Patients treated with HBP had narrow-paced QRS complexes, higher left ventricular (LV) ejection fraction, and lower rates of death and hospitalization for heart failure (HFH) if ventricular pacing (VP) burden was above 40%. Source: Vijayaraman *et al.* [54]. Reproduced with permission of Elsevier.

patients, wide range of baseline LV function, varying spectrum of underlying heart disease, and varying durations of follow-up. Few randomized trials comparing RV apical pacing with alternative RV sites have followed patients over extended periods beyond 1 year. The benefits that may accrue from RVOT pacing seem primarily related to prevention of deterioration of LV function that develops in some patients undergoing RV apical pacing, rather than improvement in function associated with RVOT pacing.

A meta-analysis of randomized trials comparing RV apical versus non-apical pacing concluded that LVEF is higher with non-apical than apical pacing (weighted mean difference of LVEF 4.27%; 95% CI 1.15–7.40%), but only in trials with follow-up of 12 months or longer and in those conducted in patients with a baseline LVEF of 40–45% or less [45]. No significant difference in LVEF was observed in trials of patients whose baseline ejection fraction was preserved. Importantly, available data for end points other than ejection fraction, including exercise capacity, functional class, quality of life, and survival, are limited and inconclusive.

Further complicating the evaluation of alternative RV pacing sites, some studies have suggested

that the hemodynamically optimal RV pacing site may vary from patient to patient and may not always reside on the RV septum [55]. One small study attempted to find the best RV pacing site, defined as the site with the shortest paced QRS duration [55]. The study found that a shorter QRS duration positively correlated with a higher LVEF, but that the RV septal pacing site did not necessarily produce the shortest QRS or consistently result in improved LV function. QRS duration was shorter in nine patients, longer in four patients, and no different in one patient between RV septal and apical pacing. Overall, the QRS duration was not significantly different between RV septal and apical pacing (156 ± 10 vs. 166 ± 18 ms, respectively). Thus, anatomical lead optimization may not be as critical as hemodynamic lead optimization, and the optimal RV site may not be anatomically defined but may vary from patient to patient.

In summary, whether the detrimental hemodynamic effects of RV apical pacing can be attenuated by selecting a more optimal RV pacing site continues to be of clinical interest, but still remains to be determined definitively. Ongoing pacemaker studies continue to evaluate these issues.

Left ventricular pacing and cardiac resynchronization therapy

CRT is an established therapy in heart failure patients with LV systolic dysfunction, and a wide QRS duration. Clinical trials have demonstrated benefits of CRT incremental to optimized medical therapy on quality of life, exercise tolerance, heart failure symptoms, functional class, and hospitalization. Moreover, CRT confers survival benefit [57,58]. Original trial populations targeted severely reduced LV systolic function, refractory heart failure, markedly prolonged QRS durations (usually due to LBBB), and no bradycardia indication for pacing. Later studies showed benefits extending to patients with NYHA class I/II level of symptoms [59]. CRT is therefore an important interventional therapy in this high-risk population.

The concept underlying CRT is that in patients with prolonged QRS duration, delayed LV activation leads to LV mechanical dysfunction but may be corrected by appropriately timed LV stimulation [60]. The hemodynamic deficit provoked by abnormal pathways of ventricular activation deviating from synchronous ventricular electrical activation (i.e. rapid impulse conduction through the His–Purkinje system) has been known for decades. Chronic effects due to LBBB (and with RV pacing, which mimics several aspects of LBBB) in heart failure are manifest by LV remodeling and symptoms of heart failure with increased mortality [61]. Mechanical dysfunction results from dyssynchronous contraction – both interventricular and intra-LV conduction delays may impair contraction. Regions of the ventricle still actively contracting while other regions are relaxing and filling in diastole (i.e. reciprocated stretching) creates mechanical inefficiency [62]. The result is that part of the contractile effort does not wholly contribute to cardiac ejection.

CRT aims to reverse this sequence of adverse events. Its effects may be assessed hemodynamically, both acutely by measurement of contractile function (e.g. ejection fraction) and chronically through remodeling (e.g. changes in LV dimension). These effects may be modulated by variations in both underlying electrical substrate and responses to pacing. CRT results in a more synchronous electrical activation sequence and mechanical contraction. CRT resynchronizes the severely uncoordinated and dysfunctional patterns of ventricular contraction in patients with prolonged native QRS complexes. CRT improves systolic function acutely within one beat of initiation of pacing, with immediate improvements in LV contractility, cardiac output, and arterial pulse pressure. Chronic therapy is required to produce reverse remodeling with reduction in end-diastolic volume and improvement in LVEF.

Atrio-biventricular pacing

Attempts to restore coordinated contraction generally use ventricular-based pacing, coordinated with atrial contraction when possible, to correct VV, intra-LV, and also AV dyssynchronies. CRT conventionally involves ventricular stimulation of both the right and left ventricles (biventricular pacing). Biventricular devices incorporate pacing leads capable of stimulating the right and left ventricles via the coronary sinus transvenously or from the epicardium surgically, in conjunction with an atrial electrode to maintain AV synchrony. Initial case reports were followed by systematic investigation and reported positive acute hemodynamic effects [63,64]. Improvements could be perceived immediately on initiation of pacing (Figure 3.37), manifest in improvements in systolic function, LV contractility, cardiac output, and arterial pulse pressure, not seen with RV pacing alone. Both LV free wall and biventricular pacing reduced end-systolic volume and increased stroke volume (Figure 3.38). These results indicated that ventricular mechanics could be improved dramatically by pre-excited LV pacing to reduce existing conduction delay. This inotropic effect was metabolically efficient as measured in terms of conversion of myocardial oxygen consumption to mechanical work [40].

Atrial synchronization by modulating AV intervals may affect LV pump function. The relationship between AV delay and LV dP/dt_{max} among patients with acute improvement in contractile response to simultaneous biventricular pacing demonstrated peak effect at approximately 50% of native PR interval [63]. Effects were diminished at very short AV delays (truncated filling times) or very long AV delays. Thus, routine optimization with acute echocardiographic measures (e.g. VTI, mitral inflow)

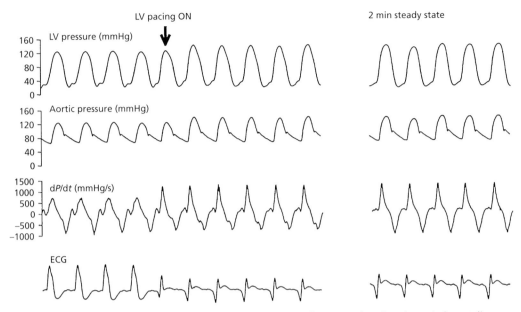

Figure 3.37 Raw data tracings before, immediately on initiation of left ventricular (LV) electrical stimulation, and after 2 min of steady-state LV stimulation in a patient with dilated cardiomyopathy and discoordinate contraction due to left bundle branch block. Stimulation of the LV free wall rapidly increased aortic and ventricular systolic pressures, aortic pulse amplitude, and maximal d*P*/d*t*. These increases changed very little after 2 min of steady-state stimulation. Source: Nelson *et al*. [40]. Reproduced with permission of Wolters Kluwer Health.

offers no significant advantage over empirical settings (100–130 ms) except in non-responders.

A further significant hemodynamic benefit of CRT observed in many patients is reduction in functional MR. The following mechanisms may be involved. Optimization of AV timing and shortening of contraction sequence prolongs diastolic filling time and reduces diastolic MR. Acutely, ventricular resynchronization may restore interpapillary muscle coordination. Ventricular remodeling effects may further improve valve function. In several large-scale trials, sustained hemodynamic improvements led to reverse volumetric LV remodeling with reduced sphericity and improvement in ejection fraction. The magnitude of reduction in end-systolic volume ranges between 10 and 30%. This remodeling process may be evident as early as 4 weeks after implementing therapy and reverses with its withdrawal [65]. Further discussion is found in Chapter 9.

Univentricular left ventricular pacing

CRT with LV-based pacing (i.e. without RV pacing) demonstrated acute hemodynamic benefits that were similar (if not superior to) biventricular pacing [64] (Figure 3.38). Resynchronization may result from fusion between a wavefront produced by intrinsic conduction down the AV node and intact right bundle and a second wavefront stimulated by LV pacing. Avoidance of RV pacing in this manner avoids the RV hemodynamic deficit seen with simultaneous biventricular pacing modes [66]. RV pacing-induced changes in activation sequence and prolongation of activation duration may all potentially perturb the normal sequential pattern of RV inflow-to-outflow contraction [67]. These alterations in RV activation and thus interventricular dyssynchrony may interfere with ventricular coupling and pump function. These effects may be avoided by LV pacing alone, with critically timed AV delays resulting in fusion of the propagated paced wavefront with intrinsic conduction via an intact right bundle. The long-term effects of univentricular LV pacing have been comparatively less well studied compared with evaluations of biventricular resynchronization pacing. Studies to date show no superiority to conventional biventricular stimulation [68]. However, maintaining fusion pacing consistently on a near beat-to-beat basis may offer long-term advantages in select patients [69,70].

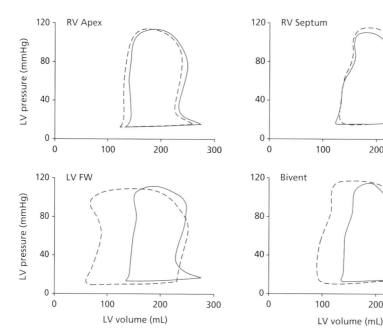

Figure 3.38 Pressure–volume loops from a patient with baseline left bundle branch block as a function of varying pacing site. Data are shown for the optimal atrioventricular (AV) interval at each site. Solid line indicates normal sinus rhythm (NRS, control); dashed line indicates VDD pacing. There was negligible effect from right ventricular (RV) apical or sensory pacing. However, left ventricular (LV) pacing produced loops with greater area (stroke work) and width (stroke volume) and a reduced systolic volume. The latter is consistent with increased contractile function and thus with elevation of dP/dt_{max}. LV FW, left ventricular free wall. Source: Kass et al. [64]. Reproduced with permission of Wolters Kluwer Health.

Left ventricular endocardial pacing

LV endocardial pacing sites usually render better hemodynamic performance than RV endocardial pacing sites and conventional epicardial sites accessed via coronary sinus tributaries [71,72]. This approach offers the advantage of access to a great variety of LV pacing sites, removing constraints of the coronary sinus tributary. The hemodynamics have been best studied experimentally. In normal hearts, pacing at the left side of the interventricular septum (LV septum) induced a near normal sequence of activation, characterized by rapid spread of depolarization from the pacing site around the LV circumference [73]. LV systolic function was near normal with minimal dyssynchrony. The rapidly conducting superficial endomyocardial layer may be responsible for this effect. Importantly, results were equivalent to biventricular pacing [74]. LV septal pacing differs greatly from RV septal pacing in electric activation and hemodynamic effects: transseptal conduction occurs rightwardly but with simultaneous circumferential LV endocardial conduction, thus reducing total LV activation time. Therefore, both the interventricular and intraventricular asynchronies are reduced. However, direct LV pacing is potentially hazardous, introducing risks during transseptal puncture, potential mitral valve trauma, thromboembolism, and infection with additional risks during an extraction. Novel techniques to deliver this pacing mode include deployment of electrodes to the LV aspect of the septum from the *right* septum with extended screws, and LV endocardial pacing utilizing a wireless LV pacing electrode [73–75]. Safety and feasibility remain to be determined, though initial pilot studies do suggest that wireless LV endocardial pacing is clinically feasible [75].

Pacing in hypertrophic obstructive cardiomyopathy

In the past some clinicians advocated a therapeutic role for cardiac pacing in selected patients with hypertrophic obstructive cardiomyopathy (HOCM).

These patients have a dynamic obstruction to LV outflow caused by hypertrophy of the interventricular septum, typically in the subaortic valve area, combined with systolic anterior motion of the mitral valve. In this select subset of patients with LV outflow tract (LVOT) obstruction and refractory symptoms despite pharmacological therapy, it was proposed that DDD pacing with a short AV delay would be of benefit. It was speculated that by producing dyssynchrony of LV contraction and paradoxical septal movement, dual-chamber pacing with ventricular pacing from the RV apex wiould reduce the degree of outflow obstruction and symptoms. An AV delay of less than 100 ms is usually necessary to ensure full RV apical preexcitation. Shorter AV delays allow for more complete apical preexcitation and minimal basal septal activation through the His–Purkinje system. Apical preexcitation with short AV delays must be maintained at higher heart rates and during exercise.

Retrospective studies suggested that AV synchronous pacing with a short AV delay decreases LVOT gradient and symptoms. An example of modest improvement in LV outflow gradient in such a patient is shown in Figure 3.39. AV delays ranging from 80 to 100 ms may be optimal for gradient reduction. Other investigators documented subjective as well as objective improvement in such parameters as oxygen consumption at peak exercise. These studies generated interest in the role of pacing in HOCM, but subsequent prospective studies of dual-chamber pacing yielded conflicting results [76,77]. Results varied from patient to patient and were inconsistent. Some patients had marginal benefit, whereas others obtained complete gradient abolition. Part of the reason for this variability may be that AV delays that are too short can be detrimental to diastolic filling and can worsen symptoms. If interatrial conduction is impaired, then short AV delays will result in LA contraction occurring after mitral valve closure, which can elevate LA pressure and promote atrial arrhythmias. Reduction in LVOT gradient may require AV interval optimization with Doppler echocardiographic guidance assessing both LV outflow gradient and mitral inflow velocities.

At least three randomized, controlled, crossover trials of pacing in HOCM patients refractory to medical therapy have been performed and found that the benefit of this therapy is less than suggested by earlier reports. These studies included a total of about 140 patients and suggested that pacing can reduce LVOT gradient and lead to a modest reduction in symptoms, but does not improve exercise capacity. The North American M-PATHY trial was a randomized, double-blind, crossover, multi-center trial of 48 patients with drug-refractory HOCM [77]. An average reduction in LVOT gradient of 40 mmHg was seen, but no significant effect was demonstrated on quality of life, exercise capacity, peak oxygen consumption, or septal wall thickness. A small subgroup of patients over the age of 65 years showed consistent improvement in functional capacity. Likewise, the European Pacing in Cardiomyopathy (PIC) study also suggested that elderly patients (>65 years) are most likely to respond to pacing [76].

A non-randomized comparison of dual-chamber pacing and septal myectomy for patients with drug-refractory symptoms analyzed LVOT gradients, symptoms, and exercise testing in 39 patients who underwent surgery or pacemaker implantation based on physician preference [78]. Although both groups showed subjective improvement, myectomy patients had a greater reduction in LVOT gradients and larger improvements in functional status.

Despite observations that some patients derive benefit, DDD pacing with short AV delays cannot be regarded as a primary treatment modality for LVOT obstruction in HOCM and is not routinely indicated for the alleviation of symptoms. There may be benefit of pacing therapy in selected subgroups, such as those older than 65 years or patients who are not candidates for myectomy or septal ablation because of comorbidities. Pacing is indicated in HOCM patients with sinus node dysfunction or AV block, and may have utility in preventing bradycardia and allowing more aggressive drug therapy with beta-blockers or verapamil. Whether incorporating DDD pacing with short AV delays into implantable defibrillators plays a role in the treatment of HOCM patients remains ill-defined. Finally, pacing therapy has not been shown to be beneficial in patients with minimal intraventricular gradients or in those with non-obstructive hypertrophic cardiomyopathy, and is not indicated in the absence of bradycardia.

Pacemaker mode selection

A logical approach to pacemaker mode selection is to choose a mode that targets the underlying bradycardia and to avoid modes that electrically stimulate chambers that have appropriate intrinsic electrical and conduction properties. Selection of the appropriate pacing mode should fit the patient's electrical and hemodynamic condition. This decision should incorporate consideration of the patient's electrical conduction status, including the atrial rhythm, AV conduction, ventricular conduction (i.e. QRS duration), chronotropic competence, and hemodynamic status, including the patient's LV systolic function and whether there is a history of heart failure. Pacemaker mode selection should be consistent with evidence from clinical trials indicating at least

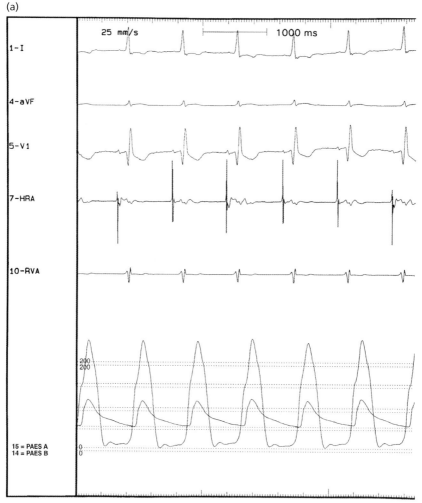

Figure 3.39 Tracings showing the impact of atrioventricular (AV) sequential pacing on left ventricular and femoral arterial pressure in a selected patient with hypertrophic obstructive cardiomyopathy. (a) The presence of a nearly 150-mmHg pressure gradient at baseline during sinus rhythm. (b) With AV sequential pacing at an AV interval of 75 ms, the pressure gradient decreases to 50–90 mmHg. The beat-to-beat variability of the measurement of this gradient is highlighted by the bottom tracing. (*Top to bottom*) I, aVF, V1, surface ECG leads; RA, right atrial intracardiac recording; RV, right ventricular intracardiac recording; femoral and left ventricular pressure tracings (in mmHg) superimposed on each other. Source: Sweeney MO, Ellenbogen KA. Implantable devices for the electrical management of heart disease: overview of indications for therapy and selected recent advances. In: Antman EM, ed. *Cardiovascular Therapeutics*, 2nd edn. Philadelphia: WB Saunders, 2002. Reproduced with permission of Elsevier.

(b)

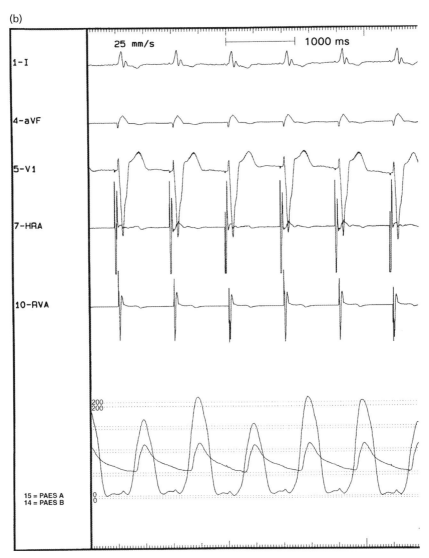

Figure 3.39 (Continued)

a lack of harm of a particular pacing mode and pref- erably supporting a potential benefit on important clinical outcomes. Striving to provide AV syn- chrony, rate modulation, and CRT when clinical evidence supports their benefits assists in this decision-making process [79]. Pacemaker mode selection algorithms in sinus node disease and AV block are shown in Figures 3.40 and 3.41.

In pure sinus node dysfunction with normal AV conduction, atrial pacing should be the primary pacing mode and RV stimulation should be avoided as much as possible. This can be accomplished either using atrial pacing (AAI) alone or with a

dual-chamber pacing (DDD) system, preferably one that incorporates an algorithm that reduces frequency of unnecessary ventricular pacing. These pacing mode selections are supported by evidence from clinical trials indicating a reduction in incidence of AF and progression to chronic AF, a lower risk of developing pacemaker syndrome, and small improvements in quality of life with atrial- based compared with single-chamber RV pacing (Table 3.2).

Preexisting PR interval prolongation (>200 ms), LBBB, or a low Wenckebach rate (<100 bpm) are pre- dictors for subsequent requirement for implantation

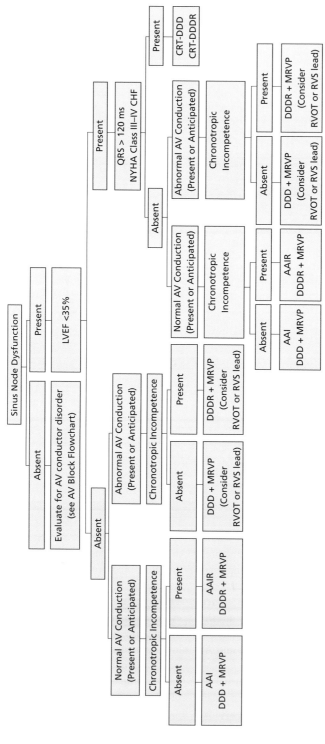

Figure 3.40 Pacemaker mode selection algorithm for sinus node dysfunction. AAI, atrial demand pacing; AAIR, atrial demand rate-adaptive pacing; AV, atrioventricular; CHF, congestive heart failure; CRT, cardiac resynchronization therapy; DDD, dual-chamber pacing; DDDR, dual-chamber rate-adaptive pacing; LVEF, left ventricular ejection fraction; MRVP, minimize right ventricular pacing; NYHA, New York Heart Association; RVOT, right ventricular outflow tract; RVS, right ventricular septal. Pacemaker codes are discussed in detail in Chapter 6.

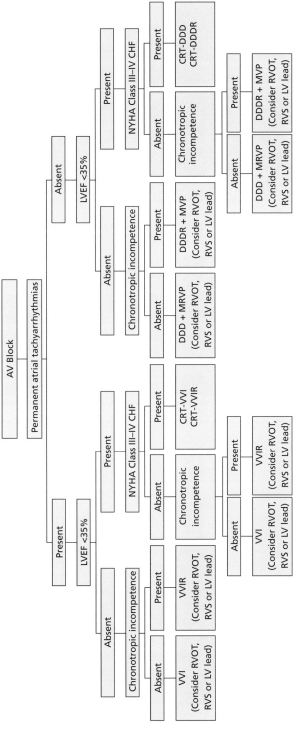

Figure 3.41 Pacemaker mode selection algorithm for atrioventricular block. AV, atrioventricular; CHF, congestive heart failure; CRT, cardiac resynchronization therapy; DDD, dual-chamber pacing; DDDR, dual-chamber rate-adaptive pacing; LV, left ventricular; LVEF, left ventricular ejection fraction; NYHA, New York Heart Association; MRVP, minimize right ventricular pacing; MVP™, Managed Ventricular Pacing; RVOT, right ventricular outflow tract; RVS, right ventricular septal; VVI, ventricular demand pacing; VVIR, ventricular demand rate-adaptive pacing. Pacemaker codes are discussed in detail in Chapter 6.

Table 3.2 Randomized controlled trials of pacemaker mode selection

Trial	Date of publication	No. of patients	Average follow-up (years)	Indication	Pacing modes	Mean age (years)	Primary end point	Summary of results; P value (hazard ratio; 95% CI)	Mortality (%/year)	AF (%/year)	Thromboembolism (%/year)
Danish [84]	1994	225	5.5	Sinus node dysfunction	AAI vs. VVI	76	Mortality, AF, thromboembolism	Mortality: 0.045 (0.66; 0.44–0.99) AF: 0.012 (0.54; 0.33–0.89) Thromboembolism: 0.023 (0.47; 0.24–0.92)	5.8 vs. 6.8	4.1 vs. 7.1	1.7 vs. 5.4
PASE [85]	1998	407	1.5	All pacemaker patients ≥65 years	DDDR vs. VVIR	76	Quality of life	No overall group differences between pacing modes	10.7 vs. 11.3	11.3 vs. 12.7	1.3 vs. 2.3
CTOPP [86]	2000	2568	6.0	All pacemaker patients	DDD/DDDR or AAI/AAIR vs. VVI/VVIR	73	Cardiovascular death or stroke	0.26 (0.91; 0.78–1.05) AF less frequent in atrial-based group	6.3 vs. 6.6	5.3 vs. 6.6	1.0 vs. 1.1
MOST [34]	2002	2010	4.5	Sinus node dysfunction	DDDR vs. VVIR	74	Death or non-fatal stroke	0.40 (0.97; 0.80–1.18) AF and heart failure reduced in DDDR	7.0 vs. 7.3	7.9 vs. 10.0	1.4 vs. 1.8
UKPACE [87]	2005	2021	4.6	AV block ≥70 yo	DDD vs. VVI/VVIR	80	Death	0.56 (0.96; 0.83–1.11)	7.4 vs. 7.2	2.8 vs. 3.0	1.7 vs. 2.1

AAI, atrial pacing; AAIR, atrial pacing with rate adaptation; AF, atrial fibrillation; AV, atrioventricular; DDD, dual-chamber pacing; DDDR, dual-chamber pacing with rate adaptation; VVI, ventricular pacing; VVIR, ventricular pacing with rate adaptation.

of a ventricular lead [80,81]. Notably, trials have not demonstrated a beneficial effect on long-term clinical outcomes comparing atrial with dual-chamber pacing. However, there is an incremental risk of a complication associated with an operative revision from single-chamber atrial to dual-chamber pacing necessitated by the development of AV block in this population. Therefore, most implanters prefer to implant a dual-chamber rather than an AAI-only pacing system in patients with sinus node disease, even in the presence of normal AV conduction. An AAI pacing system might still be considered on occasion in carefully selected younger patients who are expected to require decades of pacemaker therapy in the presence of sinus node disease, but who show no evidence of AV or ventricular conduction abnormality.

In patients with AV block, any pacing mode that provides ventricular pacing support (i.e. single-chamber ventricular, single-lead VDD, dual chamber or biventricular) will prevent bradycardia [15]. However, single-chamber ventricular pacing will not maintain AV synchrony and non-CRT pacing modes will not prevent the potential deleterious effects of long-term RV pacing. The optimal pacing mode for patients with AV conduction disease has been the subject of a number of clinical trials and remains an area of debate. Trials have investigated the need for dual-chamber rather than single-chamber ventricular pacing in elderly patients and the need for biventricular pacing in patients with LV ejection fractions above 35–40% [82,83]. In this group of patients with permanent AV block, dual-chamber pacing is preferred over single-chamber ventricular pacing because the former pacing mode preserves AV synchrony and chronotropic response driven by the sinus node rather than by an artificial rate-adaptation sensor. This may be most important in younger or more physically active patients and in those with any degree of systolic and/or diastolic dysfunction in whom the maintenance of AV synchrony is needed for optimizing hemodynamics. The atrial arrhythmia detection features in dual-chamber pacemakers may have the added benefit of detection of atrial tachyarrhythmias that may result in therapeutic interventions, including therapy for stroke prevention. Single-chamber ventricular pacing is chosen primarily for patients with AV conduction disease who have permanent AF or longstanding persistent AF if no attempt to restore sinus rhythm is

contemplated, or in whom pacing would rarely be required. Single-chamber ventricular pacing might also be appropriate for patients with paroxysmal AV block in whom only intermittent ventricular pacing for bradycardia is expected.

Because of the need for ventricular pacing support in patients with advanced AV conduction disease, alternatives to RV apical pacing should be considered to address the issue of forced ventricular desynchronization. If it is anticipated that frequent ventricular pacing will be required (>40%) in a patient with AV block and symptomatic LV dysfunction (NYHA class II–IV and LVEF ≤35%), then CRT employing either biventricular or His bundle pacing should be utilized. For patients with AV block and normal or mildly impaired LV systolic function (LVEF >35%), alternative RV pacing sites (His, RV septum) may be considered. However, existing clinical data are equivocal in support of alternative RV pacing sites; there is no evidence to suggest an increase in detrimental effects, but no definitive evidence of improved clinical outcomes over the RV apex. Notably, atrio-biventricular or His bundle pacing may be the optimal pacing mode for hemodynamic indications in patients who require frequent ventricular pacing, regardless of baseline ejection fraction.

Several trials of biventricular pacing in patients requiring pacing for bradycardia provide insight into the role of CRT in this group. In a study of patients with bradycardia and a normal ejection fraction, patients randomized to RV pacing had a lower mean LVEF (55 ± 9% vs. 62 ± 7%; $P <0.001$) and a larger LV end-systolic volume (36 ± 16 mL vs. 28 ± 10 mL; $P <0.001$) than patients in the biventricular pacing group at 12 months [82]. Results from the Biventricular versus RV Pacing in Heart Failure Patients with Atrioventricular Block (BLOCK HF) study comparing RV with biventricular pacing in patients with AV block requiring ventricular pacing and mild-to-moderate LV dysfunction and heart failure (LVEF ≤50%, NYHA class I–III) demonstrated that biventricular pacing led to a 26% reduction in the combined end point of mortality, heart failure-related urgent care, and increase in end-systolic volume index [83].

When chronotropic incompetence accompanies sinus node dysfunction or AV block, as it often does in the pacemaker population, then rate-adaptive pacing might be considered. However, the rate-adaptive pacing mode should not be programmed at the expense of a greater frequency of ventricular pacing and promotion of ventricular dyssynchrony. Rate-adaptive pacing may promote ventricular pacing, particularly if rate-adaptive AV delays are programmed. Furthermore, there is an absence of conclusive data showing that DDDR pacing is superior to DDD with regard to improved quality of life and reduced symptoms [79]. Thus, rate-adaptive pacing should not be used routinely in pacemaker patients unless there is a strong clinical need (i.e. highly symptomatic patients with inadequate chronotropic response to exercise). Furthermore, the sinus node should be given priority as the primary modulator of heart rate when its chronotropic function is unimpaired. Thus, for patients with complete AV block and preserved sinoatrial nodal function, an artificial sensor is not required for rate-adaptive pacing. The VDD and DDD pacing modes provide rate modulation and AV synchrony in this setting. Patients with sinus node dysfunction and an inadequate chronotropic response to exercise are candidates for AAIR or DDDR pacemakers, depending on AV conduction status. For patients with paroxysmal or chronic atrial arrhythmias, a rate-adaptive pacing system is often preferred. Patients with chronic AF or flutter and inappropriately slow ventricular rates during exercise are managed best with VVIR pacing.

References

1 Narahara KA, Blettel ML. Effect of rate on left ventricular volumes and ejection fraction during chronic ventricular pacing. *Circulation* 1983;67(2):323–329.

2 Linnarsson D. Dynamics of pulmonary gas exchange and heart rate changes at start and end of exercise. *Acta Physiol Scand Suppl* 1974;415:1–68.

3 Wilkoff BL, Corey J, Blackburn G. A Mathematical model of the cardiac chronotropic response to exercise. *J Electrophysiol* 1989;3(3):176–180.

4 Melzer C, Witte J, Reibis R, *et al.* Predictors of chronotropic incompetence in the pacemaker patient population. *EP Europace.* 2006;8(1):70–5.

5 Dresing TJ, Blackstone EH, Pashkow FJ, *et al.* Usefulness of impaired chronotropic response to exercise as a predictor of mortality, independent of the severity of coronary artery disease. *Am J Cardiol* 2000;86(6):602–609.

6 Lamas GA, Knight JD, Sweeney MO, *et al.* Impact of rate-modulated pacing on quality of life and exercise capacity: evidence from the Advanced Elements of Pacing Randomized Controlled Trial (ADEPT). *Heart Rhythm* 2007;4(9):1125–1132.

7 Sims DB, Mignatti A, Colombo PC, *et al.* Rate responsive pacing using cardiac resynchronization therapy in patients with chronotropic incompetence and chronic heart failure. *Europace* 2011;13(10):1459–1463.

8 Shukla HH, Flaker GC, Hellkamp AS, *et al.* Clinical and quality of life comparison of accelerometer, piezoelectric crystal, and blended sensors in DDDR-paced patients with sinus node dysfunction in the Mode Selection Trial (MOST). *Pacing Clin Electrophysiol* 2005;28(8):762–770.

9 Hauser J, Michel-Behnke I, Zervan K, Pees C. Noninvasive measurement of atrial contribution to the cardiac output in children and adolescents with congenital complete atrioventricular block treated with dual-chamber pacemakers. *Am J Cardiol* 2011;107(1):92–95.

10 Gold MR, Brockman R, Peters RW, Olsovsky MR, Shorofsky SR. Acute hemodynamic effects of right ventricular pacing site and pacing mode in patients with congestive heart failure secondary to either ischemic or idiopathic dilated cardiomyopathy. *Am J Cardiol* 2000;85(9):1106–1109.

11 Reynolds D, Wilson M, Burow R, *et al.* (ed.) Hemodynamic evaluation of atrioventricular sequential versus ventricular pacing in patients with normal and poor ventricular-function at variable heart rates and posture (Abstract). *J Am Coll Cardiol* 1983;1(2 Pt 2):636.

12 Taylor JA, Morillo CA, Eckberg DL, Ellenbogen KA. Higher sympathetic nerve activity during ventricular (VVI) than during dual-chamber (DDD) pacing. *J Am Coll Cardiol.* 1996;28(7):1753–1758.

13 Healey JS, Toff WD, Lamas GA, *et al.* Cardiovascular outcomes with atrial-based pacing compared with ventricular pacing. *Circulation* 2006;114(1):11–17.

14 Fleischmann KE, Orav EJ, Lamas GA, *et al.* Pacemaker implantation and quality of life in the Mode Selection Trial (MOST). *Heart Rhythm* 2006;3(6):653–659.

15 Gillis AM, Russo AM, Ellenbogen KA, *et al.* HRS/ACCF expert consensus statement on pacemaker device and mode selection. *J Am Coll Cardiol* 2012;60(7):682–703.

16 Meisner JS, McQueen DM, Ishida Y, *et al.* Effects of timing of atrial systole on LV filling and mitral valve closure: computer and dog studies. *Am J Physiol* 1985;249(3):H604–H619.

17 Barold SS, Ilercil A, Leonelli F, Herweg B. First-degree atrioventricular block. Clinical manifestations, indications for pacing, pacemaker management and consequences during cardiac resynchronization. *J Interv Card Electrophysiol* 2006;17(2):139–152.

18 Strohmer B, Pichler MAX, Froemmel M, Migschitz M, Hintringer F. Evaluation of atrial conduction time at various sites of right atrial pacing and influence on atrio-ventricular delay optimization by surface electrocardiography. *Pacing Clin Electrophysiol* 2004;27(4):468–474.

19 Chirife R, Pastori J, Mosto H, Arrascaite M, Sambelashvili A. Prediction of interatrial and interventricular electromechanical delays from P/QRS measurements: value for pacemaker timing optimization. *Pacing Clin Electrophysiol* 2008;31(2):177–183.

20 Sorajja D, Bhakta MD, Scott LR, Altemose GT, Srivathsan K. Utilization of electrocardiographic P-wave duration for AV interval optimization in dual-chamber pacemakers. *Indian Pacing Electrophysiol J* 2010;10(9):383–392.

21 Gorcsan J, Abraham T, Agler DA, *et al.* Echocardiography for cardiac resynchronization therapy: recommendations for performance and reporting. A report from the American Society of Echocardiography Dyssynchrony Writing Group endorsed by the Heart Rhythm Society. *J Am Soc Echocardiogr* 2008;21(3):191–213.

22 Ellenbogen KA, Gold MR, Meyer TE, *et al.* Primary results from the SmartDelay determined AV optimization: a comparison to other AV delay methods used in Cardiac Resynchronization Therapy (SMART-AV) Trial. *Circulation* 2010;122(25):2660–2668.

23 Steinberg JS, Fischer AVI, Wang P, *et al.* The clinical implications of cumulative right ventricular pacing in the Multicenter Automatic Defibrillator Trial II. *J Cardiovasc Electrophysiol* 2005;16(4):359–365.

24 Shurrab M, Healey JS, Haj-Yahia S, *et al.* Reduction in unnecessary ventricular pacing fails to affect hard clinical outcomes in patients with preserved left ventricular function: a meta-analysis. *Europace* 2017;19(2):282–288.

25 Nielsen JC, Thomsen PE, Hojberg S, *et al.* Atrial fibrillation in patients with sick sinus syndrome: the association with PQ-interval and percentage of ventricular pacing. *Europace* 2012;14(5):682–689.

26 Ellenbogen K, Wood M, Stambler B. Pacemaker syndrome: clinical, hemodynamic and neurohumoral features. In: Barold S, Mugica J, eds. *New Perspectives in Cardiac Pacing*. Armonk, NY: Futura Publishing, 1993: 85–112.

27 Link MS, Hellkamp AS, Estes NAM, *et al.* High incidence of pacemaker syndrome in patients with sinus node dysfunction treated with ventricular-based pacing in the Mode Selection Trial (MOST). *J Am Coll Cardiol* 2004;43(11):2066–2071.

28 Ellenbogen KA, Stambler BS, Orav EJ, *et al.* Clinical characteristics of patients intolerant to VVIR pacing. *Am J Cardiol* 2000;86(1):59–63.

29 Sanagala T, Johnston SL, Groot GD, Rhine DK, Varma N. Left atrial mechanical responses to right ventricular pacing in heart failure patients: implications for atrial fibrillation. *J Cardiovasc Electrophysiol* 2011;22(8):866–874.

30 Nielsen JC, Bøttcher M, Toftegaard Nielsen T, Pedersen AK, Andersen HR. Regional myocardial blood flow in patients with sick sinus syndrome randomized to long-term single chamber atrial or dual chamber pacing: effect of pacing mode and rate. *J Am Coll Cardiol* 2000; 35(6):1453–1461.

31 Sweeney MO, Hellkamp AS, Ellenbogen KA, *et al.* Adverse effect of ventricular pacing on heart failure and atrial fibrillation among patients with normal baseline QRS duration in a clinical trial of pacemaker therapy for sinus node dysfunction. *Circulation* 2003;107(23):2932–2937.

32 O'Keefe JH, Abuissa H, Jones PG, *et al.* Effect of chronic right ventricular apical pacing on left ventricular function. *Am J Cardiol* 2005;95(6):771–773.

33 Tse H-F, Lau C-P. Long-term effect of right ventricular pacing on myocardial perfusion and function. *J Am Coll Cardiol* 1997;29(4):744–749.

34 Lamas GA, Lee KL, Sweeney MO, *et al.* Ventricular pacing or dual-chamber pacing for sinus-node dysfunction. *N Engl J Med* 2002;346(24):1854–1862.

35 Sweeney MO, Bank AJ, Nsah E, *et al.* Minimizing ventricular pacing to reduce atrial fibrillation in sinus-node disease. *N Engl J Med* 2007;357(10):1000–1008.

36 Nielsen JC, Thomsen PEB, Hojberg S, *et al.* A comparison of single-lead atrial pacing with dual-chamber pacing in sick sinus syndrome. *Eur Heart J* 2011;32(6): 686–696.

37 Riahi S, Nielsen JC, Hjortshoj S, *et al.* Heart failure in patients with sick sinus syndrome treated with single lead atrial or dual-chamber pacing: no association with pacing mode or right ventricular pacing site. *Europace* 2012;14(10):1475–1482.

38 Wilkoff BL, Cook JR, Epstein AE, *et al.* Dual-chamber pacing or ventricular backup pacing in patients with an implantable defibrillator: the Dual Chamber and VVI Implantable Defibrillator (DAVID) Trial. *JAMA* 2002;288(24):3115–3123.

39 Sharma AD, Rizo-Patron C, Hallstrom AP, *et al.* Percent right ventricular pacing predicts outcomes in the DAVID trial. *Heart Rhythm* 2005;2(8):830–834.

40 Nelson GS, Berger RD, Fetics BJ, *et al.* Left ventricular or biventricular pacing improves cardiac function at diminished energy cost in patients with dilated cardiomyopathy and left bundle-branch block. *Circulation* 2000;102(25):3053–3059.

41 Sweeney MO, Shea JB, Fox V, *et al.* Randomized pilot study of a new atrial-based minimal ventricular pacing mode in dual-chamber implantable cardioverter-defibrillators. *Heart Rhythm* 2004;1(2):160–167.

42 Olshansky B, Day JD, Moore S, *et al.* Is dual-chamber programming inferior to single-chamber programming in an implantable cardioverter–defibrillator? *Circulation* 2007;115(1):9–16.

43 Olshansky B, Day JD, Lerew DR, Brown S, Stolen KQ. Eliminating right ventricular pacing may not be best for patients requiring implantable cardioverter–defibrillators. *Heart Rhythm* 2007;4(7):886–891.

44 Kaye G, Stambler BS, Yee R. Search for the optimal right ventricular pacing site: design and implementation of three randomized multicenter clinical trials. *Pacing Clin Electrophysiol* 2009;32(4):426–433.

45 Shimony A, Eisenberg MJ, Filion KB, Amit G. Beneficial effects of right ventricular non-apical vs. apical pacing: a systematic review and meta-analysis of randomized-controlled trials. *Europace* 2011;14(1):81–91.

46 Vijayaraman P, Chung MK, Dandamudi G, *et al.* His bundle pacing. *J Am Coll Cardiol* 2018;72(8):927–947.

47 Deshmukh P, Casavant DA, Romanyshyn M, Anderson K. Permanent, direct His-bundle pacing. *Circulation* 2000;101(8):869–877.

48 Zanon F, Baracca E, Aggio S, *et al.* A feasible approach for direct His-bundle pacing using a new steerable catheter to facilitate precise lead placement. *J Cardiovasc Electrophysiol* 2006;17(1):29–33.

49 Deshmukh A, Lakshmanadoss U, Deshmukh P. Hemodynamics of His bundle pacing. *Card Electrophysiol Clin* 2018;10(3):503–509.

50 Narula OS. Longitudinal dissociation in the His bundle. Bundle branch block due to asynchronous conduction within the His bundle in man. *Circulation* 1977;56(6):996–1006.

51 Barba-Pichardo R, Manovel Sánchez A, Fernández-Gómez JM, *et al.* Ventricular resynchronization therapy by direct His-bundle pacing using an internal cardioverter defibrillator. *Europace* 2012;15(1):83–88.

52 Abdelrahman M, Subzposh FA, Beer D, *et al.* Clinical outcomes of His bundle pacing compared to right ventricular pacing. *J Am Coll Cardiol* 2018;71(20):2319–2330.

53 Zanon F, Ellenbogen KA, Dandamudi G, *et al.* Permanent His-bundle pacing: a systematic literature review and meta-analysis. *Europace* 2018;20(11):1819–1826.

54 Vijayaraman P, Naperkowski A, Subzposh FA, *et al.* Permanent His-bundle pacing: long-term lead performance and clinical outcomes. *Heart Rhythm* 2018;15(5):696–702.

55 Schwaab B, Fröhlig G, Alexander C, *et al.* Influence of right ventricular stimulation site on left ventricular function in atrial synchronous ventricular pacing. *J Am Coll Cardiol* 1999;33(2):317–323.

56 Stambler BS, Ellenbogen KA, Zhang X, *et al.* Right ventricular outflow versus apical pacing in pacemaker patients with congestive heart failure and atrial fibrillation. *J Cardiovasc Electrophysiol* 2003;14(11):1180–1186.

57 Bristow MR, Saxon LA, Boehmer J, *et al.* Cardiac-resynchronization therapy with or without an implantable defibrillator in advanced chronic heart failure. *N Engl J Med* 2004;350(21):2140–2150.

58 Cleland JG, Daubert JC, Erdmann E, *et al.* The effect of cardiac resynchronization on morbidity and mortality in heart failure. *N Engl J Med* 2005;352(15):1539–1549.

59 Moss AJ, Hall WJ, Cannom DS, *et al.* Cardiac-resynchronization therapy for the prevention of heart-failure events. *N Engl J Med* 2009;361(14):1329–1338.

60 Leclercq C, Kass DA. Retiming the failing heart: principles and current clinical status of cardiac resynchronization. *J Am Coll Cardiol* 2002;39(2):194–201.

61 Baldasseroni S, Opasich C, Gorini M, *et al.* Left bundle-branch block is associated with increased 1-year sudden and total mortality rate in 5517 outpatients with congestive heart failure: a report from the Italian network on congestive heart failure. *Am Heart J* 2002;143(3):398–405.

62 Prinzen FW, Hunter WC, Wyman BT, McVeigh ER. Mapping of regional myocardial strain and work during ventricular pacing: experimental study using magnetic resonance imaging tagging. *J Am Coll Cardiol* 1999;33(6):1735–1742.

63 Auricchio A, Stellbrink C, Block M, *et al.* Effect of pacing chamber and atrioventricular delay on acute systolic function of paced patients with congestive heart failure. *Circulation* 1999;99(23):2993–3001.

64 Kass DA, Chen C-H, Curry C, *et al.* Improved left ventricular mechanics from acute VDD pacing in patients with dilated cardiomyopathy and ventricular conduction delay. *Circulation* 1999;99(12):1567–1573.

65 Yu C-M, Fung JW-H, Zhang Q, *et al.* Tissue Doppler imaging is superior to strain rate imaging and postsystolic shortening on the prediction of reverse remodeling in both ischemic and nonischemic heart failure after cardiac resynchronization therapy. *Circulation* 2004;110(1):66–73.

66 Lee KL, Burnes JE, Mullen TJ, *et al.* Avoidance of right ventricular pacing in cardiac resynchronization therapy improves right ventricular hemodynamics in heart failure patients. *J Cardiovasc Electrophysiol* 2007;18(5):497–504.

67 Varma N, Jia P, Ramanathan C, Rudy Y. RV electrical activation in heart failure during right, left, and biventricular pacing. *JACC Cardiovasc Imaging* 2010;3(6):567–575.

68 Thibault B, Ducharme A, Harel F, *et al.* Left ventricular versus simultaneous biventricular pacing in patients with heart failure and a QRS complex ≥120 milliseconds. *Circulation* 2011;124(25):2874–2881.

69 Martin DO, Lemke B, Birnie D, *et al.* Investigation of a novel algorithm for synchronized left-ventricular pacing and ambulatory optimization of cardiac resynchronization therapy: results of the adaptive CRT trial. *Heart Rhythm* 2012;9(11):1807–1814.

70 Birnie D, Lemke B, Aonuma K, *et al.* Clinical outcomes with synchronized left ventricular pacing: analysis of

the adaptive CRT trial. *Heart Rhythm* 2013;10(9): 1368–1374.

71 Derval N, Steendijk P, Gula LJ, *et al.* Optimizing hemodynamics in heart failure patients by systematic screening of left ventricular pacing sites. *J Am Coll Cardiol* 2010;55(6):566–575.

72 Ginks MR, Shetty AK, Lambiase PD, *et al.* Benefits of endocardial and multisite pacing are dependent on the type of left ventricular electric activation pattern and presence of ischemic heart disease. *Circ Arrhythm Electrophysiol* 2012;5(5):889–897.

73 Mills RW, Cornelussen RN, Mulligan LJ, *et al.* Left ventricular septal and left ventricular apical pacing chronically maintain cardiac contractile coordination, pump function and efficiency. *Circ Arrhythm Electrophysiol* 2009;2(5):571–579.

74 Strik M, Rademakers LM, van Deursen CJM, *et al.* Endocardial left ventricular pacing improves cardiac resynchronization therapy in chronic asynchronous infarction and heart failure models. *Circ Arrhythm Electrophysiol* 2012;5(1):191–200.

75 Reddy VY, Miller MA, Neuzil P, *et al.* Cardiac resynchronization therapy with wireless left ventricular endocardial pacing. *J Am Coll Cardiol* 2017;69(17):2119–2129.

76 Kappenberger L, Linde C, Daubert C, *et al.* Pacing in hypertrophic obstructive cardiomyopathy: a randomized crossover study. *Eur Heart J* 1997;18(8):1249–1256.

77 Maron BJ, Nishimura RA, McKenna WJ, *et al.* Assessment of permanent dual-chamber pacing as a treatment for drug-refractory symptomatic patients with obstructive hypertrophic cardiomyopathy. *Circulation* 1999;99(22): 2927–2933.

78 Ommen SR, Nishimura RA, Squires RW, *et al.* Comparison of dual-chamber pacing versus septal myectomy for the treatment of patients with hypertrophic obstructive cardiomyopathy: a comparison of objective hemodynamic and exercise end points. *J Am Coll Cardiol* 1999;34(1):191–196.

79 Lamas GA, Ellenbogen KA. Evidence base for pacemaker mode selection. *Circulation* 2004;109(4):443–451.

80 Nielsen JC, Kristensen L, Andersen HR, *et al.* A randomized comparison of atrial and dual-chamber pacing in 177 consecutive patients with sick sinus syndrome. *J Am Coll Cardiol* 2003;42(4):614–623.

81 Kristensen L, Nielsen JC, Pedersen AK, Mortensen PT, Andersen HR. AV block and changes in pacing mode during long-term follow-up of 399 consecutive patients with sick sinus syndrome treated with an AAI/AAIR pacemaker. *Pacing Clin Electrophysiol* 2001;24(3): 358–365.

82 Yu C-M, Chan JY-S, Zhang Q, *et al.* Biventricular pacing in patients with bradycardia and normal ejection fraction. *N Engl J Med* 2009;361(22):2123–2134.

83 Curtis AB, Worley SJ, Adamson PB, *et al.* Biventricular pacing for atrioventricular block and systolic dysfunction. *N Engl J Med* 2013;368(17):1585–1593.

84 Andersen HR, Nielsen JC, Thomsen PE, *et al.* Long-term follow-up of patients from a randomized trial of atrial versus ventricular pacing for sick-sinus syndrome. *Lancet* 1997;350:1210–1216.

85 Lamas GA, Orav EJ, Stambler BS, *et al.* for the PASE Investigators. Quality of life and clinical outcomes in elderly patients treated with ventricular pacing as compared with dual-chamber pacing. *N Engl J Med* 1998;338:1097–1104.

86 Connolly SJ, Kerr CR, Gent M, *et al.* Effects of physiologic pacing versus ventricular pacing on the risk of stroke and death due to cardiovascular causes. Canadian Trial of Physiologic Pacing Investigators. *N Engl J Med* 2000;342:1385–1391.

87 Toff WD, Camm AJ, Skehan JD, for the United Kingdom Pacing and Cardiovascular Events Trial (UKPACE) Investigators. Single chamber versus dual-chamber pacing for high-grade atrioventricular block. *N Engl J Med* 2005;353:145–155.

CHAPTER 4

Temporary cardiac pacing

T. Jared Bunch[1], Jeffrey S. Osborn[2], and John D. Day[2]
[1]Division of Cardiovascular Medicine, University of Utah School of Medicine, Salt Lake City, UT, USA
[2]Intermountain Heart Institute, Intermountain Medical Center, Salt Lake City, UT, USA

Introduction

Temporary cardiac pacing is a commonly used tool in the practice of cardiovascular and intensive care medicine. Temporary cardiac pacing is typically used to treat a bradyarrhythmia until it resolves or a permanent pacing solution can be applied. Temporary pacing can be life-saving in maintaining cardiovascular and hemodynamic function. Although temporary pacing can be used to treat tachyarrhythmias, the most common use is for symptomatic or life-threatening bradyarrhythmias. Temporary pacing is required in approximately 20% of patients presenting to the emergency department with symptomatic bradycardia [1]. This chapter will focus on the use of temporary pacing in cardiopulmonary resuscitation, on the treatment of reversible causes of bradyarrhythmias, and then highlight current temporary pacing options and approaches.

Cardiopulmonary resuscitation

Symptomatic bradycardia can present with hypotension, signs of heart failure, cardiac ischemia, or electrical instability (Figure 4.1). Current guidelines suggest that pacing be considered only in those symptomatic patients who do not respond to pharmacological approaches such as atropine,

isoproterenol, or dopamine [2,3]. Randomized trials have also failed to show a benefit of esophageal or transvenous pacing versus drug therapy during intraoperative bradycardia or bradycardic arrest [4,5].

In general, temporary pacing is not recommended for patients who present in asystolic cardiac arrest as randomized controlled trials have failed to show an improvement in survival to hospital admission or discharge with pacing (either transcutaneous or transvenous) in this patient subset [2,6–8]. In these patients pharmacological approaches remain the mainstay of therapy, but if the patient is resuscitated to a bradyarrhythmia, temporary pacing may reenter the resuscitation algorithm.

Reversible causes of severe bradycardia

Temporary pacing is indicated for symptomatic bradycardia that stems from acute and reversible causes of cardiac instability. In these scenarios, temporary pacing may serve as a bridge to placement of a permanent pacemaker, or merely provide back-up while the reversible condition resolves. There are many potential reversible and/or acute causes of bradycardia that may require temporary

Cardiac Pacing and ICDs, Seventh Edition. Edited by Kenneth A. Ellenbogen and Karoly Kaszala.
© 2020 John Wiley & Sons Ltd. Published 2020 by John Wiley & Sons Ltd.

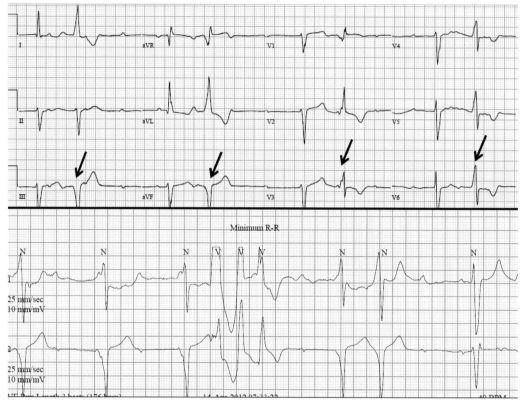

Figure 4.1 Sinus rhythm with complete heart block. (*Top*) There are coupled premature ventricular beats (arrows) in a bigeminal pattern. (*Bottom*) In the setting of severe bradycardia with prolongation of the QT interval, these premature ventricular beats can induce polymorphic ventricular tachycardia. Bradycardia-induced polymorphic ventricular tachycardia is an indication for temporary or permanent pacing independent of the presence of other symptoms.

pacing (Table 4.1). In some cases, despite removal or treatment of the offending source, long-term need for pacing may persist. Nonetheless, a careful patient history and laboratory investigation is required to exclude reversible causes of bradyarrhythmia, before committing the patient to long-term pacing. An algorithm is provided in Figure 4.2 to show our approach to a patient who presents with symptomatic bradycardia.

Patients admitted to hospital for symptomatic bradycardia due to atrioventricular (AV) block with concurrent use of antiarrhythmic or AV-blocking medications are often observed to determine if there is an improvement of conduction after drug withdrawal. In elderly patients the likelihood of significant improvement after drug withdrawal is poor [9]. In a study of 55 patients with symptomatic bradycardia and an average age of 77 years, 47 required a pacemaker during the index hospitalization. Of the eight patients discharged without a pacemaker, two had a new indication and one re-presented with syncope. In this study only five (9%) did not have a pacemaker need or indication after drug withdrawal.

Other indications

Although the vast majority of temporary pacemakers are used to treat or prevent bradycardia in the setting of sinoatrial or AV node dysfunction, there are additional indications for use. The most common is to perform rapid pacing of the ventricle to shorten the diastolic interval and improve hemodynamics in the setting of acute aortic insufficiency. Rapid pacing supports the ventricle during aortic or mitral valve valvuloplasty or transmitral or transaortic valve replacement. In the latter scenario, pacing often stabilizes the hemodynamics until aortic paravalvular leaks can be addressed.

Table 4.1 Examples of potentially reversible causes of symptomatic bradycardia

Metabolic/electrolyte

Drug-induced/toxic
  Digoxin
  Antiarrhythmic drugs
  β-Adrenergic blockers
  Calcium channel blockers
  Clonidine

Cardiac ischemia
Inflammatory or stress-mediated cardiomyopathy
Injury to the sinus node and/or AV node during cardiac surgery
Post cardiac transplant
Central nervous system injury

Infectious
  Lyme carditis
  Bacterial endocarditis
  Influenza

Trauma to the AV node or His–Purkinje system during a cardiac procedure
  Electrophysiology study catheter placement
  Catheter ablation near the sinus node, AV node, or His bundle
  Right heart catheterization
  Cardiac pacing
  Transcutaneous aortic valve placement/valvuloplasty
  Ethanol ablation for hypertrophic cardiomyopathy

Paroxysmal atrial tachyarrhythmias
Autonomically mediated syndromes
Sleep apnea

Temporary pacing options

Transcutaneous pacing

Transcutaneous pacing was first described in the 1950s by Zoll, reporting treatment of asystole in two patients with subcutaneous needle electrodes. Since the utility of the concept was established, transcutaneous pacing has been an integral part of the treatment of bradyarrhythmias in the emergency setting.

The successful application of transcutaneous pacing requires pacemaker pads and cables, a pulse generator unit, electrocardiogram patches, monitoring equipment, and analgesia/sedation medications.

Placement of the pads, as shown in Figure 4.3, is typically done by using one of two configurations. One option is an anterior and posterior placement. The anterior pad is placed on the left chest over the heart and the posterior patch immediately behind this pad on the left upper quadrant of the back. Another option is to place one pad on the right upper chest and the other pad lateral over the region of the anticipated apex of the heart.

Initially the pacing rate is often set between 70 and 80 bpm. The generator current is increased until there is capture of the myocardium and then typically increased an additional 10 mA above this capture threshold. The transcutaneous pacing threshold is variable among patients and their disease states, typically between 40 and 80 mA, and lowest in healthier individuals [10–12]. Care must be taken to confirm that capture of the myocardium has been accomplished as presence of transcutaneous pacing spikes (and polarization artifact) on telemetry does not indicate myocardial capture. Assuring adequate capture may be verified with palpation of the femoral or carotid pulse or observing arterial pressure waveform (if an arterial line is present). In patients with coexistent sepsis or hypotension, additional confirmation of pacing capture may be required with echocardiography [13]. ECG evidence of temporary transcutaneous electrical capture is shown in Figure 4.4. The common causes and management of inadequate myocardial capture with transcutaneous pacing are summarized in Table 4.2.

Transcutaneous pacing is painful. Sedation and analgesia are often required and at levels that may necessitate general anesthesia with intubation. Side effects of the sedatives can impact hemodynamic stability in an already compromised patient. In addition, there can be a mild reduction in cardiac function and stroke index due to AV dyssynchrony during transcutaneous pacing. As such, transcutaneous pacing is largely used as a temporary bridge to either permanent pacing or a more stable endovascular temporary pacing modality.

Temporary endocardial pacing

Transvenous endocardial pacing is the most stable means to provide temporary pacing. There are various types of electrode catheters available for temporary pacing. Unlike transcutaneous pacing, once transvenous pacing is initiated it is typically well tolerated and can be applied for extended periods

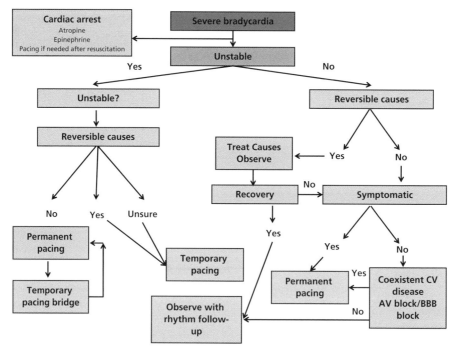

Figure 4.2 An algorithm to consider in the treatment of a patient with severe bradycardia, including when to consider temporary and/or permanent pacing. BB, bundle branch; CV, cardiovascular.

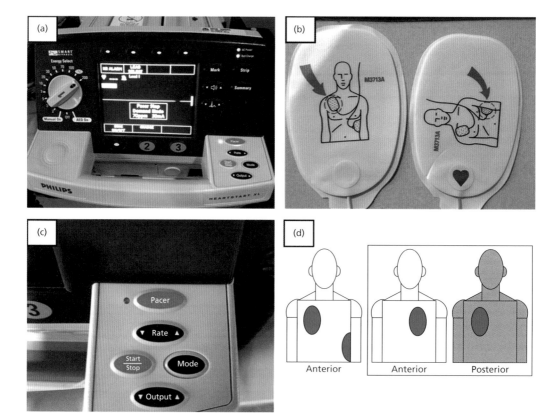

Figure 4.3 Components required for transcutaneous pacing. (a) Automated external defibrillator/pacemaker. (b) Gelatinous pads are applied to deliver transcutaneous pacing in the anticipated positions highlighted in (d). (c) A close-up view of the control panel highlighting the pacemaker function and controls to adjust rate and current delivery.

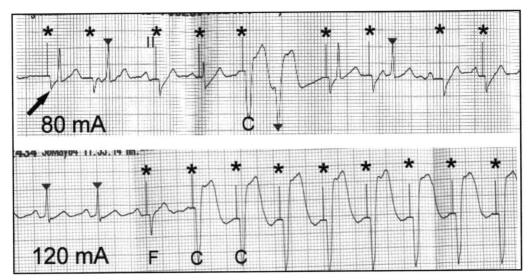

Figure 4.4 Transcutaneous pacing in an intubated 180-kg patient with recurrent episodes of sinus arrest. The tracings are obtained from the pacing generator itself. (*Top*) Subthreshold stimulation. At 80-mA output, the pacing stimuli (*) are followed by a polarization artifact (arrow), but there is no ventricular capture except for the fifth stimulus (C). The polarization artifact may be confused with an evoked QRS complex. Note the demand pacing mode with intrinsic complexes (arrowheads). (*Bottom*) At 120-mA output, ventricular capture (C) begins with the first pacing stimulus (*). This first complex shows fusion (F). Source: adapted from Wood MA. Temporary cardiac pacing. In: Ellenbogen KA, Wood MA, eds. *Cardiac Pacing and ICDs*, 5th edn. Oxford: Blackwell Publishing, 2008. Reproduced with permission of John Wiley & Sons Ltd.

Table 4.2 Common causes of failure to capture with transcutaneous pacemaker

Cause	Evaluation	Solution
Catheter dislodgement	Check morphology of surface electrocardiogram (ECG)	Reposition lead Increase output
Perforation	Check morphology of surface ECG, echocardiogram ± pericardiocentesis	Reposition lead
Local myocardial necrosis/ischemia	Rule out perforation Check ECG for acute ischemia	Reposition lead under fluoroscopy Change to an active fixation lead
Hypoxia/acidosis/electrolyte disturbance/drug effect (type Ia and Ic antiarrhythmics)	Serum electrolytes, arterial blood gas, lactate level	Correct reversible causes Increase output
Unstable electrical connections/battery failure	Assess system power source Check connections	Secure connections Change power source
Failure to sense with secondary	Check ECG/telemetry to assure capture failure is due to pacing during the ventricular refractory period	Reposition lead
Oversensing, with failure to pace	Check ECG Determine cause Assure adequate connections	Myopotentials (decrease sensitivity) Electromagnetic interference (decrease sensitivity or remove source) T or P wave oversensing:(decrease sensitivity or reposition lead)

of time Furthermore, depending on the type of electrode catheter used, these patients can remain ambulatory.

The tools required for temporary endocardial pacing continue to evolve. Initially, transvenous electrode catheters are inserted through a large vein, typically the femoral vein, using a modified Seldinger technique. The catheters can be balloon tipped to allow easier and safer navigation into the right ventricle. There are different catheter sizes and shapes that enhance their stability in the right atrium and ventricle. However, typically, an atrial catheter is not inserted as the procedure is largely viewed as temporary for a reversible condition and control of the ventricular rate provides the quickest avenue toward stability. At times dual-chamber

pacing may be helpful. These potential scenarios are discussed later in this chapter. Figure 4.5 shows the insertion of a 5-Fr balloon-tipped relatively stiff temporary electrode catheter via a transfemoral approach. In this case, the electrode catheter was placed as a precaution at the time of a transcutaneous aortic valve placement in case high-grade AV block developed during the procedure. A femoral venous approach offers rapid stable access for temporary pacing. Other venous access sites, such as the subclavian or internal jugular vein, are better options if pacing is anticipated for an extended period to allow ambulation and reduction of deep vein thrombosis and infection risk.

With electrode systems such as the one shown in Figure 4.5, the target location for the catheter is the

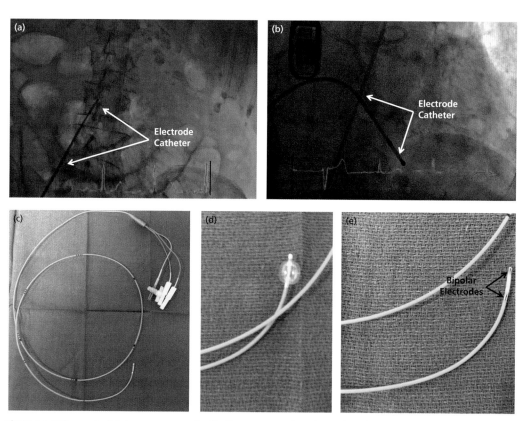

Figure 4.5 Delivery of a 5-Fr transvenous passive fixation pacing electrode catheter. (a) Initial advancement of the catheter through the common femoral and iliac veins. (b) Final location of the electrode catheter in the right ventricular apex. There is a bend in the catheter in the region of the tricuspid annulus that is consistent with the pressure required to minimize lead dislodgement. (c) The complete electrode catheter. There is a central lumen that is connected to a tip balloon that has not been inflated and two pacemaker wires at the distal end. (d) Inflated tip balloon. This balloon enhances migration through the veins and facilitates movement toward the right ventricle. (e) A magnified image of the catheter tip showing the spacing and characteristics of the bipolar system.

right ventricular apex. As shown in the figure, adequate pressure is required to create a slight bend along the region of the tricuspid annulus to minimize risk of lead dislodgement. Excessive pressure on the tip of the catheter increases risk of perforation and tamponade. The risk of perforation is variable, based on operator experience and patient characteristics, but in general it is estimated at approximately 1% or less [14]. Furthermore, despite initial proper placement of the electrode, lead dislodgement risk remains high with passively placed temporary catheters (in one series the risk was 16%) [15].

There are alternatives to consider in choosing a transvenous temporary electrode catheter in order to reduce risk of perforation or dislodgement. These alternatives share the common characteristics of active fixation technologies and

a less stiff structure. Figure 4.6a shows a 3-Fr temporary active fixation electrode. This more compliant system is delivered through a sheath that can be deformed to allow the electrode to be placed in different locations in the right atrium or ventricle. Until recently these technologies contained a rigid distal tip that when placed distally in the right ventricular apex could increase perforation risk. Recently, a balloon-guided system has been developed with a soft tip and active fixation (Figure 4.7). The balloon improves passage to the right ventricle and actively deploys stabilizing loops to achieve stable position [16]. In a study of 25 patients who underwent transcatheter valve replacement, the device was successfully implanted in 92% and used for up to 5 days post procedure without dislodgements.

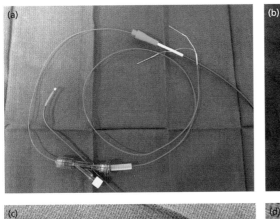
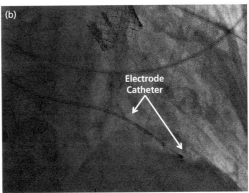
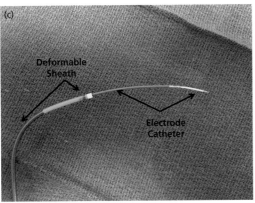
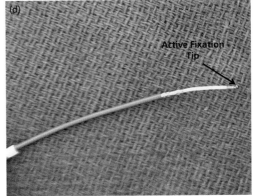

Figure 4.6 Delivery of a 3-Fr transvenous passive fixation pacing electrode catheter through the right internal jugular vein. (a) The complete system with delivery sheath and active fixation pacing electrode catheter. (b) Final location of the electrode catheter in the right ventricular apex. There is a bend in the catheter in the region of the tricuspid annulus that is consistent with the pressure required to minimize lead dislodgement. (c) A magnified image of the catheter showing the deformable delivery sheath and active fixation electrode catheter. (d) A magnified image of the electrode catheter tip showing the active fixation mechanism.

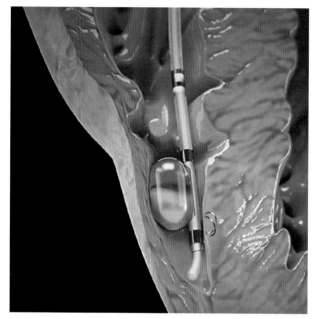 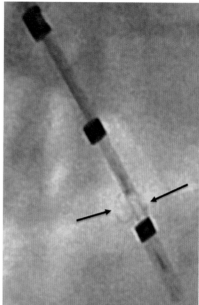

Figure 4.7 (*Left*) Simulation of the balloon-based positioning of the Tempo™ (BioTrace Medical) temporary active fixation pacemaker lead. (*Right*) Fluoroscopic image of the device in a patient who underwent a transcatheter valve replacement. Arrows show the wire loop active fixation stabilizers. Source: adapted from Webster *et al.* [16].

In patients who will require long-term pacing but who are not candidates for permanent pacemakers due to a reversible condition that may take days to weeks to resolve, we favor a more durable solution that allows the patient to fully ambulate with low risk of lead dislodgement. Figure 4.8 demonstrates such an approach. We use an externalized permanent pacemaker generator that we can resterilize after each use. We then use a permanent bipolar pacemaker lead that can be inserted into a jugular or subclavian vein through a 6–7 Fr sheath placed via a modified Seldinger technique. The lead is connected externally to a pacemaker and the complete system held in place against the chest wall using sutures and a tight sterile dressing. Since this approach uses standard pacemaker lead technologies and their respective tools that assist in placement, these leads can be placed into the right ventricle, coronary sinus, or right atrium depending on need. In a study of 49 patients who had systemic infection and urgent pacing indication, outcomes were compared between conventional temporary pacemaker and an externalized (temporary) permanent pacemaker system for safety and efficacy. On average, patients used the temporary pacemaker for 8 days. Complications (lead dislodgement, local infection) occurred less frequently in the externalized permanent pacer group (1 vs. 24 events; *P* <0.01) [17].

Temporary epicardial pacing

Epicardial pacing leads are frequently used as they are a common aspect of postoperative management of patients undergoing various types of cardiac surgery. These small, flexible, externally placed epicardial leads are typically bipolar. These leads are inserted in the epicardium in an orientation that allows easy removal with simple traction on the externalized wires. Figure 4.9 shows the placement of bipolar epicardial leads in the right atrium and ventricle during cardiovascular surgery. The pacemaker lead wires are tunneled through the skin and then connected to a temporary external transvenous pacing generator. The generators used for temporary pacemaker leads are capable of demand and asynchronous pacing modes.

Transesophageal pacing

Because of the proximity of the esophagus and left atrium, a transesophageal pacemaker lead can be used for atrial pacing. The lead requires placement through the nose or mouth. Since contact in the esophagus can be variable, capture consistency is

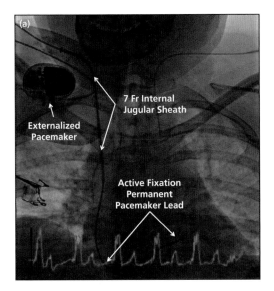

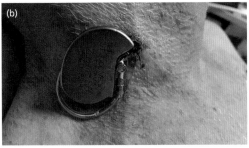

Figure 4.8 (a) X-ray image of a permanent bipolar pacemaker lead placed in the right ventricle through the right internal jugular vein. The pacemaker lead is connected to an externalized reusable pacemaker generator. (b) Photographic image of an externalized pacemaker in a different patient. Source: courtesy of Karoly Kaszala, MD.

not reliable and high current and broad pulse widths are required, which can be painful. These are uncommonly used in the adult population. In our practice transesophageal pacing approaches are largely used only for diagnostic approaches to discern the atrial arrhythmia if other non-invasive diagnostic methods have been unsuccessful.

Temporary dual-chamber pacing

Patients with an intact sinus node with high-grade AV block may develop hypotension with ventricular-only pacing (pacemaker syndrome). These are often patients who have an underlying moderate to severe impairment in diastolic function. Since the need for temporary pacing is often brief, these

patients can typically be stabilized with ventricular pacing alone but, rarely, dual-chamber pacing is required. Two venous cannulations are required, with placement of either permanent pacemaker leads in the right atrium and ventricle connected to an externalized permanent pacemaker generator or two active fixation 3-Fr leads in the right atrium and ventricle connected to an external transvenous pacing generator. Figure 4.10 shows an example of a temporary dual-chamber pacemaker system that was implanted in a patient with restrictive filling and complete heart block after placement of a transfemoral aortic valve.

Leadless pacemakers

Leadless pacemakers have emerged as an alternative to single-chamber pacemakers and do not expose patients to the risk of transvenous leads, surgical pacemaker pocket formation, or skin breakdown from long-term exposure to the pacemaker generator. In patients who undergo extraction of a prior dual- or multi-chamber device in which the extent of temporary pacing may be prolonged, temporary placement of a leadless pacemaker may be an alternative [18].

Other means of pacing

There remain other methods for temporary pacing that can be considered when all other options are not available. For example, percussion- or fist-based pacing can be attempted. This largely represents a variant of cardiopulmonary resuscitation. However, it remains a means to provide perfusion in a patient who is severely compromised. Clearly this method should only be used in those who are in or near cardiac arrest.

Complications

Although the procedure is typically indicated in an emergency situation to retain cardiovascular stability, a number of complications can be encountered, such as lead dislodgement, systemic infection, and lead perforation. A list of common complications is shown in Table 4.3. The use of current active fixation leads would likely decrease procedural complications, especially lead dislodgements. Use of an active fixation electrode allows lead placement in locations other than the right ventricular apex, and

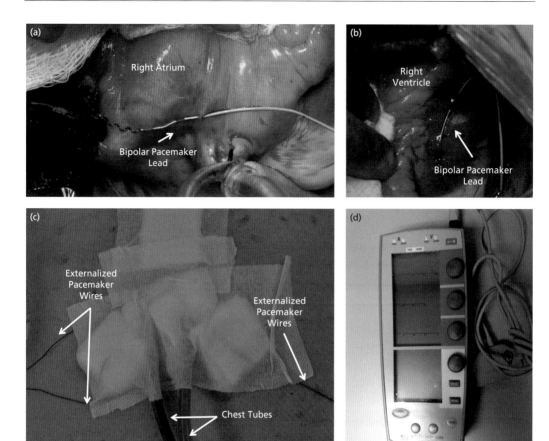

Figure 4.9 An epicardial pacing system placed during cardiac surgery. (a) Epicardial pacemaker lead in the right atrium. The bypass cannula inserted into the right atrium is seen in the lower part of the image. (b) The epicardial pacemaker lead in the right ventricle. (c) The external manifestation of the epicardial pacemaker system with the wires tunneled and externalized to be connected to a temporary transvenous pacemaker generator (d).

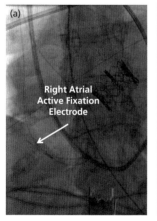
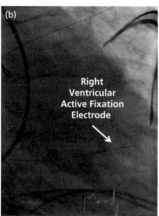
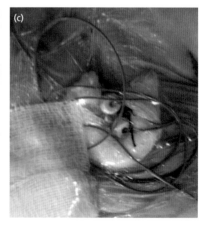

Figure 4.10 Placement of 3-Fr active fixation electrode catheters in the right atrium (a) and ventricle (b) to allow atrioventricular synchrony in a patient with heart block following transfemoral aortic valve replacement. (c) The double access and sheath placement approach in the extrathoracic subclavian vein for insertion of the two electrode catheters. The catheters are subsequently connected to a temporary transvenous pacemaker generator.

Table 4.3 Complications encountered during placement of a transvenous temporary pacing system

Pneumothorax and/or hemothorax
Hemopericardium
Lead displacement/dislodgement
Local infection
Systemic infection
Induction of ventricular fibrillation or ventricular tachycardia
Air embolism
Deep vein thrombosis
Thromboembolism/pulmonary embolism

Inadvertent arterial puncture
    Arterial pseudoaneurysm
    Arterial–venous fistula

Retroperitoneal bleed
Hematoma

likely also reduces the risk of perforation. In order to minimize further systemic infection, we try to avoid leaving a temporary pacemaker system in place for more than 1 week. Clinical management of patients often requires pacemaker troubleshooting; such may be the case with loss of capture or when unusual pacing behavior is noted. A summary of common problems and possible clinical actions are summarized in Table 4.4.

Clinical application

Table 4.5 summarizes the various temporary pacemaker technologies discussed in this chapter. For emergency situations involving cardiac arrest, transcutaneous pacing is the dominant utility given its ease of use and minimal time required for application. In patients who are more stable but require temporary pacing due to symptomatic bradycardia, the available options depend on the time required for application, dislodgement risk, and chambers that require pacing.

Table 4.4 Loss of pacing or loss of capture during transvenous temporary pacing

Problem	Cause	Evaluation	Solution
Loss of pacing	Intrinsic rate faster than programmed rate	Check ECG	Normal behavior
	Oversensing	Check pacer sensitivity	Adjust sensitivity
		Check for EMI	Eliminate source, adjust sensitivity
	Unstable lead connection, battery depletion	Check connections and power source	Secure connection, change battery
Loss of capture	Catheter dislodgement	Check ECG, CXR	Increase output, reposition lead
	Perforation	Check surface ECG, echocardiogram	Reposition lead ± pericardiocentesis
	Local ischemia/necrosis	Check ECG, rule out perforation	Increase output, reposition lead
	Hypoxia/acidosis/electrolyte disturbances/drug effect (type Ia and Ic antiarrhythmics)	Obtain serum electrolyte, arterial blood gas, lactate level	Increase output, correct reversible cause
	Unstable lead connection, battery depletion	Check connections and power source	Secure connection, change battery
Erratic pacing	Inadequate sensing	Check sensitivity	Adjust sensitivity
	Asynchronous pacing mode	Check pacing mode	Change to demand pacing
	Dual-chamber tracking mode	Check ECG, pacing mode	Change upper tracking rate

CXR, chest X-ray; EMI, electromagnetic interference.

Table 4.5 Comparison of temporary pacing technologies

Variable	Transcutaneous	Transvenous passive fixation	Transvenous active fixation	Transvenous permanent pacing lead	Epicardial
Chambers	Ventricle	Primarily ventricle	Atrium/ ventricle	Atrium/ventricle	Atrium/ventricle
Time to Initiate	Minimal	5–10 min	5–10 min	10–15 min	Minimal (CV surgery)
Training	Minimal	Moderate	Moderate– extensive	Extensive	Extensive
Stability	+	++	+++	++++	+++/++++
Long-term use	–	–	+	++	++
Infection risk	–	+	+	+	–
Perforation risk	–	++	+	+	–
Cardiac arrest	+	±	–	–	–

Table 4.6 Recommendations for temporary pacing in patients with symptomatic sinus node dysfunction or atrioventricular block

Class recommendation	Indication
Sinus node dysfunction	
IIa	Persistent hemodynamically unstable sinus node dysfunction refractory to medical therapy: temporary transvenous pacing is reasonable in order to increase heart rate and improve symptoms until a permanent pacemaker is placed or the bradycardia resolves
IIb	Sinus node dysfunction with severe symptoms or hemodynamic compromise: temporary transcutaneous pacing may be considered in order to increase heart rate and improve symptoms until a temporary transvenous or permanent pacemaker is placed or the bradycardia resolves
Atrioventricular block	
I	Transient or reversible causes of atrioventricular block: should have medical therapy and supportive care, including temporary transvenous pacing if necessary, before determination of need for permanent pacing
IIa	Second-degree or third-degree atrioventricular block associated with symptoms or hemodynamic compromise that is refractory to medical therapy: temporary transvenous pacing is reasonable in order to increase heart rate and improve symptoms
IIa	Patients who require prolonged temporary transvenous pacing: it is reasonable to choose an externalized permanent active fixation lead over a standard passive fixation temporary pacing lead
IIb	Second-degree or third-degree atrioventricular block and hemodynamic compromise refractory to antibradycardic medical therapy: temporary transcutaneous pacing may be considered until a temporary transvenous pacemaker is placed or the bradyarrhythmia resolves

Source: Kusumoto *et al.* [3]. Reproduced with permission of the American Heart Association.

Recent clinical guidelines support the application of temporary pacemaker leads in cardiovascular surgery and for stabilization in patients with symptomatic sinus node disease or AV block (Table 4.6) [3]. In our practice, for patients requiring urgent/emergent pacing due to non-reversible causes we generally implant a permanent pacemaker as the initial procedure, even during off hours, rather than initially performing temporary pacing, only for the patient to undergo permanent pacing at a later time. In our experience, with a readily available catheterization laboratory and personnel, patients can undergo a definitive procedure with minimal risk of lead dislodgement or complications from multiple procedures. In particular, this type of strategy can help to minimize the long-term infection risk associated with temporary endocardial pacing systems.

Conclusion

Temporary pacing is part of the armamentarium of emergency room, critical care, cardiovascular surgery, and cardiovascular medicine physicians. Temporary pacing can provide immediate cardiovascular stabilization in patients with severe symptomatic bradycardia. Technologies have evolved to enhance lead stability and minimize risk, allowing temporary pacing to provide a bridge to permanent pacing or until the reversible condition resolves, even when this requires weeks. Although specialized training and equipment are required, temporary pacing will remain fundamental to the care of cardiac patients.

References

1 Sodeck GH, Domanovits H, Meron G, *et al.* Compromising bradycardia: management in the emergency department. *Resuscitation* 2007;73(1):96–102.

2 Field JM, Hazinski MF, Sayre MR, *et al.* Part 1: Executive Summary: 2010 American Heart Association Guidelines for Cardiopulmonary Resuscitation and Emergency Cardiovascular Care. *Circulation* 2010;122(18 Suppl 3): S640–S656.

3 Kusumoto FM, Schoenfeld MH, Barrett C, *et al.* 2018 ACC/AHA/HRS guideline on the evaluation and management of patients with bradycardia and cardiac conduction delay: A Report of the American College of Cardiology/ American Heart Association Task Force on Clinical Practice Guidelines and the Heart Rhythm Society. *Heart Rhythm* 2019;16(9):e128–e226.

4 Smith I, Monk TG, White PF. Comparison of transesophageal atrial pacing with anticholinergic drugs for the treatment of intraoperative bradycardia. *Anesth Analg* 1994;78(2):245–252.

5 Morrison LJ, Long J, Vermeulen M, *et al.* A randomized controlled feasibility trial comparing safety and effectiveness of prehospital pacing versus conventional treatment: PrePACE. *Resuscitation* 2008;76(3):341–349.

6 Cummins RO, Graves JR, Larsen MP, *et al.* Out-of-hospital transcutaneous pacing by emergency medical technicians in patients with asystolic cardiac arrest. *N Engl J Med* 1993;328(19):1377–1382.

7 Sherbino J, Verbeek PR, MacDonald RD, *et al.* Prehospital transcutaneous cardiac pacing for symptomatic bradycardia or bradyasystolic cardiac arrest: a systematic review. *Resuscitation* 2006;70(2):193–200.

8 Ornato JP, Carveth WL, Windle JR. Pacemaker insertion for prehospital bradyasystolic cardiac arrest. *Ann Emerg Med* 1984;13(2):101–103.

9 Knudsen MB, Thogersen AM, Hjortshoj SP, Riahi S. The impact of drug discontinuation in patients treated with temporary pacemaker due to atrioventricular block. *J Cardiovasc Electrophysiol* 2013;24(11):1255–1258.

10 Zoll PM, Zoll RH, Falk RH, *et al.* External noninvasive temporary cardiac pacing: clinical trials. *Circulation* 1985;71(5):937–944.

11 Klein LS, Miles WM, Heger JJ, Zipes DP. Transcutaneous pacing: patient tolerance, strength–interval relations and feasibility for programmed electrical stimulation. *Am J Cardiol* 1988;62(16):1126–1129.

12 Kelly JS, Royster RL, Angert KC, Case LD. Efficacy of noninvasive transcutaneous cardiac pacing patients undergoing cardiac surgery. *Anesthesiology* 1989;70(5): 747–751.

13 Ettin D, Cook T. Using ultrasound to determine external pacer capture. *J Emerg Med* 1999;17(6):1007–1009.

14 Metkus TS, Schulman SP, Marine JE, Eid SM. Complications and outcomes of temporary transvenous pacing: an analysis of >360,000 patients from the National Inpatient Sample. *Chest* 2019;155(4):749–757.

15 Betts TR. Regional survey of temporary transvenous pacing procedures and complications. *Postgrad Med J* 2003;79(934):463–465.

16 Webster M, Pasupati S, Lever N, Stiles M. Safety and feasibility of a novel active fixation temporary pacing lead. *J Invasive Cardiol* 2018;30(5):163–167.

17 Braun MU, Rauwolf T, Bock M, *et al.* Percutaneous lead implantation connected to an external device in stimulation-dependent patients with systemic infection: a prospective and controlled study. *Pacing Clin Electrophysiol* 2006;29(8):875–879.

18 Kypta A, Blessberger H, Lichtenauer M, Steinwender C. Temporary leadless pacing in a patient with severe device infection. *BMJ Case Rep* 2016;pii: bcr2016215724.

CHAPTER 5

Techniques of pacemaker and ICD implantation and removal

Joseph E. Marine, Charles J. Love, and Jeffrey A. Brinker
Johns Hopkins University School of Medicine, Baltimore, MD, USA

Introduction

A conventional permanent pacing and implantable cardioverter–defibrillator (ICD) system consists of a generator and one or more leads that connect it to the endocardial or epicardial surface of the heart. Considerable evolution in technique and hardware has occurred over the past several decades, which has simplified the implantation procedure with minimal difference in technical aspects of pacemaker or ICD implantation. Associated with this evolution has been a miniaturization of the power source and circuitry of the generator, and near-universal use of smaller and more flexible transvenous leads. The newest generation of "leadless" pacing systems are entirely self-contained capsules implanted directly into the heart.

Compared with such tasks as optimization of programming and interpretation of complex pacemaker electrograms, the implantation of a modern pacemaker or ICD may now be the least challenging aspect of cardiac device therapy. However, it would be inappropriate to create the impression that all implantation is easy. Implanters should be dedicated to lifelong continuous improvement of their skills and knowledge, learning from their own challenging cases as well as those of colleagues. Moreover, innovations such as leadless cardiac pacing and His bundle pacing will continue to challenge the skills of implanters.

In this chapter, transvenous single- and dual-chamber pacemaker and ICD implantation, as well as newer techniques of leadless pacemaker and His bundle pacemaker implanation, are examined from a broad perspective that emphasizes the practical considerations influencing the safety and efficacy of this procedure. In addition, the indications for and methodology of removing implanted pacing devices are reviewed.

Physician qualifications

Pacemaker implantation is performed by physicians from a variety of specialties, including cardiothoracic surgeons, non-electrophysiology cardiologists, and electrophysiologists. Formal training in the implantation of arrhythmia management devices is most extensive in clinical cardiac electrophysiology fellowship programs. Despite the growth in numbers of trained electrophysiologists, many non-electrophysiology cardiologists continue to implant pacemakers either alone or as part of a surgical team. In addition, many electrophysiologists and cardiologists call upon their surgical colleagues for assistance in more complicated implantations, such as submammary or subpectoral dissections.

Cardiac Pacing and ICDs, Seventh Edition. Edited by Kenneth A. Ellenbogen and Karoly Kaszala.
© 2020 John Wiley & Sons Ltd. Published 2020 by John Wiley & Sons Ltd.

Procedural success and safety are determined in large part by the skill and experience of the operator. Although the degree of "surgery" required for a routine transvenous implantation is modest, good surgical technique is essential. Experience is also necessary to ensure proper positioning of leads so that optimal stability and long-term performance are obtained. A physician wishing to implant pacing systems independently should perform a sufficient number of procedures under the supervision of an accomplished operator to gain the skill and confidence necessary for independent work.

The minimal number of cases to credential a physician depends on the physician's prior familiarity with intravascular catheterization, surgical technique, and knowledge of the principles of pacing. This experience should include single- and dual-chamber systems, and use of both the subclavian/axillary and cephalic approaches for venous access. In addition to this initial training experience, an adequate number of implantations should be performed over time to maintain a level of proficiency. Guidelines for training in pacemaker implantation have been published that may serve as a general model [1,2]. The guidelines acknowledge the special training necessary for those physicians seeking credentials in biventricular pacing, defibrillator implantation, and lead extraction. Because fluoroscopic imaging is a necessary component of the implantation process, knowledge of the basics of radiation physics and safety is required to minimize risk to the patient, operator, and laboratory personnel.

Specialty assistance may be anticipated before a procedure in some cases, and appropriate consultation should be obtained. Implantation procedures are generally performed under moderate sedation, but on occasion there may be a need for the support of an anesthesiologist. Implanting physicians should be familiar with the principles of moderate sedation and the particular institutional guidelines under which they operate, including the acceptable drugs (dosages, reversibility) and the necessary support personnel, monitoring equipment, and recovery procedures.

Quality assurance has become a necessary part of every hospital's activities, and surgical operations and the physicians who perform them are most thoroughly scrutinized. It is the responsibility of all physicians to be conscious of the quality of

their work; those in administrative positions should ensure that proper databases are maintained and performance evaluations are carried out. The objective of these practices is excellence and continually improving quality of care.

Logistical requirements

The logistical requirements for pacemaker implantation are relatively modest. The procedure may be carried out in an operating room, a catheterization laboratory, or a special procedure room with no compromise of success rate or difference in complications. Implantation in the cardiac catheterization laboratory has been shown to result in a significant reduction in the cost and length of hospital stay compared with implants in the operating room by surgeons. This is probably due to the increased flexibility in scheduling in the catheterization laboratory, as well as the use of conscious sedation administered by catheterization laboratory personnel instead of anesthesia staff.

The procedure room should be adequate in size and well lit, and it should comply with all the electrical safety requirements for intravascular catheterization. The radiographic equipment should function within accepted guidelines, and appropriate radiation shielding should be available and used. The room should have appropriate temperature control and ventilation for sterile procedures.

In addition to the operator, the staff should include qualified individuals to monitor the electrocardiogram (ECG) and assist with the imaging equipment. A nurse is required to prepare and administer medications. Often a representative of a device company is present to provide technical assistance, such as with operating the pacing system analyzer or device programmer. These individuals may be a valuable source of information, but should not be considered a substitute for a nurse or laboratory technologist during the implant procedure. Laboratory personnel should also be trained in adherence to rigorous sterile techniques.

An adequate imaging system is an important requirement of the pacemaker laboratory. The fluoroscopy equipment may be portable or fixed, but must be capable of rotation so that oblique and lateral views of the areas of interest (which may extend from the neck to the groin) can be obtained.

A mechanism for magnification is helpful for situations such as confirmation of extension of the helix of active fixation leads, appropriate tine fixation of leadless pacemakers, lead removal procedures, and the identification of problems such as fracture of a conductor. Digital acquisition and storage capabilities have proven to be advantageous and are widely used. Such technology can be used to road-map or superimpose real-time fluoroscopy on a stored image. Thus, one can bring up a stored image of the subclavian venogram to document the vein patency and to serve as a target for an exploring needle being advanced under fluoroscopic monitoring (Figure 5.1).

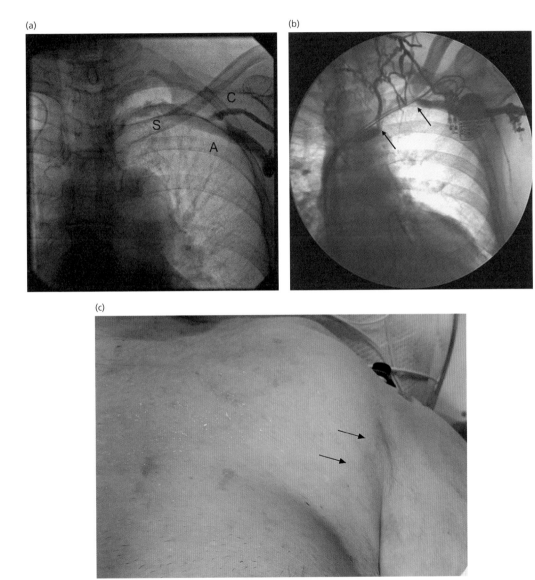

Figure 5.1 Venography may be helpful in documenting the patency of venous structures. (a) A normal left arm venogram. A, axillary portion of the vein; C, cephalic vein; S, subclavian vein. (b) Complete occlusion of the subclavian vein (between the two arrows) with extensive collateral vein formation in a patient with prior pacemaker implantation. This information would clearly be important when planning for procedures requiring new venous access. (c) The subclavian region in a patient before pacemaker implantation. Superficial collateral veins are identified (arrows) which may raise concerns about possible subclavian vein stenosis or occlusion. In this case, there was moderate subclavian vein stenosis on venography.

The use of pulsed digital fluoroscopy can reduce radiation exposure to the patient and operator, and should be used whenever possible. Frame rates of 7.5 frames per second (fps) are usually adequate for pacemaker implantation, and newer systems may use as little as 3.75 fps or less. Newer imaging systems also increase patient safety by providing on-line dose measurements that more accurately reflect radiation exposure than does total fluoroscopy time. The patient table should be flat, radiolucent, and configured in such a way that the operator may work on either side of it. The goal should always be to keep radiation dose to patient and staff "as low are reasonably achievable" (ALARA).

It is essential that the ECG be continuously monitored; a simultaneous multilead display that is easily visualized is preferable in order to assess paced QRS axis and morphology, particularly when assessing His bundle pacing capture or left ventricular (LV) pacing. Leads placed on the chest or back should consist of radiolucent electrodes and wires. The patient should be connected via radiolucent transthoracic electrode patches to an external defibrillator capable of transcutaneous pacing, cardioversion, and defibrillation in case an arrhythmia develops during the procedure. Arterial blood pressure and pulse oximetry should be monitored throughout the procedure. A portable ultrasound device may be helpful in identifying vascular structures and provide guidance for venous access.

The surgical instruments required for the procedure depend on the demands of the particular procedure and operator. A pacemaker tray may be derived from the hospital's surgical cut-down set and supplemented in accordance with the specifics of the case. Add-ons include tear-away vascular introducer sets, appropriate cables to connect to a pacing system analyzer (PSA), suction, and electrocautery. The operator should be familiar with the guidelines for electrocautery use to ensure safety, particularly when oxygen is being administered.

An adequate supply and variety of pacing hardware should be available, including not only pacemaker generators and leads, but also sheaths, stylets, and lead adaptors. It is good practice to have at least two of every necessary item on hand in case of accidental damage or loss of sterility.

The PSA measures a variety of pacing parameters (capture and sensing threshold, lead impedance, electrograms, slew rate) that assess the adequacy of lead position and integrity. A direct digital readout and the capability to print a hard copy are desirable. Equipment necessary for emergency pericardiocentesis, chest tube insertion, and temporary endocardial pacing must be at hand, and it is advantageous to have prompt access to a two-dimensional echocardiography machine. A crash cart containing resuscitative supplies (including those necessary to establish endotracheal intubation), an adequate supply of all appropriate drugs, and experienced staff should be readily available.

Assessment of the patient

The implantation process begins with a thorough evaluation of the patient. This should include reviewing medical records, obtaining a pertinent history (including current medications, especially anticoagulants and antiplatelet agents, and previous reactions to drugs and contrast media), performing a physical examination, and acquiring the basic laboratory tests.

The indication for device implantation should be documented and characterized in accordance with the American College of Cardiology (ACC)/ American Heart Association (AHA) guidelines [3–6]. In some situations, it may be reasonable to offer pacemaker therapy for conditions in which the indication for such therapy is controversial and evolving, such as recurrent neurally mediated syncope with a prominent cardioinhibitory component.

Consideration of the type of pacing or defibrillator system to be used should be part of the patient assessment. The choice of mode of pacing (e.g. atrial; ventricular; single chamber, dual chamber, biventricular, leadless, or His bundle) is made on the basis of the underlying conduction disturbance, the present and future potential need for pacing, and the hemodynamic and functional status of the patient [5,6]. Other factors that might influence the method of implantation, the operative site, or the type of hardware needed should be considered before the procedure. Examples include the need for an unusual vascular approach (e.g. iliac vein) or an epicardial lead system in a patient with a previously documented venous anomaly; and employment of an active fixation ventricular lead in a patient with severe tricuspid regurgitation or

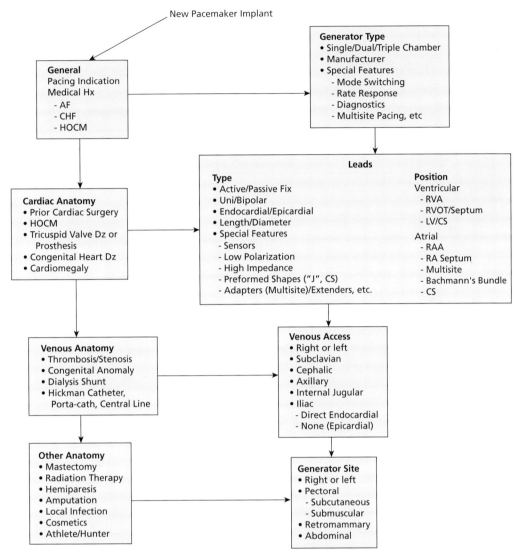

New Pacemaker Implant

General
Pacing Indication
Medical Hx
- AF
- CHF
- HOCM

Generator Type
- Single/Dual/Triple Chamber
- Manufacturer
- Special Features
  - Mode Switching
  - Rate Response
  - Diagnostics
  - Multisite Pacing, etc

Cardiac Anatomy
- Prior Cardiac Surgery
- HOCM
- Tricuspid Valve Dz or
  Prosthesis
- Congenital Heart Dz
- Cardiomegaly

Leads

Type
- Active/Passive Fix
- Uni/Bipolar
- Endocardial/Epicardial
- Length/Diameter
- Special Features
  - Sensors
  - Low Polarization
  - High Impedance
  - Preformed Shapes ("J", CS)
  - Adapters (Multisite)/Extenders, etc.

Position
Ventricular
- RVA
- RVOT/Septum
- LV/CS

Atrial
- RAA
- RA Septum
- Multisite
- Bachmann's Bundle
- CS

Venous Anatomy
- Thrombosis/Stenosis
- Congenital Anomaly
- Dialysis Shunt
- Hickman Catheter,
  Porta-cath, Central Line

Venous Access
- Right or left
- Subclavian
- Cephalic
- Axillary
- Internal Jugular
- Iliac
  - Direct Endocardial
  - None (Epicardial)

Other Anatomy
- Mastectomy
- Radiation Therapy
- Hemiparesis
- Amputation
- Local Infection
- Cosmetics
- Athlete/Hunter

Generator Site
- Right or left
- Pectoral
  - Subcutaneous
  - Submuscular
- Retromammary
- Abdominal

Figure 5.2 Flow chart for decision process surrounding a new device implant. AF, atrial fibrillation; CHF, congestive heart failure; CS, coronary sinus; Dz, disease; HOCM, hypertrophic obstructive cardiomyopathy; Hx, history; LV, left ventricle; RAA, right atrial appendage; RVA, right ventricular apex; RVOT, right ventricular outflow tract.

corrected transposition of the great vessels. These factors comprise an array of choices that should be carefully considered before the patient enters the procedure room (Figure 5.2). Thorough preparation is essential to minimize problems at implantation.

Special issues

Several issues in patient assessment and preparation merit special consideration (Table 5.1).

Infection

Implanters are frequently asked to implant permanent pacemakers semi-urgently in hospitalized patients with coexisting infectious issues. Decision-making regarding the timing of pacemaker implantation in these patients can be complex, and depends on the site of the suspected or documented infection, concern for bacteremia, and indication for cardiac pacing. For example, a patient with complete atrioventricular (AV) block who has

Table 5.1 Special issues in the assessment of the patient who requires cardiac device implantation

Clinical problem	Implant consideration
Infection	Delay implantation
Kidney disease	Increased pocket hematoma risk Increased infection risk Increased risk of contrast nephropathy
Anticoagulants and antiplatelet agents	Increased pocket hematoma risk Hold offending agent if possible Apply meticulous hemostasis

Possible venous access problems:
  Subclavian vein anomalies
  Prior central venous lines or leads present
  Prior clavicular fracture
	Preoperative venogram to evaluate patency
	Choose alternative site

Prior mastectomy	Risk of arm edema Choose alternative site

Tricuspid valve disease
  Mechanical prosthesis: RV lead contraindicated
  Severe tricuspid regurgitation
	Mechanical prosthesis: use LV lead or epicardial lead
	Severe tricuspid regurgitation: use active fixation lead

Risk for asystole (left bundle branch block, complete atrioventricular block)	Consider perioperative temporary pacer placement
History of contrast allergy	Treat preoperatively with steroid

asymptomatic bacteriuria with no fever and normal white count can usually be implanted with minimal delay while treating the potential lower urinary tract infection. On the other hand, a patient with bacterial endocarditis and mildly symptomatic sinus node dysfunction is best completely treated and cure proven prior to implantation. Patients with pneumonia without bacteremia can usually be implanted after antibiotic therapy has rendered them afebrile for 2–3 days.

A special population comprises patients with an existing infected cardiovascular implantable electronic device (CIED) that needs to be removed. Although temporary pacing may be immediately required for dependent individuals, guidelines for reimplantation of a permanent system require evaluation for infective endocarditis and negative blood cultures. In general, the minimum duration between extraction and reimplantation is 3–14 days [7]. In such difficult cases, consultation with infectious disease colleagues regarding duration of antibiotic therapy may be helpful. In considering the timing of implantation, the risk of pacemaker infection needs to be balanced against the risk of delaying pacemaker therapy and of prolonged hospitalization.

Kidney disease

Patients with chronic kidney disease also merit special consideration. For the patient with end-stage renal disease (ESRD) on dialysis, pacemaker implantation and overnight observation must be coordinated with the outpatient dialysis center to ensure that dialysis is not disrupted. Implantation is usually scheduled on a non-dialysis day and dialysis is scheduled the next day, either as an inpatient on the morning of discharge or at the outpatient center in the afternoon. In general, implantation should be performed on the side opposite to the functioning dialysis access site, due to elevation of venous pressure on that side (raising risk of bleeding) as well as risk of loss of use of the dialysis access site should subclavian vein stenosis or occlusion result from the pacemaker insertion. In cases where the ipsilateral pectoral site must be used, some advocate use of the supraclavicular or internal jugular approach to minimize these risks. A leadless pacemaker system should be considered in patients for whom single-chamber ventricular (VVI) pacing is adequate. Because the risk of infection is higher in ESRD patients, especially in those receiving catheter-based hemodialysis, some thought might be given to the implantation of an epicardial lead system in specific situations.

For patients with lesser degrees of renal dysfunction (determined by estimated creatinine clearance), the main issue is whether use of intravenous contrast is anticipated, and if so at what dose. Upper extremity venography can usually be performed with 10–20 mL of diluted contrast, which generally poses little risk. Patients undergoing biventricular pacemaker implantation may occasionally require as much as 80–100 mL of contrast when there is difficulty engaging the coronary sinus (CS) or identifying a suitable tributary for lead placement. In general, we favor use of isosmolar, non-ionic contrast for such patients and make every effort to minimize total contrast dose, using diluted contrast wherever possible. Recent consensus guidelines for prevention of contrast-induced nephropathy have emphasized use of pre- and post-procedure intravenous hydration with normal saline [8].

Anticoagulants and antiplatelet agents

Many patients requiring pacemaker implantation take oral anticoagulants for a variety of reasons, including atrial fibrillation, mechanical heart valves, and prior venous thromboembolism. Their peri-implant management is often complicated and related to the indication for anticoagulation and type of anticoagulant used. Previously used protocols which involved stopping warfarin 4–5 days prior to implantation surgery, with use of intravenous heparin or subcutaneous low-molecular-weight heparin for bridging in higher-risk patients, have been largely supplanted with use of uninterrupted or minimally interrupted oral anticoagulant therapy. For patients at low risk of thromboembolism, warfarin may be held for several days without anticoagulant bridging [9].

The most commonly used option currently for managing the patient on warfarin is to perform the procedure without reversal of the anticoagulant. Giudici et al. [10] reported excellent results with this strategy in a series of 470 patients with a mean international normalized ratio (INR) of 2.6. The authors used meticulous implantation technique and suggest that the risk of pocket bleeding is not prohibitive because hemostasis in these procedures is primarily a function of capillary vasoconstriction and platelet activity. In their study, the rate of pocket hematoma formation was 2.6% and was not significantly different from the rate in the control group of 555 patients implanted with an INR of less than 1.5 (2.2%).

Since this report was published, numerous additional studies have reported similar findings of relative safety of pacemaker implantation with continuation of therapeutic warfarin. Cheng et al. [11] conducted a randomized trial of 100 patients on warfarin undergoing pacemaker or ICD implantation, or generator replacement, comparing a strategy of continuation of warfarin with interruption, and found a strong trend toward fewer complications in the group assigned to continuous warfarin. Ghanbari et al. [12] conducted a meta-analysis of eight studies enrolling 2321 patients undergoing pacemaker or ICD implantation in which continuation of warfarin was compared with a heparin bridging strategy. This analysis found that continuation of warfarin was associated with a lower risk of postoperative bleeding and equivalent risk of thromboembolism. The results of this meta-analysis were conform in the randomized BRUISE CONTROL study of 681 patients, with 3.5% of patients assigned to continuous warfarin developing a pocket hematoma compared with 16.0% in the heparin-bridging arm [13].

It should be emphasized that pacemaker implantation in the setting of therapeutic warfarin is associated with potential risk and should be carried out by experienced operators who are confident in their implantation skills and ability to manage complications. This strategy is increasingly used, however, as the least problematic solution to the challenging situation of pacemaker implantation in a patient at high risk for periprocedural thromboembolism.

Increasingly, patients with atrial fibrillation are anticoagulated with newer agents such as the direct-acting thrombin inhibitor dabigatran and the oral factor Xa inhibitors rivaroxaban and apixaban. These agents have a prompt anticoagulation effect after being started and half-lives of 8–16 hours. Little information has been published on the safety of continuation of these agents during pacemaker implantation. In general, these agents are held for 2–3 days prior to the procedure and restarted 1–2 days afterward, depending on risk of thromboembolism, risk of bleeding, and quality of hemostasis obtained during the procedure [14].

Increasing use of prolonged dual-antiplatelet therapy in patients who receive intracoronary drug-eluting stents poses an additional challenge for the pacemaker implanter. Although low-dose aspirin alone may usually be continued when it is indicated, it is clear that the use of dual-antiplatelet therapy (i.e. aspirin plus ticlopidine, clopidogrel, or prasugrel) markedly impairs surgical hemostasis. Tompkins *et al.* [15] reviewed 1388 device implantations at a single large urban health system and found that the combination of aspirin and clopidogrel was associated with a 4.5-fold increased risk of bleeding compared with use of no antiplatelet therapy, and with a twofold increased risk compared with use of aspirin alone. Given that the recommendation for dual-antiplatelet treatment has been increased to 1 year after most placements of drug-eluting stents, and optimal duration remains undefined, implanting physicians are frequently asked to implant pacemakers and defibrillators in such patients. If the procedure cannot be postponed and dual-antiplatelet therapy cannot be held, then the pacemaker implanter will need to pay particularly careful attention to pocket hemostasis.

Subclavian vein anomalies

Patients with potential subclavian vein anomalies require additional preprocedure planning. In particular, patients with a preexisting transvenous permanent pacemaker or ICD system have an approximately 25% prevalence of subsequent ipsilateral subclavian vein stenosis or occlusion. One can usually anticipate a patent, suitable subclavian vein in a patient without prior chest surgery, pacemaker/ICD implantation, or deep venous thrombosis (DVT). Other patients should undergo upper extremity venography prior to the implantation procedure, either on a separate day or in the pacemaker laboratory prior to the sterile preparation of the patient. Management of a subclavian stenosis or occlusion, if identified, will depend on the degree of stenosis, length of occlusion, and perceived need to place the device on a particular side. If the side opposite to the venous stenosis/occlusion is felt to be unsuitable, various interventional techniques for crossing and dilating these lesions have been described [16]. Of the significant congenital anomalies of the brachiocephalic system, a persistent left superior vena cava (SVC) is the most

frequent. It is discussed in more detail in the Chapter (see section Implant Procedure; Site).

Prior mastectomy

With improved survival from breast cancer, the pacemaker implanter is more likely to encounter patients with prior mastectomy who require implantation of a CIED. In general, the side opposite to the mastectomy is used, due to concern for exacerbating arm swelling should subclavian vein stenosis or occlusion follow pacemaker implantation. However, breast surgery should not automatically preclude use of the ipsilateral pectoral site if that side is preferred for appropriate reasons. For example, a patient with a partial mastectomy and minimal or no lymph node dissection, good preservation of subcutaneous tissue, and no history of lymphedema or arm swelling could probably undergo ipsilateral implantation with little or no increased risk. If the patient has a history of arm swelling or lymphedema, that side is best avoided. In the unusual patient with bilateral mastectomies, the pectoral site with best preservation of subcutaneous tissue and least degree of ipsilateral arm swelling should be used. Preoperative upper extremity venography should also be performed in this situation.

Tricuspid valve disease

Patients with preexisting severe tricuspid regurgitation can pose a substantial challenge for the pacemaker implanter, due to both turbulent blood flow from the regurgitation and the resulting right heart enlargement. Active fixation leads are usually required to reduce the risk of dislodgement. Larger-diameter, heavier leads and stiffer stylets are often required to place the right ventricular (RV) lead. Lead stability may need to take priority over best possible lead parameters.

In patients with prosthetic tricuspid valves, it is imperative to determine the type of prosthesis. Transvenous leads cannot be placed through a mechanical prosthesis, and an alternative site for ventricular pacing must be chosen (CS or epicardial). In patients with bioprosthetic valves, transvenous RV leads have been successfully placed, although the long-term effects on prosthetic valve function are not known [17]. This is another situation in which leadless cardiac pacing may be particularly suitable for patients needing only single-chamber ventricular (VVI) pacing.

Patients at risk for asystole

The operator should consider whether a temporary pacing wire should be placed at the start of the procedure to provide back-up pacing in the event of prolonged asystole during permanent lead placement. Patients with complete left bundle branch block (LBBB) or AV block with a ventricular escape mechanism are at particular risk for this complication. Patients with isolated sinus node dysfunction without bundle branch block are generally at low risk. Operators with less experience should have a lower threshold for placing a temporary wire prior to permanent pacemaker implantation if potential for severe intraprocedural bradycardia is anticipated. Patients who are pacemaker dependent and undergoing generator replacement or system revision should generally have a temporary pacing wire placed for the procedure. All patients should be connected via adhesive electrode patches to an external defibrillator capable of emergency external pacing; however, this device should not be considered a substitute for a temporary wire in a high-risk patient.

Cost-effectiveness

More emphasis is currently being placed on the cost-effectiveness of medical care, especially those aspects of care that are procedurally centered. Ideally, attention to cost-effectiveness is accompanied by increased quality of care. Health system administrators have increasingly focused on minimizing length of stay, the cost of specific devices, and increasing the level of patient satisfaction. Mechanisms of clinical practice improvement that may reduce cost yet increase the quality of care have been used. Practice guidelines, critical pathways, and other methods of standardizing care are likely to become more widespread. Physicians should continue to play a leading role in cost constraint without compromising excellent patient care.

Informed consent

It is generally the implanting physician's responsibility to obtain informed consent from the patient (or surrogate decision-maker) before the procedure.

A candid appraisal of the anticipated risks and benefits, acute and long term, must be undertaken along with an explanation of alternatives using a shared decision-making approach which incorporates the patient's healthcare goals, values, and preferences. If the indication for pacing is controversial or investigational, more extensive counseling of the patient and documentation are usually necessary. The small but finite possibility of premature failure of the leads and/or generator should also be reviewed. Finally, physical or occupational restrictions imposed by the presence of a pacemaker should be discussed with the patient. The need for regular, lifelong follow-up evaluations should be noted, and mention should be made of the eventual need for generator replacement for an end-of-service indication. The participation of other physicians at the time of implantation or during the follow-up assessments should be described. If the pacemaker follow-up is to be performed by the referring physician, that person should be consulted in advance to help determine the most appropriate choice of pacemaker system.

Preimplantation orders

Although outpatient pacemaker implantation with same-day discharge is increasingly performed, the usual practice in most centers is to keep the patient in the hospital for overnight observation [18]. Almost all third-party payors now consider these stays as 23-hour observation periods rather than full admissions for this purpose. Routine preimplant laboratory tests may include a 12-lead ECG, a complete blood cell count (including platelet count), and measures of prothrombin time and activated partial thromboplastin time (aPTT), serum electrolytes, blood urea nitrogen and creatinine. It may be helpful to have a recent posteroanterior and lateral chest radiograph to compare with the postprocedure radiographs, particularly in patients with prior chest surgery and/or prior pacemaker or ICD implantation.

Patients usually fast for at least 8 hours before the procedure. Hydration is maintained by the establishment of an intravenous line, preferably with a large-bore cannula, in a vein of the upper extremity ipsilateral to the intended implant site. This will facilitate the injection of contrast should difficulty be encountered in achieving venous access. In general, patients are allowed to continue whatever medication they have been taking, with the possible exception of anticoagulants and antiplatelet agents, and some diuretics and antihypertensive drugs (see section Special issues). The dosage of insulin or oral hypoglycemic drugs may require temporary alteration, usually holding or reducing the dose on the morning of the procedure.

Antibiotic prophylaxis decreases the incidence of short-term and late pacemaker infection. A meta-analysis of randomized trials that used a systemic antibiotic has supported the use of a prophylactic antibiotic to prevent infection associated with permanent pacemaker implantation [19]. In an accompanying report, the same investigators have suggested that contamination by local flora cultured at the site of implant can result in delayed pacemaker-related infections presenting months later [20]. We routinely give an antibiotic active against *Staphylococcus* (cefazolin, vancomycin, or clindamycin) before the procedure. It is of obvious importance that the initial antibiotic dose be completed prior to skin incision, preferably 30–60 min before, to allow for peak tissue concentrations. There are no data to support giving prophylactic antibiotics for more than 24 hours after implantation procedures. Quality guidelines for surgical procedures generally call for stopping prophylactic antibiotics within 24 hours of clean sterile procedures, unless there are extenuating circumstances. A recent trial did not find a statistically significant reduction in infection rate by adding 2 days of postprocedural oral antibiotics to a single preoperative dose of intravenous cefazolin [21].

The implant site (typically the area from above the nipple line to the angle of the jaw bilaterally) should be cleaned just before the patient's arrival in the pacemaker laboratory. Shaving the surgical site is controversial, and guidelines have been issued recently that argue against shaving in favor of surgical hair clippers that do not abrade the skin. A reliable intravenous line is established in the preparation area, preferably ipsilateral to the implant site, and intravenous fluids administered for hydration. Mild preprocedural sedation [e.g. 5–10 mg of diazepam (Valium) and 25–50 mg of diphenhydramine (Benadryl), orally] may be given in the preparation area. Sedation is usually augmented by intravenous sedatives/analgesics during the procedure (e.g. 0.5–1 mg of midazolam, 25–50 μg of fentanyl) as needed.

Care should be taken not to oversedate patients, especially the elderly. Drugs to reverse sedation should be readily available: intravenous flumazenil in 0.2-mg increments reverses midazolam; intravenous naloxone in 0.2-mg increments reverses fentanyl and other opiates. For particular patients (such as children or adults with significant cardiopulmonary or neurological comorbidities), general anesthesia may be needed and should be arranged in advance.

Patient preparation

On entering the procedure room, the patient is placed supine on the fluoroscopy table in such a way as to facilitate access to the specific operative site. Physiological monitoring (ECG, automated blood pressure, and pulse oximetry) should be quickly established so that rhythm disturbances may be detected and treated. The operative site is thoroughly prepared with an antiseptic solution (usually chlorhexidine or iodine based), which is allowed to dry, and a plastic adhesive sterile field is applied. Disposable towels and drapes are applied to provide a large sterile workplace and to minimize the risk of accidental contamination. A separate adhesive plastic pocket is affixed to the lateral aspect of the procedure site to collect draining fluid and sponges. A sterile plastic cover is placed over the image intensifier and the leaded glass shield (if used) to avoid inadvertent contamination of the sterile field during the procedure.

Implant procedure

Site

Access to the right heart for permanent pacing has been achieved by introducing leads into several veins, including the subclavian, cephalic, internal or external jugular, and iliofemoral. Typically, the choice of venous entry site determines where the generator will be placed, although lead extenders can be used when necessary to allow for remote positioning of the device. In most cases, a cephalic, axillary, or subclavian vein is used, and the pacemaker is placed subcutaneously in the adjacent infraclavicular region. On occasion, however, the generator may be implanted under the pectoral muscle or in an abdominal position. For women in whom there is a concern about cosmetic appearance, an inframammary incision may be performed and the pacemaker placed under the breast. In such circumstances, it may be prudent to enlist the assistance of a plastic surgeon. Patients should be advised that such remote generator implantation sites may make any future lead revisions and generator changes more complicated procedures and also adversely affect the accuracy of future breast cancer screening imaging tests.

The site of implantation is influenced by the factors listed in Figure 5.2. Most often the left side is chosen because most patients are right-handed and there is a less acute angle between the left subclavian and the innominate vein than exists on the right side. A disadvantage of using the left side is the small (0.3–0.5%) incidence of a persistent left SVC with drainage into the CS, which complicates lead positioning. Suspicion of this anomaly may be raised by finding greater distension and a double *a* wave in the left jugular vein compared with that of the right vein, a left paramediastinal venous crescent on the chest radiograph, and an enlarged CS on echocardiography. Contrast echocardiography or venography will confirm the diagnosis.

Although both single-chamber ventricular and dual-chamber systems have been placed through a persistent left SVC via the CS [22], it is preferable to approach implantation from the right side when this anomaly exists (Figure 5.3). Rarely, there is a coexistent absence of the right SVC with all brachiocephalic flow entering into the CS. Such a condition should be excluded before implantation is attempted from the right side in patients with a persistent left SVC. The increasing experience with pacing from the coronary venous system, coupled with the relative ease of entering these vessels in the case of persistent left SVC, suggests that this is a reasonable alternative in the latter patients. Other options for patients with anomalous venous drainage include an iliofemoral approach or an epicardial implantation, which now may be performed through a subxiphoid or thoracoscopic approach.

Venous access

Figure 5.4 illustrates the two major easily identifiable landmarks (clavicle and deltopectoral groove) for implantation in a left infraclavicular site.

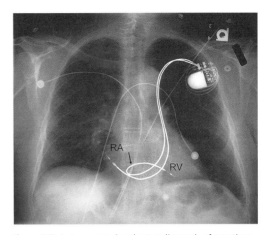

Figure 5.3 Anteroposterior chest radiograph of a patient with a dual-chamber pacemaker placed through a congenital persistent left superior vena cava. Given the circuitous course of the ventricular lead (arrow), long lead lengths are sometimes needed to reach the right ventricle. RA, right atrial lead; RV, right ventricular lead.

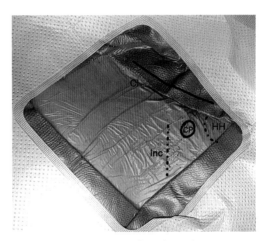

Figure 5.4 Surface landmarks from the implanter's perspective in a patient who is about to undergo a left-sided pacemaker implantation. The important skeletal landmarks include the clavicle (Cl, straight line), the head of the humerus (HH, dashed line), and the coracoid process (CP). These should be palpated as the incision line and pocket position is considered. The dashed line (Inc) indicates the planned incision line that runs parallel to the deltopectoral groove (about 1 cm medial). Access to the subclavian, axillary, and cephalic veins is possible from this region. The cephalic vein runs in the deltopectoral groove just inferior and medial to the CP.

Venous access into either the axillary/subclavian or cephalic vein is usually achieved through an incision that will also serve as the portal for subcutaneous generator placement. Local anesthetic is injected through a small-gauge needle along a line 4–6 cm long and two fingerbreadths below and parallel to the clavicle. If the cephalic vein is used, the incision begins about 0.5 cm lateral to the deltopectoral groove and is extended medially; otherwise, the incision may be placed just medial to the groove. This method provides adequate exposure for access to either the subclavian or cephalic vein.

Some operators begin with a smaller incision specifically located to achieve venous access, after which the incision is extended or a new one is made for the pocket. This is necessary when a supraclavicular approach to the subclavian vein or a jugular venous access is contemplated. In the latter situations, the leads are tunneled over the clavicle to the generator, which is placed in the usual ipsilateral infraclavicular position.

Pacing leads may be introduced through a venotomy in an exposed vein (cephalic, jugular, iliofemoral) or venous access may be achieved using the Seldinger technique. The latter approach provides easy access to a relatively large central vein, obviating the need for surgical dissection. In addition, the use of the dilator-sheath technique facilitates the introduction of multiple large leads and provides a means (via a retained guidewire) to reenter the venous system should that be necessary. Nevertheless, the subclavian puncture poses the risk of injury to nearby structures, including the artery, lung, thoracic duct, and nerves, and it is sometimes the most hazardous part of the implantation procedure. Forces exerted on leads in this position may predispose them to insulation failure and/or conductor fracture (Figure 5.5) due to crush injury.

Axillary vein approach

Adverse consequences of subclavian lead placement have led to the development of techniques to access the axillary vein instead. This method appears to be safe and effective and it is more likely to be successful than cephalic vein cut-down [23].

The introduction of the peel-away sheath has provided an effective means for the insertion of permanent pacemaker leads, and this method is now the most frequently used. The efficacy and safety of axillary and subclavian entry are increased by taking measures to distend the vein (proper hydration, leg elevation) and place it in the proper position (by placing a wedge under the patient's

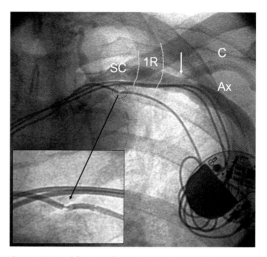

Figure 5.5 Lead fracture from "subclavian crush" seen on fluoroscopy during left arm venography. The fractured lead (dotted circle) was placed through a venous access point in the subclavian vein (SC) medial to the first rib (1R, outlined with dotted lines). The other two leads, placed more laterally in the left axillary vein (Ax), are intact. Note that the cephalic vein (C) joins the axillary vein lateral to the first rib (arrow); leads placed in the cephalic vein are generally immune from this risk. (*Inset*) Complete disruption of the insulation and outer conductor coil, and stretching of the inner conductor coil, of the fractured lead.

shoulders and by adduction of the ipsilateral upper extremity).

We find ipsilateral upper extremity contrast venography to be helpful in demonstrating patency of the vessel, ruling out any anomaly which would preclude access, and providing a "road map" for using the axillary access technique. Adequate opacification of the axillary/subclavian vein is achieved by the injection of a bolus of 10–20 mL of iodinated contrast through a large-bore cannula in an ipsilateral arm vein. This should be followed immediately by injection of a saline "chaser" to hasten the transit of the contrast solution. The amount of fluid and rate of injection are gauged by fluoroscopic observation of the course of dye into the central veins. It is important that sufficient contrast be used and that adequate time be given for the contrast to fill the subclavian vein or collateral vessels. If the vessel is patent, there is often enough lingering contrast to allow an exploring needle to be directed at it.

Our current practice is to use a smaller gauge micropuncture system for all percutaneous vascular access; this system is safer and usually less painful (Figure 5.6). The micropuncture needle, attached to a 10-mL syringe containing a few milliliters of local anesthetic or saline, is introduced through an incision that has been dissected to the underlying prepectoral fascia. The needle enters the pectoral muscle with the access needle just medial to the coracoid process on anteroposterior fluoroscopy. If a submuscular pocket is to be used, it is best to access the vein through the floor of the pocket with

the needle. This will prevent excessive angulation of the leads between the access site and the pocket. Through the floor of the submuscular pocket, the axillary vein may be extremely shallow, and care is needed to avoid entry into the pleural space or lung. The needle is then directed under fluoroscopy to the point at which the lateral border of the first rib appears to cross the inferior margin of the clavicle (Figure 5.7). The needle approach is angulated to a degree such that the first rib is struck with the

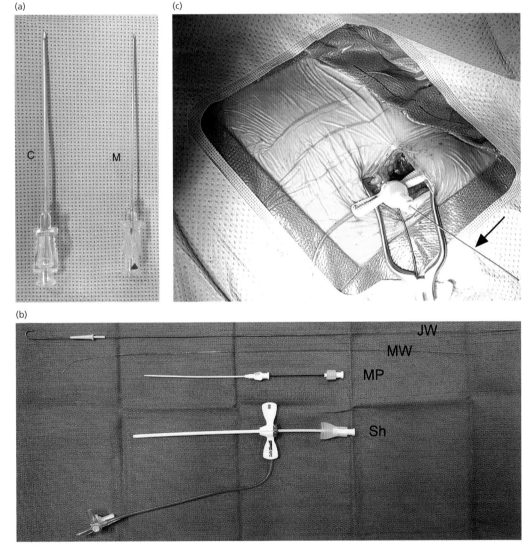

Figure 5.6 Micropuncture technique for vascular access. (a) 18-G micropuncture needle (M) is compared with a standard 21-G Cook needle (C). (b) Other components of the access equipment, including the valved peel-away sheath (Sh), standard 0.035 J-wire (JW), the 0.018 micropuncture wire (MW), and the 5.0-Fr micropuncture sheath/dilator assembly (MP). (c) The valved peel-away sheath is placed over the standard wire (arrow).

(a)

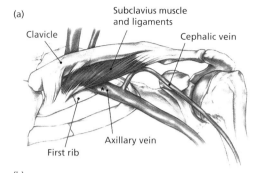

(b)

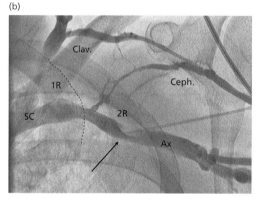

Figure 5.7 (a) Anatomy of the subclavian venous system and skeletal landmarks relevant to percutaneous access. The subclavius muscle and costoclavicular ligament complex are shown between the clavicle and first rib. Accessing the subclavian vein medially requires the lead to pass through these structures. This may be associated with a higher risk of lead fracture due to compressive forces on the lead. By accessing the cephalic vein or axillary vein (*) extrathoracically, the problems of lead entrapment are eliminated. (b) Fluoroscopic guidance for the introducer needle into the axillary vein. The peripheral venogram delineates the axillary vein (Ax) as it crosses the first rib (1R, dotted line) in anteroposterior projection. The introducer needle is seen indenting the axilllary vein (arrow) just before puncture over the second rib (2R) at a site that is far outside the thoracic cage. Ceph., cephalic vein; Clav., left clavicle; SC, subclavian vein.

needle if the vein is not entered. By walking the needle up and down the first rib on repeated passes, the axillary vein is eventually entered. Small amounts of anesthetic may be injected along this course. Negative pressure is exerted on the syringe as the needle is advanced so that blood is aspirated on entry into the vein.

After advancement, the needle should not be redirected; doing so may lacerate underlying structures. If venous entry is not obtained, the needle should be withdrawn, cleared of any obstructing

tissue, and reinserted in a slightly different direction. Inadvertent arterial entry is apparent with the appearance of pulsatile bright-red blood. Prompt withdrawal of the needle and compression at its entry site is usually all that is necessary to obtain hemostasis. Repeated unsuccessful attempts to enter the vein suggest a deviation in anatomy or occlusion of the vessel. In either situation, the risk of complication is increased with additional blind needle insertions. At this point one should consider a repeat contrast injection to determine vessel patency and to provide an updated road map.

On successful entry of the needle into a vessel, the character of the aspirated blood is examined. Dark non-pulsatile flow suggests a venous location; however, non-pulsatile flow does not exclude arterial entry, and pulsatile flow is sometimes noted from a vein (e.g. tricuspid regurgitation, right heart failure, cannon waves). Once vascular access is achieved, the syringe is detached (taking care to prevent air from entering the venous system) and a micropuncture wire is inserted through the needle and advanced under fluoroscopy to the inferior vena cava (IVC). If this is accomplished, inadvertent aortic entry is precluded; merely observing the guidewire coursing to the right of the sternum or even into a ventricular chamber does not exclude its presence in a tortuous ascending aorta or its passing retrograde into the left ventricle. It is critically important that entry into the proper venous structure is confirmed prior to advancing a dilator or sheath over the wire.

If resistance to advancement of the guidewire is encountered, the guidewire should be withdrawn through the needle with great care to prevent shearing off the distal wire by the needle tip. If any difficulty is encountered with withdrawal, both the wire and needle should be withdrawn together or, if enough wire has been passed into the vein, the needle may be withdrawn and a small-lumen plastic catheter advanced over the wire and into the vein. In the latter situation, contrast may then be injected through the catheter to identify the problem and a more torqueable wire capable of being directed appropriately can be introduced.

After the micropuncture wire has been properly placed, a 4- or 5-Fr micropuncture dilator is placed over the wire and the wire withdrawn, taking care to avoid entry of air into the vasculature. A standard

J-wire or glidewire is then placed through the micropuncture dilator and passed into the IVC. The access procedure may be repeated for as many leads as will be implanted during the procedure. Some operators prefer to use a single access site and retain the guidewire throughout the case. Although this potentially reduces the risk of vascular injury or pneumothorax, this approach may create problems with lead–lead interaction during positioning within the heart.

Once the guidewire is positioned in the IVC, a commercially available peel-away sheath–dilator combination (6–9 Fr, depending on lead size) may be advanced over the wire into the SVC, which will provide access for the introduction of pacing leads. Advancement of the device under the clavicle may be facilitated by torqueing it as if it were being screwed into place. Considerable resistance may be encountered if the subclavian vein has been entered medially through a fibrous or calcified ligament. Entrance into such a location may be a marker for future lead entrapment; thus, one may consider seeking a more lateral entry site. If the site is retained, the use of a stiffer guidewire may be advantageous in such a situation, as may the passage of initially small, then progressively larger dilators. Excessive force should not be necessary once the sheath has entered the vein. Fluoroscopic confirmation of proper alignment of dilator and wire is necessary if resistance is encountered. On occasion, countertraction on the wire while advancing the dilator is helpful. The sheath should not be allowed to slide over the tapered tip of the dilator, nor should the dilator be unprotected by a guidewire at any time during advancement.

Once it is properly positioned in the SVC, the dilator is removed while the guidewire is retained within the sheath to allow for the introduction of a second sheath if necessary. A clamp should be applied to the end of the guidewire to prevent its accidental migration into the vein. If possible, the patient should not be heavily sedated and should be instructed to avoid deep inspiration during this process. Deep breathing, and particularly snoring, greatly increases the chance of significant air embolus through an unvalved sheath. The use of peel-away sheaths with hemostatic valves is helpful in limiting bleeding and preventing air embolism, and should be used whenever possible.

The pacing lead is introduced carefully to avoid kinking the tip and advanced into the right atrium or IVC, at which time the sheath is withdrawn and peeled apart proximal to the venous entry site to prevent injury to the vessel. Some operators prefer to retain the sheath until the lead is placed in its final position in the heart. If a dual-chamber device is to be employed, the retained wire or a second access wire is used to introduce a second sheath. If only one lead is to be used, it may be helpful to retain one guidewire so that venous reentry is facilitated.

Cephalic vein approach

The cephalic vein resides in the sulcus between the deltoid and pectoral muscles. This area is readily identified by palpation and is occupied by loose connective tissue and fat, which are easily separated to reveal the underlying vein that sometimes lies fairly deep in this groove. The consistent course of this vessel, its reasonable size, and the direct path it takes to the central venous system make it useful for transvenous lead placement. On occasion, however, this vessel is small, consists of a plexus of tiny veins rather than a larger single channel, or takes a circuitous route to the subclavian vein. These conditions may make lead insertion difficult or impossible. In addition, the occasional difficulty in inserting two leads into the cephalic vein may limit the opportunity of using this approach for multilead systems in some patients.

The vein is isolated along a 1–2-cm length within the groove and ligated distally with a silk suture (Figure 5.8). A ligature is looped but not tightened around the proximal aspect of the vein for hemostasis. The vein is entered by venotomy using a straight blade, iris scissors or direct needle puncture. Using a vein pick, the tip of a 4- or 5-Fr dilator is placed in the venotomy and used to guide a floppy or hydrophilic-coated wire to secure access. Use of an angled glidewire with a torquing tool can be particularly helpful in negotiating the junction between the cephalic and axillary veins, which may form an acute angle in some patients, taking the wire peripherally down the arm rather than centrally to the thorax. A dilator–introducer sheath combination may then be used as described previously for the retained wire method in the subclavian approach.

(a)

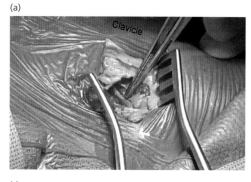

(b)

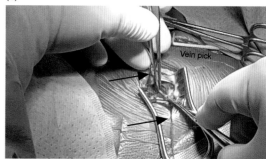

(c)

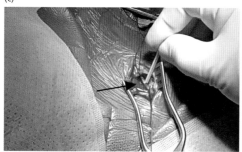

(d)

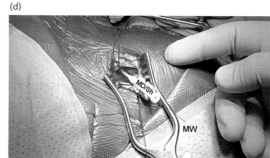

Figure 5.8 Surgical access to the left cephalic vein at pacemaker implant. (a) The incision has been carried down to the pectoralis fascia and cephalic vein dissected (marked by the tip of the forceps). (b) Ligatures are placed in the proximal (top arrow) and distal end (bottom arrow) of the dissected vein and venotomy is made in the superior wall of the vein with an iris scissor. (c) Vein pick (arrow) is placed into the incision to help with insertion of the lead directly or first inserting a J-wire (see Online Video 5.1 for failed direct lead implant due to venospasm) or (d) micropuncture wire and sheath may be used to gain central access in challenging cases due to tortuous vein or venospasm. MW, micropuncture wire; MD/Sh, micropuncture dilator/sheath assembly. Source: courtesy of Jose Huizar MD.

The greatest benefit of the cephalic approach is its margin of safety compared with that of the axillary/subclavian puncture – there is almost no risk of pneumothorax or hemothorax. Although the cephalic vein itself is often sacrificed by this hybrid procedure, there is rarely any clinical consequence. In either case, the guidewire provides virtually unlimited access to the central venous system. Tearing of the vein may result in significant bleeding from tributaries into the pocket, which may be controlled with a pursestring suture around the venous access site.

Rarely, the cephalic vein takes an aberrant course or a pectoral vein is inadvertently accessed. In such cases the guidewire may easily enter the subclavian vein, but it may not be possible to manipulate a sheath over the wire successfully, which necessitates abandoning the technique and sacrificing the vein. In other cases, the vein may spasm or invaginate by passage of the sheath, essentially grasping it and preventing its advancement or removal. Application of a vasodilator (e.g. nitroglycerin) or actually cutting the constricting vein, exposed by pulling back on the dilator, may be necessary to insert the sheath fully. Despite these potential limitations of the cephalic technique, an experienced operator can successfully implant leads by this approach in most cases when it is attempted.

Subclavian vein approach

Despite widespread use in the past, the subclavian vein approach should be used rarely in favor of the axillary and cephalic access methods already described. On occasion, when these two methods are unsuccessful, the traditional subclavian vein approach may be required and so it is described further.

Preparation of the patient is similar to that for the axillary vein approach. Contrast venography through the ipsilateral arm may be helpful to assure patency of the vein and to define its anatomical course, which may vary in different patients. Temporarily raising the patient's legs on a wedge may help to distend the vein and make puncture easier. The patient's arm should be pulled caudally to flatten the clavicle and minimize "hunching" of the shoulders.

The access needle, attached to a 10-mL syringe containing a few milliliters of local anesthetic or saline, is introduced through an incision that has been bluntly dissected to the underlying pre-pectoral fascia. The tip of the needle is advanced, bevel down, along this tissue plane at the level of the junction of the medial and middle thirds of the clavicle, and directed toward a point just above the sternal notch. The appropriate point to meet the clavicle is at the angle evident on palpation or fluoroscopy. On reaching the clavicle, the needle's angle of entry with respect to the thorax is increased until the tip slips under the bone. Alternatively, the needle is marched anterior to posterior along the clavicle using the thumb of the non-dominant hand to depress the needle or barrel of the syringe. Once under the clavicle, the needle and syringe should be maintained parallel to the floor; this prevents the needle from plunging ever more posteriorly as the needle is advanced. Negative pressure is exerted on the syringe as the needle is advanced so that blood is aspirated upon entry into the vein. Once under the clavicle, the needle should not be redirected; doing so may lacerate underlying structures. If venous entry is not obtained, the needle should be withdrawn, cleared with saline, and reinserted in a slightly different direction. The subclavian artery is cranial and posterior to the subclavian vein. Entry into the subclavian artery should lead to appropriate adjustments in the needle's trajectory. In addition, crossing under the clavicle from too lateral a position will often result in arterial access.

Once venous entry is assured, a J-wire or glidewire is passed and the procedure continued as described for axillary vein access.

Pacemaker pocket

The pacemaker is usually placed in a subcutaneous position near the site of venous entry. Generators have continued to decrease in size and can be placed easily in most patients, including those having a paucity of subcutaneous tissue. Most often, the device is placed in the infraclavicular area

through the incision used to obtain venous access. Local anesthesia is applied to the subcutaneous tissue, which is then dissected down to the pre-pectoral fascia. The pocket should be created in the plane just above this fascial layer and below the subcutaneous fat. Placing the pocket too superficially in a subcuticular pocket may lead to erosion or to a pain syndrome requiring reoperation.

A pocket directed inferomedially over the pectoral fascia and large enough to accommodate both the generator and redundant lead is made in this tissue plane by a combination of electrocautery and blunt dissection. Too small a pocket may result in tension exerted on the overlying tissue by the implanted hardware; too large a pocket invites future migration or "flipping over" of the generator. Augmentation of sedation with a rapidly acting parenteral agent is recommended during the brief time it takes for pocket creation, because this is usually the most painful part of the procedure. Attention to hemostasis is necessary, but significant bleeding rarely accompanies blunt dissection and electrocautery in the proper tissue plane. Stripping away the pectoral fascia during the dissection often leads to excessive bleeding from the denuded muscle, especially in patients taking antiplatelet agents. On completion of its formation, the pocket may be flushed with saline or antibacterial solution and temporarily packed with radiopaque sponges. All sponges used in this fashion should be accounted for in order to avoid leaving one in the pocket. Even a radiopaque sponge may be missed by fluoroscopy if it is under the generator and only casual observation is made. The use of oversized laparotomy sponges that cannot be concealed in the pocket may also avoid this problem.

In some circumstances (e.g. sparse subcutaneous tissue, large generator, impending erosion from a previous device, concerns about cosmetic appearance) the generator may be placed subpectorally or under the breast [24]. These procedures should be planned ahead of time with the assistance of appropriate personnel (e.g. a plastic surgeon) as needed. The subpectoral site is best accessed by dissecting the natural plane between the pectoralis major and minor muscles. This plane is identified by blunt dissection in the deltopectoral groove and carried inferiorly and medially. Alternatively, a muscle-splitting incision can be made in the body of the pectoralis major itself. When used, the subpectoral location should be noted in the operative report for reference for future revisions or generator changes.

A pocket located at a distance from the site of lead insertion requires that the leads (with or without extenders) be tunneled through subcutaneous tissue to its location.

Lead implantation

A variety of leads are available for endocardial placement. They differ in composition, shape, electrode configuration, and method of fixation. Passive fixation leads have tines that anchor them in the trabeculated right ventricle or atrial appendage. Active fixation leads employ a helix as the mechanism for fixing them to the endocardium. The helix may be extendable and retractable, or may be permanently fixed at the tip. In some lead models, the fixed helix is covered with an absorbable agent to facilitate passage of the lead to its site of implantation, by which time absorption of the material exposes the helix and allows it to be fixed to the heart. In general, leads with extendable–retractable helices are easier to implant and easier to remove if necessary.

Both active and passive fixation leads have advantages and disadvantages (Table 5.2) and may be used for either atrial or ventricular placement. Steroid-eluting passive fixation leads may offer some benefit in terms of lowered subacute and possibly chronic thresholds. Despite the progress in lead designs and their overall excellent performance, the failure over

Table 5.2 Lead characteristics

Active fixation lead
Easy passage
Low acute dislodgement rate
Unrestricted positioning
Easier removal of chronic implant
Higher capture thresholds

Passive fixation lead
Greater electrode variety
Lower thresholds
More difficult passage
More difficult chronic removal
Higher early dislodgement rate

time of several models of these devices remains a cause for concern [25,26].

Before their introduction, leads should be inspected for anomalies. Proper sheath selection should be made to allow passage of the lead and, if used, the retained guidewire. Active fixation leads should be tested on a clean surface to ensure that the helix extends and retracts appropriately. The connector pin of the lead should be appropriate for the selected pulse generator. For the past 25 years, the IS-1 pin connector system has been used almost exclusively for new bipolar atrial and RV pacing leads. Multipolar LV leads use the IS-4 connection, adapted by all manufacturers as industry standard. High-voltage leads may be designed with DF-1 or DF-4 connector. Attention to these details are especially important during planning for generator change to assure that the device with the right type of header is available for the procedure. Lead designs are further discussed in Chapter 2. The suture sleeve should be positioned at the proximal portion of the lead and prevented from migrating distally during lead placement.

Stylets of varying length and stiffness are used to manipulate and steer the lead in the body. Stylets should be kept clean and dry to facilitate insertion and withdrawal from the lead. Torque applied to a shaped stylet will help rotate the lead to its desired location. Steerable stylets are now available that allow for *in situ* alteration of the degree of curve they provide to the lead tip, which may facilitate atrial placement or selective-site ventricular lead placement. One 4-Fr lead model has no central lumen for a stylet and uses a steerable sheath system for implantation.

Leads are usually inserted through a valved peel-away sheath. Care should be taken to avoid damaging the lead tip when pushing it through the valve. The central venous system is usually traversed easily and the lead advanced to the low right atrium or IVC. On occasion there may be difficulty in advancing the lead through a kink in the sheath or through tortuous central vasculature. Withdrawing the sheath slightly, advancing the retained guidewire along with the lead, and sometimes withdrawing the stylet to soften the lead tip may prove helpful in these situations. When tortuous or stenosed central vasculature is encountered, a long sheath may be required for passage of the lead into the heart.

Although the retained-guidewire approach facilitates the insertion of the two leads required for dual-chamber pacing, manipulation of one lead may affect the position of the other, especially when silicone-coated leads are used. Some implanters consider that two independent sheaths should be used and not withdrawn until both leads have been positioned, or that separate venous sites (e.g. cephalic and axillary or two separate axillary entry sites) be accessed for each lead. If necessary, however, two leads may usually be inserted and positioned through the same access site by using the retained-guidewire technique. Good fluoroscopic imaging is key to successful lead implantation, and care should be taken always to image the tip of any lead as it is advanced, and with any lead manipulation in the heart. Slight withdrawal of the stylet while advancing the lead decreases the chance of mechanical trauma by the lead tip.

Ventricular lead positioning

In dual-chamber systems, the RV lead is usually positioned first because it may supply back-up pacing, its position is usually more stable than that of the atrial lead, and it is usually the most important of the leads. LV lead placement is described in Chapter 9.

Once the RV lead has been advanced to the low right atrium or IVC, the straight stylet is withdrawn a few inches to allow the lead tip to catch in the right atrium; further advancement of the lead will cause its distal portion to form a J shape, which may then be rotated toward the tricuspid valve (Figure 5.9a–f). Slight retraction results in prolapse into the right ventricle, at which time the lead can be either advanced into the pulmonary artery or directed down toward the apex by advancing the stylet while the lead is slowly pulled back. Prolapsing the lead into the right ventricle ensures that the lead is not in the CS and is not passing through the tricuspid valve apparatus. Entry into the pulmonary artery confirms that the lead has traversed the right ventricle and is neither in the atrium nor in the CS. The lead may then be pulled back as the stylet is advanced. Tined leads may become readily entangled with the tricuspid apparatus when prolapsed across the valve. Directly steering these leads through the valve may be necessary.

Once the lead tip falls toward the apex, the lead is advanced into place. This maneuver is often accompanied by ventricular ectopy, the absence of which suggests that the lead may not be in the ventricle. An alternative method of gaining entry to the right ventricle is to form the stylet into a dogleg or a J shape and to use it to direct the lead across the tricuspid valve or to facilitate prolapsing the lead from the right atrium. Once it is in the right ventricle, the shaped stylet may be replaced with a straight one to facilitate positioning at the apex. The proper fluoroscopic appearance of the RV apical lead is one in which the lead's tip is to the left of the spine and is pointing anteriorly and slightly caudal (Figure 5.9g,h). Visualization of the lead in multiple planes should be performed to confirm appropriate location of the lead.

For the patient with LBBB or AV block with a ventricular escape mechanism, special care needs to be taken when crossing the tricuspid valve to avoid bumping the right bundle branch if no temporary pacing wire is in place. The transient block in conduction may result in prolonged asystole and even death if temporary pacing cannot be quickly established. In these situations, less experienced operators may wish to place a temporary pacing wire at the outset of the procedure to avoid this complication.

In the anteroposterior projection it may not be possible to distinguish whether a lead is in a posterior coronary vein, the left ventricle, or the RV apex. Left oblique views and the 12-lead ECG pattern of ventricular activation (QRS morphology) during pacing are helpful in avoiding such lead misplacement. If a lead is inadvertently placed in the left ventricle, the paced QRS complex will usually show a right bundle branch block (RBBB) pattern, whereas positioning in the right ventricle will usually show a LBBB pattern. In patients with LV prominence and/or counterclockwise rotation of the heart, the lead tip may not appear to extend far enough to the left border of the cardiac silhouette. Imaging in the right anterior oblique (RAO) position may be helpful in such circumstances; observing the position of the lead with respect to the tricuspid valve allows an estimation of how far the lead projects into the right ventricle. Placement of the ICD lead is very similar to pacemaker lead placement but septal lead position (either in the

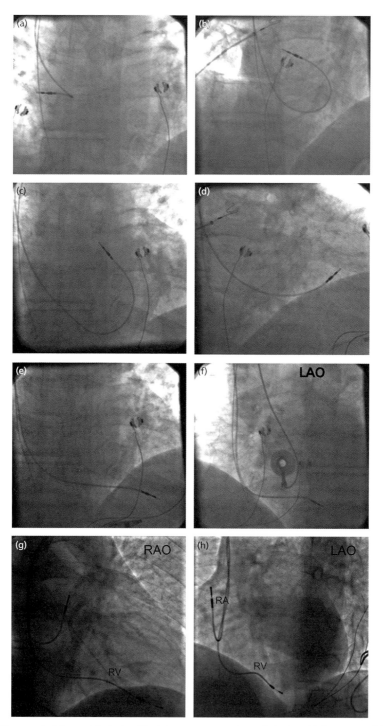

Figure 5.9 (a–f) Placement of the ventricular lead in right anterior oblique (RAO) views. (a) The lead forms a loop in the right atrium. (b) The lead is rotated and the loop advanced across the tricuspid valve. (c) The lead is advanced to pass the tip into the right ventricular outflow tract. (d) Changing from a curved to a straight stylet, the lead is withdrawn toward the apex. As the lead falls, it may be advanced slightly to engage positions suitable for septal pacing. (e) After the tip falls to the floor of the ventricle, the lead is advanced to its final position in the apex, as shown in RAO and left anterior oblique (LAO) views (f). (g) RAO and (h) LAO views of passive fixation right atrial (RA) and right ventricular (RV) apical lead positions at the time of implantation. The ventricular lead is positioned with the tip at the RV apex, well beyond the spine shadow, as shown here. The slight downward position of the tip is desirable. Some indentation of the ventricular lead at the level of the tricuspid valve is common. In LAO the lead lies against the ventricular septum. The atrial lead is positioned in the RA appendage.

apical or mid-septum) is important in order to maximize ICD shock efficacy. Pacing at 10-V output is performed to exclude diaphragmatic stimulation by the lead, which may indicate microperforation and should usually lead to repositioning of the lead.

Once the proper position has been confirmed, the active fixation mechanism, if present, should be deployed while viewed under magnified fluoroscopy. The stylet is then partly withdrawn and pacing parameters (R-wave size, pacing impedance, and capture threshold) are determined. High-output pacing is performed again. Once in place after stylet withdrawal and lead fixation, the tip should maintain a relatively stable position and not appear to bounce with cardiac contraction. A slight loop of lead (or "heel") should be retained in the right atrium to avoid tension at the tip during deep inspiration. Too large a loop may result in ectopy, lead dislodgement, or prolapse into the IVC, while too little slack in the lead creates a risk for dislodgement from mediastinal shift when the patient resumes upright posture and normal inspiration.

Although an apical RV lead position is usually preferred for reasons of stability, there are occasions when another location in the right ventricle is required (e.g. a retained ventricular lead, which might result in contact potentials). Efforts to obtain a more physiological activation sequence and a more efficient mechanical contraction from RV stimulation have led some investigators to advocate positioning the lead in the RV outflow tract (Figure 5.10), the interventricular septum (Figure 5.11) [27] or the His bundle region (discussed later). In these circumstances, the use of an active fixation lead is required. To place a lead in the outflow tract or septum, the lead is prolapsed into the pulmonary artery as described. By withdrawing the lead with a curved stylet and torque to drive the tip into the septum, the septum can be mapped and the lead fixed. The hemodynamic benefits of routinely seeking such a position compared with the stability of the traditional apical location are unproven [28], but this position may reduce the risk of free wall perforation and diaphragmatic stimulation when an active fixation lead is required.

When a reasonable position is obtained, preliminary measurements of the electrical parameters are made. This is usually accomplished with the stylet withdrawn about halfway so as not to interfere with the position of the lead tip and to facilitate movement of the lead body should that be necessary. When active fixation leads are used, such measurements may be taken before extensions of the helix, as a screen of the implant site prior to fixing the leads. If the parameters are not acceptable, an alternative position may be tried. Once a reasonable site is established, the helix is extended and the parameters remeasured. Failure to record a current of injury after deployment of active fixation leads suggests a potentially unstable lead position (Figure 5.12) [29].

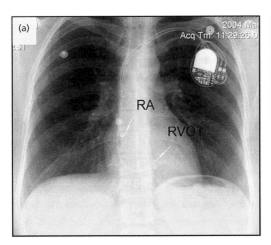
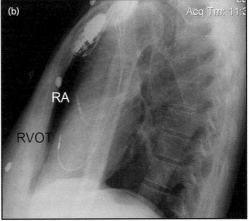

Figure 5.10 (a) Posteroanterior and (b) lateral chest radiographs of active fixation right atrial (RA) and right ventricular outflow tract (RVOT) lead positions after implantation. Stable ventricular lead placement in the RVOT usually requires an active fixation lead. The RA lead is in the right atrial appendage.

(a)

(b)

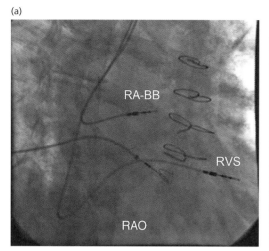

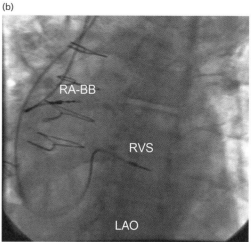

Figure 5.11 (a) Right anterior oblique (RAO) and (b) left anterior oblique (LAO) views of an atrial lead in the high right atrial septum (Bachmann's bundle) at the time of implant (RA-BB). Note that in the LAO view the lead tip is directed posteriorly as opposed to anteriorly for right atrial appendage positions (compare with Figure 5.8b). The unique position of the lead is difficult to appreciate in the RAO view. The ventricular lead (RVS) is fixed to the right ventricular septum.

(a)   (b)   (c)   (d)

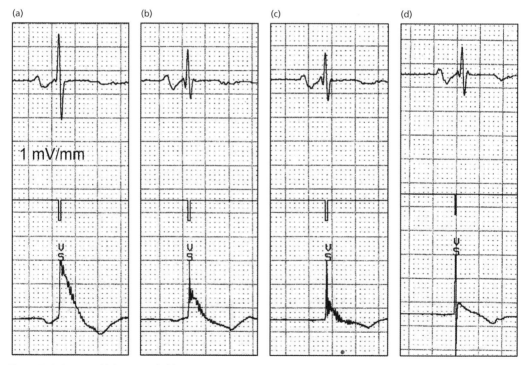

Figure 5.12 Current of injury recorded by a pacing system analyzer after extension of the helix of an active fixation ventricular lead. (a) Maximal injury current immediately after extension of the helix. (b,c) The current gradually decreasing over several minutes. (d) The final electrogram recorded through the pulse generator.

Table 5.3 Acceptable electrical parameters for new lead placement

Parameter	Atrium	Ventricle
Capture threshold[a]	<1.5 V	<1.0 V
Sensed P/R wave	>1.5 mV	>5.0 mV
Slew rate	>0.2 V/s	>0.5 V/s
Impedance	300–1000 Ω^b	300–1000 Ω^b

[a] At 0.5-ms pulse duration.

[b] High-impedance leads typically exceed these values; check with manufacturer for acceptable values.

Active fixation leads vary in the ways they interface with the heart; the helix may be electrically active, the distal ring electrode may be active, or both the helix and a distal ring electrode may be active. Adequate pacing characteristics may not be found immediately after extension of the helix: the screw may not have entered the myocardium, the site may be inadequate, or local tissue injury may have occurred due to entry of the helix. All lead positions should be confirmed by both left anterior oblique (LAO) and RAO views in the laboratory. It is common for capture thresholds and lead impedance to decrease significantly 15–30 min after active fixation.

Threshold parameters tested with a PSA define the electrical adequacy of lead position. This is accomplished using a set of connector cables, which can be configured for unipolar or bipolar leads. When testing unipolar leads, the anode is connected to tissue in the pacemaker pocket using a disk electrode or a clamp. Electrograms may be obtainable from the PSA or may be recorded using the chest (V) lead of a standard ECG machine. If satisfactory parameters (Table 5.3) are not obtained, alternative lead positions should be sought. It is important to confirm that diaphragmatic pacing does not occur by temporarily testing the lead at high-output energy (10 V).

Capture threshold may be influenced by a number of factors, including myocardial site, presence of infarction or scar, electrolyte disturbance, medications, and lead type. On occasion, optimal parameters may not be achieved, and acceptance of the best available position is necessary. However, because the short- and long-term success of the pacing system is related to the initial lead position, effort should be made to obtain the best possible initial location in terms of both stability and electrical performance. Rarely, a CS vein may prove the only site from which one may sense and/or pace the ventricle reliably [30].

Once acceptable lead parameters are obtained, the amount of lead slack should be adjusted, depending on the size of the patient. Taller and heavier patients will typically require greater lead redundancy to account for the mediastinal shift that will take place as the patient stands and inspires deeply. The lead stylet is then removed and the lead secured to the pectoral fascia with 2-0 or 0 non-absorbable suture (silk or equivalent). These sutures should be placed around a suture sleeve, and never directly to the lead insulation, which may fracture under this chronic stress.

Atrial lead implantation

The right atrial appendage has become the preferred implant site for atrial leads because of its trabeculated nature. Studies have shown that good pacing parameters may be obtained and maintained from this location. A number of studies have suggested that dislodgement is not more common with atrial leads, but reliance on an atrial appendage location may mandate the acceptance of less than ideal pacing characteristics that become unacceptable over time. Active fixation leads appear to be beneficial in this regard by allowing further exploration of the right atrium in the search for an optimal position. There is no evidence that the atrial stimulation site influences hemodynamics per se, although atrial septal pacing near Bachmann's bundle may be of some importance when atrial tachycardia algorithms are applied (see Figure 5.11). Trials of alternative or multisite right atrial pacing for prevention of atrial tachyarrhythmias have yielded mixed results.

A variety of leads (active, passive, J-shaped, straight) may be used for atrial pacing. When using active fixation leads, there are advantages and disadvantages to preformed devices. A straight active fixation lead may be easier to place in areas other than the appendage; however, dislodgement may result in the lead's falling into the right ventricle and causing competitive pacing or ectopy (Figure 5.13). The J-shaped active fixation lead may also be positioned almost anywhere in the atrium, but in some sites (e.g. the low atrium) its shape may cause undue tension at the site of

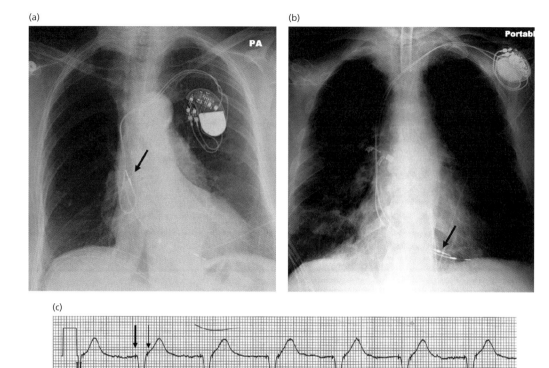

Figure 5.13 Posteroanterior radiographic views illustrating different patterns of atrial dislodgement. (a) This preformed atrial "J" lead was dislodged within 24 hours of implant and retracted into the superior vena cava (arrow), producing loss of atrial sensing and right phrenic nerve stimulation. (b) This straight active fixation lead was dislodged shortly after implantation into the right ventricle (arrow), resulting in the ECG (c) showing ventricular capture from the dislodged atrial lead (wide arrow) followed by ventricular pacing at the paced atrioventricular delay (thin arrow) without capture.

attachment to the endocardium, increasing the risk of dislodgement or cardiac perforation.

The atrial lead is inserted into the venous system with a straight stylet to facilitate negotiation of the central veins. Positioning in the atrial appendage is usually attempted first. The lead is directed toward the high anterior atrium and allowed to take its J shape either by withdrawing the straight stylet (in preformed leads) or by inserting a J stylet. Slow retraction of the preformed J-shaped lead results in the tip entering the appendage, where it will appear to catch and take on a characteristic to-and-fro motion with atrial activity (Figure 5.14). When it is well positioned, slight rotation of the lead should not dislodge the tip, and deep inspiration opens the curve to an L-shaped configuration but no further. In some patients the atrial appendage may be enlarged and trabeculae may be attenuated; in others who have received cardiopulmonary bypass,

the appendage may be oversewn. In these circumstances, placement of a passive fixation J lead may be difficult.

Although some implanters feel that previous cardiac surgery is a mandate for an active fixation atrial lead, others find passive fixation leads to be acceptable. We nearly always use active fixation atrial leads for patients with prior cardiac surgery. To place a lead on the atrial septum, allow the curve of the active fixation lead to form free in the body of the atrium and be directed anteriorly. Rotate the lead to the septum in the LAO view and pull the lead up until the roof of the atrium is encountered (see Figure 5.11). Opening the stylet to a curve of less than 180° facilitates reaching the septum.

Acceptable electrical parameters for atrial pacing are listed in Table 5.3. As seen when active fixation leads are used in the ventricle, there may be a significant improvement in the parameters during

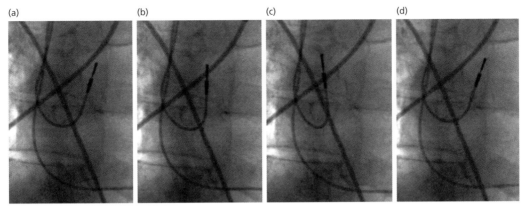

(a)   (b)   (c)   (d)

Figure 5.14 (a–d) Motion of an atrial lead placed in the right atrial appendage in a series of fluoroscopic views in the right anterior oblique projection. Typical lead motion through a single cardiac cycle is depicted.

the first 15–30 min. If borderline values are obtained initially, it may be worthwhile to perform serial measurements every 3–5 min. If poor values are obtained initially, however, it is best to search for a new position. The better the electrical characteristics, the more probable that long-term pacing will be successful. As with the ventricular lead, it is important to test for diaphragmatic pacing by temporarily stimulating the atrium at high output (10 V) and observing the right hemidiaphragm for phrenic nerve capture.

When acceptable parameters are obtained, the lead slack is adjusted, the stylet is removed, and the lead secured with non-absorbable suture. Final lead parameters are then obtained for both atrial and ventricular leads.

Epicardial lead placement

Permanent epicardial leads can be placed on the atria and ventricles at thoracotomy using a variety of surgical approaches. Newer steroid-eluting active fixation and atraumatic suture-on electrodes provide the best long-term thresholds [31]. However, chronic epicardial atrial lead performance remains problematic. These leads must be passed between or beneath the ribs and then tunneled subcutaneously to the pocket, potentially raising risk of lead fracture (Figure 5.15). In general, available epicardial lead systems demonstrate decreased longevity and worse chronic lead performance compared with endocardial pacing. Surgical epicardial placement of LV pacing leads may be needed in a small percent of patients to achieve biventricular pacing when the CS approach

is unsuitable due to unfavorable anatomy or refractory phrenic nerve stimulation. The minimally invasive thoracoscopic approach may often be employed [32].

Single-lead VDD pacing

The general principles of lead insertion are similar for the dual-chamber VDD systems that use specially arrayed proximal atrial sensing electrodes as well as a tip electrode to sense and pace the ventricle on a single lead. These devices may be useful for selected patients with AV block who have a normal sinus mechanism, because they obviate the need for a separate atrial lead. When used, it is important to have the atrial electrodes at an optimal position in the right atrium; one may have to choose among leads with varying distances between the tip and atrial electrodes. Care is necessary to ensure that there is a chronotropically intact sinus mechanism before implantation and that atrial activity is consistently sensed by the lead at implantation. Testing for atrial sensing during extremes of respiration and during cough is necessary. Although it may be necessary to accept low-amplitude P waves and program the device to a high atrial sensitivity, reasonable results have been reported over a moderately long follow-up period [33].

Inappropriate atrial sensing may become a problem for a significant proportion of patients implanted with single-lead VDD systems. Because atrial capture is rarely possible with VDD leads, the device provides only single-chamber VVI(R) function if the atrial rhythm slows below the lower rate limit and atrial undersensing occurs. Of course, the

(a)

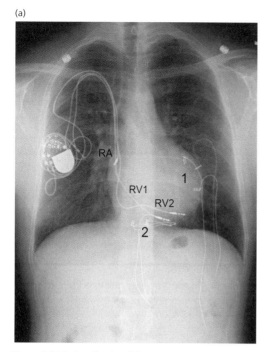

(b)

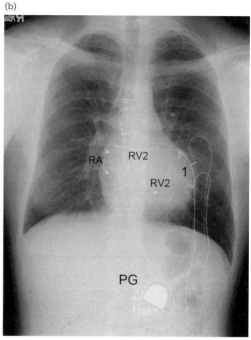

Figure 5.15 Series of epicardial pacing systems in a 34-year-old man who underwent his first pacemaker implantation at the age of 4 years due to acquired atrioventricular block. (a) Posteroanterior chest X-ray shows two sets of abandoned failed epicardial VVI systems (1 and 2). A right-sided dual-chamber transvenous system was later placed (RA and RV1). Failure of the first endocardial right ventricular (RV) lead led to its replacement (RV2). (b) Infection of the transvenous pacing leads led to complete surgical extraction of that system, followed by implantation of a third dual-chamber epicardial system, with bipolar right atrial (RA) and right ventricular (RV1 and RV2) leads tunneled to an epigastric pulse generator (PG). The second RV lead was capped for potential future use should the first lead fail. One of the old epicardial systems (2) was removed at the same operation.

VDD system is at a disadvantage if there is sinus node dysfunction, unless one is willing to sacrifice atrial synchronization and revert to VVI(R).

His bundle pacing

His bundle pacing (HBP) has recently emerged as an alternative to conventional RV pacing and, in some cases, cardiac resynchronization therapy (CRT) [34]. It has been applied successfully to patients with normal AV conduction, LBBB, and varying degrees of nodal and infra-nodal AV block [35]. The principal advantage of HBP is that it provides physiological activation of the ventricles through the normal His–Purkinje system and thereby prevents the electrical and mechanical dyssynchrony produced by other ventricular pacing methods. Disadvantages include the more challenging implantation technique, limited available leads and implantation equipment, higher acute

and chronic capture thresholds, and paucity of long-term follow-up and randomized controlled trial data (Table 5.4).

The only lead currently approved for HBP is the 3830 Select Secure MRI SureScan lead (Medtronic, Minneapolis, MN) (Figure 5.16). This lead has an outer diameter of 4.2 Fr with a 1.8-mm exposed, non-retractable active helix. The lead has a 69-cm solid core and has no lumen for stylets. It therefore requires use of a guiding catheter for placement. The two most commonly used outer guiding catheters are the C315His sheath and the C304-69 sheath (both Medtronic).

The C315His sheath (Figure 5.17) is 43 cm long with a fixed primary curve designed to reach the tricuspid valve region and a fixed secondary curve directed toward the septum. It has a 5.5-Fr inner diameter and 7.0-Fr outer diameter. The C304-69 sheath is deflectable with a single primary curve, an inner diameter of 5.7 Fr, and outer diameter of 8.4 Fr. The primary deflectable curve may be helpful in more challenging anatomical situations, such as a dilated right atrium, but the lack of a secondary septal curve is a disadvantage.

To implant a HBP lead, the patient is prepared with a 12-lead ECG set up through the electrophysiology (EP) recording system and prepared and draped in the usual fashion [36,37]. A diagnostic EP catheter may be placed in the His bundle region from a femoral vein in order to mark the target site

Table 5.4 Advantages and disadvantages of His bundle pacing

Advantages

- Normal activation of His–Purkinje system
- Avoidance of electrical and mechanical dyssynchrony
- Single ventricular lead versus RV and LV leads for cardiac resynchronization therapy
- May avoid tricuspid valve dysfunction

Disadvantages

- More difficult implantation technique
- Lower implant success rate, learning curve
- Limited available leads/implant equipment
- Higher acute/chronic pacing threshold
- Potential far-field P-wave oversensing/other programming challenges
- Little long-term follow-up/randomized controlled trial data

for pacing. Axillary or subclavian venous access is obtained in the usual way and a 7-Fr peel-away sheath is placed over the wire. The C315His sheath is then advanced over a long wire to the right atrium and the guidewire is then removed (Figure 5.18). The tip of the sheath will tend to then point toward the His bundle region, although some advancement and torquing may be required. The 3830 pacing lead is then advanced into the sheath until the helix is just inside the tip. Unipolar recording is then set up through the EP recording system or PSA and the helix is used to map the His bundle. Some further advancement and/or torquing of the sheath–lead combination may be required to identify a high-frequency His bundle recording (Figure 5.19a).

Once a suitable His bundle electrogram is recorded, usually with an atrial to ventricular ratio of 1 : 3 or smaller (smallest atrial signal to largest ventricular signal is desired), unipolar pacing is performed, typically starting with an output of 5 V/ms, and the paced 12-lead ECG is assessed for selective or non-selective His bundle capture (Figure 5.20). Selective His bundle capture is identified by a paced QRS identical to the native narrow QRS and a stimulus–QRS interval equal to the intrinsic His–ventricular (HV) interval. With non-selective His capture, a shorter stimulus–QRS interval and some fusion with local ventricular septal myocardial capture is apparent.

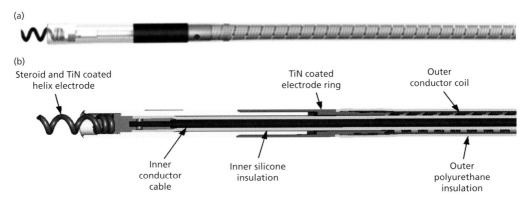

(a)

(b)

Steroid and TiN coated
helix electrode

TiN coated
electrode ring

Outer
conductor coil

Inner
conductor
cable

Inner silicone
insulation

Outer
polyurethane
insulation

Figure 5.16 MDT 3830 lead used for permanent His bundle pacing. (a) Photograph of the 3830 lead (Medtronic, Minneapolis, MN, USA). (b) Schematic overview of 3830 lead design. The bipolar lead has a 4.1-Fr outer diameter with a 1.8-mm fixed helix and a solid lumenless design. The inner cable conductor to the helix electrode is surrounded by a layer of silicone, which is surrounded by the outer conductor coil to the ring electrode. The outer insulation is polyurethane. Source: Reproduced with permission of Medtronic.

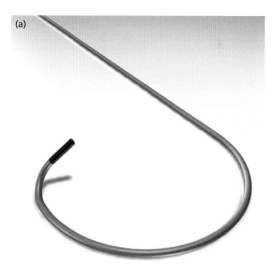
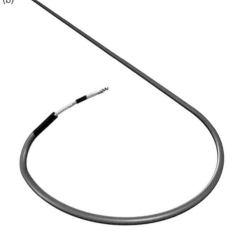

Figure 5.17 MDT C315His guiding catheter used for placing the 3830 lead in the His bundle position. (a) Photograph of the C315His guiding catheter (Medtronic, Minneapolis, MN, USA) showing fixed primary and secondary curves. The valved, braided, splittable catheter has a 7-Fr outer diameter, 5.4-Fr inner diameter, and 43-cm working length. (b) The C315His guiding catheter with the 3830 pacing lead positioned inside. Source: Reproduced with permission of Medtronic.

After a suitable paced QRS complex is identified, the lead is fixed by applying slow clockwise rotation to the lead approximately five times while holding the sheath steady with the left hand, with magnified fluoroscopy in the LAO position (Figure 5.21). As the lead is fixed, the operator should see the sheath pull back from the lead tip and feel some slight recoil of the lead toward the end of the fixation process. Once the helix is presumed to be fixed, the sheath is slowly pulled back while the lead is slightly advanced to allow a loop to form. Electrical recording is then repeated, which may show a His bundle injury current in about 50% of cases (see Figure 5.19b). Pacing is then performed in both unipolar and bipolar configurations looking for either selective or non-selective His bundle capture and a target threshold of 2 V/ms or less. If sensing or pacing parameters are unacceptable, the lead is unfixed through counterclockwise torque and the mapping and fixation process is repeated. If several attempts with the C315His sheath are unsuccessful, the 7-Fr peelaway introducer sheath may be replaced with a 9-Fr introducer sheath and the procedure repeated using the C304-HIS deflectable sheath.

Once an acceptable lead location has been found, the guiding sheath is split, the introducer sheath is peeled away, and the lead is secured to the pectoral fascia with 0 silk. Additional leads may then be placed in standard intracardiac locations as needed and the procedure is completed in the usual fashion (Figure 5.22). Final interrogation should be performed to assess for selective and non-selective His bundle capture threshold and final programming is performed, taking care to note some idiosyncrasies of programming for HBP leads [38].

Generator insertion

After the leads have been placed in acceptable positions, stability is confirmed with fluoroscopic observation during deep inspiration and cough. There should be enough intravascular lead to prevent undue tension at the tip with inspiration. The suture sleeve is carefully advanced distally, with care taken not to pull on the lead. The lead is tied down to the underlying muscle with two or three non-absorbable sutures. Sutures should never be tied around the unprotected lead; an excessively tight suture may compromise lead integrity even in the presence of a suture sleeve. However, the sutures should be tight enough to avoid lead migration. Electrical parameters and fluoroscopic position should be rechecked after suturing; if they are

(a)

(b)

(c)

(d)

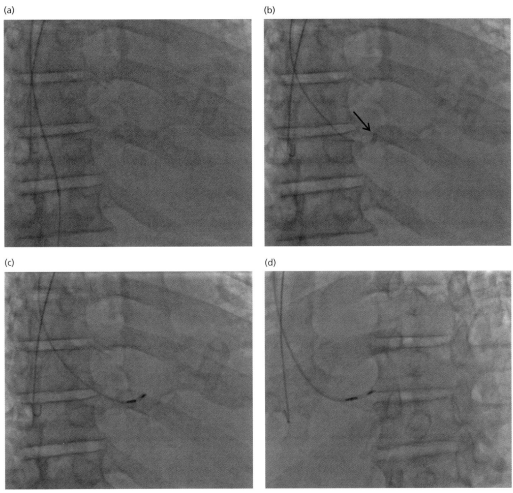

Figure 5.18 Stages of permanent His bundle pacing lead implantation I. (a) C315His sheath is placed over a wire. (b) As the wire and dilator are withdrawn, the C315His sheath primary and secondary curves form and position the tip of the sheath (arrow) near the septal tricuspid valve region. The 3830 lead is then inserted with helix at the tip ofb the sheath in right (c) and left (d) anterior oblique positions.

not optimal, the sutures may be removed and the lead repositioned.

Once the leads have been secured, any sponges that had been placed in the subcutaneous pocket are removed and the area is irrigated and checked for hemostasis and foreign matter. The pacemaker should be preprogrammed to the desired initial settings while still in its sterile package, after which it is given to the operator for implantation. For dual-chamber devices it is important that the atrial and ventricular leads be correctly identified and connected properly to the generator (Figure 5.23).

The lead pins should be cleaned and dried prior to insertion into the generator. The screwdriver should be inserted through the sealing plug over the screw to enhance air release ("burping") as the lead pin is inserted in order to minimize post-implant noise due to air. The distal connector pin of the lead should be seen to pass the set-screw(s) of the generator and remain there after tightening. Care should be taken that the screws are not over-torqued when tightened. A slight tug on the lead will confirm a tight connection. For in-line bipolar leads, both screws (when present) must be set correctly. Some pacemakers (i.e. unipolar) may not

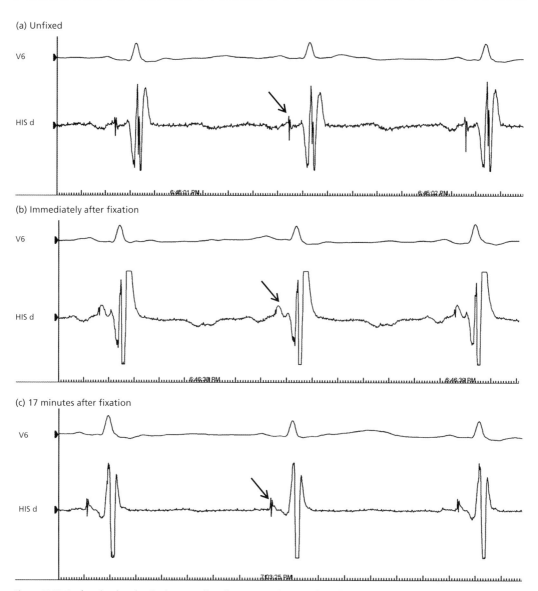

Figure 5.19 Surface lead and unipolar recording from the helix of the 3830 pacing lead at various stages of permanent His bundle pacing lead implantation. (a) Lead tip positioned in the His bundle region without fixation. Favorable characteristics include a prominent sharp His bundle electrogram (arrow) and very small atrial electrogram. (b) Immediately after lead fixation showing His bundle electrogram injury current. (c) Near 20 min after lead fixation, the His bundle current of injury is resolving.

function as programmed until the generator (functioning as the anode) is placed within the pocket.

The generator is carefully placed in the pocket, coiling redundant leads along the sides of the device or underneath it to avoid acute angulations. Extra leads should not be placed above the generator, as this will complicate generator replacement or lead revision in the future. We generally tie the generator down to the pectoralis fascia with a 0-silk suture through the tie-down hole in the header of the generator. This serves to limit migration of the generator and to defend against patient "twiddling" of the device (Figure 5.24). Once in place, evidence of proper pacemaker function should be observed, with placement of a sterile magnet or programming head if necessary. Fluoroscopic examination

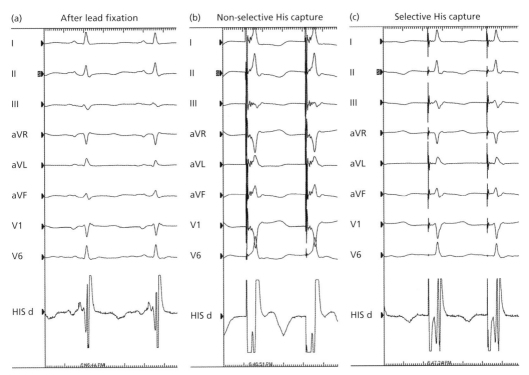

(a) After lead fixation (b) Non-selective His capture (c) Selective His capture

Figure 5.20 Surface ECG leads and His bundle recordings after lead fixation (a), pacing at 2 V/ms showing non-selective His capture, representing a fusion of His bundle and local ventricular myocardial capture (b), and pacing at 0.7 V/ms showing selective His capture, with QRS identical to sinus rhythm (c).

of the entire system should be performed before pocket closure.

The pocket is closed in two to three layers using 2-0 to 4-0 resorbable suture. Care must be taken to avoid piercing a lead with the suture needle. The skin edges may be approximated with skin sutures, resorbable subcuticular sutures, or surgical staples. A sterile dressing is then applied.

Before the patient leaves the pacemaker laboratory, the system is non-invasively interrogated to confirm adequacy of function and is programmed so that it temporarily overdrives the intrinsic heart rate. A 12-lead ECG is obtained to demonstrate the configuration of the paced rhythm, and then final programming of the pacemaker is performed.

In some centers, when the patient has reached the recovery room or the hospital floor, an over-penetrated anteroposterior chest radiograph is performed to document the lead position and the absence of a pneumothorax. In other centers, an immediate post-operative chest X-ray is not performed unless there is clinical suspicion of a complication. A sling may help

discourage excessive movement of the ipsilateral upper extremity during the first 12–24 hours. A thorough operative report should be generated immediately to include the manufacturer, model, and serial numbers of all hardware implanted, abandoned, or explanted, as well as any difficulties encountered during the case.

Revision of the implanted pacemaker system and pulse generator change

Revision of an implanted pacing system may involve replacement of the pulse generator, the pacing leads, or both (Figures 5.15 and 5.25). The uncomplicated generator change is usually a straightforward procedure; however, the preparation is in some ways more involved than for a new implant (Figure 5.26). The indication for generator change should be confirmed and documented, and the system evaluated non-invasively to identify any problems with the leads. In addition, pacemaker generator change provides an opportunity for the physician to evaluate the indications for pacing to

(a)

(b)

(c)

(d)

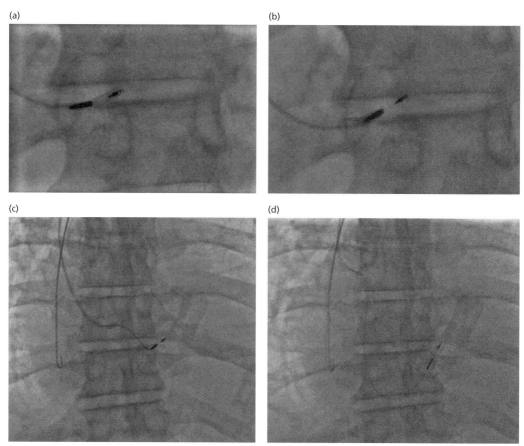

Figure 5.21 Stages of permanent His bundle pacing lead implantation II. (a) Beginning of 3830 lead fixation in the His bundle region in magnified left anterior oblique view. (b) Completion of lead fixation after five clockwise turns of the lead. Note that the tip of the sheath has been pushed back to the proximal electrode in the process. (c) After lead fixation, the guiding sheath is pulled back to form a loop of lead. (d) After satisfactory lead testing, the sheath is split, leaving the lead with suitable loop in the right atrium.

ensure that the existing hardware is appropriate for the patient's needs. In some cases, addition of atrial or LV pacing leads may be appropriate. In other cases, the patient may have developed an indication for revision of the system to an ICD.

For lead failure or system revision, the procedure itself is often more complex than a new implant (usually due to issues of venous access) and again requires preoperative investigation into the cause of the lead failure to prevent its recurrence. If a lead replacement is anticipated, the patency of the ipsilateral upper extremity venous system should be confirmed by venography. The decision to extract malfunctioning or abandoned leads should be made beforehand so that appropriate preparations can be made (see section Lead extraction). Even if the leads are known to function preoperatively, they may be damaged or found to be compromised on surgical exposure. Therefore, the patient and operator should be prepared for revision of any or all of the pacemaker leads at the time of generator replacement. One of the most critical aspects in preparing for a lead or generator change is ensuring mechanical and electrical compatibility between the new and retained components, as well as any new components that may be added to the system (Figure 5.26). Over the years, pacemaker systems have been manufactured with a variety of lead connector pins and generator header ports that may not be interchangeable. Currently, all new pacing systems conform to standard designs for these components (IS-1, IS-4 or DF-1

(a)

(b)

(c)

(d)

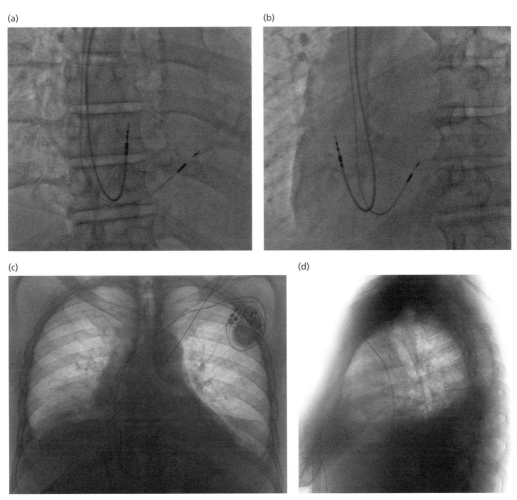

Figure 5.22 Stages of permanent His bundle pacing lead implantation III. Final position of right atrial and His bundle pacing leads in right (a) and left (b) anterior oblique views. Posteroanterior (c) and lateral (d) chest X-rays taken the following day show final lead positions. The pleural effusions (related to congestive heart failure) were present prior to the procedure.

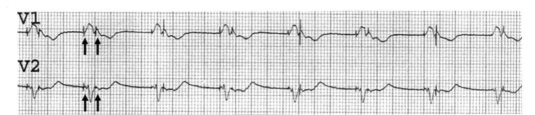

Figure 5.23 Continuous rhythm strip of a patient with a dual-chamber pacemaker in whom the leads were inadvertently reversed at the generator. There is atrioventricular sequential output from the generator (arrows) with the first stimulus capturing the ventricle and the second stimulus to the atrium occurring late in the QRS complex. This problem can be averted at implantation by double-checking appropriate lead placement in the header by serial number and documenting appropriate pacemaker activity prior to closing the pocket.

(a)

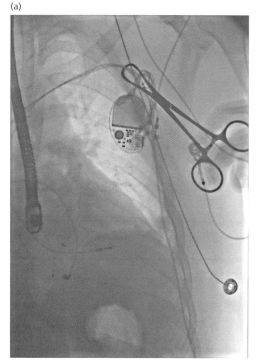

(b)

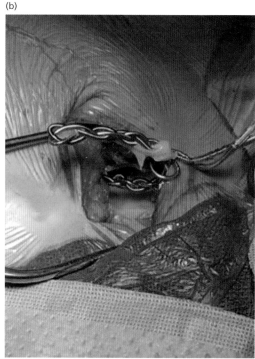

Figure 5.24 Preoperative X-ray (a) and photograph (b) obtained at the time of operative intervention to extract leads due to twiddler's syndrome. The lead can be seen to be tightly twisted upon itself. Although this tangle can be straightened, the stresses imparted to both the conductor and the insulation make it unsafe to reuse this lead. Source: courtesy of Richard Sheppard MD.

and DF-4 standard). Older systems may have pacemaker lead designs that are incompatible with new generators or have a serviceable generator that is not compatible with new leads.

During generator exchange or pacemaker revision surgery, particular care should be taken for sterility and infection prevention, as studies have shown higher rates of infection and other complications comparing with *de novo* CIED implantation. In addition, the clinical consequences of acute infection after generator exchange or system revision are usually greater, as lead extraction (rather than simple removal) is usually required. A recent randomized trial found that use of an antibacterial envelope in such procedures reduced the infection rate compared with standard care (0.7% vs. 1.2%; hazard ratio 0.60, 95% CI 0.36–0.98; $P = 0.04$) [39].

One infrequent but potentially challenging situation which may be encountered during otherwise uncomplicated generator replacement or system revision is the "frozen lead" that will not easily disengage from the header. Estimated to occur in 1–2% of generator replacements, this situation may be caused by a stripped set-screw or when some component of the lead pin has melted or otherwise fused with the header or vice versa. When firm traction is applied to the point where lead integrity may be compromised, an alternative solution should be sought. Potential solutions include use of silicone lubricants, application of surgical or dental drills, or use of orthopedic bone cutters to reveal the distal end of the pin, allowing it to be pushed through the header [40]. Rarely, if no solution is available, the lead may have to be cut from the header, then capped and replaced. The problem of the frozen lead, though infrequent, points to the value of having a temporary wire placed for generator replacement and system revisions in pacemaker-dependent patients.

For the lead to fit into the generator, the lead diameter, pin length, and presence or absence of sealing rings must be accommodated by the pulse

(a)

(b)

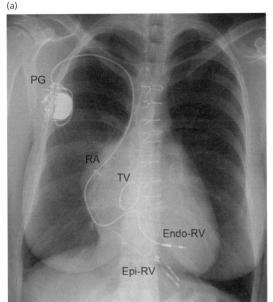

Figure 5.25 (a) Posteroanterior and (b) lateral chest X-ray of a 38-year-old woman with Ebstein's anomaly and complete atrioventricular block. In childhood, she had undergone implantation of a dual-chamber unipolar epicardial system using a transmyocardial right atrial lead (RA) and epicardial ventricular lead (Epi-RV). She later had tricuspid valve replacement with a bioprosthesis. By age 21 she had developed ventricular lead failure and generator. In addition, one manufacturer (Guidant/permanent atrial fibrillation, leading to placement of a single-chamber transvenous pacemaker (Endo-RV) with a subpectoral pulse generator (PG). At age 30, her tricuspid valve bioprosthesis had failed and was replaced with a mechanical prosthesis (TV). The transvenous right ventricular (RV) lead was placed outside the sewing ring of the prosthesis. This lead can now be extracted only by an open surgical route.

generator. In addition, one manufacturer (Guidant/ Boston Scientific) introduced a proprietary LV-1 pin configuration for some of its CS leads, although few likely remain in service. In addition, newer quadripolar CS leads utilize the IS-4 connector pin. Certain leads can be made compatible with new generators by the use of adaptors. Most manufacturers continue to provide generator models to fit some of the discontinued lead styles. In addition, some pacemakers require unique leads to perform specialized functions or special tools to free the leads from the device. The importance of identifying the lead and pacemaker connector configuration before surgery cannot be overstated. Manufacturers can provide the needed information about compatibility between components.

During the operative procedure, electrocautery may cause failure of output in generators near their end of service. For this reason and because leads may be damaged during generator removal, temporary pacing should be established in pacemaker-dependent patients (see Chapter 4). Meticulous attention to surgical technique is mandatory to prevent damage to implanted hardware and to reduce the risk of infection. If lead replacement is required but the ipsilateral vein is occluded, abandoning the entire system for another site or recanalization of the vein by lead extraction (see section Lead extraction) will be necessary. Occasionally, isolated outer insulation defects in silicone leads can be repaired, but the integrity of the conductors remains questionable. If leads are capped and abandoned in the pocket, it is advisable to suture the lead to the floor of the pocket to prevent migration or erosion of the free end. Some operators prefer to cut the proximal portion of abandoned leads to reduce the hardware remaining in the pocket. This may be problematic for active fixation leads since retraction of the helix may not be possible, complicating extraction should that be needed in the future. Cutting a lead too short may predispose to retraction of the lead into the venous system.

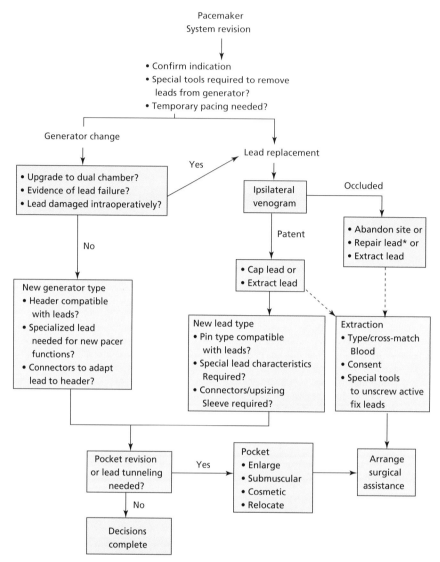

Figure 5.26 Flow chart for decisions surrounding revision of a previously implanted pacemaker system. All decisions should be thoroughly considered and the necessary equipment secured before the patient enters the operating room. (* Repair of an isolated outer insulation defect can be performed on an exposed section of some silicone insulation leads using a repair kit. The integrity of the lead conductors is not assured, however.)

Finally, replacement of a lead or generator also provides the opportunity to revise the pocket, consider alteration of device site for comfort, reimplant the generator submuscularly, or revise the surgical scar as indicated. All these factors should be evaluated and plans made for any contingency before the surgical procedure begins.

Leadless cardiac pacemaker implantation

Implantable cardiac pacemakers have shown remarkable technological improvements over the past 60 years. However, there remain significant complications related to the pacemaker pocket and the leads. Leadless pacemakers have been designed to eliminate pocket- and lead-related complications (Table 5.5). Currently, one model, the Medtronic Micra® transcatheter pacing system (TPS) has been approved by the Food and Drug Administration (FDA) for use in the USA [41].

The Micra has a length of 26 mm, diameter of 6.67 mm (20 Fr), volume of 0.8 cm³, and weight of 2 g. It is designed to be placed transvenously in the

Table 5.5 Advantages and disadvantages of leadless cardiac pacing

Advantages

- No risk of pneumothorax or subclavian artery/vein injury or thrombosis
- No lead crossing the tricuspid valve
- No pacemaker pocket
- Potentially lower risk of endovascular device infection

Disadvantages

- Single-chamber VVI(R) pacing only
- No ability to revise system if pacing/ICD needs change
- Uncertain ability to retrieve chronic device
- Risk of device embolization
- Very large (27 Fr) femoral sheath required
- Higher cost
- Battery longevity highly dependent on pacing output/capture threshold

right ventricle via a femoral vein approach. It uses tines for passive fixation and provides VVI(R) pacing via accelerometer. The system consists of an introducer, a delivery system, and a leadless pacemaker (Figure 5.27).

To place the Micra TPS, the patient is prepared and draped under sterile conditions in the EP lab for a femoral access procedure [42]. Biplane fluoroscopy is preferred, if available. Femoral venous access (usually right-sided) is obtained in standard fashion, preferably using micropuncture technique and ultrasound guidance. Because of the large size of the introducer sheath, particular care should be taken to avoid vascular access complications.

After a standard J-wire is placed, a standard 6–8 Fr sheath may be placed for venography to ascertain normal anatomy and absence of excessive tortuosity or venous anomaly. A long stiff guidewire is then placed up to the SVC. Serial dilators of 12–18 Fr are then used to prepare the vessel to accept the

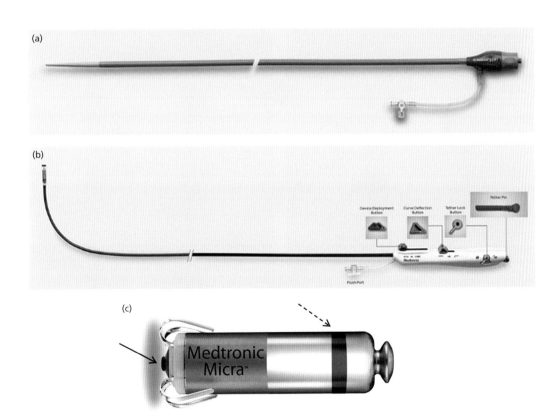

Figure 5.27 Micra® transcatheter pacing system (TPS). (a) The 27-Fr introducer sheath. (b) Micra delivery system. (c) The Micra leadless pacemaker showing the tip (solid arrow) and ring (dashed arrow). Source: Reproduced with permission of Medtronic.

27-Fr outer diameter Micra introducer sheath, which should be carefully advanced with the radio-paque ring marker to the mid-right atrium (Figure 5.28a). The wire and dilator are then withdrawn, and the sheath is carefully aspirated and then flushed with sterile saline. The side port of the introducer should be continuously flushed with constant-flow heparinized saline drip to minimize risk of clot formation. A low-dose heparin bolus of 2000–5000 units may also be considered.

The Micra delivery system is then prepared and flushed according to manufacturer instructions. The system is placed into the introducer and advanced under fluoroscopy until the device is just inside the end of the introducer. The introducer sheath is then pulled back to the IVC–right atrial

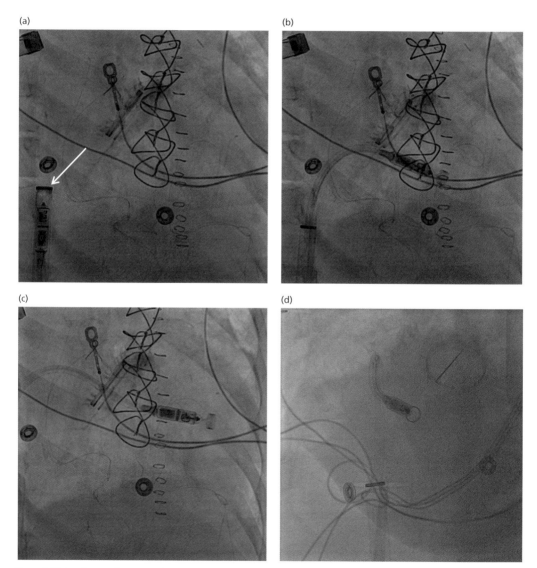

(a)

(b)

(c)

(d)

Figure 5.28 Leadless cardiac pacemaker implantation I: initial positioning. The patient is a 60-year-old woman s/p mitral valve replacement and tricuspid valve annuloplasty with postoperative atrioventricular block. (a) Placement of the 27-Fr introducer sheath from the right femoral vein to the mid-right atrium (arrow). (b) After slight withdrawal of the introducer sheath to expose the end of the delivery system, the system is deflected toward the tricuspid valve and advanced into the right ventricle. With slight reduction in deflection and advancement with clockwise torque, the tip of the system is placed on the mid-right ventricular apical septum in right (c) and left (d) anterior oblique projections.

junction to expose the Micra device and the distal end of the delivery system. The delivery system is then curved using the deflection button on the handle in order to direct the pacemaker to the tricuspid valve and right ventricle (Figure 5.28b). This process should be observed in RAO and LAO to ensure direction through the center of the tricuspid valve.

Once the device has been advanced through the tricuspid valve, the curve may be released slightly to prevent directing the pacemaker to the floor

of the right ventricle. The mid-apical septum is usually targeted initially, advancing the system forward while applying mild clockwise torque to direct the device septally. When contact with myocardium has been made, a small amount of additional forward pressure is exerted to create a "goose-neck" appearance of the delivery system (Figure 5.28c,d). Diluted contrast is then injected to ensure the device is seated against a trabeculated portion of the RV apical septum (Figure 5.29a,b).

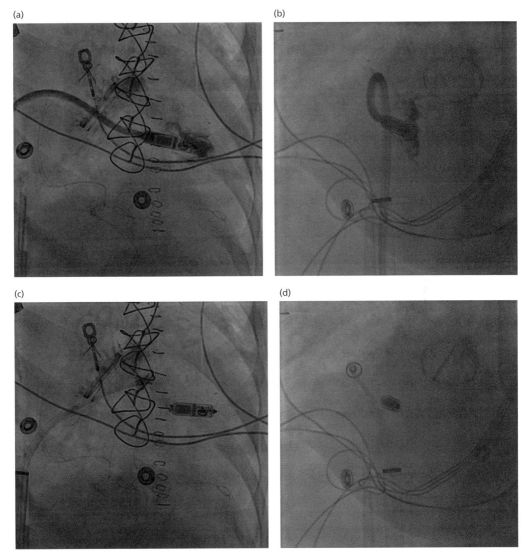

(a)

(b)

(c)

(d)

Figure 5.29 Leadless cardiac pacemaker implantation II: contrast ventriculography and initial release. Contrast is injected through the delivery system showing muscular trabeculations at the mid-apical septum in (a) right anterior oblique (RAO) and (b) left anterior oblique (LAO) projections. The leadless pacemaker is then deployed from the end of the system while retaining the tether, shown in RAO (c) and LAO (d) projections.

The Micra pacemaker is then deployed by first unlocking the tether and removing the tether pin from the handle. While maintaining adequate tip pressure, the pacemaker device is deployed halfway out of the delivery system, exposing the tines to the trabeculated myocardium. Forward pressure is then relieved by gentle withdrawal of the delivery system while completing the deployment (Figure 5.29c,d).

Initial electrical testing via the programmer is performed to assess for adequate parameters (R wave >5 mV, impedance 400–1500 Ω, capture threshold <1–1.5 V at 0.24 ms). Fixation testing is then performed by gently pulling and holding the tether while observing the tines on magnified cinefluoroscopy. Proper fixation is marked by observing at least two tines open during the pulling

phase (Figure 5.30a,b). Electrical testing is then repeated to ensure adequate sensing and pacing parameters. Ensuring an adequate capture threshold is particularly important since battery life of the device is highly dependent on pacing output. If electrical parameters or fixation are deemed to be inadequate, the pacemaker should be recaptured and redeployed in a slightly different location.

Once a final satisfactory position and electrical parameters have been obtained, the tether is removed, first bringing the recapture cone close to the Micra device to create support. The tether is gently pulled back and forth to observe mobility. The tether with higher tension is cut and retracted slowing while observing absence of movement of the Micra device on fluoroscopy (Figure 5.30c,d). The delivery system can then be withdrawn

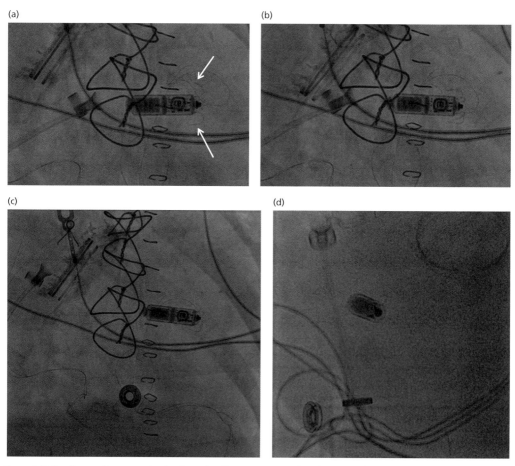

Figure 5.30 Leadless cardiac pacemaker implantation III: tug test and final release. Using magnified fluoroscopy in right anterior oblique projection, a gentle pull on the tether shows splaying of two of the tines (arrows), indicating appropriate fixation in the myocardium. With release of the tether (b), the tines assume normal position. The tether is then cut and removed, releasing the leadless pacemaker, shown in right (c) and left (d) anterior oblique projections.

through the introducer. After a final test of pace-maker electrical parameters, the introducer sheath is removed and hemostasis obtained with a figure-of-eight suture and direct pressure.

Subcutaneous ICD

As with conventional pacemakers, the lead of an ICD system is the component most vulnerable to failure and complications, which include dislodg-ment, cardiac perforation, conductor fracture, insulation breach, and infection. To address these limitations of transvenous leads, the totally subcu-taneous ICD (S-ICD) was developed, tested in clinical trials, and approved by the FDA in 2013 [43,44] (Figure 5.31). Important advantages and limitations of the S-ICD are shown in Table 5.6.

After passing preprocedure ECG screening, the patient is brought to the EP laboratory in the fasting postabsorptive state. We prefer general anesthesia for patient comfort and need to maintain the left arm in an extended position on an arm board without movement. The landmarks of the chest, including xiphoid process, midsternal line, and ster-nal notch, are marked with a marking pen. We posi-tion a model of the generator and lead on the chest to confirm landmarks with fluoroscopy, anticipating the desired final positions (Figure 5.32). The chosen

Table 5.6 Advantages and disadvantages of S-ICD vs. transvenous ICD

Advantages

- Absence of intravascular or intracardiac foreign body
- Decreased risk of endocarditis or endovascular infection
- No risk of pneumothorax, hemothorax, other vascular or thoracic injury during implantation
- Extremely low risk of lead failure
- Lower risk of system extraction

Disadvantages

- No bradycardia or CRT pacing
- No antitachycardia pacing
- Higher rate of oversensing
- Lowest VT rate cutoff 170 bpm
- Larger generator size
- Shorter battery longevity
- Higher risk of oversensing
- Need for ECG screening with 10% failure rate

CRT, cardiac resynchronization therapy; VT, ventricular tachycardia.

site for pulse generator implantation and incision sites are then additionally marked. The chest is extensively prepared and draped (Figure 5.33a–c).

(a)

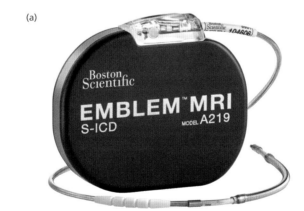

(b)

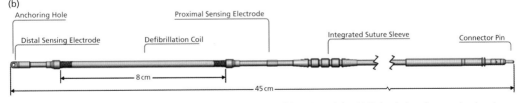

Figure 5.31 S-ICD system hardware (a) S-ICD generator and lead. (b) Design of the S-ICD lead, showing proximal and distal sensing electrodes, 8-cm defibrillating coil, and single terminal connector pin.

(a)

(b)

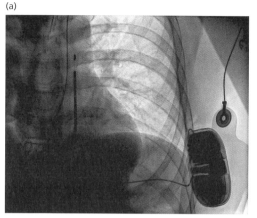
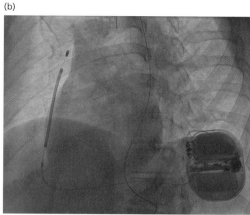

Figure 5.32 Fluoroscopy showing (a) posteroanterior and (b) steep left anterior oblique views of S-ICD system after implantation. Note the left parasternal position of the shocking electrode of the lead and relatively posterior position of the S-ICD generator, ensuring adequate "sandwiching" of the heart between the two defibrillating electrodes of the system.

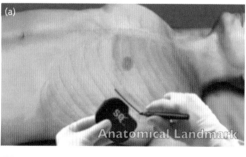
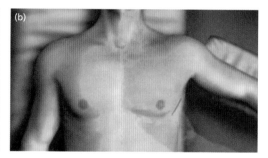
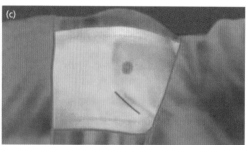
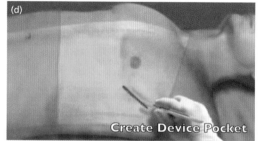
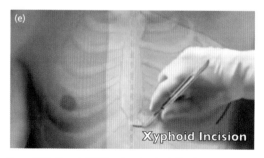
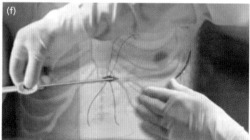

Figure 5.33 Steps in S-ICD system implantation I.
(a) Anatomical landmarks are marked with marking pen and incisions planned. (b) A wide sterile preparation of the chest, neck, left axilla, and upper arm is performed. (c) The chest is draped to allow exposure of left pectoral, inframammary, and sternal regions. (d) The generator pocket is made in the anterior-mid axillary region near the fifth to sixth ribs. (e) A smaller incision is made just lateral to the xiphoid process and two 0-silks are tied to the fascia. (f) The tunneling tool is guided along the fascia plane into the generator pocket.

The incision for the generator is made in the fifth to sixth intercostal space in an inframammary position in the anterior axillary area, usually parallel to the course of the ribs (Figure 5.33d). The pocket for the pulse generator is then made, dissecting carefully along the fascial plane of the serratus anterior. To provide adequate cardiac defibrillation, it is important to make the pocket for the generator as posterior as possible, which usually requires extension of the pocket to the latissimus dorsi muscle. After complete hemostasis has been obtained, the large pocket may be packed with a laparotomy sponge.

Next, a small incision is made in the xiphoid region just lateral to the midsternal line and carried down to the fascial plane (Figure 5.33e). Two 0-silk sutures are then tied to the fascia in the incision to be later tied to the lead anchoring sleeve. The S-ICD lead is brought on the field after tying an 0-silk suture in the end hole at the tip of the lead. The tunneling tool is then inserted into the small xiphoid incision and carefully pushed through along the fascial plane into the generator pocket (Figure 5.33f). The silk suture on the end of the lead is then tied to the end of the tunneling tool and the lead pulled through to the surface through the xiphoid incision, leaving the connector pin in the lateral pocket. The tie-down sleeve is then tied with free 0-silk securely to the lead 0.5–1.0 cm proximal to the proximal electrode (Figure 5.34a,b).

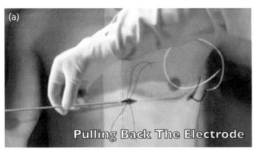
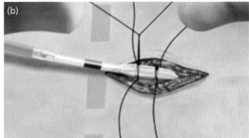
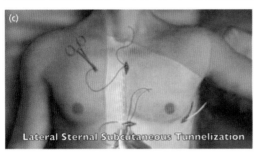
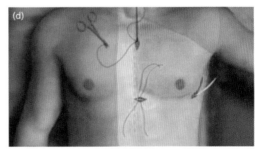
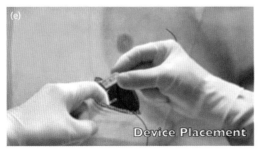
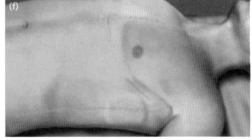

Figure 5.34 Steps in S-ICD system implantation II. (a) The S-ICD lead is tied with 0-silk to the tunneling tool and then pulled through the xiphoid incision. (b) The anchoring sleeve is tied to the lead insulation with 0-silk 5–10 mm proximal to the proximal sensing electrode. (c) With the traditional three-incision technique, a small incision is made near the suprasternal notch and the lead is tunneled superiorly to it just lateral to the mid-sternal line along the fascial plane. (d) The anchoring sleeve is tied down to the fascia in the xiphoid incision, and the distal lead is tied down in the upper sternal incision, attempting to the keep the distal lead straight along the parasternal region. (e) The terminal lead pin is cleaned and connected to the S-ICD generator, which is placed in the pocket with excess lead below and then anchored to the fascia with 0-silk. (f) All three incisions are closed in standard fashion.

When the traditional three-incision technique is used, a small incision is then made just below the suprasternal notch and 1 cm left of the midsternal line, estimating where the tip of the S-ICD lead will lie when pulled through (Figure 5.34c). A single 0-silk suture is tied to the fascia at this incision. The tunneling tool is then carefully pushed up from the xiphoid incision to the suprasternal incision, taking care to stay just above the fascial plane and about 1 cm left of and parallel to the midsternal line. If the tunneling course is too superficial, higher defibrillation thresholds and greater risk of lead erosion may result. When the tip of the tunneling tool emerges, the suture is cut, the tunneling tool removed, and the lead is pulled through with the suture attached to the end of the lead. The lead is then anchored in the xiphoid incision with the prepared fascial sutures to the anchoring sleeve. The tip of the lead is then tied to the fascia in the upper sternal incision, attempting to keep the distal lead and defibrillating coil straight along the parasternal line (Figure 5.34d).

More recently, a two-incision technique has been developed and widely adopted by experienced S-ICD implanters [45]. In this technique, the upper sternal incision is omitted. An 11-Fr non-valved peel-away sheath is placed over the tunneling tool, which is inserted along the parasternal route from the xiphoid incision as already described. The tool is removed, leaving the peel-away sheath in place. The lead is then placed into the sheath, which is peeled away leaving the distal lead in place. The lead is then anchored in the xiphoid incision as described.

Attention is then turned to the generator pocket. All sponges are removed and the pocket carefully irrigated and inspected for hemostasis. The lead pin is cleaned and dried and inserted into the S-ICD generator, which is placed in the pocket, coiling any extra lead under the generator (Figure 5.34e,f). Because of the large size and dependent position of the generator, it should be anchored with 0-silk in the pocket using at least one of the anchoring holes in the header to prevent migration and rotation. The incisions are then closed in layers and defibrillation testing is performed. Final programming and selection of the optimal sensing vector is performed in the recovery area with the patient in the supine and upright posture. Two-zone tachy therapy programming is strongly advised in order to reduce the risk of inappropriate ICD shocks. A chest X-ray may be performed prior to discharge to document the final lead and generator positions (Figure 5.35).

Postprocedure management

Elective generator replacement is most often accomplished on a same-day outpatient basis. While there is increasing interest in performing same-day de-novo pacemaker implantation, most procedures involving lead placement or revision continue to involve in-hospital observation for at least one night. For such new implants, ECG telemetry is usually obtained for 12–24 hours [18]. The following morning, an ECG is performed. Prior to discharge, posteroanterior and lateral chest radiographs are performed to document lead positions and exclude delayed pneumothorax.

Longer hospitalization may be required because of ancillary medical problems or as a result of complication. Analgesia may be necessary, but it is rarely needed after the first few days. The patient is advised to limit motion of the ipsilateral upper extremity for a time – specifically, to avoid raising it high above shoulder level or subjecting it to marked abduction for approximately 2 weeks. However, patients should not excessively restrict motion of the arm, as this may cause a frozen shoulder and delay ultimate rehabilitation. The incision should be kept dry for 3–7 days.

Even the most skillfully implanted permanent pacemaker system will provide limited benefit if it is not programmed properly. Before discharge, the device should be programmed in accordance with the patient's specific needs and a complete non-invasive assessment of the pacing system performed. Programming of the pacemaker is guided by two principles: (i) optimization of the patient's hemodynamic state, and (ii) maximal conservation of battery energy expenditure. When these two factors are in opposition, the first should take precedence; however, opportunities to achieve the second should not be overlooked. This might include programming a longer AV interval to avoid fusion beats, a lower resting minimal heart rate, and lower stimulation outputs (within an acceptable safety margin). In general, higher outputs are programmed at initial implant to accommodate the possibility of acute threshold rise.

(a)   (b)

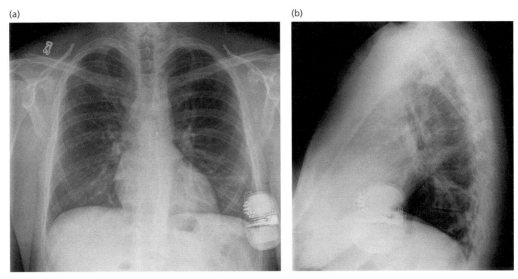

Figure 5.35 Posteroanterior (a) and lateral (b) chest X-rays after S-ICD lead implantation.

Outputs are then lowered to maximize battery longevity 6–12 weeks after implantation.

A number of studies have indicated the importance of avoiding unnecessary RV pacing, especially in patients with heart failure and LV dysfunction [46]. Such patients with preserved AV conduction should be programmed with long AV delays and/or a non-tracking mode (such as DDI).

Rate-adaptive parameters may be set before the patient is discharged or during a follow-up visit. This is commonly done empirically and is tested by having the patient perform walking exercises, if necessary. The adequacy of pacing response may be judged by real-time telemetry or by using rate histograms stored in the pacer. Follow-up evaluation and possibly adjustment of programmed parameters, including rate adaptation, will be necessary.

Some of the newer pacemaker generators have a mechanism for automatic capture threshold detection. These devices may allow for the programming of a lower pacing output with the recognition that the algorithm will increase pacing output if it detects a rise in threshold. Care should be taken to ensure that these devices have acceptable evoked response amplitudes acutely and at follow-up assessments, especially in pacemaker-dependent patients, who may experience syncope with even a rare transient failure of the algorithm. A copy of the programmed parameters should be given to the patient to keep, in addition to the device registry card.

It is important that the physician or pacemaker field technician registers the generator and leads appropriately so that the patient may be tracked should a device advisory occur. Arrangements for follow-up care should be made by the implanting physician, and the patient should be counseled as to the importance of having the system checked at regular intervals. While there was previously some controversy as to the need for endocarditis prophylaxis, current guidelines do not recommend routine antibiotic prophylaxis for patients with endocardial leads.

Complications of implantation

Inherent to pacemaker therapy is the potential for the occurrence of an untoward event. Skill, experience, and technique are all mitigating factors, but every operator should anticipate that they will have to manage a complication eventually. Thus, the implanting physician must be concerned not only with measures to avoid complications, but also with their recognition and treatment [47]. Such untoward events associated with the introduction and physical presence of the generator and leads may be classified according to their etiology (Tables 5.7 and 5.8).

In the Pacemaker Selection in the Elderly (PASE) study, 6.1% of the 407 patients receiving dual-chamber pacing systems had a complication of implantation [48]. There were nine lead dislodgements (2%), eight instances of pneumothorax (2%), and four cardiac perforations (1%). A repeat surgical procedure was required in 18 (4.4%) of the patients. In a single-center study of more than 1300 permanent pacemaker implants reported by Tobin *et al.* [49], complications were noted in 4.2% of patients. Lead dislodgement occurred in 2.4%,

significant pneumothorax in 1.5%, pericardial tamponade in 0.2%, and hemothorax leading to death in one patient (0.08%). The economic consequences of a complication were substantial, with the average incremental cost of \$14 547 for a lead dislodgment, \$10 052 for a pneumothorax, and \$32 472 for a tamponade. There was an inverse relationship between the incidence of acute complication and operator case volume and experience. Although the acute implant complications associated with DDD pacing are no different from those with single-chamber pacing, the total complication rate associated with dual-chamber pacing over time is higher than that with VVI or single-lead VDD due to the presence of the additional lead.

Although neither elective generator replacement nor revision of a VVI system to a dual-chamber device is usually considered to be a dangerous procedure, both are associated with potential complications. Harcombe *et al.* [50] found that the rate of late complications (those occurring later than 6 weeks after the procedure) was higher for elective replacement (6.5%) than for initial system implantation (1.4%). These were primarily erosion and infection related to the pacemaker pocket. Complications were more common with inexperienced operators, suggesting that technique as well as physiological substrate play important etiological roles. Revision of a VVI device to a dual-chamber or biventricular

Table 5.7 Acute complications of pacemaker implantation

Venous access by needle puncture
Secondary to Seldinger technique
Pneumothorax
Hemothorax
Other (e.g. injury to thoracic duct, nerves)
Secondary to sheath insertion:
Air or foreign body embolism
Perforation of the heart or central vein
Inadvertent entry into artery

Lead placement
Bradyarrhythmia or tachyarrhythmia
Perforation of heart or vein
Damage to heart valve
Damage to lead

Generator
Improper or inadequate connection of lead
Pocket hematoma

Table 5.8 Delayed complications of pacemaker therapy

Lead related	Generator related	Patient related
Intravascular thrombosis and/or embolization	Pain	Manipulation of the incision
Intravascular stenosis (i.e. superior vena cava obstruction)	Erosion	Twiddler's syndrome
Macro- or micro-lead dislodgement	Infection of pocket	
Fibrosis at electrode–myocardial interface (exit block)	Migration	
Infection: endocarditis	Premature failure	
Lead failure:	Damage from extrinsic energy (e.g. radiation, electrical shock)	
Insulation failure (inner/outer)		
Conductor fracture		
Retention wire fracture		
Chronic perforation		
Pericarditis		

system carries the potential for all the complications associated with venous access and lead placement (which may be confounded by the preexisting lead and associated vascular abnormalities), as well as an increase in risk of late pocket infection and skin erosion. Revision procedures are often longer in duration than a *de-novo* dual-chamber implantation. This may be related to difficulty isolating the generator and lead in the pocket due to adhesion formation, difficulty with venous access, interference with the existing lead, or a combination of these factors.

Venous access

By its very nature, the axillary/subclavian venous puncture has the potential for complication, the risk of which depends on both operator skill and the patient's anatomy. Inadvertent damage by the exploring needle to structures that lie in proximity to the vein (e.g. lung, subclavian artery, thoracic duct, and nerves) is the most frequent cause of significant complications encountered during the implantation process. Knowledge of subclavian venous anatomy by venography may be helpful in accessing the vessel and avoiding complication.

Pneumothorax is often asymptomatic and discovered on the routine postprocedure chest radiograph (Figure 5.36). Rarely, it may be the cause of severe respiratory distress intraprocedurally. Pleuritic pain, cough (especially if productive of blood-tinged sputum), and difficulty in breathing suggest the diagnosis. The aspiration of air into the syringe during attempted venous puncture may also raise concern about this possibility, but it is neither a sensitive nor specific sign. The presence of apical cystic lung disease, variations in the relationship between the clavicle and subclavian vein, and an uncooperative patient may increase the risk for this complication, and repeated unsuccessful attempts at venous puncture certainly do. Respiratory symptoms arising during the procedure should prompt assessment of pulse, blood pressure, oximetry, and perhaps blood gas analysis. Fluoroscopic examination of both lung fields should also be performed.

Treatment of pneumothorax depends on its severity and associated symptoms. Respiratory distress during the procedure may necessitate the urgent/emergency insertion of a chest tube. The

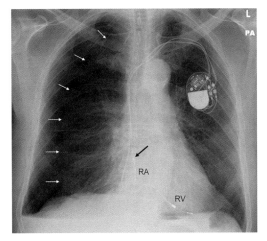

Figure 5.36 Right pneumothorax after left-sided pacemaker implantation in an elderly man with emphysema. The pleural line is indicated by the white arrows. This unusual complication probably results from microperforation of the active fixation right atrial lead (black arrow). Note the mediastinal shift to the left. RA, right atrial lead; RV, right ventricular lead.

completion of the implantation will depend on the patient's status and the progress already made. Although there may be some controversy as to the need for evacuation of an asymptomatic pneumothorax seen on chest radiograph, if its extent is greater than 10% a chest tube should be considered. If a small pneumothorax does not resolve or enlarges on serial radiographs, evacuation is indicated. Inspiration of 100% oxygen by facemask may help to resolve a small pneumothorax.

Hemothorax, a less common complication of the axillary/subclavian approach, results from injury to the subclavian artery, vein, or other intrathoracic vessel. Penetration of the subclavian artery by the exploring needle is usually harmless if the needle is withdrawn and pressure is applied at the site of entry under the clavicle. Significant complication may occur, however, if the artery is lacerated by the cutting edge of the needle or if a large-bore dilator or sheath is inadvertently introduced. If a large sheath is mistakenly inserted into the artery, it should probably be left in place, pending a prompt definitive management decision, since removal may result in significant bleeding. Options include surgical repair, endovascular treatment using a prolonged balloon inflation or a stent graft, or an attempt at sheath withdrawal with external compression. If the latter option is considered, there are several case reports of using vascular closure devices to assist with hemostasis. Use of both a collagen-based system (Angio-Seal; St. Jude Medical, St Paul, MN, USA) and a suture-based system (Perclose; Abbott Laboratories, Redwood City, CA, USA) has been described.

Opinions from an interventional radiologist and a vascular surgeon should be obtained if possible. A quick angiogram may determine whether an important branch vessel (e.g. internal mammary graft or vertebral artery) is involved or might be excluded by a covered stent. Because of the risk of thrombus formation around the sheath, it should be withdrawn to the subclavian artery itself to prevent embolization of clot to the cerebrovascular system. The likelihood of a bleeding complication is increased if the coagulation system is impaired either intrinsically by coexisting disease or by pharmacological therapy. Angiographic evaluation and possible repair should be considered for severe or persistent bleeding from an uncertain source.

Air embolism can occur when a central vein is accessed by a sheath, regardless of the technique used to introduce it. This complication may be signaled by a hiss as air is sucked into the sheath by negative intrathoracic pressure and may occur suddenly when a heavily sedated, snoring patient deeply inspires at a time when control over the sheath's orifice is not adequate. Air may be fluoroscopically tracked into the right ventricle and pulmonary outflow tract. In most instances, the amount of air introduced is small and well tolerated, but respiratory distress, chest pain, hypotension, and arterial oxygen desaturation may occur if there is significant blockage of pulmonary flow. Infrequently, introduced air may cross a patent foramen ovale or atrial septal defect and cause a stroke or coronary air embolus. Treatment of symptomatic air embolism includes supplemental oxygen, attempted catheter aspiration, and inotropic support if necessary. These supportive measures will usually suffice until the air embolism breaks up and absorption occurs. Preventive measures are listed in Table 5.9. The most important of these is routine use of valved sheaths.

Rare complications of venous access include laceration of the thoracic duct leading to chylothorax, and damage to the internal mammary artery, which

Table 5.9 Avoidance of air embolism

1	Increase central venous pressure: Hydrate well Elevate legs (Trendelenburg position) Have patient perform Valsalva maneuver when sheath is open
2	Awaken patient and caution against deep inspiration
3	Use smallest sheath compatible with task
4	Pinch or occlude neck of sheath if there is no hemostatic valve
5	Use of sheaths with hemostatic valves
6	Timing of critical parts of sheath manipulation with respiratory cycle in uncooperative patients

may cause acute ischemia when this conduit has been used as a coronary arterial graft.

Lead placement

The introduction, manipulation, and positioning of the pacemaker leads in the heart may give rise to a number of complications.

Arrhythmia

Arrhythmia may be a manifestation of the patient's underlying disease, or it may be procedurally related (Table 5.10). In a pacemaker-dependent patient, accidental interference with a preexisting pacing system, whether temporary or permanent, may cause asystole or symptomatic bradycardia. Other causes of a bradyarrhythmia include a vagal reaction, excessive local anesthetic, and injury to the conduction system during lead manipulation (e.g. trauma to the right bundle branch in a patient with LBBB). The use of transcutaneous pacing and/or the administration of atropine or isoproterenol may be helpful in these situations until a means of effective pacing can be established. For patients at risk of asystole during permanent pacemaker implantation, revision, or generator change, a preoperative temporary pacing wire should be considered.

Tachyarrhythmia may also occur during implantation; it is usually the result of stimulation of myocardium by a lead or guidewire. Supraventricular arrhythmias are most likely to occur in patients with atrial enlargement, heart failure, pulmonary disease, or other predisposing conditions such as sick sinus syndrome; they are usually transient.

Table 5.10 Causes of arrhythmia during pacer implantation

Bradyarrhythmia

Patient's underlying electrophysiological disorder
Vagal reaction
Lead trauma to the conduction system
Inadvertent disruption of a pacing system
Suppression of escape rhythm by anesthetic

Tachyarrhythmia

Atrial/ventricular
Underlying electrophysiology
Irritation by lead/wire
Ischemia, anesthesia, hypoxia

Atrial fibrillation occurring before or during atrial lead placement may be problematic, in that atrial parameters cannot be tested unless the rhythm terminates either spontaneously or by chemical or electrical cardioversion. An atrial lead may be placed in the presence of atrial fibrillation occurring at the time of implantation using the criterion of intracardiac fibrillatory amplitude of 1.0 mV or greater. This reduces implantation time compared with the option of intraprocedural cardioversion, which may also lead to postoperative stroke [51].

Ventricular arrhythmia is common as the lead is manipulated in this chamber, but it is rarely sustained. Predisposing factors to more malignant arrhythmia include hypoxia, ischemia, pharmacological therapy (e.g. sympathomimetics), and asynchronous pacing. Removal of the lead from an irritating position almost always terminates the ectopy. In a susceptible patient, however, wire- or lead-induced ventricular ectopy may induce sustained ventricular tachycardia or fibrillation, and the implanting team should be prepared for this possibility and ready to defibrillate the patient if needed. Because the attention of the implanter may be focused on the fluoroscopic image during lead placement, another individual, usually the nurse or anesthetist, should be assigned to monitor the ECG during this time. On occasion, a retained guidewire or a temporary ventricular pacing lead is displaced and serves as an occult source of ventricular irritation that is not resolved by retraction of the permanent pacing lead. Rarely, a permanent ventricular (or prolapsing atrial) pacing lead will be the cause of recurrent ventricular ectopy post implantation.

Perforation

The heart may be perforated internally (into another cardiac chamber) or externally (into the pericardial space) by the pacing lead; such perforations may be acute or delayed [52]. RV perforations are probably more common than reported because clinical sequelae may not occur. Poor sensing or capture thresholds may prompt withdrawal of the lead back into the ventricle with "self-sealing" of the perforation. On occasion, however, life-threatening tamponade may occur, and progressive hypotension during or after lead placement should be considered tamponade until proven otherwise. If access to an echocardiogram is not readily available or not feasible due to rapid deterioration in hemodynamic status, fluoroscopy in LAO projection to assess the cardiac silhouette excursion is helpful for evaluating pericardial fluid collection and allowing expedited pericardiocentesis [53]. Older age, female gender, steroid therapy, recent RV infarction, prior use of temporary pacing wire, and the use of stiff leads (or stylets) may be considered risk factors for perforation [54]. Pericarditis, tamponade, and even pneumothorax have been reported as complications caused by active fixation atrial lead placement due to the helix protruding through the atrial myocardium.

Interference with normal coagulation predisposes the patient to pericardial tamponade. Thrombolytics should be considered contraindicated in the immediate post-implant period. If symptoms suggestive of tamponade occur, echocardiographic confirmation should be obtained unless the condition dictates emergency pericardiocentesis. Every effort should be made to obtain an echocardiogram in the latter situation as soon as possible. Pericardiocentesis with catheter drainage will rapidly reverse the pathophysiology of tamponade and may be the only therapy necessary, since the perforation is frequently self-sealing. In some cases tamponade may occur with the acute accumulation of only a small amount of pericardial fluid. In such cases inexperienced providers may find it difficult to access the pericardial space with a needle, necessitating emergency surgical consultation. Less frequently, a more slowly accumulating effusion may develop over several days as a reaction to a relatively small amount of bleeding into the pericardial space or irritation from a subclinically perforated lead. This may follow signs and/or symptoms of pericarditis or present as *de-novo* tamponade. Drainage may be necessary if hemodynamic stability is threatened; otherwise, non-steroidal anti-inflammatory agents and observation may be used.

Suspicion of perforation without tamponade may be aroused by an extreme distal location of the lead tip at the cardiac apex (especially if it seems to curve around the apex, tenting up the cardiac silhouette), or by the presence of a pericardial friction rub, chest pain, an ECG pacing pattern of RBBB, or an upright unipolar electrogram recorded from the lead tip. Poor pacing and sensing thresholds may be seen. In such situations, fluoroscopy or computed tomography scanning may be helpful in localizing the lead tip (Figure 5.37) [55]. If perforation is confirmed, the lead should be withdrawn under hemodynamic monitoring at a time and facility capable of emergency surgical drainage if necessary.

A transvenous pacing lead may enter the left heart through a communication between the atria, through the membranous septum separating the right atrium from the left ventricle, or through the muscular interventricular septum. The permanent pacing lead may also be inadvertently introduced into an artery and passed retrograde across the aortic valve into the left ventricle. The anteroposterior radiographic image of a lead positioned in the left ventricle may not be distinguishable from an image of one placed in the RV apical position. Oblique or lateral views, however, will demonstrate the posterior location of a LV lead (Figure 5.38). In addition, pacing from the left ventricle will result in a RBBB QRS pattern on

(a)

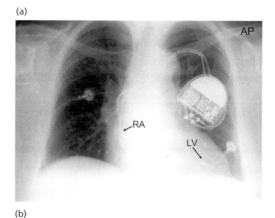

(b)

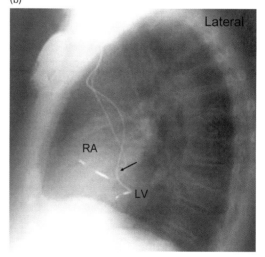

Figure 5.38 Chest radiographs of a patient after implantation of a dual-chamber pacemaker with inadvertent left-sided ventricular lead placement. The paced QRS complex on 12-lead ECG showed a right bundle branch block pattern. (a) On anteroposterior view, the ventricular lead appears to be positioned near the right ventricular apex. (b) Lateral chest radiograph shows a posterior diversion of the ventricular lead at the atrial level (arrow). Passage of the lead across a patent foramen ovale, across the mitral valve, and into the left ventricle was later confirmed. Treatment options include removal of the lead or chronic anticoagulation to prevent thromboembolus. This problem can be avoided by careful fluoroscopy of the leads in multiple views and observation of an appropriate 12-lead paced QRS complex at the time of implantation. LV, ventricular lead in the left ventricle; RA, right atrial lead.

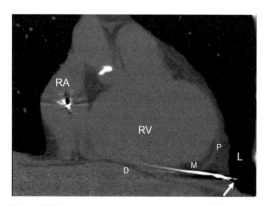

Figure 5.37 Reconstructed computed tomographic image in right anterior oblique view showing perforation of an active fixation ventricular lead through the right ventricular apex and pericardium into the lung parenchyma. This problem may present with loss of ventricular sensing and capture, pneumothorax, pericardial effusion, and/or stimulation of the diaphragm or chest wall. The lead was later withdrawn uneventfully in the operating room. D, diaphragm; L, left lung; M, right ventricular myocardium; P, pericardium; RA, right atrium; RV, right ventricle.

ECG. This combination of techniques should always be performed during lead implantation to exclude this important and preventable complication.

Early recognition of a lead in a systemic chamber should prompt its immediate repositioning because of the danger of thrombus formation and systemic embolization. A review of the literature has found that 10 of 27 patients with systemic pacing leads had thromboembolic complications, including three patients on antiplatelet drugs [56]. Options for management of patients with chronically implanted left heart endocardial leads include long-term anticoagulation, lead removal at thoracotomy, or percutaneous lead removal. The latter has been thought to be associated with excessive risk of systemic embolization, but a number of successful procedures have been reported.

Other lead complications

The presence of a pacing lead across the tricuspid valve orifice ordinarily results in little or no valvular dysfunction. On occasion, however, this structure may be compromised or damaged, resulting in tricuspid regurgitation [57]. During insertion, the tines of a passive fixation lead may become entangled with the chordae tendineae, and rupture of the latter may result if vigorous lead withdrawal is attempted. Occasionally, extrication of the lead from the tricuspid apparatus may require use of a locking stylet (with or without an extraction sheath) to transmit the force of traction to the lead tip rather than merely stretching the lead. The valve may be chronically injured by the lead's passage across it and by the resultant fibrosis. Thrombus and adhesions may form between the two and serve as a nidus for infection. Recurrent endocarditis on an RV lead has been associated with the development of tricuspid stenosis and insufficiency.

The pacing lead itself may be damaged by the physical forces exerted upon it during the process of implantation, by entrapment in the musculoskeletal system, by retention ligatures, and by the stresses placed on it by the beating heart. Loss of integrity of the insulation (either inner or outer) is usually manifested by a low pacing impedance that causes a high current drain; conductor fracture is associated with a high pacing impedance. Rarely, lead fracture may be recognized radiographically (see Figure 5.5). A defect in the insulation between the conductor wires of a bipolar lead may produce contact potentials resulting in oversensing and transient inhibition of pacemaker output. Detection of such intermittent dysfunction may require the performance of provocative maneuvers such as raising, abducting, or adducting the ipsilateral upper extremity. Prolonged contact between the conductors can result in a short circuit, preventing current from reaching the electrodes and depleting the battery. Both lead fracture and loss of insulation integrity may lead to clinical symptoms and adverse events in pacemaker-dependent patients.

The most common complication of lead placement is its subsequent dislodgement (see Figure 5.13). This may be obvious on fluoroscopy or radiography (macro-) or accompanied by no obvious change in position (micro-) and usually occurs early after implantation, before adhesion and fibrosis act to anchor the device further. Dislodgement rates are inversely related to the experience of the implanter, which suggests that inadequate initial positioning, allowance of lead slack, and/or anchoring are significant risk factors. Patient-related factors may include variant anatomy, right atrial/ventricular enlargement, and tricuspid regurgitation, especially when passive fixation leads are utilized.

An additional clinical scenario, termed "sagging heart syndrome," may be seen in patients with marked caudal mediastinal shift with upright posture, resulting in loss of what appeared to be adequate lead slack in the supine posture during lead implantation. This problem has been described in obese patients and in patients who have undergone significant weight loss.

A unique cause of lead dislodgement is known as Twiddler's syndrome. In these cases, the patient twists the pacemaker generator in the pocket (usually subconsciously), turning it in such a way that the leads are wound around it and are gradually withdrawn from the heart (see Figure 5.24). A similar problem may occur when the generator is not sutured to the underlying pectoralis fascia. In this scenario, a generator lying in the subcutaneous tissue (or in a submuscular space) may gradually descend through this space and exert traction on the lead.

The incidence of lead dislodgement has been reduced with refinement of both active and passive fixation devices; it is now less than 2–3%. The risk of this complication is lessened by ensuring a stable position at implant, leaving a proper amount of intravascular lead slack so that tension is not exerted at the tip by respiration or arm motion, adequately anchoring the suture sleeve to underlying tissue, and limiting abduction and elevation of the ipsilateral upper extremity for a short time after implantation.

Early recognition of lead dislodgement (often by deterioration in pacing parameters or the occurrence of ectopy) should result in attempts at repositioning as soon as possible. This is usually accomplished with minimal effort when the lead has not fibrosed to endocardium or venous endothelium. Deterioration in the performance of one or more chronic leads may present a more difficult problem and it is often necessary to implant a new lead.

Venous thrombosis

The presence of one or more intravascular leads may incite DVT of the subclavian vein. Although asymptomatic thrombosis appears to be common,

its relationship with the number and type of leads remains controversial. Clinically significant pulmonary embolization is rare. Symptomatic thrombosis of the subclavian, axillary, or cephalic veins occurs on occasion and presents as a swollen painful upper extremity, usually within a few weeks of implantation. Extension of the thrombus to involve the innominate vein, SVC, contralateral structures, or the cerebral venous sinus may occasionally occur. Venography will reveal the extent of thrombus and the state of development of collateral pathways (Figure 5.39). Symptomatic thrombosis that is limited to the subclavian or axillary veins may be treated conservatively, with heparin acutely, upper extremity elevation, and then oral anticoagulation for 3–6 months. In selected patients with highly symptomatic acute DVT with proximal extension, thrombolytic therapy may be considered.

Silent DVT is common. Routine venography at the time of elective generator replacement has shown an approximately 25% incidence of severe stenosis or occlusion of the ipsilateral subclavian

(a)

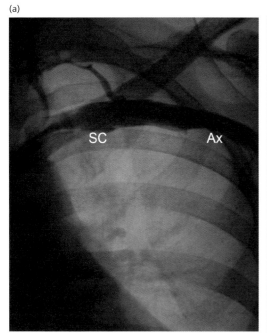

(b)

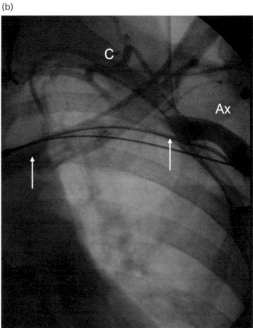

Figure 5.39 Deep venous thrombosis (DVT) during pacemaker implantation. (a) Preprocedure left upper extremity venogram shows patent axillary (Ax) and subclavian (SC) veins. (b) A second intraprocedural venogram was performed due to an inability to access the vein for a third left ventricular lead after placement of the right ventricular and atrial leads. Acute occlusion of the subclavian vein between the two arrows is demonstrated, along with the appearance of collateral venous circulation (C).

vein [58]. No risk factors for thrombotic or fibrotic venous occlusion have been unequivocally identified, although some studies have suggested that an increased number of leads and systemic infection predispose to venous occlusion. In most patients, asymptomatic venous occlusion becomes a problem only when attempts are made to reenter the vessel for lead revision or placement of additional leads. It is not necessary to treat asymptomatic chronic occlusions. Pacemaker leads inserted by the transfemoral route may be associated with femoral and iliac thrombosis and significant pulmonary embolization, necessitating lead extraction, anticoagulation, and possibly insertion of an IVC filter.

Complete or partial occlusion of the SVC has been reported as a complication of pacemakers. This has been attributed to both thrombosis and fibrosis, and may be treated with balloon dilation or surgical reconstruction if it becomes symptomatic. Acute or subacute occlusion may be treated with anticoagulants and/or thrombolytic agents. Chronic occlusion is more problematic and is, in general, resistant to pharmacotherapy. In some situations of total occlusion of the SVC, endovascular reconstruction may be complicated by an inability to pass a guidewire through the obstruction. In such cases it may be possible to remove the existing leads and use the extraction sheath as a means of gaining entrance through the occluded venous system. Dilation and stenting may then be considered. Stenting should not be performed over indwelling pacemaker leads. In cases in which endovascular repair is not possible, a surgical approach that enlarges the venous channel with a patch graft has been used with some success.

The true incidence of lead-associated thrombosis is uncertain, since transesophageal echocardiography (TEE) is usually performed only if there is a clinical indication. Such thrombus in the presence of infection would be termed a "vegetation." In general, the chance finding of a thrombus on a lead does not, in itself, mandate therapy; however, if it is very large, consideration should be given to anticoagulation. Anticoagulation therapy would be indicated if there is evidence of thromboembolism. A pedunculated thrombus on a pacing lead may occlude the tricuspid orifice and cause symptoms similar to those of a myxoma. Treatment of lead-associated atrial thrombus with thrombolytic therapy has been reported.

Generator

The function of a pacing system depends on a proper connection between the leads and the generator. The terminal lead pins are inserted into the connector block of the generator and are fixed into position by some mechanism, usually set-screws. If this procedure is not performed properly, the pin may either lose contact altogether (i.e. have no electrical continuity, an "open circuit") or intermittently contact the pacemaker terminal and produce spurious potentials that may be sensed by the pacemaker as intrinsic electrical activity, which will cause inhibition of pulse generator output. When dual-chamber systems are used, it is essential that the atrial and ventricular leads be connected correctly to their corresponding terminals (see Figure 5.23).

Care should be exercised when using electrocautery, since its application in the vicinity of the generator may lead to inhibition of pacing or to abnormal tracking. Reprogramming of the device to a reversion mode may also result. Exposure to other sources of energy, such as direct-current defibrillation, magnetic resonance imaging (MRI), and high-dose radiation therapy, may also affect pacemaker function. In some cases, pacemaker function can be restored by use of a special engineering programmer; in other situations, the device may be permanently damaged and require replacement.

The generator is usually well tolerated in its subcutaneous pocket, but on occasion its presence may be associated with pain. Most often this occurs because the pocket is small and tension is exerted on the overlying tissue. A chronic indolent infection may also be a source of pain. Pain attributed to neuralgia has been treated successfully with steroid injections and with pocket revision. Movement of the pacemaker may occur if the pocket is large, the surrounding tissue lax, and the device not secured. Swelling of the pocket may be caused by infection, seroma, or hematoma. Aspiration of the effusion should be discouraged because of the possibility of introducing infection. A strong suspicion of infection should prompt surgical exploration.

Migration of the pacemaker under the breast or into the axilla may place tension on the leads or result in the assumption of a position that is uncomfortable or is predisposed to erosion. Erosion of pacing hardware is caused by pressure necrosis of overlying tissue or infection. This event is usually signaled by a preceding period of "pre-erosion," during which there is discomfort and discoloration of thinning tissue tensely stretched over a protrusion of the pacing apparatus (Figure 5.40). The risk factors for erosion include a paucity of subcutaneous tissue, the mass and configuration of the pacemaker, need for extra hardware (e.g. lead adaptor) in the pocket, the pocket's construction, and irritation caused by activity or

physical manipulation or by articles of clothing. Identification of pre-erosion allows the possibility of salvage of the pacing system, as the hardware may be repositioned under the pectoralis muscle or in an abdominal location.

If erosion occurs, the system is considered contaminated and current practice is removal of the generator and leads.

Bleeding into the pocket may occur when hemostasis is inadequate, when there is a coexistent

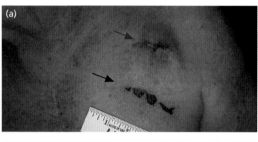
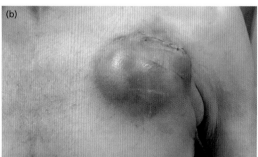
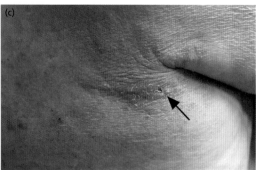
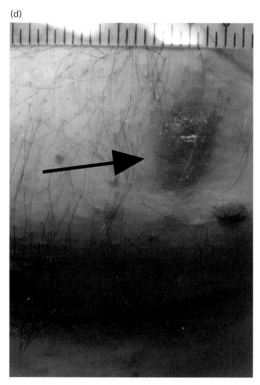

Figure 5.40 Examples of device pocket abnormalities. (a) Severe skin reaction to tape (black arrow) inspected several days after device implant. Incision (blue arrow) is healing normally, with some ecchymosis present around it. (b) Large hematoma formation in a patient with a new biventricular device implant treated with dual anticoagulation agents. Because of risk factors, these agents were not stopped preoperatively. The hematoma healed with conservative management. (c) Erythema at the incision site soon after an implant most likely due to a stitch abscess. The patient was treated with 2 weeks of oral antibiotics and followed closely until the incision fully healed. (d) Near-erosion of a device pocket 13 months after an ICD generator change at a referral hospital. The patient had three prior generator changes (this was the fifth device) over more than 20 years. This presentation is consistent with a smoldering infection. Patient eventually underwent a difficult lead and generator explantation. Source: courtesy of Karoly Kaszala MD.

coagulopathy, or when anticoagulant or thrombolytic therapy is begun soon after implantation. On occasion, this may compromise the pocket's integrity and may be a risk factor for infection. Hematoma progression, excessive pain, and stress on the suture line may require hematoma evacuation and search for a bleeding site.

Although not a complication of implantation per se, a generator may prematurely and without warning fail or may revert to an unsafe pacing mode. The former may relate to a defect in the power supply and the latter is a function of unrecognized problems with circuit design. The incidence of pacemaker failure has steadily declined over the years with improvement in design, and in 2006 the risk was estimated to be approximately 1.4 per 1000 devices [59]. Despite the decrease in absolute risk over the years, public concern over this issue has increased in the wake of several highly publicized device advisories.

Infection

Even a non-eroded pacemaker implantation site may become infected. Diabetes mellitus and postoperative hematoma appear to be predisposing factors. Acute infections (usually with *Staphylococcus aureus*) become manifest within the first few weeks of implantation and are often associated with the accumulation of pus. A more indolent infection caused by a less virulent agent such as *S. epidermidis* may present months or years after implantation. A fungal infection may also occur in the pocket and present as an indolent process with relatively scant growth of the organism. Infections with less virulent organisms may present as a small area of erythema, a pimple-like lesion, or a draining sinus. Some cases of indolent infection appear as cellulitis or pre-erosions. One-third to half of acute infections complicate new implants; the remainder are associated with reoperation for generator replacement or lead repositioning. Pocket infections are generally considered to result from organisms introduced from the skin's surface [20]. Superficial infections of the suture line that do not extend to the pocket itself may be treated conservatively.

Staphylococci, and presumably other pathogens, adhere to the plastic insulation of pacing hardware and form colonies that become covered with a secreted substance protecting the organism from host defense and antimicrobial drugs. Antibiotic therapy alone is rarely sufficient to eradicate these infections, and removal of the pacing system is usually indicated. In patients with erosions or localized pocket infections who have been on antimicrobial therapy and have negative blood cultures, it may be possible to place a new pacing system at a different site at the time of removal of the suspect hardware. Most of the time, however, it is prudent to use a two-step approach with temporary pacing (if the patient is pacer dependent) used to bridge the time between explantation and new device implantation a few days later. After device removal, the infected pocket may be partially closed and a drain inserted, or packed with wet-to-dry dressings and left open to heal by secondary intention.

Vacuum-assisted wound closure is a technique introduced in 1997 to assist in wound healing through the application of continuous negative pressure, resulting in removal of toxic products, devitalized tissue, and secretions, and increased lymphatic and blood flow. This technique accelerates healing and may allow for delayed surgical closure. Applied successfully to cases of orthopedic, diabetic, and sternal wound infections, it has been used to promote wound healing after pacemaker and ICD explantation in which the wound must be left open. Small case series have been published in which the technique has been used to salvage an infected pocket site without lead extraction in patients deemed to be at prohibitive risk or who refuse extraction [60]. However, there are currently no controlled trials showing that vacuum-assisted wound closure is superior to standard therapy for either indication.

Less frequently, a pacemaker patient may develop bacteremia without localizing signs, in which case endocarditis associated with a pacing lead should be considered. Lead endocarditis generally occurs later than pocket infection. It may be related to an organism introduced at implantation, but is more often thought to be secondary to a transient bacteremia, often from an undefined source. The diagnosis of lead endocarditis can be made when a vegetation is detected by echocardiography in the presence of other signs of infection (Figure 5.41). TEE may be helpful if transthoracic examination is non-diagnostic. One report has

(a)

(b)

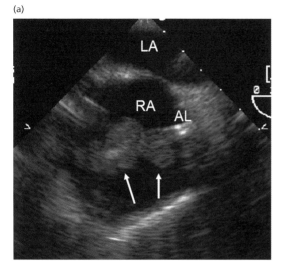

Figure 5.41 Pacemaker lead infection in transesophageal echocardiographic images from a patient presenting with signs and symptoms of subacute endocarditis. Blood cultures grew *Staphylococcus epidermidis*. (a) The right atrium (RA) showing two large vegetations (arrows) attached to the right atrial lead (AL). LA, left atrium. (b) The right ventricle (RV) showing the ventricular lead (VL) encased in fibrinous infectious material (arrows). The pacemaker system was extracted with an open surgical procedure and an epicardial pacing system was placed.

suggested that pacemaker-associated endocarditis constitutes 4.6% of the entire population with infective endocarditis and occurs with an incidence of about 0.6% in patients with pacemakers. Staphylococcal species predominate, with about two-thirds being coagulase negative [61]. Lead extraction should be strongly considered if *Staphylococcus* bacteremia or antibiotic-resistant occult Gram-negative bacteremia is present.

Diagnosis of pacemaker lead infection necessitates the removal of all pacing hardware after antibiotics have been started [62]. In these situations, adequate time between explantation and implantation of a new permanent system is necessary for antibiotic therapy to sterilize the blood. Generally, this interval is related to the duration of previous antibiotic treatment and the confirmation of negative blood cultures, usually 3–10 days [7]. The antibiotic therapy is selected on the basis of the organism cultured from the blood or hardware, and treatment duration should be similar to that of non-pacemaker-associated infective endocarditis with the same organism.

Complications of biventricular pacing

Implantation of a coronary venous lead is the major procedural difference between biventricular and simple dual-chamber pacemakers. It is subject to all the complications associated with dual-chamber systems plus those unique to LV pacing [63]. The LV lead must be placed in a lateral wall CS tributary vein. The technical challenge of this procedure has decreased with improvement in lead design and delivery equipment. Inability to achieve LV lead placement by a transvenous approach ranges from 2 to 10%.

Unique complications include CS dissection (2–4%) and coronary venous perforation (2%), complications mainly related to CS venography. CS perforation may lead to pericardial tamponade requiring urgent drainage. With better leads and delivery equipment, and greater operator experience, lead placement has been facilitated and the procedure times as well as the significant complication rate reduced. Extracardiac stimulation from the LV lead (diaphragm and phrenic nerve) may also be problematic and should be sought at the time of implantation. Its occurrence should prompt the search for another lead implant site. This problem may also first appear after implantation and can sometimes be corrected with reprogramming, although lead revision may be required. Newer lead design, such as the quadripolar lead configuration, may reduce the risk of this problem and allow more options for "electronic repositioning."

Lead extraction

General principles

Removal of existing "permanent" endocardial leads is a commonly performed procedure, and in experienced hands can be done safely and with a high degree of success. There continues to be an increasing need for the procedure due to (i) the increasing rate of CIED infection, (ii) the large number of defibrillator leads exhibiting premature failure, and (iii) the presence of an occluded vessel with a need to "upgrade" systems from pacemaker to ICD or CRT device. The tools and techniques for lead removal have matured and are associated with very high clinical success rates (usually in excess of 97%). The complication rate in experienced hands is around 1.5% or less, with a mortality rate less than 0.3%. The mortality rate is likely to be even lower now since the introduction of the SVC occlusion balloon (see Table 5.17).

The ease of accomplishing lead removal and the associated risks are strongly related to the time the lead has been implanted. Thus, a lead that has been in place for 6–12 months or less is usually easily removed, whereas one in place for longer periods may well present difficulties due to fibrosis, which may occur at a number of sites in the heart and central veins with which the lead has contact (Figure 5.42). The concept of "lead management" has come into vogue, and includes consideration of the risk of lead abandonment versus the risk of extracting the lead(s). Limiting the number of intravascular leads to those actively providing a service to the patient and removing non-functional, superfluous or potentially problematic leads at an earlier time allows for the procedure to be performed with lower risk and higher success rates as opposed to potentially performing the procedure at a later time when it would be more difficult.

Lead extraction is defined as removal of a lead that has been implanted for more than 1 year, when it is less than 1 year old and specialized tools (e.g. sheaths, locking stylets, snares) are needed, and/or when the lead is removed from a site other than that of original venous access. The term "lead explant" is used for the removal of leads having an implant duration of less than 1 year with only the tools used in a typical implantation along with manual traction. These definitions have some

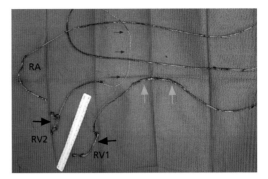

Figure 5.42 A newly extracted active fixation atrial (RA) and two ventricular leads (RV1, RV2) with numerous adherent fibrous vascular attachments (black and yellow arrows). The active fixation helix has been retracted into the tip of the leads. It is these fibrous vascular adhesions, which may form anywhere along the length of the lead (black arrows indicate right ventricular adhesions, yellow arrows superior vena cava adhesions), that can make lead extraction physically challenging and potentially hazardous due to the risk of vascular or cardiac injury. Lead RV2 suffered significant structural damage during the extraction process (red arrows) with extension and uncoiling of the inner electrodes. All leads were extracted without any remnants. Source: courtesy of Karoly Kaszala MD.

importance in terms of the requisite qualifications of physicians performing the respective procedures (see section Techniques) [64]. Although most of this discussion is directed at lead "extraction," it is relevant to physicians performing lead "explantation" also.

There are two general approaches for the removal of transvenous pacing leads: percutaneous and transthoracic. In most cases, the percutaneous route is preferred due to lower morbidity. Certainly, simple traction on the lead is easy, straightforward, and logistically undemanding. If all leads would safely yield to this treatment there would be little debate as to the threshold for lead extraction. Unfortunately, chronic leads are not so readily removed and, even with the variety of tools available to assist in the percutaneous technique, the procedures may be long, difficult, and associated with a low but finite mortality as well as morbidity.

The risks of lead removal should influence the aggressiveness with which one should pursue this approach as chronic lead implants reveal intense fibrosis and encapsulation, especially involving the ventricular portion of the lead, and may include the tricuspid valve and its supporting apparatus. Wherever the lead is relatively stationary, such as against a vein wall or the myocardium, thrombus develops that is eventually infiltrated by fibroblasts with the development of fibrous encapsulation. Over time, this tissue may calcify, commonly seen in younger patients and hemodialysis patients.

Contemporary leads are of low profile and they do not tolerate the physical forces that may be necessary to extract them by simple traction in the presence of significant fibrosis. The current generations of coradial leads are even less robustly constructed with regard to tensile strength. A variety of tools have been developed to facilitate the extraction of these leads via the concept of traction and countertraction [65]. The basic process was developed in the late 1980s and utilizes two components. First, a stylet (when possible) is placed into the lead, locking at the tip or along the length of the lead. This provides stability and stiffness to the lead. The second component is a sheath that is passed over the lead body and which cuts, avulses, or encapsulates the fibrous attachments. The current methods are based on these principles with advancements in sheath technology.

The specific adverse events that might complicate lead extraction mostly pertain to the physical forces used to separate the lead from the venous and cardiac structures. Catastrophic events, when they occur, usually result from either laceration of a central vein by an extraction tool or avulsion of the heart at the site of tip fixation. Embolization of a vegetation or thrombus to the pulmonary artery may also cause hemodynamic compromise or, rarely, death. Damage to the tricuspid valve, or embolization of a lead fragment to the lung may also occur. If a patent foramen ovale or atrial septal defect is present, embolic material may cross into the systemic circulation with major consequences. Although most complications become evident during or shortly after the extraction procedure, some, such as a hemothorax, pulmonary embolism, or pericardial tamponade, may be delayed in presentation. Because of the risks involved, it is essential that adequate informed consent be obtained from the patient and that the reasons for performing lead extraction, the potential risks and benefits, and alternatives (including lead abandonment) are thoroughly discussed with the patient and family by the operator in a shared decision-making process.

Indications

Consensus indications for lead removal have been developed by the Heart Rhythm Society (HRS) [64] (Table 5.11). This classification system primarily addresses the nature of the risk to the patient of not removing a lead, but it does not approach the risk of extracting a chronically implanted lead in a specific patient. Issues such as the presence of CIED-related infection would generally result in a decision to extract even if the lead was very old, while removing a non-functional lead in an elderly patient might not justify the risk if the vessel was patent. Each patient and lead scenario is unique, and the risk of abandonment versus extraction needs to be considered based on the individual patient and lead characteristics.

A number of factors have been shown to influence the risk of lead extraction and these have been included in the indication guidelines [66]. These parameters relate to the patient (age, gender, overall health), anatomy (presence of calcification and vegetations associated with the lead), lead (number, construction, and condition), operator (physician training, experience, and case volume), and the wishes, goals, and values of the patient.

An infected CIED system (whether localized or systemic) provides the strongest indication for lead removal. In nearly all cases, complete removal of all prosthetic material has been shown to be necessary for eradication of the infection. In a large case series, 123 patients underwent pacemaker or ICD system extraction due to documented infection [67]. About one-third of patients had bacteremia, whereas most of the remainder had pocket infections. Staphylococci were the dominant infectious agents. One hundred and seventeen patients (95%) had complete system removal. Of the remaining six patents, three (50%) had relapse of infection, whereas only one of the 117 successfully extracted patients had relapse, and this single relapse resulted from reuse of an infected pocket. It is critical to note that delay in extracting an infected CIED in a bacteremic patient will increase the risk of death despite an uncomplicated lead extraction.

The microbiology of pacemaker and ICD infections in a published series of 412 patients is presented in Table 5.12 [61]. As in previous reports, infections with staphylococci predominate, representing over 80% of infections. In addition, 10% of cases were polymicrobial and in 12% no organism could be identified. Of note, in this recent series,

Table 5.11 HRS consensus indications for transvenous lead extraction

Recommendations for lead extraction apply only to those patients in whom the benefits of lead removal outweigh the risks when assessed based on individualized patient factors and operator-specific experience and outcomes

Infection
Class I

1 Complete device and lead removal is recommended in all patients with definite CIED system infection
2 Complete removal of epicardial leads and patches is recommended for all patients with confirmed infected fluid (purulence) surrounding the intrathoracic portion of the lead
3 Complete device and lead removal is recommended in all patients with valvular endocarditis without definite involvement of the lead(s) and/or device
4 Complete device and lead removal is recommended for patients with persistent or recurrent bacteremia or fungemia, despite appropriate antibiotic therapy and no other identifiable source for relapse or continued infection

Chronic pain
Class IIa

1 Device and/or lead removal can be useful for patients with severe chronic pain at the device or lead insertion site or believed to be secondary to the device, which causes significant patient discomfort, is not manageable by medical or surgical techniques, and for which there is no acceptable alternative

Thrombosis or venous stenosis
Class I

1 Lead removal is recommended for patients with clinically significant thromboembolic events attributable to thrombus on a lead or a lead fragment that cannot be treated by other means
2 Lead removal is recommended for patients with SVC stenosis or occlusion that prevents implantation of a necessary lead
3 Lead removal is recommended for patients with planned stent deployment in a vein already containing a transvenous lead, to avoid entrapment of the lead
4 Lead removal as part of a comprehensive plan for maintaining patency is recommended for patients with SVC stenosis or occlusion with limiting symptoms

Class IIa

1 Lead removal can be useful for patients with ipsilateral venous occlusion preventing access to the venous circulation for required placement of an additional lead

Other
Class I

1 Lead removal is recommended for patients with life-threatening arrhythmias secondary to retained leads

Class IIa

1 Lead removal can be useful for patients with a CIED location that interferes with the treatment of a malignancy
2 Lead removal can be useful for patients if a CIED implantation would require more than four leads on one side or more than five leads through the SVC
3 Lead removal can be useful for patients with an abandoned lead that interferes with the operation of a CIED system

Class IIb

1 Lead removal may be considered for patients with leads that due to their design or their failure pose a potential future threat to the patient if left in place
2 Lead removal may be considered for patients to facilitate access to MRI[a]
3 Lead removal may be considered in the setting of normally functioning non-recalled pacing or defibrillation leads for selected patients after a shared decision-making process
4 Lead abandonment or removal can be a useful treatment strategy if a lead becomes clinically unnecessary or non-functional

[a] Removal of leads to prevent their abandonment, removal of broken or abandoned leads, or removal of leads to allow implantation of an MRI-conditional system.

Class I, general agreement for transvenous removal; class II, situations in which leads are often removed but with some divergence of opinion; class III, general agreement that removal is unnecessary or that an alternate approach should be considered.

CIED, cardiac implantable electronic device; SVC, superior vena cava.

Source: Kusumoto *et al.* [64]. Reproduced with permission of Elsevier.

Table 5.12 Microbiology of pacemaker/ICD infections

Staphylococcus epidermidis	44%
Staphylococcus aureus	36%
Enteroccoci	5%
Streptococcus viridans	2%
Other Gram-positive aerobes	1%
Gram-negative bacilli	9%
Anaerobic organisms	1%
Fungi/mycobacteria	1%
Polymicrobial infections	10%
No organism identified	12%

Source: data from Chua [67].

50% of *Staphylococcus* species isolated were resistant to methicillin. The overall rate of relapsed infection was 1.9%, and was slightly higher in patients reimplanted during the same hospitalization.

Retained non-infected but non-functioning hardware generally poses little immediate risk to the patient, but may complicate the placement of additional pacing leads, either by adding to the venous obstruction (and the risk of thrombosis/embolization) or by generation of spurious mechanical potentials between leads. A small but definite increase in the risk of infection has been shown with lead abandonment. In patients with a longer life expectancy, the late risks of retained abandoned leads, especially ICD leads, may include higher risk of infection and venous thrombosis. Abandoned leads also create a potential barrier to accessing MRI, which is needed at a rate of about 5% per year in such patients. Since complications of extraction increase with time elapsed since lead implantation, some argue for routine extraction, rather than abandonment, of unused leads in these patients [68]. In the absence of clear data supporting one point of view, clinicians will need to balance risks and benefits of this approach on a case-by-case basis [69]. In the 2017 HRS Consensus Statement, extraction of abandoned functional or non-functional leads, in the absence of another specific indication, is a class IIb indication [64].

Risks

The risk of a lead extraction procedure is highly dependent on the individual circumstances of the patient and lead system implanted. Just as importantly, the experience, competency, and preparedness of the extracting physician and team strongly impacts the risk of mortality and major adverse events. In a multicenter study of 1684 patients at 89 US centers, lead extraction of pacing and ICD leads using modern tools was associated with a 0.8% risk of death and a 1.9% risk of major complications, such as pericardial tamponade, hemothorax, and pulmonary embolus (Table 5.13) [70]. Ten percent of patients had incomplete (3%) or failed (7%) transvenous extraction. Of the 13 patients who died in this registry, five died from pericardial tamponade, three from hemothorax, one from pulmonary embolus, and one from innominate arteriovenous fistula.

The LExICon study reported on outcomes of 1449 consecutive patients at 13 centers who underwent laser-assisted extraction of 2405 leads [71]. Leads were completely removed in 96.5% of cases. Procedural failure was more likely with leads implanted for more than 10 years. Major adverse events occurred in 1.4% of cases, and the procedural mortality rate was 0.28% (four patients: three vascular tears and one RV tear). In centers with higher procedure volumes, clinical success rates were higher and major adverse event rates were lower. As noted later in this section, the now routinely used venous occlusion balloon has the potential to lower the mortality rates for highly lethal SVC tears by approximately 80%.

Table 5.13 Risks of lead extraction

Major	
Death	0.8%
Pericardial tamponade	1.4%
Hemothorax	0.4%
Pulmonary embolus	0.1%
Lead fragment migration/embolization	0.1%
Total major complications	1.9%
Minor	
Perforation without tamponade	0.4%
Myocardial avulsion	0.1%
Venous avulsion	0.1%
Other	0.9%
Total minor complications	1.4%

Source: data from Byrd *et al.* [70].

Increasing operator experience (>50 procedures performed) appears to reduce the risk of complications, and some highly experienced operators have reported complication rates lower than those reported in multicenter series. Acknowledging the well-documented association between complications and operator experience, current guidelines for the qualification of physicians have proposed a minimum of 40 lead extractions under supervision before start of independent practice [1,64]. To maintain skills, "extractionists" should extract at least 20 leads per year. Though these small numbers are truly minimums that should be met, it is obvious that achieving procedure numbers alone may not result in an acceptable level of competency.

There are several patient-specific features that predict major complications, including female gender, low body surface area, number of leads in place, and implant duration. Extraction of any chronically implanted lead should be undertaken only after careful consideration of the risk–benefit ratio, including patient age, overall health, presence of calcification or vegetations involving the leads, duration of implant, and patient preferences, goals of care, and values. It is also important to consider that following successful lead extraction for sepsis, there is an overall 1-year mortality of 15–25% [61,64]. These late deaths are probably related to underlying comorbidities as well as more extensive infectious complications in a chronically ill population. Note that mortality rate is even higher in infected patients if extraction is not performed or significantly delayed [64].

Technique

The extraction process begins with gathering relevant clinical information (Table 5.14). A chest radiograph should be performed to exclude the presence of undocumented hardware and assess for calcification. If a systemic infection is present or suspected, TEE should be performed to assess for presence of vegetations (class I recommendation) [64]. TEE has been shown to be twice as sensitive for detection of lead-related vegetations as transthoracic echocardiography. Blood should be typed and cross-matched in case transfusion is needed. It is necessary to know whether complete removal of all leads is necessary, and whether a new device will be implanted as part of the same procedure. Based on these data, a plan of action is devised. Availability of all the tools and equipment that may be needed should be confirmed before the patient is taken to the procedure room.

Lead extraction may be performed in either a specialized EP laboratory or in a cardiac surgical operating room [72]. At this time, standard practice is that if the procedure is performed in an EP laboratory, it should be capable of supporting open heart surgery. Thus, the concept of the "hybrid" laboratory is of particular relevance to lead extraction. Poor C-arm fluoroscopy units cannot show the detail needed to perform extraction procedures safely and effectively, especially if snaring of small fragments of leads becomes necessary. On the other hand, although an EP laboratory typically has excellent imaging, if a major complication occurs there is no time to move a patient to a cardiac operating room if exsanguination or other catastrophe is occurring. Regardless of the venue, the equipment

Table 5.14 Pre-explant information

Device	Patient	Laboratory
Site(s) of venous access	Degree of pacemaker dependency	Complete blood cell count, INR, aPTT,
Number and types of leads	and need for temporary pacing	platelet count, sample to blood bank
Method used for fixation	Risk for sedation/anesthesia	with type and cross-match
of leads	Comorbidities/medications	Blood chemistries
Difficulties encountered in	Special considerations (e.g.	ECG
prior procedures	vascular anomaly or occlusion;	Chest radiograph (PA and lateral)
Information on previously	IVC filter, bleeding diathesis)	and/or lead fluoroscopy
abandoned leads		

aPTT, activated partial thromboplastin time; ECG, electrocardiogram; INR, international normalized ratio; IVC, inferior vena cava; PA, posteroanterior.

and personnel needed to perform emergency thoracotomy and cardiopulmonary bypass must be immediately available. If the procedure is not being performed by a cardiac surgeon, such a surgeon needs to be available and knowledgeable about the types of injuries that occur with extraction, and should be prepared to perform the rescue procedure quickly should the need arise.

A cardiac anesthesiologist is preferred, in most cases with the patient under general anesthesia. A TEE probe should be in the room, and preferably inserted into the patient at the start of the procedure. This allows for initial screening of the LV ejection fraction, presence of tricuspid insufficiency, presence of a pericardial effusion, and evidence of an interatrial septal defect and/or right-to-left shunting. Should a drop in blood pressure occur, TEE can be very helpful in determining the presence of a new or expanding pericardial effusion, pleural effusion, or a left ventricle that is either underfilled or hypokinetic. An assistant for these procedures (either a fellow or second attending physician) is helpful due to the amount of equipment that must be controlled during the case. Recommended personnel for lead extraction are listed in Table 5.15. We have developed a pre-extraction checklist that is used following the standard "time-out" (Table 5.16).

The routine preparation for lead extractions involves placement of one or two large-bore venous lines in the femoral vein (usually the right). The femoral venous sheath provides for rapid fluid administration, emergent passage of a temporary pacing wire, and ability to upgrade to a femoral approach to extraction should such be needed. Especially in high-risk cases, we use the second femoral access for insertion of a stiff guidewire to the jugular or innominate vein as a "rail" to position a venous occlusive balloon to the SVC in case of a venous tear. This balloon (Bridge™, Philips Medical) is 8 cm long, has low compliance, and is intended to stem rapid blood loss from the SVC into the pericardium, right pleural or mediastinal space should a vascular tear occur. Recently, use of the balloon in the setting of SVC tear has been reported to increase survival from the 50% range to nearly 90% [73].

A radial arterial line may be used for monitoring purposes or alternatively a small femoral arterial

Table 5.15 Recommended personnel for lead extraction procedures

Primary operator: physician performing the lead extraction who is properly trained and experienced in device implantation, lead extraction, and the management of complications
Cardiothoracic surgeon well versed in the potential complications of lead extraction and techniques for their treatment, on site and immediately available (may also be the primary operator)
Cardiac anesthesia support, also trained in transesophageal echocardiography
Personnel capable of operating fluoroscopic equipment
"Scrubbed" assistant (nurse/technician/physician)
Non-"scrubbed" assistant familiar with the procedure, location and identification of extraction tools
Cardiopulmonary perfusionist (with bypass machine immediately available)
Echocardiographer (may also be the anesthesiologist)
Additional cardiac surgery support (physician's assistant, fellow or other surgeon) available

Source: adapted from Kusumoto et al. [64].

Table 5.16 Lead extraction checklist

• Cardiothoracic surgeon covering the case and immediately available (verified by direct phone contact)
• Typed and cross-matched blood (4 units) in the room
• Operating room nurse from cardiothoracic surgery available
• Cardiac perfusionist service aware and on stand-by with pump ready
• Proper extension tubing for femoral sheaths available
• All relevant phone numbers on the dry-erase board
• Extraction cart is in room and fully stocked
• Laser extraction generator in room, near head of bed, calibration checked
• Sterile defibrillator patches, placed on patient anterior and posterior
• Temporary pacing lead and working temporary pacemaker in the room
• 60-mL syringe filled with 15 mL contrast and 45 mL of saline with stopcock on table
• Amplatz 260-cm stiff guidewire to preposition in venous system
• SVC occlusion rescue balloon and 12 F introducer ready

line on the side opposite to the venous line may be used to facilitate the placement of femoral–femoral bypass in an emergency.

The chest, abdomen, and femoral regions are prepared with chlorhexidine- or iodine-based antiseptic solutions such that emergent thoracotomy could be performed. Drapes are placed so that a large sterile field is maintained from the neck to the thighs. If the patient is pacemaker dependent, a temporary pacing wire is inserted. We prefer the femoral approach for temporary pacing during the procedure, as it is not uncommon for the lead to be dislodged. Having the lead readily accessible from the femoral vein allows for rapid repositioning should that be needed. If prolonged temporary pacing (>24–48 hours) will be needed (as in the case of an infected system in a pacemaker-dependent patient), we employ an externalized "permanent" active fixation lead as the temporary device via the contralateral internal jugular vein for added security during the postoperative treatment period until a new permanent system is placed (see also Chapter 2).

A variety of tools are available to assist with lead extraction and a partial list of equipment which should be available to the operator is given in Table 5.17. Lead extraction tools include the locking stylets and different types of sheaths. These are supplemented by a variety of other tools (e.g. various snares, guidewires, compression devices, sutures, lead extenders, and biopsy forceps). The operator should have on hand all of the tools that may be needed in a complex case, whether their use is anticipated or not. All the equipment and personnel necessary for emergent heart surgery (including cardiopulmonary bypass) should be readily available. The extraction procedure cannot start unless a designated surgeon is confirmed to be available for emergency assistance, if such is needed.

The pocket is usually entered through the previous incision line, although this may be altered to include a site of erosion or skin necrosis. With a combination of sharp and blunt dissection, the generator and leads are freed. Electrocautery is essential in freeing leads that are often extensively fibrosed to each other and to subcutaneous tissue. The lead is traced to the venous entry point, the suture sleeve is identified, and all retention sutures are cut and removed. The lead is disconnected

Table 5.17 Tools and equipment for lead extraction

General equipment
Standard lead stylets
Fluoroscopy
Pacemaker tray
Pericardiocentesis tray
Chest tube insertion kit
Emergency thoracotomy tray with appropriate sternal saw
Temporary pacing lead and pacemaker
Venous occlusion balloon

Superior approach
Locking stylets
Laser generator and laser extraction sheaths
Rotating mechanical extraction sheaths
Polypropylene telescoping sheaths
Lead extender
Compression coil
Long sutures

Femoral approach
Byrd femoral workstation
Needle's Eye snare (Cook Vascular)
Selection of intravascular snares (Amplatz gooseneck, EN Snare, etc.)
Deflecting tip wires
Deflecting guide catheter
Biopsy forceps

from the generator and its internal integrity is accessed by passing a standard stylet to the tip. In most cases, an initial attempt at gentle traction is worthwhile, but care must be taken not to damage the lead during this process. Observation under fluoroscopy during gentle traction also gives an idea about possible sites of lead attachment to the surrounding tissue.

Passive leads are usually more difficult to extract than active leads, presumably because the tines incorporated on these leads provide a greater surface area for fibrous adhesion. For active fixation leads, one should attempt to retract the helix in order to facilitate removal and possibly reduce the risk of cardiac perforation. If the retraction mechanism is not effective (or if it is a non-retractable helix), an attempt should be made to rotate the entire lead counterclockwise to unscrew the tip from the heart. This may be impossible in situations where the body of the lead is extensively fibrosed to the heart and veins. While extraction of an active fixation ventricular lead with the helix extended is not likely to be a problem, an atrial lead may come free with a small full-thickness piece of the atrial wall, resulting in pericardial bleeding and potential tamponade.

Techniques for lead extraction can be broadly categorized into the superior approach (utilizing a locking stylet and telescoping sheaths placed over the lead to provide traction and countertraction) and the femoral approach (using different types of grasping snares and wires to remove leads).

Superior approach

A stepwise approach is followed, reassessing the adherence of the lead, the integrity of the lead, the condition of the patient, and the risk of proceeding. If a lead is not easily removable by simple direct traction or traction with rotation (with or without a standard stylet inserted), the stylet (if present) should be

withdrawn and the lead cut close to the terminal pin with a lead cutter. The central lumen of the lead is identified and is exposed by removing a portion of the outer coil (when present). The central coil is inspected for burrs and roundness and, if needed, carefully dilated with a coil-expander tool. Depending on the type of locking stylet to be used, the diameter of the lumen may need to be determined by the insertion of a series of gauge pins. Some locking stylets are "universal" and do not require sizing. An appropriate locking stylet is then advanced through the lumen to the lead tip. This device is essential to focus the force of traction as close to the lead tip as possible, and to distribute traction along the length of the lead. Without the locking stylet, the lead would simply uncoil as traction is applied.

Several types of locking stylets are available (Figure 5.43), which vary in the way they grip the inner core of the lead. The operator needs to be familiar with the specific directions for each of the

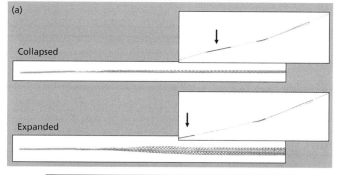

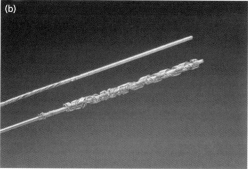

Figure 5.43 Locking stylets for lead extraction. (a) Spectranetics LLD locking stylet (Spectranetics, Colorado Springs, CO, USA) has an expandable mesh over the stylet body that binds the lumen of the lead along its length. (*Top*) With the mesh retracted, the entire length of the stylet is isodiametric with the stylet tip for insertion into the lead. (*Bottom*) Once inside the lead to be extracted, the operator slides the locking mechanism (arrow) forward, expanding the mesh, which provides a broad distribution of force along the lead when traction is applied. (b) The Cook stylet (Cook Vascular, Leechburg, PA, USA) has a small wire mesh wound at the tip that unravels and binds at the distal end of the lead lumen.

locking stylets before they are used. It may be difficult or impossible to reverse the locking mechanism and remove these devices once they are inserted into the lead. Some leads are designed with additional "cables," such as those in ICD leads or the lumenless 3830 SelectSecure™ lead (Medtronic). By tying a suture to these cables and to the body of the lead, the tension on the lead is distributed over more components of the lead (Figure 5.44). As an alternative, use of a compression coil (e.g. One-Tie™; Cook Medical, Bloomington, IN, USA) that binds all the components of the lead together can be used (Figure 5.45).

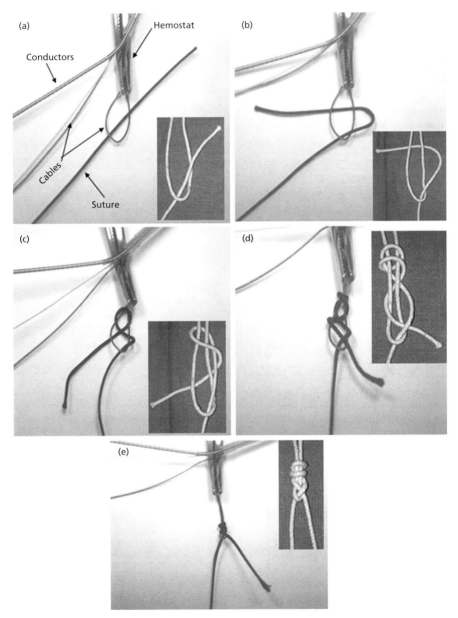

Figure 5.44 Tying to the "cables" of defibrillator leads. A modified sheet bend is used. (a) A loop is formed with the exposed end of the cable and held in place with a small hemostat. A 0-silk suture is passed through the loop from below. (b) The silk tie is passed behind the loop of cable. (c) The silk is passed in front of the loop of cable and then behind again two to three times, wrapping around the neck of the loop. (d) The end of the silk is passed under itself but over the loop of cable. (e) The ends of the silk are pulled to complete the knot. The long end of the silk tie is tied to the end of the locking stylet to provide traction on the cable.

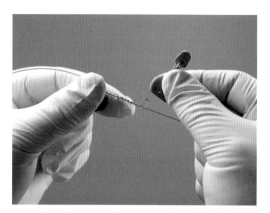

Figure 5.45 Cook Medical One-Tie compression device. This is a circular loop of wire that is used to wrap around the lead body, thereby compressing all the internal components and insulation together. This helps to provide a single traction unit.

The use of a lead extender (Bulldog™, Cook Medical) may also be helpful in cases of a lumenless lead or for a lead that will not accept a locking stylet. In patients with inner conductor failure, the inner lumen of the lead may be interrupted, making it impossible to pass a locking stylet. In this case the femoral approach may be required.

A variety of plastic, metal, fiberoptic (laser), and rotating mechanical (hand or battery powered) dilating/dissecting sheaths are available to advance over the lead body and free it from fibrous adhesions (Figure 5.46). Most of these sheaths are provided with a slightly shorter "outer" sheath that can be advanced coaxially in a telescoping fashion to aid in the extraction process. This larger outer sheath helps to prevent kinking of the inner sheath, and may be useful for advancing over larger fibrotic

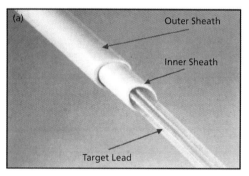

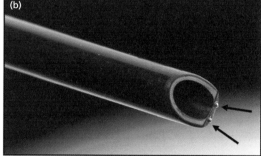

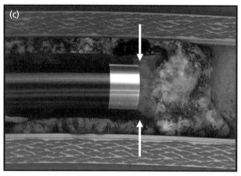

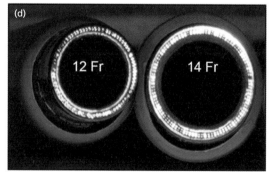

Figure 5.46 Different types of sheath used in lead extraction. (a) Simple telescoping sheaths over a lead. The outer sheath provides support as the inner sheath (with beveled edge) is gradually advanced over the lead to separate it from fibrous vascular adhesions by blunt dissection. (b) The Electrosurgical Dissection System (EDS, Cook Medical) utilizes an inner sheath with bipolar electrocautery/radiofrequency energy delivered between two poles on the tip of the sheath.

Ablative energy is limited to approximately one-quarter of the circumference of the sheath. (c) Laser-assisted sheath (Spectranetics) consists of a series of parallel fiberoptic cables wound around a flexible inner sheath and terminating at the tip of the sheath (arrows). (d) When activated, the tip of the sheath emits pulses of high-energy ultraviolet light along the entire circumference of the sheath, vaporizing fibrous adhesions in direct contact with the tip.

adhesions attached to the lead. In many cases, applying considerable pressure and torque to the sheath is necessary to separate the lead from fibrous adhesions. To minimize the risk of perforation or venous tear by the sheaths, fluoroscopic monitoring must be used during sheath advancement to ensure that the proper coaxial alignment of the dilator sheath and the lead is maintained. Traction on the lead via the locking stylet facilitates the processes by creating a "rail" over which the sheaths may be more safely advanced. Correct positioning of the sheath provides a mechanism for countertraction to be applied to the lead tip, localizing the stress to the area just around the attachment site to facilitate extraction. By advancing the outer sheath to the lead tip at the endocardial surface, the sheath applies counterpressure to pin the myocardium in place and allows traction on the lead without invaginating or tearing the myocardium (Figure 5.47).

One of the benefits of extraction is that it allows access through chronically occluded veins, thus sparing the contralateral veins from possible thrombotic complications. Access for a new lead may be retained by placing one or more guidewires through the extraction sheath after a lead has been extracted. Care should be taken to avoid air embolus as the wire is passed through the large empty extraction sheath.

The process of lead extraction with the use of early-generation unpowered tools was difficult and complete removal of a lead was achieved in only 85–95% of cases. The evolution of technology and introduction of the excimer laser sheath as well as powered mechanical sheaths have greatly facilitated lead extraction by the superior approach (Figure 5.47). The laser sheath has optical fibers arrayed circumferentially in the lining of the sheath, which is attached to the excimer laser generator (Philips Medical, Colorado Springs, CO, USA). Laser energy photoablates the fibrous adhesions as the sheath is advanced (see Figure 5.46). Complete removal of leads using this approach may be anticipated in well over 90% of patients, with partial removal in another 3% [70,71]. Though the laser sheath approach is effective in many cases, rotating mechanical sheaths are more effective if binding lesions are calcified. Although all powered sheaths have improved efficacy, they have not conclusively demonstrated a decrease in major adverse events from the procedure.

The introduction of powered mechanical sheaths has offered another option, especially for extraction of calcified leads. The EvolutionRL (Cook Medical) is a second-generation hand-powered device that has a metal tip which is very effective in cutting through difficult lesions. The system is powered b pulling on the handle. Each time the handle is r leased completely, the next pull results in turning the sheath in the opposite direction (hence the RL or right–left designation). The ability of the newer iteration to reverse when desired helps to reduce the risk of "lead wrap." If the handle of the EvolutionRL is not released fully to the resting position, the following pull of the handle will result in rotation in the same direction as the previous pull, which at times will allow for more effective dissection of difficult tissues.

Another hand-powered mechanical tool is the TightRail™ (Philips Medical). Though it too is powered by pulling a handle, this device has a flexible non-rotating shaft with a small dissection blade just inside the end of the sheath. With each pull of the handle, the blade extends slightly (but within the inner circumference of the sheath) and rotates around the lead. This system is also useful for dissecting through dense and/or calcified lesions. Most recently, the TightRail™ Guardian (Philips Medical) battery-powered version of this sheath has been introduced. This is similar to the TightRail in design, but an electric motor is added to minimize arm fatigue. In the protected mode, the rotating dissection blade does not extend beyond the end of the sheath. This is thought to be helpful in "high-risk" regions such as the bend from the innominate vein into the SVC. The extended mode is useful for more difficult binding sites and for getting through the dense tissues in the subclavicular region. Both the EvolutionRL and the TightRail are available in shorter, stiffer versions (Shortie and Sub-C, respectively) that are useful for punching through from the device pocket into the subclavian vein (Figure 5.48).

Femoral approach

Although the femoral approach is used by some extractors as a primary method, most physicians utilize it as a bail-out [74]. With this method, a large (16 Fr) sheath with a hemostatic valve is used as a "workstation" through which any of a number

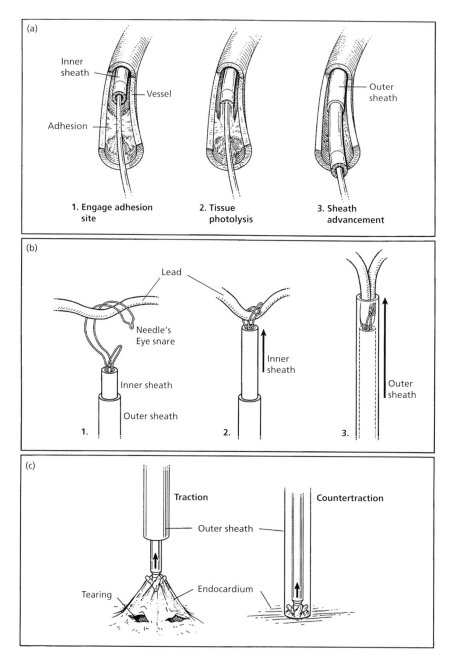

Figure 5.47 Basic techniques of lead extraction. (a) Lead extraction from the superior approach using the Spectranetics laser sheath apparatus. As the telescoping sheath apparatus encounters fibrous adhesions, the inner end-firing laser sheath is used to lyse the fibrosis. The larger outer sheath may then be advanced to apply countertraction at the lead tip. (b) Lead extraction from the femoral approach using the Cook Intravascular Needle's Eye Snare apparatus. The snare is deployed from telescoping sheaths in the femoral vein. The lead is entrapped in the snare and then secured against the inner sheath. The larger outer sheath may then be advanced to apply countertraction at the lead tip. (c) The concept of countertraction is illustrated. When unmodified traction is applied to the lead, the heart wall may invaginate and tear the myocardium around the lead tip. Using countertraction, the outer sheath holds the myocardium in place, thus minimizing deformity and tearing of the myocardium.

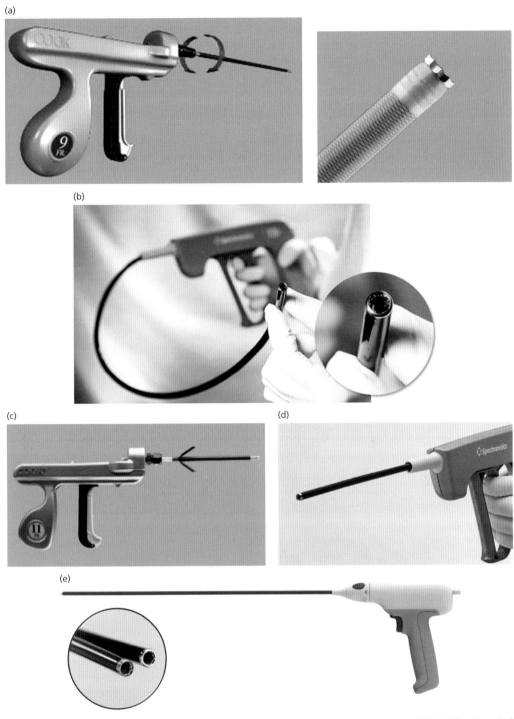

Figure 5.48 (a) Cook Medical EvolutionRL hand-powered mechanical sheath with bidirectional rotating sheath inside an outer sheath. The tip of the inner sheath has a metal tip that provides cutting and dissecting of tissues. (b) Philips (previously Spectranetics) hand-powered extraction sheath. A dissecting blade is recessed in the flexible sheath and rotates slightly outward and circumferentially to dissect tissues. (c) Cook Shortie and (d) Philips Sub-C. Both are shorter, stiffer and more aggressive versions of the hand-powered tools for getting through the difficult tissues and calcifications under the clavicle. (e) TightRail Guardian™ (Philips Medical) battery-powered mechanical extraction tool.

of devices designed to grasp the lead body may be introduced. Recently, it has been found that the introducer sheath for the leadless pacemaker system also provides an excellent workstation. Many different tools and snares may be used to grab and pull the leads down through the workstation sheath. These include smaller sheaths/catheters, a Dotter helical retrieval basket, a tip-deflecting guidewire, a Needle's Eye Snare (Cook Vascular, Leechburg, PA, USA), Amplatz gooseneck snares, triple loop EN Snare, or a variety of other catheters, snares, and bioptomes. Using a deflectable sheath such as the Agilis™ (Abbott) may facilitate positioning of the snare inside the heart (Figure 5.49).

With the femoral technique, if a free end of the lead is not available, one must grasp the lead body, which can be done with a single device (the Needle's Eye Snare) or with two devices, such as a tip-deflecting wire or deflectable catheter used for EP studies, and an Amplatz gooseneck snare. The Needle's Eye device is contained in a 12-Fr sheath. There are two independently moving mechanisms that can be advanced from the sheath: a hook-shaped wire loop (needle's eye) and a narrower "threader" that is designed to pass within the hook of the needle's eye. The goal is to place the device so that the lead body is trapped between the needle's eye and threader. This is usually accomplished by

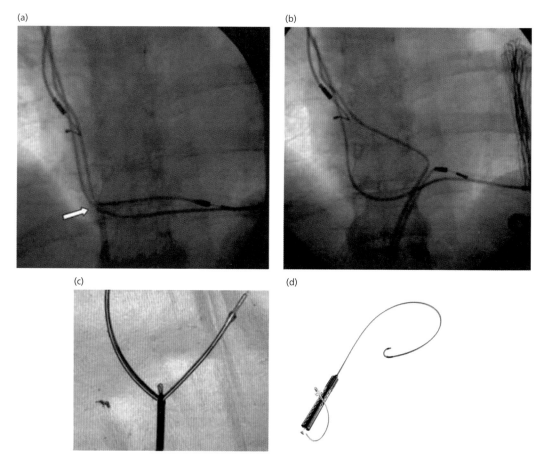

(a) (b) (c) (d)

Figure 5.49 Fluoroscopic images of ventricular lead extraction by the femoral approach. (a) The ventricular lead has been captured with the Needle's Eye snare apparatus at the point of the arrow and the redundancy of the lead retracted into the low atrium. (b) With traction, the lead tip is dislodged from the ventricle and the folded lead body is withdrawn into the large outer sheath. (c) The completely extracted lead. (d) The Agilis™ sheath can be used to help position the less steerable snares into the correct position within the vasculature and heart structures.

first placing the sheath in the low right atrium with the devices retained inside. The needle's eye is advanced out of the sheath and rotated so that it hooks around the lead body. The threader is then advanced so that it passes through the distal portion of the needle's eye so that the lead is held between the devices (Figure 5.49).

The sheath is then advanced over the ensemble, trapping and fixating the captured lead. Once this is accomplished, traction is applied by the sheath pulling the proximal lead down the SVC. The captured lead may be prolapsed into the workstation, which can be used as a countertraction device as it is advanced over the distal lead; however, this may not be feasible with many larger ICD leads. In the latter instance, simply withdrawing the proximal free end of the lead into the heart or IVC and then disengaging the needle's eye will allow it to be captured by a gooseneck snare and more easily removed through the workstation. The workstation may be advanced over the lead into the ventricle to supply countertraction if necessary.

The femoral technique has been found to be safe and effective, with a complete extraction success rate of 87% in a population that included patients who had failed prior extraction via the superior approach [75]. A similar procedure may be performed with a deflecting wire (or catheter) and snare. In this situation, both the wire and snare are situated in the right atrium through the workstation. A J curve is placed on the deflector wire, which is used to catch the lead body. The snare is then advanced to tightly grasp the tip of the deflecting wire. This effectively forms a loop around the lead body, which can act to retract the lead after the proximal portion is cut from the original access site. Once captured, the free end of the lead can be snared and then pulled into the workstation, or it may be removed as described previously with the Needle's Eye device.

Although it is always best to withdraw the lead through the workstation, there are times when this cannot be done and the workstation has to be removed with the lead inside. If multiple leads must be removed, we sometimes leave a second long wire in the femoral vein at the time of original access. This retained guidewire technique allows us to reenter the same venous site repeatedly if necessary. Once all the leads are out of the body, the femoral

workstation is removed and manual pressure to the femoral access site (and often a hemostatic suture) is applied for hemostasis.

The femoral workstation technique is safe and quite successful. It avoids having to free up adhesions in the central veins because the proximal lead is often more easily pulled through fibrous vascular attachments from below. On occasion, the proximal lead may be trapped within the subclavian vein and will not yield to femoral traction. In these cases, use of an extraction sheath from the insertion site superiorly can be very helpful in freeing up the proximal lead, allowing it to be extracted through the femoral workstation. The workstation has a large lumen and blood coagulates easily within it. A large thrombus may form and be pushed into the circulation during the manipulation of devices through the sheath. We routinely attach a pressurized continuous flush to the sidearm of the device to help prevent such thrombus formation.

Variations on the femoral approach include a hybrid procedure, in which the femoral workstation is used as described to pull the proximal lead into the heart. At this point a snare introduced from the internal jugular vein is used to catch the free end of the lead and pull it out using countertraction from a long sheath placed via the internal jugular vein. The entire procedure might be performed using an internal jugular vein approach, which has been favored by some, since the direction of force exerted during sheath advancement is parallel to the course of the lead.

The utility, safety, and efficacy of the femoral approach versus the superior approach using a laser sheath were compared in a multicenter study involving 459 patients [76]. In this study, rates of successful extraction and complications were similar between the two groups, while the femoral approach was associated with longer procedure and fluoroscopy times. The decision about which approach or approaches to use depends on the discretion of the operator, the condition of the leads, and the course of the procedure.

Extraction of coronary venous leads

With the increased use of biventricular pacing for CRT, there has been some concern that removal of chronically implanted leads from the coronary venous system will be associated with high complication rates because of the risk of disruption of the thin-walled coronary veins. The experience thus far for removal of these devices has generally not been associated with complications. However, these series include only a small number of leads with long implant duration [77,78]. With chronic CS leads, various extraction sheaths may be used to free the lead from venous adhesions. Careful passage of a sheath into the CS appears to be safe as well. However, passage of a sheath into a cardiac vein may result in a tear with resultant hemopericardium. Fortunately, in series reported to date, fibrous adhesions of these leads have generally been seen outside of the CS.

The largest series of CS lead extractions reported to date included 125 CS lead removals in 115 patients with a mean implant duration of 1.5 years (range 8 days to 8.2 years) [78]; 91% of leads were removed with simple traction, including 97% of leads implanted within 1 year. Three patients (2.4%) required use of a snare, two (1.6%) required a locking stylet alone, and six (4.8%) required a locking stylet and laser sheath; one of these six cases required laser application within the body of the CS, which was performed without complication. Nearly all leads (124 of 125, 99%) were successfully removed. Eleven patients (8.8%) had a CS stenosis or dissection from the extraction or reimplantation procedure, while non-CS complications were low and similar to those in other reported series. One patient died due to RV perforation during extraction of an ICD lead.

An exception to the general safety of CS lead removal is the Starfix® (Medtronic) active fixation coronary venous lead. This lead has plastic "lobes" that are deployed to prevent movement of the lead. Fibrous tissue can grow between the lobes and firmly attach the lead to the vein wall. Tear of the CS vein has been reported with resulting pericardial tamponade. This area of the tear is typically on the posterior surface and may be difficult for a surgeon to access and repair. In cases involving this particular lead model, extreme care must be used, since there is considerable risk of tearing a coronary vein.

Thoracotomy for lead extraction

There has been a natural reticence even among surgeons to remove leads at thoracotomy. There are no randomized data comparing the techniques of percutaneous versus open chest extraction. Surgery may be the only alternative in situations in which percutaneous techniques have failed and there is an absolute indication for lead removal, or if infected epicardial leads are components of the system. Since most transvenous extraction series demonstrate a 3–8% rate of failure to remove all lead material completely, a role for surgical lead extraction remains. Primary thoracotomy should also be considered when there is a large lead vegetation (>2.5 cm) and perhaps when there is a vegetation and a right-to-left intracardiac shunt. Close collaboration and discussion between physicians who perform extractions and cardiothoracic surgeons who can perform surgical extraction and assist with management of complications of transvenous extraction are vital components of a lead extraction program.

Lead abandonment

The alternative to extraction is lead abandonment and (usually) insertion of a new lead. This is not an option in cases of infection, where failure to remove all hardware results in an unacceptable risk of reinfection despite vigorous treatment with antibiotics. One may abandon the lead by detaching it from the generator and applying an insulating cap to the connector pin. The lead may then be placed under the generator or elsewhere in the pocket, reserving the option for future use (for a functional lead) as well as lead extraction should that prove necessary (e.g. the subsequent occurrence of infection). Some operators prefer to cut some pacing leads and electrically isolate them by pulling the silicone insulation over the exposed end and tying a ligature tightly around the insulation cuff. The lead is then sutured to the underlying tissue to prevent its retraction into the vascular space. Enough lead is left in the pocket to allow for future extraction if that proves necessary. Active fixation leads should generally not be cut, because this precludes retraction of the helix of the lead if extraction should ever be needed. A major problem occurs when a lead is cut and allowed to retract into the central circulation. This not only makes future extraction much more challenging, but in the case of an infected lead may allow continued seeding of the blood from bacteria harbored within the lumen of the lead. Leaving a lead in a condition that will permit future extraction and prevent retraction into the vessel is considered a class I recommendation [64].

Summary

- Extraction can be performed with a high level of efficacy and low morbidity and mortality.
- Higher-volume extractors and centers have better results.
- With rare exceptions, any patient with a CIED-related infection should have the entire system, including the leads, removed.
- Lead abandonment is not without risk and consequence.
- No single extraction tool will allow for the best result in all patients.
- Immediate availability of cardiac surgery rescue along with proper use of the SVC occlusion balloon can prevent mortality in the majority of patients with SVC and myocardial complications.

Medicolegal aspects of implantation and extraction

As with many invasive procedures, the patient's expectations for pacemaker therapy may exceed the results obtained. As already noted, there is ample opportunity for even the most skilled and experienced operator to encounter a misadventure. The risk of litigation is real and may focus on any of several areas of physician responsibility (Table 5.18). Avoiding conflict requires not only that the highest of standards be maintained, but also that a good rapport be established with the patient and the patient's family.

The best defense against litigation is full documentation in the patient's medical record of every aspect of the implantation (or extraction) process.

Table 5.18 Responsibilities of an implanting physician

1	Establish and document accepted indications
2	Obtain fully informed consent/shared decision-making (including the option of not implanting or extracting)
3	Implant an indicated system
4	Avoid undue delay (especially in the case of extraction of infected systems)
5	Conform to accepted technique and standards
6	Obtain expert consultation when appropriate
7	Provide for follow-up care

This should include the indication for the procedure, documentation of a shared decision-making process, the signed informed consent forms, a complete procedure note to include the pacing parameters achieved and any difficulties encountered, evidence of postprocedure evaluation, and arrangements for follow-up care. The removal of preexisting hardware and its disposition (e.g. returned to manufacturer for evaluation) should also be documented.

Performance of CIED implantation and extraction implies a great deal of physician responsibility. As with any implantable device, there is continued risk to the patient as long as he or she has the device. Somewhat specific to implantable antiarrhythmic devices is the knowledge that the power source has limited life and will eventually need to be replaced. The HRS, ACC, and AHA have provided a service to physicians and the public by creating guidelines to assist in patient treatment.

References

1 Calkins H, Awtry EH, Bunch TJ, *et al.* COCATS 4 Task Force 11: Training in arrhythmia diagnosis and management, cardiac pacing, and electrophysiology. *J Am Coll Cardiol* 2015;65(17):1854–1865.

2 Zipes DP, Calkins H, Daubert JP, *et al.* 2015 ACC/AHA/HRS advanced training statement on clinical cardiac electrophysiology (a revision of the ACC/AHA 2006 update of the clinical competence statement on invasive electrophysiology studies, catheter ablation, and cardioversion). *J Am Coll Cardiol* 2015;66(24):2767–2802.

3 Kusumoto FM, Schoenfeld MH, Barrett C, *et al.* 2018 ACC/AHA/HRS guideline on the evaluation and management of patients with bradycardia and cardiac conduction delay: executive summary. *Circulation* 2019; 140(8):e333–e381.

4 Al-Khatib SM, Stevenson WG, Ackerman MJ, *et al.* 2017 AHA/ACC/HRS guideline for management of patients with ventricular arrhythmias and the prevention of sudden cardiac death. *J Am Coll Cardiol* 2018;72(14):e91–e220.

5 Gillis AM, Russo AM, Ellenbogen KA, *et al.* HRS/ACCF expert consensus statement on pacemaker device and mode selection. *Heart Rhythm* 2012;9(8):1344–1365.

6 Tracy CM, Epstein AE, Darbar D, *et al.* 2012 ACCF/AHA/HRS focused update of the 2008 guidelines for device-based therapy of cardiac rhythm abnormalities. *J Am Coll Cardiol* 2012;60(14):1297–1313.

7 Baddour LM, Epstein AE, Erickson CC, *et al.* Update on cardiovascular implantable electronic device infections and their management. *Circulation* 2010;121(3):458–477.

8 Fähling M, Seeliger E, Patzak A, Persson PB. Understanding and preventing contrast-induced acute kidney injury. *Nat Rev Nephrol* 2017;13(3):169–180.

9 Douketis JD, Spyropoulos AC, Kaatz S, *et al*. Perioperative bridging anticoagulation in patients with atrial fibrillation. *N Engl J Med* 2015;373(9):823–833.

10 Giudici MC, Barold SS, Paul DL, Bontu P. Pacemaker and implantable cardioverter defibrillator implantation without reversal of warfarin therapy. *Pacing Clin Electrophysiol* 2004;27(3):358–360.

11 Cheng A, Nazarian S, Brinker JA, *et al*. Continuation of warfarin during pacemaker or implantable cardioverter-defibrillator implantation: a randomized clinical trial. *Heart Rhythm* 2011;8(4):536–540.

12 Ghanbari H, Phard WS, Al-Ameri H, *et al*. Meta-analysis of safety and efficacy of uninterrupted warfarin compared to heparin-based bridging therapy during implantation of cardiac rhythm devices. *Am J Cardiol* 2012; 110(10):1482–1488.

13 Birnie DH, Healey JS, Wells GA, *et al*. Pacemaker or defibrillator surgery without interruption of anticoagulation. *N Engl J Med* 2013;368(22):2084–2093.

14 Stewart MH, Morin DP. Management of perioperative anticoagulation for device implantation. *Card Electrophysiol Clin* 2018;10(1):99–109.

15 Tompkins C, Cheng A, Dalal D, *et al*. Dual antiplatelet therapy and heparin "bridging" significantly increase the risk of bleeding complications after pacemaker or implantable cardioverter–defibrillator device implantation. *J Am Coll Cardiol* 2010;55(21):2376–2382.

16 McCotter CJ, Angle JF, Prudente LA, *et al*. Placement of transvenous pacemaker and ICD leads across total chronic occlusions. *Pacing Clin Electrophysiol* 2005;28(9):921–925.

17 Eleid MF, Blauwet LA, Cha Y-M, *et al*. Bioprosthetic tricuspid valve regurgitation associated with pacemaker or defibrillator lead implantation. *J Am Coll Cardiol* 2012; 59(9):813–818.

18 Osman F, Krishnamoorthy S, Nadir A, *et al*. Safety and cost-effectiveness of same day permanent pacemaker implantation. *Am J Cardiol* 2010;106(3):383–385.

19 Da Costa A, Kirkorian G, Cucherat M, *et al*. Antibiotic prophylaxis for permanent pacemaker implantation. *Circulation* 1998;97(18):1796–1801.

20 de Oliveira JC, Martinelli M, Nishioka S, *et al*. Efficacy of antibiotic prophylaxis before the implantation of pacemakers and cardioverter–defibrillators. *Circ Arrhythm Electrophysiol* 2009;2(1):29–34.

21 Krahn AD, Longtin Y, Philippon F, *et al*. Prevention of arrhythmia device infection trial. *J Am Coll Cardiol* 2018;72(24):3098–3109.

22 Biffi M, Bertini M, Ziacchi M, *et al*. Clinical implications of left superior vena cava persistence in candidates for pacemaker or cardioverter–defibrillator implantation. *Heart Vessels* 2009;24(2):142–146.

23 Calkins H, Ramza BM, Brinker J, *et al*. Prospective randomized comparison of the safety and effectiveness of placement of endocardial pacemaker and defibrillator leads using the extrathoracic subclavian vein guided by contrast venography versus the cephalic approach. *Pacing Clin Electrophysiol* 2001;24(4):456–464.

24 Kistler PM, Eizenberg N, Fynn SP, Mond HG. The subpectoral pacemaker implant. *Pacing Clin Electrophysiol* 2004;27(3):361–364.

25 Brinker JA. Endocardial pacing leads: the good, the bad, and the ugly. *Pacing Clin Electrophysiol* 1995;18(5):953–954.

26 Hauser RG, Hayes DL, Kallinen LM, *et al*. Clinical experience with pacemaker pulse generators and transvenous leads: an 8-year prospective multicenter study. *Heart Rhythm* 2007;4(2):154–160.

27 Giudici MC, Thornburg GA, Buck DL, *et al*. Comparison of right ventricular outflow tract and apical lead permanent pacing on cardiac output. *Am J Cardiol* 1997; 79(2):209–212.

28 Stambler BS, Ellenbogen KA, Zhang X, *et al*. Right ventricular outflow versus apical pacing in pacemaker patients with congestive heart failure and atrial fibrillation. *J Cardiovasc Electrophysiol* 2003;14(11):1180–1186.

29 Saxonhouse SJ, Conti JB, Curtis AB. Current of injury predicts adequate active lead fixation in permanent pacemaker/defibrillation leads. *J Am Coll Cardiol* 2005;45(3): 412–417.

30 Bilchick KC, Judge DP, Calkins H, Marine JE. Use of a coronary sinus lead and biventricular ICD to correct a sensing abnormality in a patient with arrhythmogenic right ventricular dysplasia/cardiomyopathy. *J Cardiovasc Electrophysiol* 2006;17(3):317–320.

31 Ector B, Willems R, Heidbüchel H, *et al*. Epicardial pacing: a single-centre study on 321 leads in 138 patients. *Acta Cardiol* 2006;61(3):343–351.

32 Jutley RS, Waller DA, Loke I, *et al*. Video-assisted thoracoscopic implantation of the left ventricular pacing lead for cardiac resynchronization therapy. *Pacing Clin Electrophysiol* 2008;31(7):812–818.

33 Huang M, Krahn AD, Yee R, Klein GJ, Skanes AC. Optimal pacing for symptomatic AV block: a comparison of VDD and DDD pacing. *Pacing Clin Electrophysiol* 2004;27(1):19–23.

34 Vijayaraman P, Chung MK, Dandamudi G, *et al*. His bundle pacing. *J Am Coll Cardiol* 2018;72(8):927–947.

35 Zanon F, Ellenbogen KA, Dandamudi G, *et al*. Permanent His-bundle pacing: a systematic literature review and meta-analysis. *Europace* 2018;20(11):1819–1826.

36 Devabhaktuni S, Mar PL, Shirazi J, Dandamudi G. How to perform His bundle pacing. *Card Electrophysiol Clin* 2018;10(3):495–502.

37 Vijayaraman P, Dandamudi G. How to perform permanent His bundle pacing: tips and tricks. *Pacing Clin Electrophysiol* 2016;39(12):1298–1304.

38 Vijayaraman P, Dandamudi G, Zanon F, *et al.* Permanent His bundle pacing: recommendations from a Multicenter His Bundle Pacing Collaborative Working Group for standardization of definitions, implant measurements, and follow-up. *Heart Rhythm* 2018;15(3):460–468.

39 Tarakji KG, Mittal S, Kennergren C, *et al.* Antibacterial envelope to prevent cardiac implantable device infection. *N Engl J Med* 2019;380(20):1895–1905.

40 Fisher JD, Lapman P, Kim SG, *et al.* Lead stuck (frozen) in header: salvage by bone cutter versus other techniques. *Pacing Clin Electrophysiol* 2004;27(8):1136–1143.

41 Tjong FVY, Reddy VY. Permanent leadless cardiac pacemaker therapy. *Circulation* 2017;135(15):1458–1470.

42 El-Chami MF, Roberts PR, Kypta A, *et al.* How to implant a leadless pacemaker with a tine-based fixation. *J Cardiovasc Electrophysiol* 2016;27(12):1495–1501.

43 Lewis GF, Gold MR. Safety and efficacy of the subcutaneous implantable defibrillator. *J Am Coll Cardiol* 2016; 67(4):445–454.

44 Chue CD, Kwok CS, Wong CW, *et al.* Efficacy and safety of the subcutaneous implantable cardioverter defibrillator: a systematic review. *Heart* 2017;103(17):1315–1322.

45 Knops RE, Olde Nordkamp LRA, de Groot JR, Wilde AAM. Two-incision technique for implantation of the subcutaneous implantable cardioverter–defibrillator. *Heart Rhythm* 2013;10(8):1240–1243.

46 Wilkoff BL, Cook JR, Epstein AE, *et al.* Dual-chamber pacing or ventricular backup pacing in patients with an implantable defibrillator: the Dual Chamber and VVI Implantable Defibrillator (DAVID) Trial. *JAMA* 2002; 288(24):3115–3123.

47 Mulpuru SK, Madhavan M, McLeod CJ, Cha Y-M, Friedman PA. Cardiac pacemakers: function, troubleshooting, and management. *J Am Coll Cardiol* 2017;69(2): 189–210.

48 Link MS, Estes NA III, Griffin JJ, *et al.* Complications of dual chamber pacemaker implantation in the elderly. Pacemaker Selection in the Elderly (PASE) Investigators. *J Interv Card Electrophysiol* 1998;2(2):175–179.

49 Tobin K, Stewart J, Westveer D, Frumin H. Acute complications of permanent pacemaker implantation: their financial implication and relation to volume and operator experience. *Am J Cardiol* 2000;85(6):774–776.

50 Harcombe AA, Newell SA, Ludman PF, *et al.* Late complications following permanent pacemaker implantation or elective unit replacement. *Heart* 1998;80(3):240–244.

51 Wiegand UKH, Bode F, Bonnemeier H, *et al.* Atrial lead placement during atrial fibrillation: is restitution of sinus rhythm required for proper lead function? Feasibility and 12-month functional analysis. *Pacing Clin Electrophysiol* 2000;23(7):1144–1149.

52 Ellenbogen KA, Wood MA, Shepard RK. Delayed complications following pacemaker implantation. *Pacing Clin Electrophysiol* 2002;25(8):1155–1158.

53 Nanthakumar K, Kay GN, Plumb VJ, *et al.* Decrease in fluoroscopic cardiac silhouette excursion precedes hemodynamic compromise in intraprocedural tamponade. *Heart Rhythm* 2005;2(11):1224–1230.

54 Mahapatra S, Bybee KA, Bunch TJ, *et al.* Incidence and predictors of cardiac perforation after permanent pacemaker placement. *Heart Rhythm* 2005;2(9):907–911.

55 Henrikson CA, Leng CT, Yuh DD, Brinker JA. Computed tomography to assess possible cardiac lead perforation. *Pacing Clin Electrophysiol* 2006;29(5):509–511.

56 Gelder BM, Bracke FA, Oto A, *et al.* Diagnosis and management of inadvertently placed pacing and ICD leads in the left ventricle: a multicenter experience and review of the literature. *Pacing Clin Electrophysiol* 2000;23(5):877–883.

57 Chang JD, Manning WJ, Ebrille E, Zimetbaum PJ. Tricuspid valve dysfunction following pacemaker or cardioverter–defibrillator implantation. *J Am Coll Cardiol* 2017;69(18):2331–2341.

58 Rozmus G, Daubert JP, Huang DT, *et al.* Venous thrombosis and stenosis after implantation of pacemakers and defibrillators. *J Interv Card Electrophysiol* 2005;13(1):9–19.

59 Maisel WH, Moynahan M, Zuckerman BD, *et al.* Pacemaker and ICD generator malfunctions. *JAMA* 2006;295(16):1901.

60 Poller WC, Schwerg M, Melzer C. Therapy of cardiac device pocket infections with vacuum-assisted wound closure: long-term follow-up. *Pacing Clin Electrophysiol* 2012;35(10):1217–1221.

61 Tarakji KG, Chan EJ, Cantillon DJ, *et al.* Cardiac implantable electronic device infections: presentation, management, and patient outcomes. *Heart Rhythm* 2010; 7(8):1043–1047.

62 Henrikson CA, Brinker JA. How to prevent, recognize, and manage complications of lead extraction. Part III: Procedural factors. *Heart Rhythm* 2008;5(9):1352–1354.

63 van Rees JB, de Bie MK, Thijssen J, *et al.* Implantation-related complications of implantable cardioverter–defibrillators and cardiac resynchronization therapy devices. *J Am Coll Cardiol* 2011;58(10):995–1000.

64 Kusumoto FM, Schoenfeld MH, Wilkoff BL, *et al.* 2017 HRS expert consensus statement on cardiovascular implantable electronic device lead management and extraction. *Heart Rhythm* 2017;14(12):e503–e551.

65 Smith MC, Love CJ. Extraction of transvenous pacing and ICD leads. *Pacing Clin Electrophysiol* 2008;31(6):736–752.

66 Roux J-F, Pagé P, Dubuc M, *et al.* Laser lead extraction: predictors of success and complications. *Pacing Clin Electrophysiol* 2007;30(2):214–220.

67 Chua JD. Diagnosis and management of infections involving implantable electrophysiologic cardiac devices. *Ann Intern Med* 2000;133(8):604–608.

68 Maytin M, Epstein LM. Lead extraction is preferred for lead revisions and system upgrades: when less is more. *Circ Arrhythm Electrophysiol* 2010;3(4):413–424.

69 Henrikson CA. Think before you pull: not every lead has to come out. *Circ Arrhythm Electrophysiol* 2010;3(4): 409–412.

70 Byrd CL, Wilkoff BL, Love CJ, Sellers TD, Reiser C. Clinical study of the laser sheath for lead extraction: the total experience in the United States. *Pacing Clin Electrophysiol* 2002;25(5):804–808.

71 Wazni O, Epstein LM, Carrillo RG, *et al.* Lead extraction in the contemporary setting: the LExICon study. *J Am Coll Cardiol* 2010;55(6):579–586.

72 Wood M, Ellenbogen K. Defining the appropriate venue for lead extraction: a place for everything.… *Heart Rhythm* 2011;8(7):1006–1007.

73 Azarrafiy R, Tsang DC, Boyle TA, Wilkoff BL, Carrillo RG. Compliant endovascular balloon reduces the lethality of superior vena cava tears during transvenous lead extractions. *Heart Rhythm* 2017;14(9):1400–1404.

74 Belott PH. Lead extraction using the femoral vein. *Heart Rhythm* 2007;4(8):1102–1107.

75 Klug D, Jarwe M, Messaoudene SA, *et al.* Pacemaker lead extraction with the Needle's Eye Snare for countertraction via a femoral approach. *Pacing Clin Electrophysiol* 2002;25(7):1023–1028.

76 Bordachar P, Defaye P, Peyrouse E, *et al.* Extraction of old pacemaker or cardioverter–defibrillator leads by laser sheath versus femoral approach. *Circ Arrhythm Electrophysiol* 2010;3(4):319–323.

77 Williams SE, Arujuna A, Whitaker J, *et al.* Percutaneous lead and system extraction in patients with cardiac resynchronization therapy (CRT) devices and coronary sinus leads. *Pacing Clin Electrophysiol* 2011;34(10):1209–1216.

78 Sheldon S, Friedman PA, Hayes DL, *et al.* Outcomes and predictors of difficulty with coronary sinus lead removal. *J Interv Card Electrophysiol* 2012;35(1):93–100.

CHAPTER 6

Pacemaker timing cycles and special features

Jose F. Huizar

Arrhythmia and Device Clinic, Hunter Holmes McGuire VA Medical Center, VCU School of Medicine, Richmond, VA, USA

Introduction

Since the development of implantable cardiac pacemakers in 1960, the features and functions built into these devices has continued to change as the cardiac field evolves. Pacemakers have become highly complex due to the addition of multiple specialized features in an attempt to treat different cardiac conditions, such as sick sinus syndrome with or without chronotropic incompetence, cardioinhibitory vasovagal syndrome, and paroxysmal atrial arrhythmias, and avoid some adverse effects of chronic pacing, such as heart failure and induction of atrial and supraventricular arrhythmias. Thus, a deep understanding of the different pacing modes, pacemaker timing cycles, and special features is paramount in identifying normal versus abnormal pacemaker function.

Timing cycles are based on cardiac events such as atrial- and ventricular-sensed and -paced events. Thus, appropriate pacemaker function depends on the ability of these devices to properly recognize atrial- and ventricular-sensed events. Timing cycles include different blanking periods, refractory periods, and intervals. The number and complexity of these timing cycles depend and vary based on the number of leads, pacing mode, and/or rate sensor. Accurate examination of timing cycles and pacemaker behavior requires device interrogation and analysis of "event markers" as they provide the actual pacemaker interpretation and response to different cardiac signals. For the rest of the chapter, the following abbreviations are used to describe common pacemaker marker events: P, native atrial depolarization; A, an atrial-paced event; R, a native ventricular depolarization, and V, a ventricular-paced event.

Pacing nomenclature

The basic function of pacemakers is denoted as a generic five-letter code (Table 6.1) [1]. However, this five-letter code does not describe the specific or unique functional characteristics of each device.

The *first position* reflects the chamber or chambers in which stimulation occurs. "A" refers to the atrium, "V" indicates the ventricle, and "D" denotes dual chamber (or both atrium and ventricle).

The *second position* refers to the chamber or chambers in which sensing occurs. The letter designators are the same as those for the first position. Some manufacturers also use "S" in both the first and the second positions to indicate that the device is capable of pacing only a single cardiac chamber.

The *third position* refers to the mode of sensing, or how the pacemaker responds to a sensed event. An "I" indicates that a sensed event inhibits the pacing stimulus and causes the pacemaker to reset or reinitiate one or more timing cycles. A "T" means

Cardiac Pacing and ICDs, Seventh Edition. Edited by Kenneth A. Ellenbogen and Karoly Kaszala.
© 2020 John Wiley & Sons Ltd. Published 2020 by John Wiley & Sons Ltd.

Table 6.1 Revised NASPE/BPEG generic code for bradycardia, adaptive-rate, and multisite pacing

Position				
I	*II*	*III*	*IV*	*V*
Chamber(s) paced	*Chamber(s) sensed*	*Response to sensing*	*Rate modulation*	*Multisite pacing*
O = None	O = None	O = None	O = None	O = None
A = Atrium	A = Atrium	T = Triggered	R = Rate modulation	A = Atrium
V = Ventricle	V = Ventricle	I = Inhibited		V = Ventricle
D = Dual (A + V)	D = Dual (A + V)	D = Dual (T + I)		D = Dual (A+V)

BPEG, British Pacing and Electrophysiology Group; NASPE, North American Society of Pacing and Electrophysiology.
Source: modified from Bernstein *et al.* [1]. Reproduced with permission of John Wiley & Sons Ltd.

that an output pulse is triggered in response to a sensed event. Similar to the first two positions, a "D" means that there are dual modes of response. This designation is restricted to dual-chamber systems. An event sensed in the atrium inhibits atrial output but triggers ventricular output, also referred to as P-synchronous pacing. Unlike the single-chamber triggered mode, in which a pacing output is triggered immediately on sensing an event from the same chamber, a delay occurs between the sensed atrial event and the triggered ventricular pacing output to mimic the normal PR interval. Finally, if a native ventricular signal or R wave is sensed, it inhibits ventricular output and possibly even atrial output, depending on where sensing occurs.

The *fourth position* of the code reflects sensor rate modulation. An "R" indicates that the pacemaker incorporates a sensor to control the rate independently of intrinsic electrical activity of the heart, so-called rate-modulated pacing.

The *fifth position* indicates whether multisite pacing is not present (O) or present in the atrium (A), ventricle (V), or both (D). Multisite pacing is defined for this purpose as stimulation sites in both atria, both ventricles, more than one stimulation site in any single chamber, or any combination of these. The letter designators are the same as those for the first position. This fifth position has become relevant with the introduction of biventricular devices.

Pacing modes

Pacing modes have evolved with technology and each pacing mode has specific and general indications, as well as unique advantages and disadvantages (Table 6.2). The timing cycles of each of these pacing modes are discussed in the following section.

Single- or dual-chamber asynchronous pacing (AOO, VOO, DOO)

Ventricular asynchronous (VOO) pacing is the simplest of all pacing modes because there is neither sensing nor mode of response, and lower rate limit (LRL) is the only timing cycle available (Figure 6.1a). Atrial asynchronous (AOO) pacing behaves exactly like VOO, but pacing occurs in the atrial chamber. Dual-chamber or sequential atrioventricular (AV) asynchronous pacing (DOO) occurs at the LRL in the atrium, followed by the ventricle after completion of the atrioventricular interval (AVI), irrespective of any cardiac events. This pacing mode may be transiently used in pacemaker-dependent patients to avoid inappropriate pacing inhibition during interventions or surgeries associated with noise (Table 6.2).

Single-chamber (atrial or ventricular) inhibited pacing (AAI, VVI)

Pacemakers with an atrial lead can be programmed AAI, whereas devices with a ventricular lead can be programmed VVI (Figure 6.1b,c). AAI pacing mode denotes atrial pacing (A), atrial sensing (A), and inhibition (I) of pacing output in response to an atrial-sensed event (P wave), whereas VVI pacing mode indicates ventricular pacing (V), ventricular sensing (V), and inhibition (I) of pacing output in response to a ventricular-sensed event (R wave).

Single-chamber triggered mode (without inhibition) pacing (AAT, VVT)

Single-chamber triggered mode pacing (AAT, VVT) will deliver pacing output every time a native

Table 6.2 Indications, advantages, and disadvantages of commonly used pacing modes

Pacing mode	Indication/advantages	Disadvantages
Asynchronous pacing (AOO, VOO, DOO)	Pacemaker-dependent patients exposed to noise (e.g. electrocautery during surgery) Avoids oversensing and asystole	Pacing regardless of intrinsic events Potential risk for proarrhythmia
Single-chamber inhibited pacing (AAI, VVI)	AAI: sick sinus syndrome with intact AV node; preserves AV synchrony VVI: atrial fibrillation with slow VR and single-lead ICDs AAI/VVI require a single lead and increase battery longevity	AAI lacks ventricular pacing in the event of intermittent AV block VVI is associated with AV dyssynchrony (may manifest as pacemaker syndrome). VVI has a higher incidence of atrial arrhythmias [31]
Single-chamber triggered without inhibited pacing (AAT, VVT)	Historically used in pacemaker-dependent patients to assure pacing with lower probability of arrhythmia induction	Shortens battery life due to chronic pacing
DDD, DDDRV (CRT)	Preserves AV synchrony (less pacemaker syndrome) Low incidence of atrial arrhythmias and improved hemodynamics	Requires at least a two-chamber lead system and has a shorter battery longevity
DDI	Functions as two different pacemakers (AAI and VVI) Used as mode switch to avoid tracking atrial tachyarrhythmias	Same as DDD Possible AV dyssynchrony and pacemaker syndrome (does not track atrial-sensed events)
VDI	Used for mode switch purposes as it functions as a VVI (non-tracking pacing mode) with additional atrial sensing	Similar to VVI, as it is associated with AV dyssynchrony and potential atrial arrhythmias
VDD	Appropriate sinus node function with AV node disease, e.g. MDT RV lead model 5038; dual chamber with high atrial pacing threshold to minimize battery depletion	Lack of atrial pacing Potential AV dyssynchrony at lower rate limit
DVI	Severe sinus bradycardia/standstill and atrial lead malfunction (oversensing)	Asynchronous atrial pacing Potential AV dyssynchrony For both atrial and ventricular stimuli to be inhibited, the sensed R wave must occur during the VAI

For acronyms, see Table 6.3.

Source: modified from Huizar JF, Kaszala K, Ellenbogen KA. Cardiac pacing modes and terminology. In: Sakena S, Camm AJ, eds. *Electrophysiological Disorders of the Heart*, 2nd edn. Philadelphia, PA: Elsevier Saunders, 2012: 441–456. Reproduced with permission of Elsevier.

event is sensed or the LRL interval is reached. As it deforms the native signal, it may compromise electrocardiogram (ECG) interpretation. This pacing mode can serve as an excellent marker for the site and time of sensing within a complex in an ECG tracing. Historically, this pacing mode was used to prevent inappropriate inhibition from oversensing in a patient without a stable native escape rhythm. In contrast to asynchronous pacing (AOO or VOO), this pacing mode is less likely to induce arrhythmias as it will pace within refractoriness of myocardial tissue when the intrinsic cardiac event is sensed.

(a)

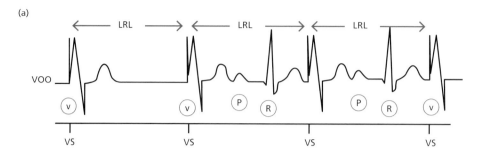

(b)

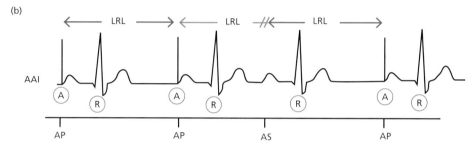

(c)

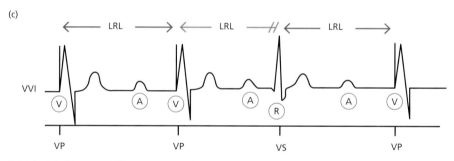

Figure 6.1 (a) VOO, (b) AAI, and (c) VVI pacing modes. Event markers represent the pacemaker's interpretation of different cardiac events. See text for details. A, atrial-paced event (AP); LRL, lower rate limit; P, intrinsic P wave (AS); R, intrinsic R wave (VS); V, ventricular-paced event (VP).

Source: modified from Huizar JF, Kaszala K, Ellenbogen KA. Cardiac pacing modes and terminology. In: Sakena S, Camm AJ, eds. *Electrophysiological Disorders of the Heart*, 2nd edn. Philadelphia, PA: Elsevier Saunders, 2012: 441–456. Reproduced with permission of Elsevier.

However, arrhythmias could be initiated if non-cardiac signals are inappropriately sensed.

Dual-chamber pacing and sensing with inhibition and tracking (DDD)

This can also be referred to as AV sequential (D) pacing, dual-chamber sensing (D) with inhibition, and P-synchronous pacing (D). DDD mode refers to atrial and ventricular pacing and sensing with dual response (inhibited and triggered pacing) to an intrinsic atrial-sensed event or a ventricular-sensed event (Figure 6.2a). In this pacing mode, the pacemaker will pace both the atrium and the ventricle (AV sequential pacing), with programmed AV delay if the intrinsic atrial and ventricular rates are below the LRL. If the atrial rate is slower than the LRL, the device will pace the atrium while *inhibiting* ventricular pacing if an intrinsic ventricular event is sensed within a predetermined AV delay. If an atrial-sensed event is faster than the LRL without an intrinsic ventricular event, the pacemaker *inhibits* atrial pacing but *triggers* ventricular pacing (P-synchronous pacing) after a predetermined AV delay (Figure 6.2a). However, tracking an atrial-sensed event will only occur up to a programmable maximum tracking rate (MTR),

(a)

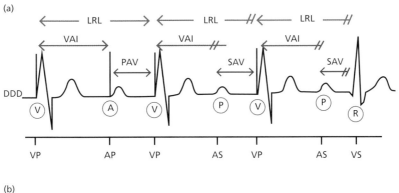

(b)

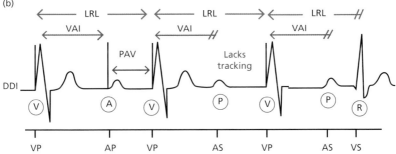

(c)

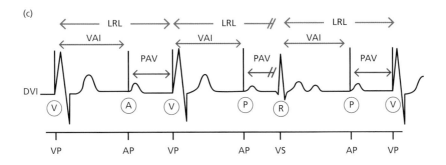

(d)

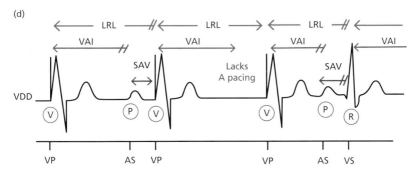

Figure 6.2 (a) DDD, (b) DDI, (c) DVI, and (d) VDD pacing modes. Event markers represent pacemaker's interpretation of different cardiac events. See text for details. A, atrial-paced event; LRL, lower rate limit; P, intrinsic P wave; PAV, paced AV interval; R, intrinsic R wave; SAV, sensed AV interval; V, ventricular-paced event; VAI, ventriculoatrial interval. Source: modified from Huizar JF, Kaszala K, Ellenbogen KA. Cardiac pacing modes and terminology. In: Sakena S, Camm AJ, eds. *Electrophysiological Disorders of the Heart*, 2nd edn. Philadelphia, PA: Elsevier Saunders, 2012: 441–456. Reproduced with permission of Elsevier.

which will prevent the pacemaker from tracking atrial dysrhythmias beyond a certain rate (see section Upper rate behavior). Finally, pacing will be completely *inhibited* if the intrinsic atrial and ventricular rates are above the LRL (unless a short AV delay is programmed). This pacing mode is the most commonly used in dual-chamber devices (DDD or DDDR) and biventricular pacemakers (DDDOV or DDDRV).

Dual-chamber pacing and sensing with inhibition but without tracking (DDI)

This can also be referred to as AV sequential pacing (D) with dual-chamber sensing (D) and inhibition (I) *without* P-synchronous pacing. This pacing mode is similar to DDD without tracking atrial-sensed events or P-synchronous pacing. Because P-wave tracking does not occur with the DDI mode, the ventricular-paced rate is never greater than the programmed LRL regardless of the atrial rate (Figure 6.2b). AV sequential pacing will only occur at LRL if no intrinsic ventricular event is sensed after atrial pacing. The main advantage and indication of DDI is in the presence of paroxysmal atrial arrhythmias such as atrial fibrillation and/or flutter (Table 6.2). This pacing mode is commonly programmed as a mode switch to avoid tracking of these atrial tachyarrhythmias.

Ventricular pacing with inhibition and dual-chamber sensing (VDI)

VDI pacing mode gives ventricular pacing (V), while sensing both chambers (D), and inhibits ventricular pacing if an intrinsic R wave is sensed. This pacing mode allows atrial sensing but does not provide P-synchronous pacing (non-tracking mode). In addition, it lacks atrial pacing for which it cannot provide AV sequential pacing. Thus, in sinus rhythm, there is AV dissociation in VDI mode regardless of rate. It can be used as an alternative pacing mode to avoid tracking of atrial fibrillation and flutter, and it is available as a mode switch feature in some pacemakers.

Atrioventricular sequential, ventricular-inhibited pacing (DVI)

DVI mode provides pacing in both the atrium and the ventricle (D), while only sensing and inhibiting

pacing in the ventricle (V). Pacing is only inhibited (I) and reset by ventricular-sensed events, but ignores all intrinsic atrial complexes. The difference between DVI and DDI is that the former lacks atrial sensing. Thus, DVI pacing may demonstrate asynchronous atrial pacing at LRL (Figure 6.2c). Similarly to DDI, ventricular pacing will never be greater than programmed LRL. DVI was used in first-generation pacemakers but it is still programmable in many available dual-chamber pacemakers. Nowadays, DVI can be used as a bail-out in patients with marked sinus bradycardia or atrial arrest with atrial lead malfunction (oversensing) in which AV synchrony is desired and lead revision is deferred (Table 6.2).

Ventricular pacing, dual-chamber sensing with P-synchronous ventricular pacing and inhibition (VDD)

VDD mode delivers ventricular pacing only (V), senses both the atrium and ventricle (D), while it inhibits ventricular pacing (I) and tracks (T) atrial-sensed events (P-synchronous pacing; Figure 6.2d). The most common use of this pacing mode is in devices with a single-pass lead which integrates an atrial-sensing electrode with a ventricular-pace/sense electrode. This system has been used in subjects with appropriate sinus node function who require ventricular back-up pacing due to high-degree AV block or during biventricular pacing. It can also be used in dual-chamber pacemakers with appropriate sensing of normal sinus node with high atrial pacing threshold in an attempt to maximize battery longevity [2,3] (Table 6.2).

Timing cycles

A given timing period or interval can continue until it completes its cycle; completion results in either the release of a pacing stimulus or the initiation of another timing cycle. Alternatively, a given period or interval can be reset by an intrinsic cardiac event, at which point it restarts the timing period again or initiates another timing period.

Blanking and refractory periods

All pacing modes that can sense cardiac events must include *blanking and refractory periods* in their basic timing cycle. The presence or absence of these periods depends on the pacemaker system as well as the pacing/sensing mode. These periods are essential to the appropriate pacemaker function as they prevent sensing of known but clinically inappropriate signals, such as the evoked potential and repolarization. The blanking and refractory periods of a pacemaker are analogous to the absolute and relative refractory periods of the heart, respectively. The blanking period (BP) is equivalent to an absolute refractory period, during which the sensing amplifier is "off" or "blind" to any cardiac event and thus cannot be detected. Once this period ends, the sense amplifier becomes alert and is receptive to the detection of native signals. During the refractory period (RP) cardiac events can be sensed and counted, but it usually does not trigger or reset timing cycles. In contrast to BPs, RPs allow detection of rapid cardiac events (Figure 6.3). In dual-chamber pacing, BP is also used to prevent cross-talk (see section Atrioventricular interval, cross-talk, and safety pacing).

Timing cycles based on pacing mode

Cardiac events and timing cycles are based on single, dual, or biventricular pacemaker systems and programmed pacing modes (Table 6.3).

Asynchronous pacing modes (AOO, VOO, DOO) pace the assigned chamber at LRL (only timing cycle), which is not reset by any intrinsic cardiac event due to lack of sensing. In dual-chamber or AV sequential asynchronous (DOO) pacing, the interval from atrial to ventricular pacing (AVI) and the interval from ventricular pacing to the subsequent atrial pacing – the ventriculoatrial interval (VAI) also referred to as the atrial escape interval (AEI) – are fixed.

Atrial inhibited pacing (AAI) consists of the atrial blanking period (ABP), atrial refractory period (ARP), and LRL (A–A interval). ABP and ARP initiate after a paced or sensed atrial event in order to avoid oversensing of evoked potentials, atrial repolarization, or ventricular depolarization. During ABP, signals are not sensed. In contrast, ARP allows sensing of rapid atrial signals (included in the counter); however, these signals are ignored as they will not reset timing cycles (but there are exceptions) (Figure 6.4a). Atrial pacing will occur after the LRL times out, but pacing will be inhibited and LRL reset after an atrial event is sensed (Figure 6.5a). Nevertheless, an A–A interval (programmed LRL) could be inappropriately reset by a far-field R wave oversensing

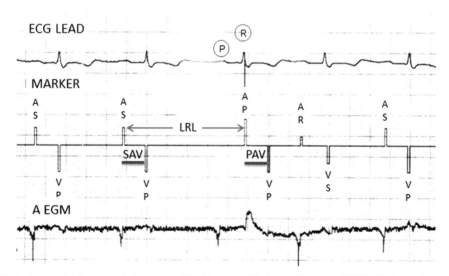

Figure 6.3 Blanking and refractory periods. Inappropriate AV sequential pacing (AP–VP) occurs after the lower rate limit expires despite sinus rhythm with intrinsic AV conduction due to the lack of atrial and ventricular sensing [third P wave (P) and QRS (R), respectively]. Lack of atrial sensing occurs due to a small atrial signal (A EGM), while ventricular undersensing (third QRS) is coincidental as it falls within the post-atrial ventricular blanking period (PAVB). The fourth P wave (labeled AR, atrial refractory) occurs within the post-ventricular atrial refractory period (PVARP) and does not initiate an AV interval. Therefore, P-synchronous ventricular pacing (triggered pacing) never occurs. AP, atrial paced; AS, atrial sensed; LRL, lower rate limit; PAV, paced AV interval; SAV, sensed AV interval; VP, ventricular paced; VS, ventricular sensed.

Table 6.3 Acronyms and description of cardiac events and timing cycles in a single-chamber, dual-chamber, and biventricular pacemakers/devices

Cardiac events/timing cycles (abbreviation)	Description
Single chamber (atrial or ventricular) pacemaker	
Atrial-sensed event (P/AS)	Sensed a native Atrial depolarization (P wave)
Atrial-paced event (A/AP)	Delivered Atrial Pacing output
Ventricular-sensed event (R/VS)	Sensed native Ventricular depolarization (QRS complex)
Ventricular-paced event (V/VP)	Delivered Ventricular Pacing output
Atrial blanking period (ABP)	Atrial-sensing amplifier is "blind" and will not detect or respond to any atrial-sensed event
Ventricular blanking period (VBP)	Ventricular-sensing amplifier is "blind" and will not detect or respond to any ventricular-sensed event
Atrial refractory period (ARP)	An atrial-sensed event will be noted but ignored, without affecting the pacemaker timing cycle
Ventricular refractory period (VRP)	A ventricular-sensed event will be noted but ignored, without affecting the pacemaker timing cycle
Lower rate limit (LRL)	Minimum pacing rate
Upper rate limit (URL)	Maximum pacing rate
Maximum sensor rate (MSR)	Maximum pacing rate by rate-modulated sensor
Dual-chamber (atrial and ventricular) pacemaker	
Atrioventricular sequential pacing (AV)	Atrial-paced event followed by paced ventricular event
P-synchronous V pacing (PV)	Atrial-sensed event followed by paced ventricular event
VA interval (VAI)	Interval from ventricular-sensed or -paced event to atrial-paced event
PR	Atrial-sensed event followed by ventricular-sensed event (native intrinsic atrial and ventricular events)
AR	Atrial-paced event followed by ventricular-sensed event
AV interval or delay (AVI)	Programmed atrioventricular pacing interval
Paced AV interval (paced AVI)	AV interval/delay from atrial-paced event (A) to ventricular-paced event (V)
Sensed AV interval (sensed AVI)	AV interval/delay from atrial-sensed event (P) to ventricular-paced event (V)
Maximum or upper tracking rate (MTR)	Maximum ventricular pacing rate allowed in response to high sensed atrial rates
Post-atrial ventricular blanking period (PAVB)	Period where ventricular sensing is "off" after an atrial-paced event
Post-ventricular atrial blanking period (PVAB)	Period where atrial sensing is "off" after a ventricular-paced or -sensed event
Post-ventricular atrial refractory period (PVARP)	Period after ventricular event where the device can sense an atrial event but does not track it
Total atrial refractory period (TARP)	Sum of AVI and PVARP
Rate-modulated AV delay [RMAVD; also referred to as rate-responsive AV delay (RRAVD)]	AV delay that adjusts by shortening as the rate increases

Table 6.3 (Continued)

Cardiac events/timing cycles (abbreviation)	Description
Cardiac resynchronization therapy/pacemakers	
RV post-atrial ventricular blanking	Period where RV sensing is "off" immediately after atrial pacing (avoids oversensing atrial signals)
LV post-atrial ventricular blanking period (LV-PAVB)	Period where LV sensing is "off" immediately after atrial pacing (prevents oversensing atrial signals)
RV refractory period (RVRP)	An RV-sensed event may be noted but ignored, without affecting the pacing timing cycle
LV refractory period (LVRP)	An LV-sensed event may be noted but ignored, without affecting LV pacing timing cycle
LV protection period (LVPP)	Period after a ventricular-paced or -sensed event that prevents inappropriate pacing during the vulnerable period
Biventricular pacing interval or LV offset	Timing gap between RV and LV pacing (RV–LV interval)

Source: modified from Huizar JF, Kaszala K, Ellenbogen KA. Cardiac pacing modes and terminology. In: Sakena S, Camm AJ, eds. *Electrophysiological Disorders of the Heart*, 2nd edn. Philadelphia, PA: Elsevier Saunders, 2012: 441–456. Reproduced with permission of Elsevier.

in the atrial channel after ABP and ARP have expired (Figure 6.5b).

Ventricular inhibited (VVI) pacing, the ventricular counterpart of AAI pacing, incorporates the same timing cycles, with the obvious differences that pacing and sensing occur in the ventricular channel and pacing output is inhibited by a sensed ventricular event (Figure 6.4b). A ventricular-paced or -sensed event initiates a ventricular blanking period (VBP) and a ventricular refractory period (VRP) during which the pacemaker will not reset the ventricular timer or LRL after a ventricular-sensed event (Figure 6.6).

DDD pacing mode embraces all timing cycles described on AAI and VVI pacing modes. In addition, LRL is divided into two sections: the VAI or AEI, and the AVI, as depicted in Figure 6.4c. The VAI initiates after a ventricular-sensed or -paced event and does not terminate until an atrial event is sensed; however, atrial pacing will occur if the VAI expires without sensing an intrinsic atrial event. The AVI begins with an atrial-sensed or -paced event and extends to a ventricular event. Similarly, ventricular pacing will occur if the AVI elapses without the presence of an intrinsic ventricular event.

Furthermore, a paced atrial event initiates a post-atrial ventricular blanking period (PAVB) (Figure 6.4c). During the PAVB, the ventricular channel is refractory and will not reset timing cycles

even in the presence of another native ventricular event. Ventricular pacing occurs only at the end of the AVI or later [see section Upper rate behavior (Wenckebach-like behavior)]. A paced ventricular event initiates a post-ventricular atrial blanking period (PVAB). The PVAB prevents sensing of a far-field ventricular-paced event on the atrial channel.

A sensed or paced ventricular event also initiates a refractory period on the atrial channel, referred to as the post-ventricular atrial refractory period (PVARP). The difference between PVAB and PVARP is that while the first one occurs only after VP event, PVARP occurs after either VS or VP event. The PVARP is designed to prevent ventricular tracking of a retrograde P wave (see discussion of PVARP in section Pacemaker-mediated tachycardia). The combination of the PVARP and the AVI establishes the total atrial refractory period (TARP). TARP is the limiting factor for the upper rate limit (URL) or so-called MTR in P-synchronous dual-chamber pacing modes (see sections Upper rate behavior and Total and post-ventricular atrial refractory periods).

DDI pacing mode includes the nearly identical timing cycles described for DDD mode except that it would not trigger ventricular pacing after atrial-sensed events (it lacks P-synchronous ventricular pacing; Figure 6.3b).

In contrast to DDD pacing mode, *DVI pacing mode* cannot trigger ventricular pacing in response

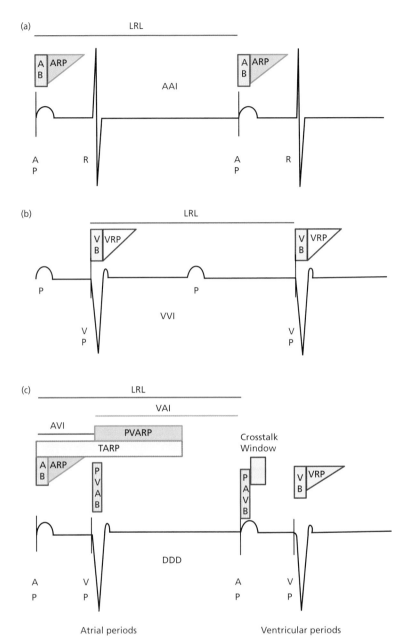

Figure 6.4 Timing cycles found on (a) AAI, (b) VVI, and (c) DDD pacing modes. See text and Table 6.3 for abbreviations. Source: modified from Huizar JF, Kaszala K, Ellenbogen KA. Cardiac pacing modes and terminology. In: Sakena S, Camm AJ, eds. *Electrophysiological Disorders of the Heart*, 2nd edn. Philadelphia, PA: Elsevier Saunders, 2012: 441–456. Reproduced with permission of Elsevier.

to atrial events since it lacks atrial sensing. Furthermore, DVI pacing mode lacks timing cycles that involve atrial sensing, such as ABP, ARP, PVAB and PVARP, and TARP (Figure 6.3c). For instance, a sensed R wave during the VAI (ventricular ectopy) will reset the VAI, delaying atrial pacing in DVI mode.

VDD pacing mode lacks atrial pacing (Figure 6.3d). Thus, the PAVB and cross-talk window (found on DDD and DDI pacing modes) are absent.

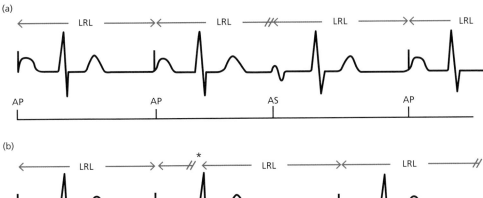

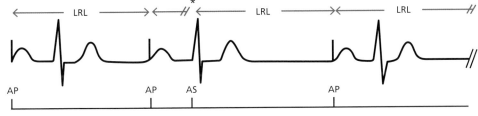

Figure 6.5 AAI pacing mode. (a) Atrial pacing (AP) occurs at the end of the lower rate limit (LRL) in the absence of an atrial-sensed (AS) event. If an intrinsic AS event occurs, LRL is restarted from that point. (b) Even though the LRL is programmed to 60 bpm (1000 ms), the interval between the second and third paced atrial events (AP) is >1000 ms.

Examination of the event markers (pacemaker's interpretation) demonstrate that the QRS complex has been inappropriately sensed on the atrial-sensing channel (far-field R-wave sensing beyond blanking and refractory periods), resetting the LRL.

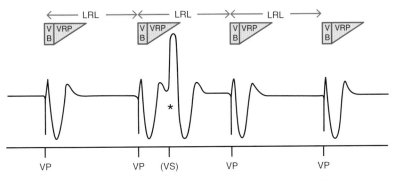

Figure 6.6 Ventricular refractory period (VRP) in VVI pacing mode. A premature ventricular contraction (PVC, *) occurs during VRP, initiated after a ventricular-paced event (VP). Since PVC (VS, ventricular-sensed event) falls within the VRP, the lower rate limit (LRL) is not interrupted or reinitiated. VB, ventricular blanking period.

A sensed atrial event initiates the AVI. If an intrinsic ventricular event occurs before termination of the AVI, ventricular output is inhibited, and the LRL timing cycle is reset. Similarly, a P-synchronous ventricular pacing at the end of the AVI will reset the LRL. A ventricular-sensed or -paced event will initiate PVARP and VAI. If no atrial event occurs, the pacemaker escapes with a paced ventricular event at the LRL (pacemaker behaves as VVI in the absence of a sensed atrial event at the base rate).

Overall, pacemaker behavior depends on the programmed pacing mode and base rate behavior. However, other programmable features may affect device behavior (Table 6.4). These are discussed throughout the chapter.

Atrioventricular interval, cross-talk, and safety pacing

AVI refers to a programmable interval initiated by a sensed or paced atrial event (P or A event, respectively) followed by ventricular pacing after the time

Table 6.4 Features that may affect device behavior[a]

Device behavior	Pacing features/algorithms
Intrinsic rate slower than programmed base rate	Rate/scan hysteresis
	Sleep or rest rate
	Sinus preference
	Special algorithms (e.g. +PVARP after PVC)
	Atrial-based timing in DDD after PVC
Base rate (AV, AR) higher than programmed rate	Sensor-driven rate
	Rate smoothing
	Fallback
	Mode-switching response rate
	Sudden bradycardia/rate drop response
	Atrial overdrive suppression
	Special algorithms (e.g. +PVARP after PVC)
	Magnet mode rate
	Atrial and ventricular auto-threshold test
Intrinsic AVI (PR, AR) longer than programmed paced or sensed AVI	AV or PV hysteresis
	Algorithms to allow intrinsic AV conduction
	Sinus rate with intact AV conduction exceeding MTR
Paced or sensed AVI shorter than programmed paced or sensed AVI	Rate-modulated or dynamic AV delay
	Negative AV or PV hysteresis
	Safety pacing
	Managed ventricular pacing (MVP, AAI ↔ DDD)
	Non-competitive atrial pacing (NCAP)
	Auto-threshold test
Loss of atrial tracking (DDD)	Automatic mode switch
	MSR > MTR

[a] Device behaviors are not necessarily continuous; the effects can be seen on a single cycle or during a brief period.
PVC, premature ventricular contraction; for other acronyms, see Table 6.3.

interval expires (Figure 6.7). If a ventricular event is sensed before the time interval is completed, the AVI will terminate and initiate the VAI. At the beginning of the AVI, the atrial channel is briefly blind (ABP) followed by an ARP to allow detection of abnormal rapid atrial signals during the AVI (Figure 6.8).

The potential exists for signals other than those of intrinsic ventricular activity to be sensed during the AVI and inhibit ventricular output. Thus, atrial pacing artifact inappropriately sensed by the ventricular-sensing amplifier could result in ventricular pacing inhibition, or a ventricular pacing artifact sensed by the atrial channel is referred to as *cross-talk*. To prevent cross-talk, atrial pacing also initiates a PAVB to avoid ventricular oversensing of

atrial-paced events (Figure 6.7b) and PVAB following a ventricular event to prevent atrial oversensing. The blanking period is traditionally of short duration to optimize subsequent sensing.

Even though the atrial pacing artifact is effectively ignored because of the PAVB, the trailing edge of the atrial pacing artifact occurring after the PAVB can occasionally be sensed on the ventricular channel. In a pacemaker-dependent patient, inhibition of ventricular output by cross-talk results in ventricular asystole. To prevent such a catastrophic outcome, DDD pacing mode has a safety mechanism called the "ventricular triggering period" or the "cross-talk sensing window" (Figure 6.7c). If activity is sensed on the ventricular-sensing amplifier during the initial part of AVI

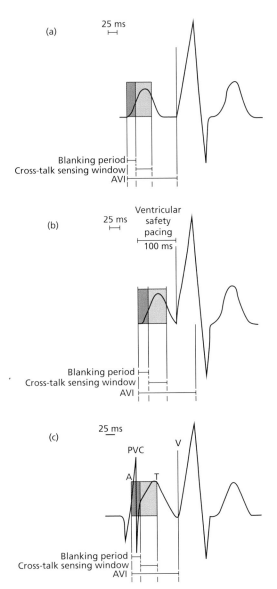

Figure 6.7 Representation of atrioventricular interval (AVI). (a) AVI corresponds to a programmed value following a paced or sensed atrial beat before a ventricular pacing artifact is delivered. The post-atrial ventricular blanking period (PAVB) is found in the initial portion of the AVI, followed by the cross-talk sensing window. (b) If the ventricular-sensing amplifier senses any event during the cross-talk sensing window, ventricular safety pacing is delivered, usually 100–110 ms after the atrial event. (c) An intrinsic ventricular event [such as a premature ventricular contraction (PVC)] during the PAVB period is not sensed by the ventricular-sensing amplifier; thus ventricular pacing is delivered at the programmed AVI.

(possible cross-talk present), a ventricular output is triggered (safety pacing). This early ventricular pacing typically occurs with a short (100–120 ms) or programmed AVI. Occurrence of cross-talk and safety pacing should be suspected if AV pacing is noted at a shorter than programmed AVI on ECG (Figure 6.9). Elimination of AV cross-talk can be achieved by extending the PAVB, decreasing atrial output, or reducing the ventricular sensitivity. If true intrinsic ventricular activity occurs during the cross-talk sensing window, safety pacing will result in a fusion beat. Although the safety pacing phenomenon accompanying a late-cycle premature ventricular contraction (PVC) has been interpreted as a sensing failure, it actually reflects normal sensing.

Differential atrioventricular interval

The differential AVI is an attempt to provide an intra-atrial conduction time of equal duration whether atrial contraction is paced or sensed. The PV interval initiated with atrial sensing, referred to as sensed AV delay (SAV), commences only when the atrial depolarization is detected by the pacemaker, and commonly occurs 20–60 ms after the onset of the P wave on a surface ECG. Conversely, the AVI initiated with atrial pacing, referred to as paced AV delay (PAV), commences immediately with the pacing artifact. Therefore, in general, the AVI that follows a sensed atrial event should be shorter than one that follows a paced atrial event in an effort to achieve similar functional AVIs (Figure 6.10). Most dual-chamber pacemakers allow the paced and sensed AV delays to be programmed independently with differences of up to 100 ms (Figure 6.11).

Dynamic or rate-adaptive atrioventricular interval

Pacemaker algorithms may be used in dual-chamber pacing modes to shorten the AVI as the atrial rate increases, either by an increase in sinus rate or sensor-driven paced rate (Figure 6.12). Dynamic AVI is intended to optimize cardiac output by mimicking the normal physiological decrease in the PR interval that occurs in the normal heart as the atrial rate increases. The rate-related shortening of the AVI can be useful for improving atrial sensing, and enhancing atrial tracking at faster rates by

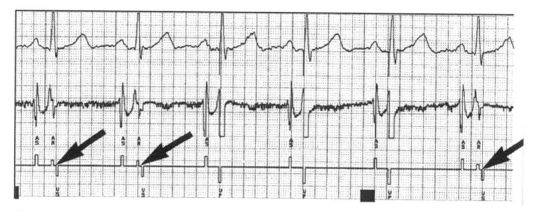

Figure 6.8 Far-field R-wave oversensing. The R wave is inappropriately sensed during the atrial refractory period (ARP) by the atrial amplifier. Surface ECG, atrial electrogram, and event markers (arrows) demonstrate occasional atrial refractory (AR) events due to far-field R-wave sensing within the ARP. AR events coincide with the QRS complex, but are detected on the atrial channel before being detected by the pacemaker on the ventricular channel (VS).

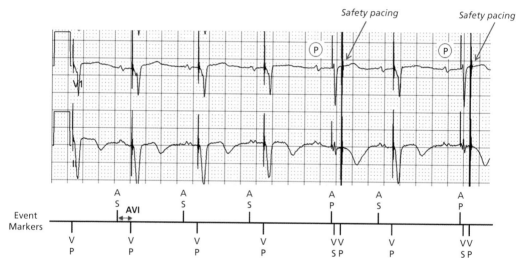

Figure 6.9 ECG demonstration of safety pacing due to atrial undersensing in DDD pacing mode. As noted by event markers, P-synchronous ventricular pacing occurs in the first four ventricular-paced events (VP) with a programmed sensed and paced AV interval (AVI) of 160 and 190 ms, respectively. The fourth and sixth P waves (P) are not sensed (fail to terminate VAI and initiate AVI), yet they demonstrate intrinsic AV conduction with a ventricular-sensed event (VS) briefly after atrial pacing (AP) (lower rate limit of 60 bpm expires). Safety pacing (fifth and seventh VP, shorter AV delay 110–120 ms) occurs as a VS event is sensed during the cross-talk sensing window.

shortening the TARP (AVI + PVARP) and thereby extending the atrial-sensing window.

The rate-adaptive AVI algorithm varies according to the pacemaker and manufacturer. A common method allows linear shortening of the AVI from a programmed baseline AVI to a programmed minimum AVI. Another method allows a limited number of stepwise shortenings of the AVI, which may or may not be programmable.

Atrioventricular interval hysteresis

The term AVI hysteresis has been used variably, but most commonly describes alterations in the paced AVI relative to the patient's intrinsic AV conduction. For example, a longer paced AVI is permitted to allow maintenance of intrinsic AV conduction, previously referred to as *positive hysteresis*. Nowadays, several algorithms have been developed to avoid the deleterious effects of chronic right

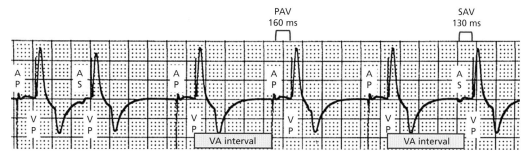

Figure 6.10 ECG tracing demonstrates differential atrioventricular interval (AVI). An AVI initiated by a sensed event and those initiated by a paced event show consistent differences. Thus, the most likely explanation is a differential AVI. The paced AVI is 50 ms longer than the PV or sensed AV intervals. Source: *Relay Models 293-03 and 294-03. Intermedics Cardiac Pulse Generator Physician's Manual*. Angleton, TX: Intermedics, 1992. Reproduced with permission of Intermedics.

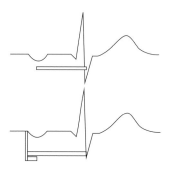

AV delay hysteresis = AR interval – PR interval

Figure 6.11 Schematic of automatic calculation of differential atrioventricular interval (AVI), designated "AV delay hysteresis." When an atrial-paced event occurs, the AR interval is measured. When an atrial-sensed event follows an atrial-paced event, a new PR interval is measured. The AV delay hysteresis is set equal to the maximum value (AR or PR) minus the PR interval. Source: modified from *Chorus II Model 6234, 6244. Dual Chamber Pulse Generator Physician's Manual*. Minnetonka, MN: ELA Medical, 1994. Reproduced with permission of ELA Medical.

ventricular (RV) pacing (see section Algorithms to minimize right ventricular pacing), including abnormal ventricular activation sequence and heart failure symptoms [4]. In contrast, the *negative hysteresis* feature is intended to temporarily shorten the AVI (to 10–150 ms) if an intrinsic ventricular event is sensed in the AVI, which could be relevant in biventricular pacing or treatment of hypertrophic cardiomyopathy.

Ventriculoatrial interval

The VAI interval is only present in dual-chamber pacing modes, regardless of tracking feature (DDD, DDI, DVI). This interval has also been called the atrial escape interval. The VAI is initiated after a sensed or paced ventricular event and reset by an intrinsic atrial or ventricular event. If no atrial- or ventricular-sensed event occurs during the VAI, an atrial pacing stimulus will occur after conclusion of this interval. The sum of VAI and AVI determines the LRL. The VAI is variable in (i) rate-modulated pacing modes [the sensor-indicated rate (SIR) will increase based on VAI shortening]; and (ii) atrial-based timing (see sections Rate-modulated pacing and Base-rate behavior).

Total and post-ventricular atrial refractory periods

The PVARP is a programmable interval in dual-chamber pacing modes with atrial sensing (DDD, DDI, VDD), initiated after a sensed or paced ventricular event. This period is intended to avoid inappropriate tracking of sensed signals due to retrograde P waves. If an atrial event occurs during PVARP, timing cycles (VAI, LRL) are not reset. Nevertheless, sensing of atrial signals during PVARP allows proper mode switch (non-tracking pacing mode) when atrial fibrillation, flutter, or tachycardia occurs (see section Mode switch).

In a P-synchronous pacing mode, PVARP should be extended to include retrograde P waves to avoid pacemaker-mediated tachycardia (PMT, also referred to as endless-loop tachycardia; see section Pacemaker-mediated tachycardia). Appropriate PVARP programming is also important for reducing tracking of atrial arrhythmias.

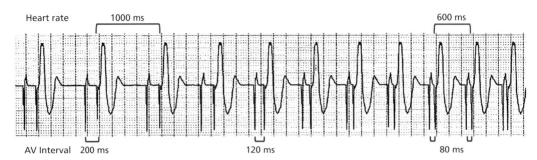

Figure 6.12 Dynamic atrioventricular (AV) delay. As heart rate increases, AV delay shortens from 200 ms to 80 ms. Source: Hayes DL, Ketelson A, Levine PA *et al*. Understanding timing systems of current DDDR pacemakers. *Eur J Cardiac Pacing Electrophysiol* 1993;3:70–86. Reproduced with permission of the Mayo Foundation.

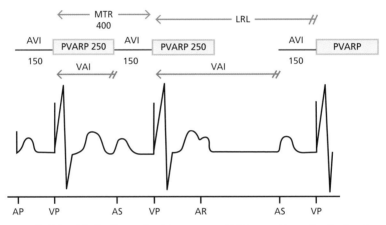

Figure 6.13 Upper rate limit (URL) limited by total atrial refractory period (TARP). In DDD pacing mode, the atrioventricular interval (AVI) and post-ventricular atrial refractory period (PVARP) are programmed at 150 ms and 250 ms, respectively (TARP 400 ms). Thus, pacemaker limits maximum tracking rate (MTR) up to 150 bpm (400 ms). After the first paced ventricular complex, an intrinsic P wave (AS) is sensed immediately after the completion of the PVARP. This AS event initiates AVI and upon completion, ventricular tracking occurs. However, the subsequent P wave (AR) is sensed within the PVARP and therefore VAI is not ended and the P wave is not tracked with ventricular pacing. Ventricular tracking (VP) will only occur until the next intrinsic P wave (AS) occurs outside PVARP.

The total atrial refractory period is the sum of the AVI and PVARP. TARP is the limiting factor for the URL (maximum tracking or sensor rate) in which the pacemaker can pace and track P waves or atrial-sensed events (Figure 6.13). For example, if the AVI is 150 ms and the PVARP is 250 ms, the TARP is 400 ms or 150 bpm. In this case, a 250-ms PVARP initiates after a ventricular-paced event, and only after this interval has expired can an atrial event be sensed. If an atrial event is sensed immediately after termination of the PVARP, it initiates an AVI of 150 ms. After the AVI ends, a paced ventricular event will occur in the absence of an intrinsic R wave, resulting in a V–V cycle length of 400 ms or 150 bpm. Thus, programming a long PVARP limits the MTR and maximum sensor rate (MSR).

Dynamic PVARP

In current pacemakers, a heart rate- or SIR-determined dynamic PVARP adjustment may be enabled. In tracking pacing modes (DDDR, DDD, VDD), PVARP is extended during lower heart rates in order to protect against PMT (see section Pacemaker-mediated tachycardia), while it is shortened at higher rates to allow P-synchronous ventricular pacing at faster rates (allows the programming of a higher MTR) and to reduce the likelihood of competitive atrial pacing. In non-tracking pacing modes

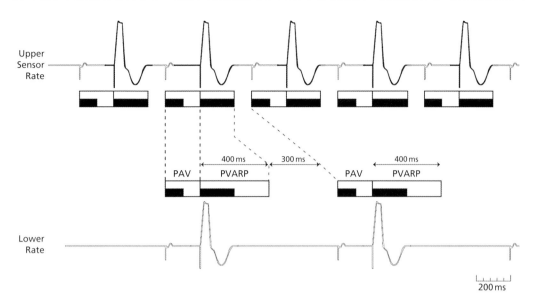

Figure 6.14 Dynamic post-ventricular atrial refractory period (PVARP) in DDDR, DDD, and VDD pacing modes. PVARP is extended to 400 ms (adjusted to maintain a 300-ms sensing window) at low heart rates, while it shortens to a minimum of the programmed post-ventricular atrial blanking period (PVAB, solid bar) at upper or maximum sensor or tracking rates (MSR, MTR). When the pacemaker is operating in the DDIR mode, the sensor-varied PVARP is approximately 400 ms at low rates and the programmed PVAB at high rates. Source: A *dapta, Versia and Sensia Manual*. St. Paul, MN: Medtronic, Inc. Reproduced with permission of Medtronic, Inc.

(DDI, DDIR), PVARP is extended to prevent inhibition of atrial pacing by an atrial event early during the VAI, and shortened at high SIR to reduce the likelihood of competitive atrial pacing (Figure 6.14).

Rate-modulated pacing

The "sensor function" of a pacemaker refers to the modulation of the paced rate in response to an input signal other than the presence or absence of native depolarization. Nowadays, there is a wide variety of sensors that may provide input to pacemakers based on (i) motion (either acceleration or vibration); (ii) changes in impedance as a measure of minute ventilation and/or contractility (Closed Loop Stimulation, Biotronik, Germany) [5]; and (iii) duration of the QT interval.

The sensor input to the pacing system temporarily adjusts the rate of the pacemaker. If the patient is active and rate modulation is enabled, the heart rate is determined by either the native rate or the SIR, whichever is faster. The SIR behaves in a manner identical to the programmed base rate. In essence, the sensor-driven pacing rate acts as if the LRL has been increased. SIR is also a unique term

found in rate-modulated pacing only, and refers to the pacing rate based on the sensor input. If the native rate is faster than the SIR, the pacemaker is either inhibited or tracks the atrial complexes. If the SIR is faster than the intrinsic rate, the heart rate is controlled by the pacemaker. Rate modulation requires a programmed URL, referred to as the maximum sensor rate.

Single-chamber inhibited and rate-modulated pacing

Single-chamber rate-modulated pacing modes (AAIR, VVIR) have the same timing cycles as their non-rate-modulated counterparts. The difference lies in the variability of the V–V or A–A intervals (Figure 6.15).

Long programmed refractory periods should be avoided when rate-modulated pacing is enabled, since it could prevent appropriate sensing of rapid intrinsic events functioning inadvertently with an asynchronous pacing behavior. Most pacemakers have a rate-dynamic/variable refractory period, which depends on the SIR and allows appropriate sensing of intrinsic events when the cycle length shortens.

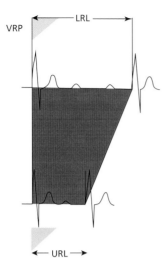

Figure 6.15 The VVIR timing cycle consists of a lower rate limit (LRL), an upper rate limit (URL), and a ventricular refractory period (VRP, represented by blue triangles). As indicated by sensor activity, the V–V interval shortens accordingly (red area represents the range of sensor-driven VV interval). In most VVIR pacemakers, the VRP remains fixed despite the changing VV cycle length. In selected VVIR pacemakers, the VRP shortens as the cycle length shortens.

Single-chamber and dual-chamber rate-modulated asynchronous pacing

The asynchronous pacing modes (i.e. AOO, VOO, DOO, as explained previously) have fixed intervals that are insensitive to all intrinsic events and timers that are never reset. If rate modulation is incorporated in an asynchronous pacing mode, the basic cycle length is altered by sensor activity. In the rate-modulated asynchronous pacing modes (AOOR, VOOR, DOOR), any alteration in cycle length is attributable to sensor activity or input signal and not to the sensing of intrinsic cardiac events (P or R wave). In the DOOR pacing mode, the AVI may be programmed in some devices to shorten progressively as the rate increases, whereas in other units it remains fixed at the initial programmed setting.

Dual-chamber rate-modulated pacing (DDDR, DDIR)

Dual-chamber rate-modulated pacing modes (DDDR, DDIR) are similar to the previously described DDD and DDI modes, respectively, except that paced rates can exceed the programmed LRL through sensor-driven activity. In addition to P-synchronous pacing as a method for increasing the heart

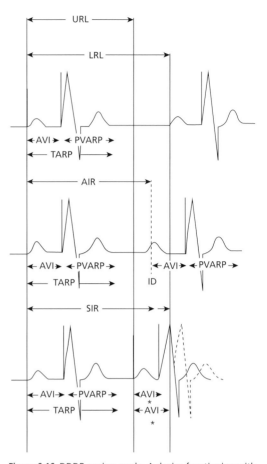

Figure 6.16 DDDR pacing mode. A device functioning with heart rates above the programmed lower rate limit (LRL) is explained on the basis of the atrial-indicated rate (AIR) or sensor-indicated rate (SIR). (*Top*) AV sequential pacing at the LRL as the patient is inactive and no intrinsic R wave is sensed after the atrioventricular interval (AVI) expires. (*Middle*) P-synchronous ventricular pacing occurs, tracking the AIR since the patient's atrial or sinus rate increases above the LRL and SIR. (*Bottom*) Atrial pacing based on the SIR (above the AIR), reaching the upper rate limit (URL). Rate-adaptive or rate-variable AVI allows shortening of the AVI as the SIR increases. Because a rate-modulated AV delay (*) is incorporated, the total atrial refractory period (TARP) may shorten by virtue of the changing AVI even though the post-ventricular atrial refractory period (PVARP) does not change at faster rates.

rate (DDD only), the sensor incorporated in the pacemaker may also increase the heart rate. Therefore, the rhythm may be sinus driven (alternatively called "atrial driven" or "P synchronous") or sensor driven (Figure 6.16). The basic cycle length may shorten from the programmed LRL up to the MSR.

Although the MSR and MTR are closely related, they are not identical. The tracking rate refers to the rate at which the pacemaker is sensing and tracking intrinsic atrial activity. The MTR is the maximum ventricular-paced rate that is allowed in response to sensed atrial rhythms. The MTR may result in fixed block, Wenckebach, fallback, or rate-smoothing responses, depending on the design of the system (see sections Upper rate behavior and Rate enhancements). The sensor-controlled rate or SIR is the rate of the pacemaker that is determined by the sensor input signal. The MSR is the maximum rate that the pacemaker is allowed to achieve under sensor control. If the SIR is higher than the intrinsic atrial rate, it will determine pacing rate. In contrast, if the SIR is lower than the intrinsic atrial rhythm, the pacemaker will track atrial events up to the MTR. Thus, the pacing rate may be in part sensor driven and in part sinus driven (P-wave tracking), and not purely one or the other (Figure 6.17), depending on the sinus node function and programmed pacemaker and sensor parameters.

In DDDR pacing mode, the MSR can be programmed above, equal to, or below the MTR. If the MSR is programmed above the MTR, P-synchronous pacing (tracking) will only occur with atrial rates up to the MTR. If the SIR is above the MTR, the device will behave as DDIR, allowing AV sequential pacing but lacking P-synchronous pacing between the MTR and MSR. For example, in a DDDR pacing mode programmed with LRL, MTR, and MSR of 60, 120, and 130 bpm, respectively, AV sequential pacing will occur between 60 and 130 bpm, but P-synchronous ventricular pacing will only occur between 60 and 120 bpm. In contrast, if the MTR is programmed above the MSR, AV sequential pacing will not occur above the MSR, but P-synchronous pacing (tracking) will occur above the MSR and up to the MTR. For example, in a DDDR programmed with LRL of 60 bpm, MTR of 130 bpm, and MSR of 120 bpm, AV sequential

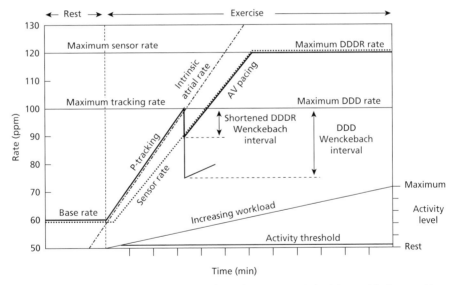

Figure 6.17 Rate response of the DDDR pacemaker and its behavior at both maximum tracking and maximum sensor rate (MSR). The dashed–dotted line represents the intrinsic atrial rate (P-synchronous tracking), and the diagonal dashed line represents the sensor-indicated rate during progressively increasing workloads. The heavy black line shows the ventricular paced rate, assuming complete heart block, as it progresses from the P-tracking mode to atrioventricular (AV) sequential pacing through a period of Wenckebach-type block.

The DDD Wenckebach interval is shortened by sensor-driven pacing, i.e. "sensor-driven rate smoothing." Maximum shortening of the Wenckebach period is accomplished by optimal programming of the sensor rate–response variables (threshold and slope programming for an activity-driven sensor).
Source: Higano ST, Hayes DL, Eisinger G. Sensor-driven rate smoothing in a DDDR pacemaker. *Pacing Clin Electrophysiol* 1989;12:922–929. Reproduced with permission of John Wiley & Sons Ltd.

pacing will occur at an SIR between 60 and 120 bpm, whereas P-synchronous pacing can occur at atrial rates between 60 and 130 bpm.

Frequently, the MSR is programmed equal to the MTR. An MSR above the MTR could be useful in unique clinical scenarios, such as (i) undersensed paroxysmal atrial tachyarrhythmias (flutter/fibrillation) that prevent or delay appropriate mode switch, resulting in inappropriate tracking of these arrhythmias (see section Mode switch), yet rate response is desired at higher rates than the programmed MTR; and (ii) sick sinus rhythm with chronotropic incompetence, intermittent paroxysmal atrial tachycardia, and inappropriate or undesired tracking at higher atrial rates.

Another dynamic component of *DDDR timing cycles* is the atrial-sensing window (ASW). The ASW is the portion of the RR cycle that is not part of the PVARP or the AVI. It is the period during which the atrial-sensed events are tracked. If the PVARP or AVI (or both) is extended, there may effectively be no ASW (i.e. TARP limits increased tracking rate) and then even a DDD pacemaker functions as a DVI system. Conversely, in DDDR pacing mode with an SIR higher than the MTR, it may appear that there is P-wave tracking at rates greater than the MTR. Sensed atrial events in this case would inhibit sensor-driven atrial pacing, but ventricular pacing would take place at the SIR irrespective of the atrial event (functioning as DDIR) [6].

Base-rate behavior

A dual-chamber pacemaker will obey the rules centered on the base-rate behavior and adjust its response based on sensed events. Base-rate behavior is non-programmable and varies among manufacturers and even among different models from the same manufacturer. Dual-chamber pacemakers have historically been designed with a ventricular- or atrial-based timing system. Nowadays, most pacemakers have a combination of both ventricular- and atrial-based systems, referred to as hybrid-based behavior. Hybrid-based timing is designed specifically to avoid the potential rate variations or limitations that could occur with either a pure atrial- or ventricular-based timing system.

Designation of a pacemaker's timing system as atrial- or ventricular-based gained increased importance with the advent of rate-adaptive pacing. The difference between atrial- and ventricular-based dual-chamber pacemakers was of little clinical importance in non-rate-adaptive pacemakers, although the difference created some minor confusion in the interpretation of paced ECGs. Thus, understanding base-rate behavior will help distinguish between appropriate or inappropriate pacemaker function.

Ventricular-based timing

The ventricular-based timing system is distinguished by a "fixed" VAI. A ventricular-sensed event occurring during the VAI will reset this timer (restarting the VAI again), while a ventricular-sensed event during the AVI terminates the AVI and initiates a fixed VAI. Thus, the AR interval (atrial stimulus to sensed R wave) is shorter than the programmed AVI in the presence of intrinsic AV conduction after an atrial-paced event. Since the VAI is fixed regardless of the presence or absence of AV conduction, the resultant atrial pacing rate (AA interval) and intrinsic RR interval are shorter than the programmed LRL, given as the difference between the AR and AV intervals (Figure 6.18a). When a native R wave occurs during the VAI, such as a ventricular premature beat, the fixed VAI is reset. This results in an RR interval rate equal to the LRL, determined by the sum of the VAI and AVI (Figure 6.19a). In both cases, a ventricular-sensed event resets the VAI, regardless of where it occurs.

Atrial-based timing

An atrial-based timing system is characterized by a "fixed" AA interval, regardless of AV conduction and VA interval. As long as the LRL pacing remains stable, there is no discernible difference between the two timing systems. In contrast to a ventricular-based system, an atrial-based timing system will not reset the basic AA timing if a sensed R wave occurs during the AVI (either intrinsic AV conduction or PVC). Hence, the atrial pacing rate will remain at the programmed LRL (Figure 6.18b). However, a PVC during the VAI (after the AVI has ended) can reset the AA timing, resulting in a longer AA interval and PVC–R interval than the

(a)
Ventricular based

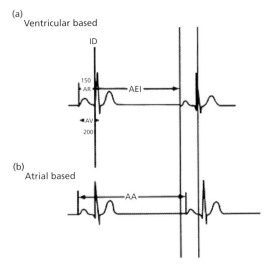

(b)
Atrial based

Figure 6.18 (a) Ventricular-based timing: fixed ventriculoatrial interval (VAI), the so-called atrial escape interval (AEI), is initiated by intrinsic R wave [intrinsic atrioventricular (AV) conduction] after an atrial-paced event (AR interval). The base pacing interval consists of the sum of the AR and the AEI; thus, it is shorter than the programmed minimum rate interval. The tracing represents a pacemaker programmed to a lower rate limit (LRL) of 60 bpm (pacing interval of 1000 ms) with an AVI of 200 ms, resulting in a fixed AEI of 800 ms (AEI = LRL − AVI). If AV nodal conduction occurs at 150 ms (AR interval = 150 ms), the conducted or sensed R wave inhibits ventricular pacing and initiates the 800-ms fixed AEI. Thus, the resulting atrial pacing and RR intervals are shorter than the programmed LRL by the difference between the AR and the AVI (950 ms or 63 bpm). (b) The atrial-based timing in patients with intact AV nodal conduction after an AR interval inhibits ventricular output but does not reset the basic AA timing interval. Thus, atrial pacing occurs at the programmed base rate. Source: Levine PA, Hayes DL, Wilkoff BL, Ohman AE. Electrocardiography of rate-modulated pacemaker rhythms. Sylmar, CA: Siemens-Pacesetter, 1990. Reproduced with permission of St. Jude Medical, Inc.

programmed LRL (Figure 6.19b). Thus, the LRL may be violated in atrial-based timing, mimicking the compensatory pause commonly seen in normal sinus rhythm with ventricular ectopy.

Comparison of atrial- and ventricular-based systems

A difference between these two base rate systems is noticed in some circumstances, such as 2 : 1 AV block and rate-modulated pacing.

Intermittent 2 : 1 AV block at the lower rate will result in alternating heart rates between sequential

AV pacing at programmed LRL and atrial-pacing ventricular inhibition (AR) with a slightly faster rate than the LRL (Figure 6.20a). Although ventricular-based timing may result in an increase in the paced rate during AR pacing (see section Effects of ventricular- and atrial-based timing systems on rate-modulated pacing modes), the LRL is never violated.

In contrast, an atrial-based timing system will demonstrate the alternation of the longer AVI with the shorter AR interval, which results in alternating faster and slower ventricular rates than, but never the same as, the programmed LRL (Figure 6.20b). When an AV complex follows an AR complex, the effective paced ventricular rate for that cycle is lower than the programmed LRL. In this scenario, atrial-based timing violates programmed LRL.

Interpretation of an ECG from a patient with a dual-chamber pacemaker is helped by knowing whether the pacemaker has atrial- or ventricular-based timing. A ventricular-based timing system can be identified (using calipers) as a fixed VAI measured backwards from an atrial-paced event to the point of ventricular sensing, since a ventricular event (paced or sensed) always initiates a VAI (Figures 6.18a and 6.19a). In contrast, an atrial-based timing system is identified as the fixed AA interval measured backwards from the atrial-paced event to the point of atrial sensing or ventricular sensing if a ventricular event occurs during the VAI (Figure 6.19b). However, this could be potentially challenging as inappropriate ventricular sensing, such as T-wave oversensing, could be responsible for resetting the AA interval, which can only be proven by simultaneous acquisition of event markers (interpretation of cardiac events).

Effects of ventricular- and atrial-based timing systems on rate-modulated pacing modes

In a ventricular-based timing with enabled rate modulation, the effective atrial-paced rate theoretically may be considerably higher than the programmed MSR if AR conduction were present (Figure 6.21a). This is possible since the VAI shortens as the sensor input increases to the same extent, regardless of intrinsic AV conduction. For instance, a device programmed with an MSR of 150 bpm (400 ms) and an AVI of 200 ms will have

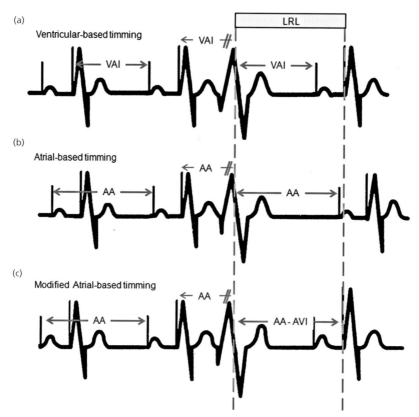

Figure 6.19 Different responses to premature ventricular contraction (PVC) depending on base-rate behavior. (a) Ventricular-based timing resets the ventriculoatrial interval (VAI) after PVC, so that the subsequent ventricular pacing (VP) interval is equal to the programmed base rate [PVC–VP interval equal to lower rate limit (LRL)]. (b) In contrast, atrial-based timing resets the AA interval after PVC, resulting in violation of the LRL due to the addition of the atrioventricular interval (AVI) (PVC–VP interval is longer than LRL). (c) After PVC, the modified atrial-based timing subtracts the AVI from the AA timing, resulting in a similar response (PVC–VP interval equal to LRL) to ventricular-based timing. Source: Levine PA, Hayes DL, Wilkoff BL, Ohman AE. Electrocardiography of rate-modulated pacemaker rhythms. Sylmar, CA: Siemens-Pacesetter, 1990. Reproduced with permission of St. Jude Medical, Inc.

a 200-ms VAI at the MSR. If AV conduction is intact with an AR interval of 150 ms, the actual A–A pacing interval would be 350 ms (AR interval + VAI, or 150 + 200 ms) or 171 bpm, which is markedly higher than the programmed MSR of 150 bpm. Although this potentially faster rate may not be a problem or may even be advantageous for some patients, it could create problems for other patients. In contrast, atrial-based timing does not violate the MSR as intrinsic AV conduction (shorter AVI) does not affect or disturb the AA interval (Figure 6.21b).

Rate acceleration in a DDDR ventricular-based timing can be minimized by incorporating a rate-modulated AV delay. As the sinus or sensor-driven rate progressively increases, the rate-modulated AV delay causes the AVI to progressively shorten (Figure 6.21c). Shortening the AVI at faster rates (in response to sensor input) results in a shorter TARP (shorter AVI + PVARP), which increases the intrinsic atrial rate that can be sensed and reduces the likelihood of both a fixed-block upper rate response and functional atrial undersensing. Furthermore, the enabled rate-modulated AV delay will add to the VAI the time subtracted from the AVI, so that the ventricular rate drive is ruled by the sensor. Thus, rate-modulated AV delay provides a more physiological AVI at the faster rate and minimizes the degree of rate increase over the programmed MSR if AR conduction is intact.

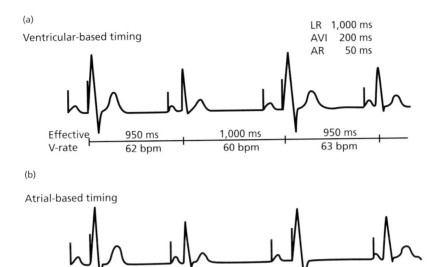

(a)

Ventricular-based timing

LR 1,000 ms
AVI 200 ms
AR 50 ms

Effective V-rate	950 ms	1,000 ms	950 ms
	62 bpm	60 bpm	63 bpm

(b)

Atrial-based timing

Effective V-rate	950 ms	1,050 ms	950 ms
	63 bpm	57 bpm	63 bpm

Figure 6.20 Schematic representations of 2 : 1 AV block during different base-rate behaviors. (a) With a ventricular-based timing system, the interval between consecutive AV- and AR-paced complexes (VR interval) is slightly faster (62 bpm) than the programmed LRL (60 bpm), while the interval between consecutive AR- and AV-paced complexes (RV interval) results in an effective ventricular rate at the lower rate limit (LRL) for that pacing cycle. (b) In an atrial-based timing system, the effective ventricular-paced rate alternates between rates that are faster and slower than the programmed rate. The cycle between an AR and AV complex results in a ventricular rate (RV interval) that is slower (57 bpm) than the programmed LRL. Meanwhile, the cycle between an AV and an AR complex causes the ventricular rate (VR interval) to be faster (63 bpm) than the programmed LRL. While the effective atrial pacing rate is stable at the programmed LRL regardless of base-rate behavior, the effective ventricular rate (that induces cardiac output) varies depending on base-rate behavior. Source: Levine PA, Hayes DL, Wilkoff BL, Ohman AE. Electrocardiography of rate-modulated pacemaker rhythms. Sylmar, CA: Siemens-Pacesetter, 1990. Reproduced with permission of St. Jude Medical, Inc.

Another option available in some devices is a forced extension of the VAI, which extends the VAI to avoid violation of the programmed MSR if intrinsic AV conduction is present (Figure 6.21d).

Hybrid-based timing

Hybrid-based systems are intended to avoid the heart rate variations noted with pure atrial- or ventricular-based timing systems noted previously (Figures 6.18 and 6.20) [2]. These systems use primarily an atrial-based timing, whereby an atrial-sensed or -paced event will reset the timing cycle (much like the sinus node itself), while ignoring a sensed R wave during stable AR pacing, and eliminating the rate acceleration in ventricular-based timing designs. To avoid drawbacks of atrial-based timing, the device will change to ventricular-based timing after PVCs or during intrinsic

AV conduction (Figure 6.22a), whereas some other devices will demonstrate modified atrial-based timing after PVC (Figure 6.19c). Once an intrinsic R wave occurs (return of AV conduction) before the AVI expires, atrial-based timing is restored, but only after the AVI is first subtracted (Figure 6.22b). Interpretation of pacemaker ECGs are further complicated by the increasing use of algorithms to promote intrinsic AV nodal conduction (Figure 6.23).

Upper rate behavior

As the sinus rate increases (shorter PP interval) in a P-synchronous ventricular pacing mode (DDD, VDD), the atrial-sensed event terminates the VAI, inhibits atrial pacing, and starts an AVI. If the intrinsic AV conduction is shorter than the set AV delay, ventricular pacing is completely inhibited.

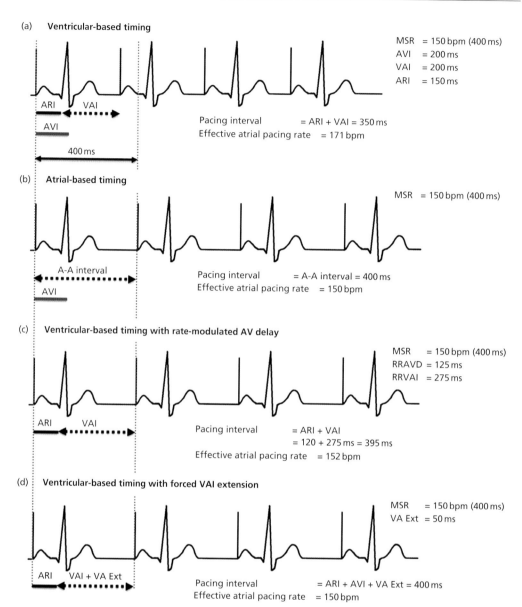

Figure 6.21 Effect of different base-rate behavior systems on rate-modulated pacing in patients with intact stable atrioventricular (AV) nodal conduction. (a) Ventricular-based timing. Even though the maximum sensor rate (MSR) is programmed at 150 bpm (400 ms), the effective atrial pacing rate achieved is 171 bpm. This can be explained since the effective atrial pacing rate is the sum of the interval from atrial stimulus to sensed R wave [AR interval (ARI)] and the ventriculoatrial interval (VAI), i.e. 150 + 200 = 350 ms (171 bpm). (b) Atrial-based timing. The R wave sensed during the AV interval (AVI) does not alter or reset the AA timing and atrial pacing rate occurs at the sensor-indicated rate (SIR). (c) Rate-modulated AV delay (RMAVD) in the ventricular-based timing system. RMAVD minimizes the increase in the paced atrial rate above the programmed SIR. A programmed RMAVD of 125 ms in ventricular-based timing (a) causes the AVI to shorten to 125 ms when the SIR reaches the MSR (75 ms subtracted from the programmed AVI of 200 ms). Subsequently, the 75 ms subtracted from the AVI are added to the VAI [rate responsive VAI or rate-modulated AV delay (RMVAI) of 275 ms], maintaining the programmed MSR of 150 bpm. However, if intact AV conduction (ARI) is present at 120 ms (5 ms faster than RMAVD), the overall AA pacing interval will be shorter by only 5 ms (395 ms or 152 bpm). (d) Forced extension of VAI in ventricular-based timing. A programmed VA extension (50 ms) is added to the VAI (AA timing = AR + VAI + VA extension) as a function of sensor input, providing an alternative (if available) to maintain pacing at MSR. Source: (c) Levine PA, Hayes DL, Wilkoff BL, Ohman AE. Electrocardiography of rate-modulated pacemaker rhythms. Sylmar, CA: Siemens-Pacesetter, 1990. Reproduced with permission of St. Jude Medical, Inc.

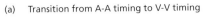

(a)   Transition from A-A timing to V-V timing

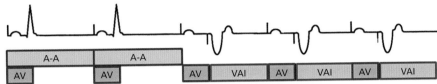

(b)   Transition from V-V timing to A-A timing

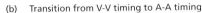

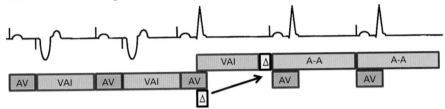

Figure 6.22 Hybrid base-rate behavior. (a) Timing changes from atrial- to ventricular-based behavior when intrinsic atrioventricular (AV) nodal conduction is no longer present. (b) Timing changes from ventricular- to atrial-based behavior after a ventricular-sensed event is noted (Δ, difference between PR interval and AV interval in the first cycle during which intrinsic conduction occurs). Δ is applied to the next VA interval (VAI) to provide a smooth transition without affecting VV intervals. Source: modified from Huizar JF, Kaszala K, Ellenbogen KA. Cardiac pacing modes and terminology. In: Sakena S, Camm AJ, eds. *Electrophysiological Disorders of the Heart*, 2nd edn. Philadelphia, PA: Elsevier Saunders, 2012: 441–456. Reproduced with permission of Elsevier.

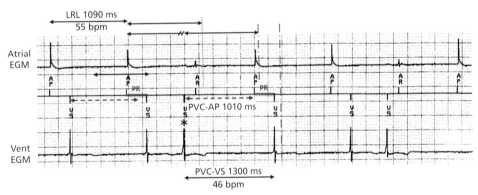

Figure 6.23 Modified atrial-based timing in managed ventricular pacing (MVP, Medtronic). MVP mode (AAI ↔ DDD pacing mode) demonstrates atrial pacing at a lower rate limit (LRL) of 55 bpm (1100 ms) even with a PR interval (AP–VS) of 280–300 ms. A premature ventricular contraction (PVC, *) is followed by a retrograde P wave that falls in the PVARP (AR, lacks resetting AA timing). In MVP mode, the PVC terminates the AA interval and reinitiates a modified AA timing which postpones the initially scheduled AP event (horizontal red dashed line). Modified atrial-based timing is calculated as AA interval = LRL – 80 ms (1090 – 80 = 1010 ms) to minimize violation of the LRL. In a pure atrial-based timing, a new AA interval after a PVC would have resulted in a PVC–AP event at 1090 ms (left blue dash–dotted line) with substantial violation of the LRL (PVC–VS of 1400 ms = 42 bpm; right blue dash–dotted line).

However, P-synchronous ventricular pacing occurs in a 1 : 1 relationship between the programmed LRL and the programmed MTR if the intrinsic AVI is longer than the programmed sensed AVI.

MTR determines the upper rate behavior or maximum paced ventricular rate in a P-synchronous pacing mode. MTR has also been referred to as "upper rate limit" and "ventricular tracking limit." MTR is limited by the TARP (AVI + PVARP; see Figure 6.13). P-synchronous ventricular pacing (tracking) is delivered at the end of the AVI only if the MTR has been completed. If the MTR interval has not yet been completed at the end of the AVI, the release of the ventricular output pulse is delayed until the MTR interval ends (Figure 6.24). This delay has the functional effect of lengthening the PV interval and places the ensuing ventricular-paced beat closer to the next P wave. Eventually, a P wave will fall within the PVARP with lack of ventricular tracking as the AVI is never initiated. Thus, an atrial or sinus rate exceeding the programmed MTR can demonstrate an AV nodal Wenckebach-like behavior, as ventricular pacing can occur with a progressive lengthening of the PV interval with intermittent pauses and a group beating pattern on the ECG. This can be summarized by the equation: Wenckebach interval = MTR interval − TARP (Figure 6.25a).When the PP interval (sinus rate) is shorter than the TARP, those P waves falling into the PVARP will not be tracked by ventricular pacing and an abrupt fixed-block behavior (2 : 1, 3 : 1, etc.) will occur (Figure 6.25b). Thus, upper rate behavior can demonstrate Wenckebach-like behavior or fixed block (e.g. 2 : 1) and may cause serious symptoms in pacemaker-dependent patients.

DDDR pacing systems further increase the complexity of the upper rate behavior. Between the programmed LRL and MSR, the pacemaker can be driven by intrinsic atrial activity to cause P-synchronous ventricular pacing, or by a sensor with an input signal that is not identifiable on the ECG, or by both, to result in AV sequential or AR pacing (see Figure 6.17). The eventual upper rate also depends on the type of sensor incorporated into the pacemaker and how the sensor is programmed.

Rate enhancements

Several pacemaker algorithms are now available in pacemakers that may alter the pacing rate from either the programmed lower rate or sinus-driven or sensor-driven rates. These features are described in Table 6.5.

Base rate during mode switch/fallback

During paroxysms of atrial fibrillation, pacemakers have automatic algorithms to switch pacing mode to a non-tracking mode (DDI, VDI, VVI), which avoids tracking high atrial rates (see section Mode switch). The programmed LRL in a non-tracking pacing mode could be too low if heart rate is too slow during atrial fibrillation and higher heart rates may be needed to compensate for the loss of atrial transport. For this reason, devices have the ability to program a different LRL when mode switch occurs. For example, a pacemaker can be programmed DDD with an LRL of 60 bpm during sinus rhythm, whereas a higher base rate may be programmed to 70–80 bpm during mode switch to DDI, VDI, or VVI pacing mode. If rate modulation were also activated, any increase in sensor-driven rates would start at the appropriate base for the functional pacing mode at the time.

Fallback mode is a feature available in some pacemakers. This feature becomes active immediately after mode switch has occurred. The fallback mode (non-tracking pacing mode) will slowly and progressively decrease the pacing rate throughout a

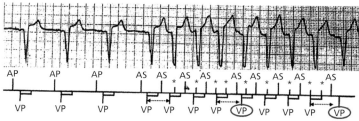

Figure 6.24 Upper rate behavior during non-sustained atrial tachycardia/flutter. As illustrated by the event markers, the ECG tracing represents initial atrioventricular (AV) sequential pacing (AP–VP) at the lower rate limit (55 bpm), followed by non-sustained atrial flutter. Rapid atrial signals are sensed (AS) and tracked with ventricular pacing (VP) at maximum tracking rate (MTR, dashed arrows). However, several atrial signals (*) fall within the post-ventricular atrial refractory period (PVARP) (represented by rectangles after VP). A 2 : 1 pacemaker behavior is noted in the first beats, while the fourth and eighth beats (ringed) demonstrate a 3 : 1 behavior since the prior two signals occurred during the post-ventricular blanking period (PVAB) and PVARP. Source: Levine PA, Hayes DL, Wilkoff BL, Ohman AE. Electrocardiography of rate-modulated pacemaker rhythms. Sylmar, CA: Siemens-Pacesetter, 1990. Reproduced with permission of St. Jude Medical, Inc.

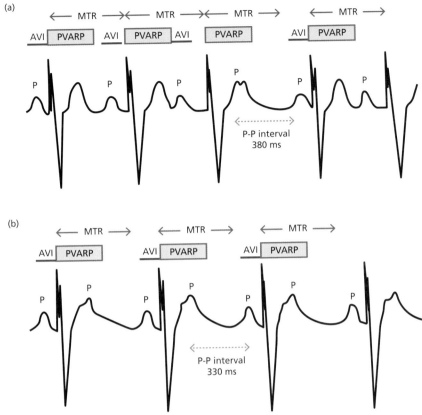

Figure 6.25 Wenckebach-like and 2 : 1 pacemaker behavior. A pacemaker is programmed with an atrioventricular interval (AVI) of 125 ms, a post-ventricular atrial refractory period (PVARP) of 225 ms and a maximum tracking rate (MTR) of 400 ms (Wenckebach interval = MTR – AVI + PVARP = 400 – 125 + 225 = 50 ms). (a) A Wenckebach-like behavior is noted since atrial rates or PP intervals are between 350 and 400 ms (50-ms Wenckebach interval). An atrial signal sensed within the atrial-sensing window (after completion of the PVARP) will initiate an AVI. Despite completion of the AVI (125 ms), P-synchronous ventricular pacing will not be delivered until the MTR is met with a PP interval of 380 ms (faster than the MTR of 400 ms), resulting in a longer than programmed AVI. This gradual prolongation of the PV interval [atrial sense (AS) to ventricular paced (VP) interval] ensures that ventricular pacing occurs closer to the next P wave, until the atrial event falls within the PVARP (the fourth P wave does not initiate an AVI). (b) In contrast, the pacemaker demonstrates a 2 : 1 AV block with PP intervals of 330 ms (PP interval faster than TARP = 125 + 225 = 350 ms), as AVI is not initiated in those P waves falling within the PVARP.

fallback programmable time from MTR (P-synchronous ventricular pacing while mode switch counter is met) to a programmable fallback LRL (Table 6.5). Fallback mode is intended to avoid a sudden heart rate drop from the MTR to the LRL or intrinsic ventricular rate that otherwise would occur without fallback (Figure 6.26). After fallback time has been completed, fallback LRL will be maintained in programmed fallback pacing mode, but it does not avoid heart rate variability between fallback LRL and maximum pacing rate, a special attribute of ventricular rate regularization (see section Rate smoothing/stabilization).

Rate smoothing/stabilization

These features were developed and are now available to avoid sudden and marked atrial and/or ventricular interval variability. Some of these features include *rate smoothing, atrial and ventricular rate stabilization* (ARS, VRS), and *ventricular rate regularization* (VRR). These algorithms have a slightly different function and programmability between manufacturers, as noted in Table 6.5.

One of the first algorithms, rate smoothing, uses the most recent RR interval, whether intrinsic or paced, to calculate an allowable increase or decrease in cycle length based on a programmable rate smoothing

Table 6.5 Rate smoothing/stabilization and fallback algorithms

Algorithm	Device	Function/programmability	Indications	Notes/comments
Rate smoothing (RS) [7,8] (Figure 6.27)	GDT, BS	Allows a percentage programmable increase or decrease (3–24% with 3% increments) in atrial and/or ventricular cycle length between LRL and MTR (P-synchronous pacing mode), MSR (adaptive pacing mode) or URL (non- P-synchronous or single-chamber pacing modes)	Symptomatic variations of ventricular rate, e.g. sick sinus syndrome, AF/flutter, PACs, PVCs, and pacemaker Wenckebach-like behavior Pause-dependent induction of torsades de pointes	RS is not active if rate is above MTR or MSR and during VRR, search hysteresis, ATR fallback, PMT termination and sudden brady response
Atrial and ventricular rate stabilization (ARS, VRS) [16] (Figure 6.28)	MDT	ARS and VRS intend to eliminate long pauses after PAC or PVC, respectively. They do not respond to sustained tachyarrhythmias. VRS operates when the rate that corresponds to the RR median interval is less than or equal to a fixed rate of 85 bpm. Medial RR interval is the median value of the last 12 measured ventricular intervals (maximum rate, interval increment)	Symptomatic pause after PVC or PAC and pause-dependent induction of polymorphic VT (Td)	ARS is suspended during mode switch and detected arrhythmia. ARS and VRS cannot be enabled if rate hysteresis is programmed "on"
Ventricular rate regularization (VRR) [7] (Figure 6.26b)	GDT, BS	Operates between LRL and programmable VRR max pacing rate (60–150 bpm). Continually active in single-chamber pacing modes. Active only after mode switch (non-tracking pacing mode) has occurred in dual-chamber pacing modes	Increase biventricular pacing in CRT during AF/flutter Symptomatic variations of ventricular rate during atrial arrhythmias (AF/flutter) Pause-dependent induction of polymorphic VT (Td)	Updates VRR-indicated pacing rate on each cardiac cycle (pacing interval estimated on a weighted sum of the current V–V cycle length and previous VRR-indicated pacing intervals)
Fallback [7,8] (Figure 6.26)	GDT, BS	Occurs automatically after switch mode, gradually decreasing pacing rate to ATR/VTR fallback LRL, VRR rate (if enabled) Fallback mode (non-tracking pacing mode) Fallback time (how quickly paced rate will decrease to ATR)	Symptoms related to sudden drop in heart rate from MTR (while counters are met for mode switch to occur) to LRL or SIR	Only available when programmed to a dual-chamber pacing mode RS, rate hysteresis, AV search and PVARP extension are disabled during fallback mode

AF, atrial fibrillation; ATR, atrial tachycardia response; BS, Boston Scientific; CRT, cardiac resynchronization therapy; GDT, Guidant; PAC, premature atrial contraction; PMT, pacemaker-mediated tachycardia; PVC, premature ventricular contraction; SIR, sensor-indicated rate; for other acronyms, see Table 6.3.

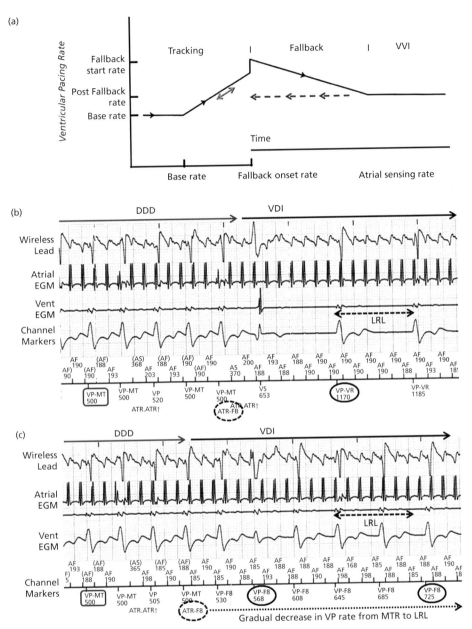

Figure 6.26 Fallback mode and ventricular rate regularization features. (a) Diagram illustrating the fallback mode feature. P-synchronous pacing (DDD mode) occurs between the base rate and up to the maximum tracking rate (MTR). Once the atrial rate exceeds the mode switch rate (also referred to as the fallback onset rate), pacing mode will switch from DDD to a programmable non-tracking pacing mode (DDI, VDI, VVI). The fallback (FB) feature prevents sudden drop on ventricular pacing (VP) from the MTR to the lower rate limit (LRL). When fallback time is enabled, the device will slowly decrease the VP rate from the MTR to the LRL in the time frame instructed. Once atrial rate decreases below the mode switch rate, the device will return back to DDD pacing mode. (b) DDD pacing mode initially tracks an atrial flutter of 300 bpm (3 : 1 block) at an MTR of 120 bpm (VP–MT 500 ms; blue square) until mode switch counters are met and the pacing mode switches to VDI [atrial tachycardia response (ATR)-FB, dashed oval] at the LRL of 50 bpm (1200 ms). A sudden drop in VP rate (from MTR 120 to 52 bpm) occurs since fallback is not enabled. The VP rate occurs slightly higher than the programmed LRL of 50 bpm (VP–VR 1170 ms or 52 bpm, ringed with a solid oval) due to ventricular rate regularization (VRR, maximum rate 100 bpm) after an intrinsic R wave at 653 ms. (c) Fallback is enabled with a 15-s fallback time in the same patient as in (b). After the mode switch rate counter is met and the device switches from DDD to VDI pacing mode (ATR-FB), the VP rate gradually decreases (VP–FB, solid circles) from the MTR to the LRL (dashed arrow), avoiding the sudden drop in VP rate.

percentage [7] (Figure 6.27). For example, if the VV cycle length is stable at 900 ms during P-synchronous pacing with rate smoothing enabling at 6% increase, the subsequent VV cycle cannot accelerate by more than 54 ms (846 ms) if sinus rate suddenly accelerates.

ARS and VRS have a similar rationale as rate smoothing. However, ARS and VRS work only during premature atrial contractions (PACs) and PVCs, respectively, and are rendered non-operational during sustained tachyarrhythmias (Table 6.5 and Figure 6.28). VRR is a variant of rate smoothing; however, it will only function during mode switch (Figure 6.26b).

Rate-modulated pacing (sensor input to base rate pacing)

DDDR pacing can result in a type of rate smoothing. If the sensor is optimally programmed, then as the atrial rate exceeds the MTR (during exercise), the RR interval displays minimal variation between sinus-driven and sensor-driven pacing. As shown in Figure 6.29, the variation in RR interval is markedly lessened with the sensor "on" (DDDR) rather than "passive" (DDD). In the DDDR mode, the RR interval is allowed to lengthen only as much as the difference between the MTR and the sensor-indicated rate.

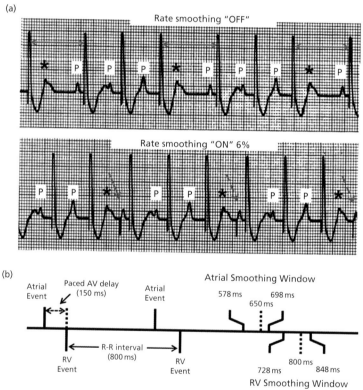

Figure 6.27 Rate smoothing. (a) ECG demonstrates a Wenckebach-like behavior (P-synchronous ventricular pacing) with significant pauses (solid red arrows) due to an atrial rate above the maximum tracking rate (MTR). P waves gradually occur sooner after ventricular pacing (VP) until a P wave falls within the post-ventricular atrial refractory period (PVARP, *), failing to initiate AVI and lacking P-synchronous ventricular pacing. An enabled rate smoothing down (6% of the preceding RR interval) will minimize pauses by delivering atrioventricular (AV) sequential pacing (dashed red arrows) after P wave during PVARP (*), allowing the VV interval to lengthen by only 36 ms over the preceding VV interval at an MTR of 100 bpm. (b) Calculation of atrial and ventricular smoothing windows. With a previous RR interval of 800 ms, programmed AV delay of 150 ms, and enabled rate smoothing up and down (9% and 6%, respectively), the ventricular smoothing window is 728–848 ms (800 – 9% or 72 ms to 800 + 6% or 48 ms = 728–848 ms), whereas the atrial smoothing window is 578–698 ms (ventricular smoothing window – AV delay = 728 – 150 ms to 848 – 150 ms = 578–698 ms). Sources: (a) Boston Scientific Corporation. Reproduced with permission of Boston Scientific. (b) Cognis™ 100-D device manual. Reproduced with permission of Boston Scientific.

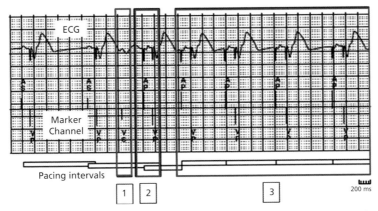

Figure 6.28 Ventricular rate stabilization. A short coupled premature ventricular contraction (1, VS) causes atrioventricular (AV) sequential pacing at the previous V–V interval plus interval increment (2), with (3) a gradual prolongation of AV sequential pacing. Source: *Entrust ICD system: Reference Manual*. St. Paul, MN: Medtronic, Inc. Reproduced with permission of Medtronic, Inc.

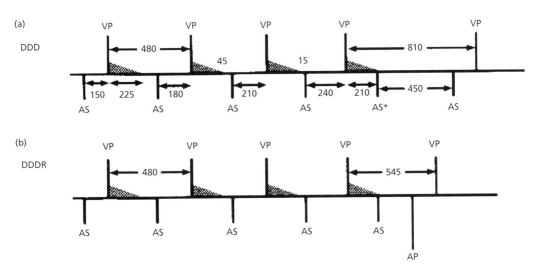

Figure 6.29 Rate modulation (DDDR pacing mode) acting as rate smoothing. (a) DDD pacing mode demonstrates Wenckebach behavior as the atrial rate (450 ms, 133 bpm) is higher than the maximum tracking rate (MTR) (125 bpm). The fifth atrial-sensed event (AS, *) [210 ms after the preceding ventricular-paced event (VP)] is sensed but does not trigger ventricular pacing [the atrioventricular interval (AVI) is not initiated] since it falls within the post-ventricular atrial refractory period (PVARP) (225 ms). The resultant VP–VP interval is 810 ms (74 bpm), significantly longer than the preceding cycles of 480 ms (125 bpm). (b) DDDR pacing mode [with otherwise identical programmed intervals as in (a)] avoids the prolonged VP–VP interval, due to a sensor-driven pacing rate of 545 ms (110 bpm). Thus, only a 65-ms difference exists between the programmed upper rate limit (URL) and the sensor-indicated rate, a minor difference in cycle lengths. Source: modified from Markowitz TH. Dual chamber rate responsive pacing (DDDR) provides physiologic upper rate behavior. *Physio Pace* 1990;4:1–4. Medtronic, Inc. Reproduced with permission of Medtronic, Inc.

Algorithms to allow intrinsic sinus rate

Different algorithms exist to search for and allow the intrinsic sinus rate to predominate (Table 6.6). These algorithms may be responsible for intrinsic or pacing rates below the SIR and/or the LRL.

Rate hysteresis (first-generation algorithm) allows prolongation of the first pacemaker escape interval to a programmed hysteresis rate only after a sensed intrinsic event occurs above a programmed LRL (Figure 6.30a). In contrast, *scan*

Table 6.6 Algorithms to allow intrinsic sinus rate (SR)

Algorithm	Settings	Search/trigger	Intervention	Notes/comments
Rate hysteresis (MDT, SJM, BS) (Figure 6.30a)	Hysteresis rate or offset (HyR)	A sensed event above base rate or LRL will trigger HyR	Pacing rate is lowered from the base rate or SIR to the HyR as long as intrinsic events are sensed	First occurrence of a pace event at HyR will reestablish pacing rate to base rate or LRL. Available in single (AAI® or VVI®) or dual-chamber pacing modes
Search hysteresis (SJM, BS)	Hysteresis rate or offset (HyR) Search interval	A sensed event above base rate or LRL will trigger HyR. Some devices (SJM, BS) provide a search interval to lower the pacing rate to HyR, looking for an intrinsic event	Pacing rate is lowered from the base rate or SIR to the HyR as long as intrinsic events are sensed	First occurrence of a pace event at HyR will reestablish pacing rate to base rate or LRL. Available in single (AAI® or VVI®) or dual-chamber pacing modes
Scan hysteresis (BTK) (Figure 6.30b)	Hysteresis rate (HyR) Number of cycles (1–10)	After 180 paced cycles, the pacing rate is lowered to HyR for a programmed number of cycles	If no SR is sensed above HyR, pacing will be restored at LRL or SIR. Intrinsic rate will be allowed if SR is sensed above HyR	
Sinus preference (SP) [10] (MDT) (Figure 6.30c)	SP zone Search interval	Sinus search: after search interval expires, a gradual drop from SIR to SP zone limit will occur until SR is sensed or rate drops to SP zone limit. If no AS events are noted for eight paced beats at SP zone limit, a gradual increase to SIR will occur	If AS is noted, SR is allowed to predominate below SIR unless or until it drops below SP zone limit	Second modality: sinus breakthrough operation initiates only if SR is detected above SIR, tracks SR within the SP zone limit, but never below the LRL. Cannot be enabled with MVP (AAIR DDDR) [10]
Sleep rate [10] (MDT)	Bed time Wake time Sleep rate	During 30 min following bed time, pacing rate gradually decreases from LRL to sleep rate. During 30 min following wake time, pacing rate gradually restored to LRL	Suspends LRL and replaces with a slower rate than LRL (sleep rate)	In rate-modulated modes, SIR increases in the presence of sensor-indicated activity
Rest rate (SJM)	Rest rate	Device analyzes activity data for a 7-day period. Triggered if sensor detects inactivity or rest >15–20 min	LRL decreases to rest rate. Heart rate increases to base rate when activity is sensed	This setting is operational regardless of day time
Night rate program (BTK)	Night rate Night begins Night ends	Programmable schedule for any time of the day or night (nominally begins at 10:00 p.m.)	LRL is lowered to a programmable night rate	In rate-modulated modes, the night program is temporarily suspended during accelerometer-indicated activity

AS, atrial sensed; BS, Boston Scientific; BTK, Biotronik; MDT, Medtronic; SJM, St. Jude Medical; SIR, sensor-indicated rate; for other abbreviations, see Table 6.3.

(a)

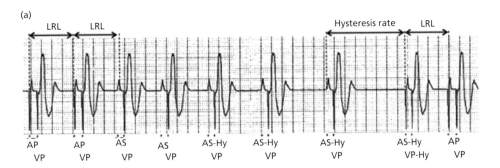

(b)

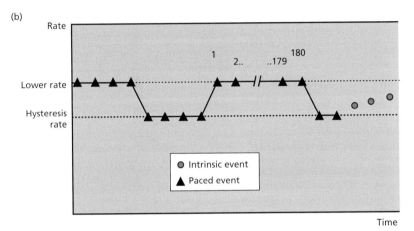

(c)

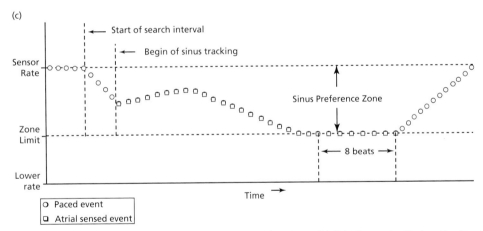

Figure 6.30 Algorithms to allow intrinsic sinus rate. (a) Rate hysteresis, (b) scan hysteresis, (c) sinus preference. Refer to Table 6.6 for details on function of these pacemaker features. Sources: (a) *Insignia I Ultra System Guide, models 1190/1290/1291*. St Paul, MN: Guidant Corporation, 2006. Reproduced with permission of Medtronic, Inc. (b) *Cylos Pacemaker Feature Handbook*, section 2.2.2, p. 33, last published 3 April 2009 (Reference MN010). Lake Oswego, OR: Biotronik. Reproduced with permission of Biotronik. (c) *Adapta, Sensia, Versa Pacemaker Reference Guide*. St Paul, MN: Medtronic, Inc., 2006. Reproduced with permission of Medtronic, Inc.

hysteresis (Figure 6.30b), *search hysteresis*, and *sinus preference* (Figure 6.30c) automatically lower pacing rate after determined paced beats or interval to a programmed hysteresis rate or sinus preference zone, respectively, searching for an intrinsic sinus rate.

Rest rate is intended to reduce paced rhythm during rest, including sleep, in order to mimic physiological decrease in heart rate during physical inactivity. Other contemporary pacemakers offer a "circadian response," or *sleep rate*, that allows a lower rate to be programmed for the approximate time during which the patient is sleeping. A separate, potentially faster LRL may then be programmed for waking hours. For example, the LRL during waking hours may be programmed to 70 bpm and during sleeping hours to 50 bpm. This feature is tied to a clock, and the usual waking and sleeping hours are programmed into some pacemakers, while other pacemakers require an additional verification of inactivity by sensor to allow decrease in the LRL to occur.

These algorithms have different programmable settings, search and trigger thresholds, and interventions (Table 6.6). Overall, these features are believed to lower battery drain and increase longevity, particularly in patients with high pacing thresholds.

Algorithms for cardioinhibitory neurogenic syncope

Different algorithms have been developed to respond to the sudden drop in intrinsic heart rate observed in subjects with severe cardioinhibitory neurogenic syncope. Some of these algorithms include hysteresis rate, sudden bradycardia response (SBR), and rate drop response (RDR). Algorithm features vary in the trigger and response in this clinical scenario (Table 6.7).

Hysteresis rate (described in the previous section) has been proposed as a strategy to prevent a sudden decrease of heart rate in cardioinhibitory neurogenic syncope (Figure 6.31) only if "advanced functions" (cycle count, intervention rate and duration, recovery time) are enabled [5,8,9]. This algorithm intervenes if the patient's intrinsic rate falls below the hysteresis rate for a period longer than the cycle count setting, pacing at the intervention rate for a period stipulated by the intervention duration setting. The device will return to the programmed base rate setting as instructed by the recovery time parameter.

Similarly, RDR or SBR reacts to a defined drop in heart rate by pacing at an elevated rate in both chambers for a specific programmed duration (Figure 6.32) [8–10]. At the conclusion of the programmed duration, the pacing rate gradually returns to the programmed lower rate (Table 6.7).

Most recently, sensors that assess beat-to-beat contractility (Closed Loop Stimulation, Biotronik) are being used to prevent cardioinhibitory neurogenic syncope, with the rationale that they can detect early changes in autonomic tone and contractility preceding syncope. Thus, these sensors can react accordingly with a proportional increase in pacing rate to prevent inappropriate drop in heart rate [5].

Overall, there are limited and controversial clinical data supporting the beneficial effect of these algorithms in the prevention of cardioinhibitory neurogenic syncope [3,11–13].

Mode switch

The mode switch feature indicates that the pacemaker is capable of automatically reprogramming itself from one pacing mode to another as a result of an inappropriate rapid atrial rhythm [14,15]. The change in pacing mode occurs after specific criteria for atrial arrhythmia have been met. Mode switch occurs between a baseline P-synchronous (tracking) pacing mode [DDD(R), VDD(R)] to a nontracking pacing mode [DDI(R), VVI(R), VDI(R)].

Mode switch is particularly useful for patients with paroxysmal supraventricular arrhythmias; otherwise rapid ventricular pacing may occur in DDD or DDDR pacing mode (see section Upper rate behavior). This feature avoids inappropriate tracking of atrial tachyarrhythmias and pacemaker Wenckebach-like behavior while an atrial arrhythmia is present (Figure 6.33).

Mode switch algorithms have become more refined and have slight variations between pacemaker manufacturers and models (Figure 6.34). Most pacemakers have a programmable mode switch rate. Only until the atrial mode switch rate is met for a specified number of intervals (often a non-programmable counter) or time duration, the pacemaker is automatically reprogrammed to a non-atrial tracking mode and remains in this mode until a specified number of long intervals have occurred and altered the counter, at which point mode switching reverts to an atrial tracking mode (Figure 6.33b). Because a counter must be met before mode switching occurs, short transient

Table 6.7 Algorithms for cardioinhibitory neurogenic syncope

Feature	Trigger	Response/intervention	Comments
Rate hysteresis with advanced functions (SJM, BTK) (Figure 6.31)	Heart rate falls below *hysteresis rate* for a period longer than *cycle count*	DDD pacing at *intervention rate* setting for the time specified in *intervention duration*	Device returns to LRL after *recovery time* is completed
Rate drop response (RDR) (MDT) (Figure 6.32A)	Two triggers available: 1 Drop detection: if sensed or paced ventricular rate drops by the programmed *drop size* or more to below the programmed *drop rate* within the programmed *detection window* 2 Low rate detection: if atrium or ventricle is paced at LRL for a consecutive number of *detection beats*	Pacing at *intervention rate* for a programmed *intervention duration*. When intervention duration expires, pacing slowly decreases in approximately 5-bpm steps until the intrinsic rate is sensed or LRL is reached	Low rate detection is only applicable to DDI pacing mode If the intrinsic ventricular rate drops too slowly to meet the RDR drop detection criteria, the pacemaker paces at LRL if the intrinsic rate drops below the programmable lower rate
Sudden bradycardia response (SBR) (BS) (Figure 6.32b)	SBR is confirmed after continuously sensed atrial rate for a programmable time (*SBR detect time* 1–15 min) suddenly decreases such that atrial pacing occurs at the LRL or SIR for a programmable *number of beats* (1–8 cycles)	Pacing occurs in DDD(R) mode at the greater of either (i) the previous average atrial rate plus the SBR *therapy rate offset*, not to exceed the MTR, or (ii) SIR (DDDR mode only) Therapy rate offset is calculated by using average atrial rate before bradycardia and adding programmable positive offset	SBR minute ventilation (MV) sensor provides ability to inhibit SBR if SBR rate and duration criteria are met but patient's current MV sensor input is lower than a programmed value (MV offset) Rate smoothing is not available if SBR is enabled

BS, Boston Scientific; BTK, Biotronik; MDT, Medtronic; SJM, St. Jude Medical; SIR, sensor-indicated rate; for other acronyms, see Table 6.3.

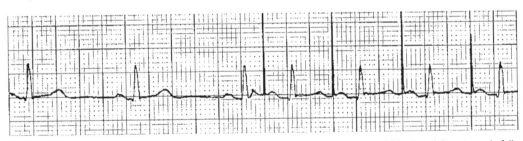

Figure 6.31 Advanced rate hysteresis. DDD pacing mode at 100 bpm (intervention rate) occurs in response to a drop in heart rate (63 bpm) below a programmed hysteresis rate of 65 bpm. After 256 cycles of pacing at 100 bpm, pacing is suspended for the pacemaker to "search" for the intrinsic lower rate. If the lower rate is greater than the hysteresis rate, pacing is inhibited until the rate again falls below the hysteresis rate. Source: Lloyd MA, Hayes DL, Friedman PA. Programming. In: Hayes DL, Lloyd MA, Friedman PA, eds. *Cardiac Pacing and Defibrillation: A Clinical Approach.* Armonk, NY: Futura, 2000; 247–323. Reproduced with permission of the Mayo Foundation.

bursts of atrial arrhythmias may still be tracked, and other algorithms, such as rate smoothing (see section Rate enhancement), may be needed to minimize palpitations.

The non-tracking mode to which the mode switch occurs is frequently a programmable option. It is most commonly DDIR and, less commonly, VDIR or VVIR. DDIR may be the preferable

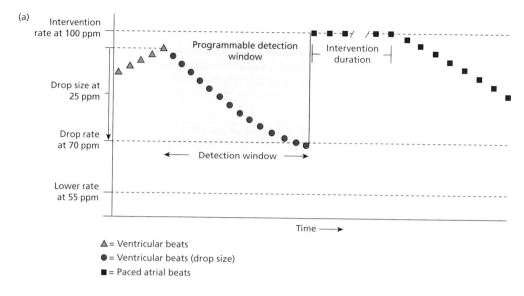

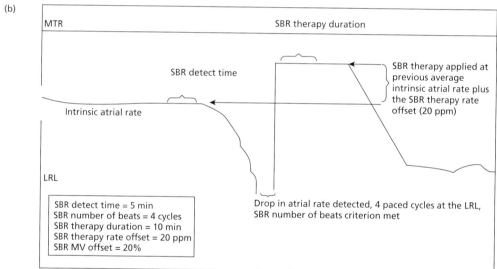

Figure 6.32 (a) Rate drop response. Algorithm detects a heart rate drop based on a programmed drop size of 25 bpm and a drop rate at 75 bpm with a 1-min detection window. Thus, the device responds by pacing at 100 bpm (intervention rate) for a programmable period of time. (b) Sudden bradycardia response (SBR) intervenes by pacing at 20 bpm above the intrinsic atrial rate (SBR therapy rate offset) for a total of 10 min (SBR therapy duration) in response to a drop in the atrial rate, meeting the SBR criteria (after 5-min detection time, a drop in heart rate occurs, pacing four cycles at the lower rate limit (LRL)]. MV, minute ventilation, see Table 6.7 for details. MTR, maximum tracking rate. Sources: (a) *Adapta, Versia and Sensia Manual.* St. Paul, MN: Medtronic, Inc. Reproduced with permission of Medtronic, Inc. (b) *Altrua Pacemaker Manual.* Reproduced with permission of Boston Scientific.

non-tracking mode switch as it will allow maintenance of AV synchrony after the atrial tachyarrhythmia has terminated, but before mode switching has been declared completed.

Appropriate mode switch depends on proper sensing of high atrial rates. Thus, identifying

rapid atrial events that occur during the refractory period is essential. In many dual-chamber pacemakers, this period includes the terminal portion of the AV delay and the latter portion of the PVARP. The first part of the PVARP (absolute portion), referred to as the PVAB, prevents sensing

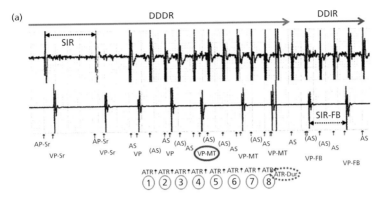

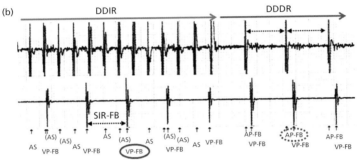

Figure 6.33 Mode switch. (a) Pacing mode changes from DDDR to DDIR after the mode switch duration criteria [eight events – atrial tachycardia response (ATR)] are met (ATR-Dur, dotted blue oval). The initial tracing demonstrates atrioventricular (AV) sequential pacing at the sensor-indicated rate (SIR, AP-Sr and VP-Sr). After the second beat, atrial flutter starts spontaneously tracking atrial-sensed (AS) events [outside the post-ventricular atrial refractory period (PVARP)] at the programmed maximum tracking rate (MTR) (VP-MT, solid blue oval) while the DDDR pacing mode continues. Once a mode switch criterion is met, right ventricular (RV) pacing will occur at the programmed mode switch/fallback heart rate (SIR-FB) without tracking AS events (DDIR). (b) The same patient demonstrates ventricular pacing (VP) at the fallback rate (VP-FB) while the patient is in atrial flutter. After sudden termination of his atrial flutter, AV sequential pacing occurs at the fallback rate (AP-FB and VP-FB), returning to DDDR pacing mode once the criterion is met.

of the far-field R wave. However, some pulse generators are limited by atrial events that fall within the TARP (AVI + PVARP) and rely on algorithms to detect atrial tachyarrhythmias (see section Algorithms for atrial arrhythmia detection and atrial pace/sense competition).

To ensure sensing of pathological atrial tachyarrhythmias whose signal amplitudes may fluctuate and may be very small, the atrial channel is usually programmed to a highly sensitive value (e.g. low value for atrial sensitivity: 0.15–0.35 mV). High atrial sensitivity, together with R waves after the PVAB, can predispose the detection of ventricular signals on the atrial channel. The pacemaker may label these ventricular signals as "P" waves and thus respond as if the atrial rate were high when the

rhythm is actually normal sinus rhythm. The result is a form of double-counting, resulting in a "false" mode switch (Figure 6.35). To prevent far-field R-wave sensing, the PVAB can be programmed (from 50 to 250 ms) in most devices. There is an inverse relationship between the duration of the PVAB and the detection of atrial arrhythmia, with the shorter PVABs allowing detection of higher atrial rates (increased sensitivity to atrial tachyarrhythmias). However, increasing the PVAB increases the specificity of rhythm detection and minimizes inappropriate mode switch. The PVAB may also limit the ability to detect atrial arrhythmias, particularly atrial flutter and tachycardias, since an atrial deflection may occur just after the paced or sensed ventricular event, creating the so-called "2 : 1 lock-in" phenomenon (see section Algorithms for atrial arrhythmia detection and atrial pace/sense competition).

However, far-field R-wave sensing (intrinsic AV conduction) with subsequent inappropriate

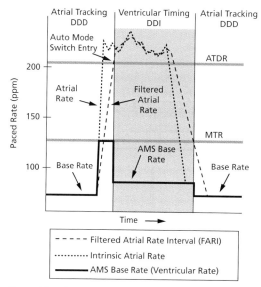

Figure 6.34 Diagram illustrates switching from atrial tracking to a non-tracking mode (DDI). During DDI pacing a separate base rate may be programmed in some devices. After the atrial arrhythmia has terminated, the mode will switch back to the DDD mode. ATDR, atrial tachycardia detection rate; MTR, maximum tracking rate. Source: *Bradycardia Devices: Help Manual*. Sylmar, CA: St. Jude Medical, Inc. Reproduced with permission of St. Jude Medical, Inc.

mode switch can occur even with an extended PVAB if the intrinsic ventricular signal is detected on the atrial channel before the ventricular channel of the pacemaker (PVARP and PVAB will be initiated only after ventricular signal is detected in the ventricular channel). This scenario is illustrated in Figure 6.8.

Algorithms for atrial arrhythmia detection and atrial pace/sense competition

Algorithms have been developed to identify rapid atrial-sensed events, including PACs and supraventricular arrhythmias (including atrial flutter and fibrillation) (Table 6.8). Frequently, these algorithms are available only in DDD(R) pacing mode. Appropriate identification of these atrial arrhythmias is important not only to allow appropriate mode switch when they persist (avoid tracking these arrhythmias), but also to avoid short coupling atrial pacing within the atrial vulnerable period that could result in the induction of other atrial arrhythmias.

Blanked flutter search

Blanked flutter search (Medtronic) monitors for AA intervals that may indicate 2 : 1 blanking of atrial events. If an AS event is "blanked," the device will extend PVARP and VAI to uncover AS. A second AS event noted above mode switch rate will be added to the counter for mode switch.

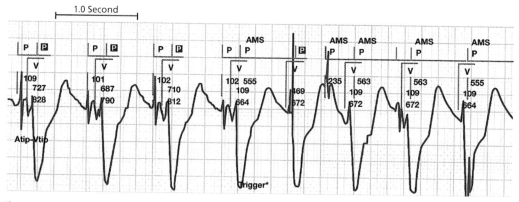

Figure 6.35 Inappropriate or false mode switch. Summed (Atip–Vtip) electrogram demonstrates oversensing of ventricular pacing by the atrial channel after the post-ventricular atrial blanking period (PVAB) has expired, resulting in double counting and inappropriate atrial mode switch (AMS) to a non-tracking pacing mode (VVI) at a higher AMS base rate.

Table 6.8 Atrial arrhythmia detection and atrial pace/sense competition algorithms

Feature	Trigger	Response/intervention	Comments
Blanked flutter search (MDT)	Monitors for eight consecutive AA intervals that are less than twice the total atrial blanking period (SAV + PVAB) and where one half of the AA interval is less than the detect rate interval	Extend PVARP and the VAI to uncover any blanked AS events. If AA interval is shorter than the detect rate interval, 2 : 1 sensing of an atrial tachyarrhythmia is assumed	Once rapid consecutive A–A intervals or 2 : 1 blanking of AS events are detected, the detect duration delay timer is started. Mode switch will occur once this timer expires
2 : 1 Lock-in protection algorithm (BTK) (Figure 6.36)	Evaluates VAIs when rate >100 bpm, and after eight beats with a rate of >100 bpm	Extends AV delay to uncover intrinsic AS events hidden previously by atrial blanking	Immediately mode switches (without meeting the X/Z out of eight criterion) to terminate the 2 : 1 lock-in
Atrial protection interval (API) (SJM)	High atrial pacing rates	Provides a 125-ms alert period at the end of PVARP and prior to next atrial pacing (non-competitive atrial pacing window) at high atrial pacing rates. If an intrinsic P wave is sensed during this 125-ms period, atrial pacing is inhibited	Non-programmable feature, only available in dual-chamber pacing modes
Atrial flutter response (AFR) (GDT, BS) (Figure 6.37)	AS event detected inside PVARP	Initiates a programmable AFR window (130–230 bpm), which is subsequently reset or restarted if another AS event is noted. Paced atrial events scheduled inside an AFR window will be delayed until the AFR window has expired	If there are fewer than 50 ms remaining before ventricular pacing (LRL expires), atrial pacing is inhibited for the cycle. Ventricular pace is not affected by AFR and will take place as scheduled by LRL or SIR. Available in DDD(R) and DDI(R) modes
Non-competitive atrial pacing (NCAP) (MDT) (Figure 6.38)	AS event that occurs within PVARP	Initiates programmable NCAP interval (200–400 ms, 50-ms increments), which will delay atrial pacing until NCAP ends, even if programmed VAI expires. Another NCAP will be initiated if a second AS event occurs during NCAP interval	NCAP can result in subsequent shortening of AV interval to avoid violation of the LRL or SIR (minimum paced AVI allowed is 30 ms)

AS, atrial sensed; BS, Boston Scientific; BTK, Biotronik; MDT, Medtronic; SJM, St. Jude Medical; SAV, sensed AV delay; SIR, sensor-indicated rate; for other acronyms, see Table 6.3.

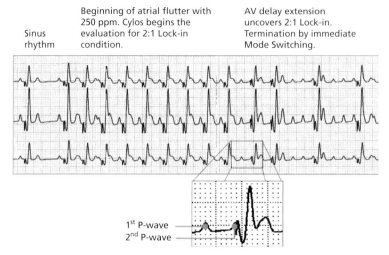

Sinus rhythm

Beginning of atrial flutter with 250 ppm. Cylos begins the evaluation for 2:1 Lock-in condition.

AV delay extension uncovers 2:1 Lock-in. Termination by immediate Mode Switching.

1st P-wave
2nd P-wave

Figure 6.36 2 : 1 Lock-in protection algorithm. Initial tracking of an atrial flutter with a 2 : 1 P-synchronous ventricular pacing occurs since every other P wave (after ventricular pacing) falls within a post-ventricular atrial blanking period (PVAB) and is not included in the mode switch counter. After eight beats of atrial rates above 100 bpm, this algorithm extends atrioventricular (AV) delay, allowing sensing of the second P wave previously "hiding" within the PVAB. Source: *Cylos Pacemaker Feature Handbook*. Lake Oswego, OR: Biotronik. Reproduced with permission of Biotronik.

2 : 1 Lock-in protection algorithm

This 2 : 1 lock-in protection algorithm (Biotronik) prevents the failure to mode switch due to the sensing of every other atrial flutter wave, the so-called "2 : 1 lock-in" response. After eight beats with a rate of greater than 100 bpm, the AV delay is extended to uncover intrinsic atrial events hidden previously within the PVAB (Figure 6.36).

Atrial flutter response

This feature initiates a programmable atrial flutter response (AFR, Boston Scientific) window or interval (130–230 bpm, 10-bpm increments) if an atrial-sensed event is detected inside the PVARP. If a second atrial-sensed event is detected within the AFR interval, this interval will be reset and the atrial-sensed event will not be tracked as it is considered refractory (Figure 6.37). High-rate atrial sensing may continuously retrigger the AFR window, effectively resulting in mode switch.

Non-competitive atrial pacing

Non-competitive atrial pacing (NCAP, Medtronic) allows delay in atrial pacing if this is scheduled to be delivered within a given interval after an atrial-sensed event (Figure 6.38). If an atrial-sensed event occurs within the PVARP (which will not terminate

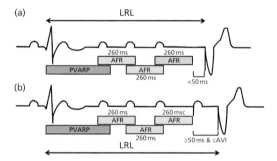

(a)

LRL

260 ms AFR
260 ms AFR
PVARP
AFR
260 ms
<50 ms

(b)

260 ms AFR
260 msc AFR
PVARP
AFR
260 ms
≥50 ms & ≤AVI
LRL

Figure 6.37 Atrial flutter response (AFR). Atrial detection inside the post-ventricular atrial refractory period (PVARP) starts a 260-ms AFR interval, which is reset if another atrial event is detected within the AFR window. (a) A ventricular pace (VP) stimulus will take place on the scheduled lower rate limit (LRL) interval or sensor-indicated rate. (b) An atrial pace will only occur if the AFR window expires at least 50 ms before the scheduled VP. This prevents competitive pacing. Source: *Altrua 20 and Altrua 40 Multiprogrammable Pacemakers*. St Paul, MN: Boston Scientific Corporation. Reproduced with permission of Boston Scientific.

the VAI or reset timing cycles), a programmed NCAP interval will begin. Atrial pacing will not occur even if the programmed VAI ends; it will be delayed until the NCAP interval expires. If a second atrial refractory-sensed event occurs during the NCAP interval, a new NCAP interval will be initiated. Thus, short coupling atrial pacing (within the

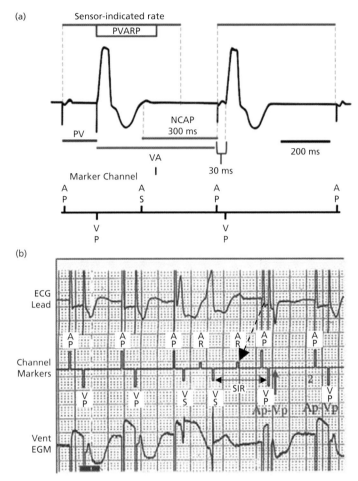

Figure 6.38 Non-competitive atrial pacing (NCAP). (a) A 300-ms NCAP window is initiated after an atrial-sensed (AS) event occurs within the post-ventricular atrial refractory period (PVARP). Even though the sensor-indicated rate (SIR) has expired, atrial pacing will not occur until the NCAP window is completed and then only if at least a 30-ms atrioventricular (AV) interval is allowed between atrial and ventricular pacing (AP, VP). (b) Premature ventricular contraction (VS) results in retrograde VA conduction. The second retrograde P wave (dashed arrow) labeled "AR" is not tracked with VP as it was sensed during the PVARP (it does not initiate an AV interval). The scheduled AP event is delayed by 300 ms (until the NCAP interval expires), resulting in a foreshortening of the AV delay (60 ms) to avoid violating the SIR. Sources: (a) modified from *Adapta, Sensia, Versa Pacemaker Reference Guide*. St Paul, MN: Medtronic, Inc. Reproduced with permission of Medtronic, Inc. (b) Courtesy of S. Serge Barold, MD.

atrial vulnerable period) is prevented, avoiding potential induction of atrial tachyarrhythmias. However, this can result in subsequent shortening of the AVI to avoid violation of the LRL or SIR (minimum allowed paced AVI is 30 ms). This algorithm becomes more important with enabled rate modulation (DDDR) as the SIR may indicate pacing at faster rates. NCAP is applicable when the device is operating in the DDDR or DDD mode [16].

Atrial protection interval

Atrial protection interval (API, St. Jude Medical) is a feature to minimize competitive atrial pacing. This feature provides a 125-ms alert period at the end of the PVARP (non-competitive atrial pacing window) and prior to the next atrial pacing event to allow an intrinsic P wave to be sensed, which subsequently will inhibit atrial pacing during high atrial pacing rates [9].

Despite these algorithms, some patients may present with inappropriate sensing of atrial arrhythmias and atrial sense/pace competition. In this situation, reprogramming bradycardia parameters or adding dynamic PVARP can assist in avoiding induction of atrial arrhythmias due to short coupled atrial pacing. For example, pacing parameters providing a 300-ms interval between the end of the ARP and the next scheduled atrial pace will prevent atrial sense/pace competition. This can be accomplished by lowering the upper sensor rate (USR), shortening the paced AVI, and shortening the PVARP to force a 300-ms interval with no atrial pacing after the PVARP. However, shortening the PVARP can potentially result in PMT (see section Pacemaker-mediated tachycardia). On the other hand, dynamic PVARP allows a longer PVARP at the LRL, and a shorter PVARP at a faster intrinsic rate or SIR (see Figure 6.13). This promotes AV synchrony and prevents atrial pacing if an atrial event is sensed early in the VAI.

Algorithms to prevent atrial fibrillation

Numerous atrial fibrillation (AF) prevention algorithms have been developed based on the concept that atrial pacing may decrease the occurrence of atrial premature beats that will trigger AF [17]. These algorithms include pace conditioning/rate soothing (Figure 6.39), PAC suppression, post-PAC response, post-exercise response, and post-AF response. The rationale, triggers, and intervention of each of these algorithms are described in Table 6.9. Overall, they are designed to promote atrial pacing above the sinus rate (shortening VA or AA interval) after a PAC, exercise, atrial tachyarrhythmia (mode switch), and/or even a sinus beat.

These algorithms are utilized in some commercially available pacemakers. Unfortunately, contradictory data exist with regard to the efficacy of these algorithms to prevent recurrent AF [17–20]. For instance, the Atrial Dynamic Overdrive Pacing Trial (ADOPT) [18] demonstrated that AF suppression (rate smoothing) decreased symptomatic AF burden in patients with sick sinus syndrome and AF. However, the AT500 verification study [21] (atrial rate stabilization, atrial preference pacing, and post-mode switch overdrive pacing plus termination algorithms), the Atrial Therapy Efficacy and Safety Trial [22] (ATTEST, AT500 pacemaker), and the Atrial Septal Pacing Efficacy Clinical Trial (ASPECT) [23] did not demonstrate improvement in median AF frequency or in overall AF burden. Most recently, the Study for Atrial Fibrillation Reduction (SAFARI) [24] demonstrated that all these prevention pacing therapies (Table 6.9) are safe and effective in reducing AF burden, particularly in subjects with an AF burden of greater than 6%.

Algorithms to minimize right ventricular pacing

Over the past few years, several algorithms (Table 6.10) have been developed and refined in order to avoid deleterious effects of chronic RV pacing, such as increase in heart failure, impair-

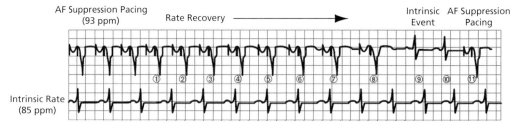

Figure 6.39 Atrial fibrillation (AF) suppression algorithm. The intrinsic heart rate is 85 bpm with enabled AF suppression (rate 93 bpm). Paced beat 1 (representing the final cycle of overdrive pacing) marks the initiation of rate recovery of this algorithm, adding 12 ms to each cycle through the eighth cycle. The interval is extended to 729 ms (83 bpm) and a P wave (at 85 bpm) is detected (beat 9). This is followed by another P wave in the tenth cycle (the second of two intrinsic events). This signals the device to resume AF suppression pacing in the 11th cycle. Source: *Bradycardia Devices: Help Manual*. Sylmar, CA: St. Jude Medical, Inc. Reproduced with permission of St. Jude Medical, Inc.

Table 6.9 Algorithms to prevent atrial fibrillation

Algorithm	Commercial name	Trigger/rationale	Response/intervention	Comments
Pace conditioning	Dynamic atrial overdrive (SJM), atrial preference pacing (GDT, BTK, MDT)	Trigger: sinus-sensed beat. Attempts to decrease likelihood of PAC by increasing heart rate upon PAC detection	Limited increase in atrial pacing rate by 15 bpm above physiological sinus rate to resume atrial pacing	Results in significant percentage of atrial pacing
Rate soothing	AF suppression (SJM) (Figure 6.39)	Trigger: 1–2 sinus-sensed beats. Prevent atrial arrhythmias by atrial overdrive pacing just above pacing rate	Increase atrial pacing at rate by 3 bpm and slowly decrease pacing rate until sinus rhythm is sensed or LRL is reached	Similar to pace conditioning but without large (15 bpm) pacing rate increase
PAC suppression	ProACT (GDT)	Trigger: atrial event classified as PAC. Decrease possibility of PAC by increasing heart rate upon PAC detection	Pacing rate is increased by 15 bpm for a certain duration	
Post-PAC response	Atrial rate stabilization (MDT)	Trigger: beat classified as PAC. Avoid pauses after PAC	First beat after PAC is delivered at average cycle length of PAC rate and physiological rate, and subsequent beat is delivered at physiological rate	Beneficial if significant pauses precede AF initiation
Post-exercise response		Trigger: post-exercise heart rate drop. Avoids abrupt bradycardia following exercise	Post-exercise pacing rate slowly increases to 90% of physiological rate. If heart rate decreases abruptly after exercise, pacing rate is increased at post-exercise pacing rate	Useful in vagal- and exercise-induced AF
Post-AF response	Post-mode switch overdrive pacing (MDT)	Trigger: termination of preceding atrial tachyarrhythmia	Programmable high rate atrial pacing rate (70–100 bpm) with gradual decline until sinus rhythm is sensed or LRL is reached	Potential benefit in patients with immediate recurrence of AF

AF, atrial fibrillation; BS, Boston Scientific; BTK, Biotronik; GDT, Guidant; SJM, St. Jude Medical; PAC, premature atrial contraction; for other acronyms, see Table 6.3.

Table 6.10 Algorithms to minimize ventricular pacing

Algorithm	Initial mode	Trigger	Intervention	Return to initial pacing settings	Advantage/disadvantage/notes
Search AV hysteresis (GDT/BS) (Figure 6.40a)	DDD(R)	VS event after AVI prolongs to programmable AVI hysteresis (extension) for up to eight consecutive cycles. Search is initiated after a programmable number (32–1024) of consecutive paced cycles (VP only)	Remains in DDD(R). AVI hysteresis as long as intrinsic R wave is sensed	AVI hysteresis (extension) remains in effect until a *single* VP occurs during the AVI extension period	*Advantages:* Does not allow blocked P waves *Disadvantages:* AVI extension is limited by TARP. P-synchronous VP may occur with a very long AVI. Fusion of VP and intrinsic R may occur at the end of AVI extension
Search AV+ (GDT/BS)	DDD(R)	Same as Search AV hysteresis. Search of intrinsic R wave initiates after a programmable number of both *paced and sensed* cycles (VS and VP)	Remains in DDD(R). Same as Search AV hysteresis	AVI extension remains in effect until a 2 of 10 VP occurs during the AVI extension period	*Advantages:* Same as search AV hysteresis. Allows for a more frequent search and more time with AVI extension than Search AV hysteresis *Disadvantages:* Same as Search AV hysteresis
AV hysteresis (BTK)	DDD(R)	AVI extends to a programmable AVI hysteresis delay for two scan cycles every 59 cycles with preset AVI; trigger criteria are met if three of the previous four scan sequences reveal intrinsic conduction	AVI hysteresis delay (extension) remains as long as intrinsic R wave is sensed	Five VP during the previous eight cardiac cycles will switch to initial preset AVI	*Advantages:* Same as Search AV+ *Disadvantages:* Same as Search AV hysteresis
Ventricular intrinsic preference (VIP) (SJM) (Figure 6.40b)	DDD(R)	AVI will be periodically extended (search interval) to an additional programmable delta (VIP extension) for a programmed number of cycles searching for VS event	AVI + delta (VIP extension) persists as long as VS is sensed. Remains in DDD(R)	If no intrinsic AV conduction is noted after AVI + delta, AV pacing will reset to initial preset AVI	*Advantages:* Same as Search AV hysteresis *Disadvantages:* Same as Search AV hysteresis

Feature	Mode	Trigger criteria	Switch behavior	Assessment	Advantages/Disadvantages
Managed ventricular pacing (MVP) (MDT) (Figure 6.41a)	AAI(R)	Persistent loss of AV conduction (two of four recent non-refractory AA intervals without an R event or blocked P wave)	Back-up P-synchronous VP at 80 ms is delivered if AA interval occurs without VS event. Switches to DDD(R) once trigger criteria are met	Periodic one-cycle assessment of AV conduction. First one occurs after 1 min, and subsequently at progressively longer intervals (2, 4, 8... min) up to 16 h, and then occur every 16 h thereafter. AAI mode is restored when intrinsic AV conduction is noted	*Advantages*: Regardless of PR interval, intrinsic conduction is allowed after AP or AS. Allows physiological AV nodal Wenckebach. *Disadvantages*: Do not allow 2 : 1 AV block
AAISafeR2 (Sorin) (Figure 6.41b)	AAI(R)	1 Two consecutive blocked Ps 2 >3 blocked out of 12 AP/AS 3 Pause > programmed duration (2–4 s) 4 >6 abnormal PR/AR intervals > programmed duration (PR >350 ms and AR >450 ms)	Switches to DDD(R) once trigger criteria are met		*Advantages*: Same as MVP. Most aggressive algorithm to allow and maintain intrinsic conduction. Programmability, different triggers for mode switch. Allows 2 : 1 AV block to persist. *Disadvantages*: Potential for symptomatic 2 : 1 AV block
RythmIQ (BS) (Figure 6.41c)	AAI and back-up VVI 15 bpm slower than LRL (lowest and fastest 30 and 60 bpm)	Three slow ventricular beats of 11 in rolling window. Slow beat is defined as: 1 Ventricular paced beat 2 VS at least 150 ms slower than AAI LRL or SIR	Switches to DDD(R) once trigger criteria are met	AV Search+ (see above) is activated at programmed settings and if AVI extension continues for at least 25 cardiac cycles, and fewer than two of the last 10 cycles are VP, then the device automatically switches the pacing mode back to AAI(R) with VVI back-up	*Advantages*: Regardless of PR interval, intrinsic conduction is allowed after AP or AS. Does not require drop in ventricular beat. *Disadvantages*: Pacemaker syndrome (AV dyssynchrony) while on AAI/back-up VVI. Frequent PVCs can easily trigger switch to DDD(R)

AP, atrial-paced event; AS, atrial-sensed event; AV, atrioventricular; AVI, AV interval; BS, Boston Scientific; BTK, Biotronik; GDT, Guidant; MVP, managed ventricular pacing; PVC, premature ventricular contraction; SIR, sensor-indicated rate; SJM, St. Jude Medical; VIP, ventricular intrinsic preference; VP, ventricular-paced event; VS, ventricular-sensed event; for other acronyms, see Table 6.3.

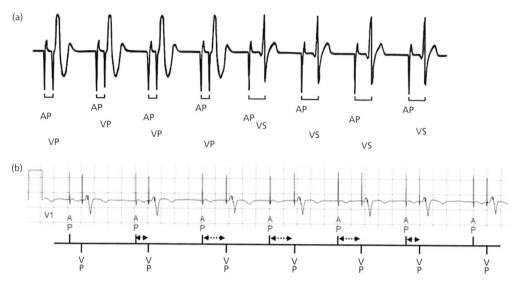

Figure 6.40 Algorithms to promote intrinsic atrioventricular (AV) conduction: Part I. (a) AV hysteresis: intrinsic R waves are sensed after the AV interval (AVI) is lengthened (programmable AV extension) allowing intrinsic AV conduction. (b) Ventricular intrinsic preference (VIP): paced AVI (200 ms) is extended to programmable delta for three beats (dashed arrows, AVI + delta = 200 + 140); however, no intrinsic R wave is sensed at extended AVI (340 ms) and sequential AV pacing resumes with the initial preset AVI. Source: (a) adapted from *Insignia I Ultra System Guide, models 1190/1290*. St Paul, MN: Guidant Corporation, 2006. Reproduced with permission of Boston Scientific.

ment of functional status, left ventricular (LV) dilation, and deterioration of LV systolic function [4]. Patients with underlying LV dysfunction appear to have the greatest hemodynamic deterioration with RV pacing. These algorithms clearly can be beneficial in patients with intact AV conduction. Some of the initial algorithms minimize pacing by extending the AVI by a programmed additional *delta* interval (AV hysteresis, Search AV+, VIP). These algorithms are frequently limited to a maximum AVI extension (limited by TARP) and may result in some ventricular pacing and fusion with intrinsic conduction. The most recent algorithms (Managed ventricular pacing, SafeAAIR [2], and RhythmIQ) use a single atrial pacing mode (AAI/AAIR) that switches to a dual-chamber pacing mode in the event of transient AV block (second-degree or high-degree AV block) (Figures 6.40 and 6.41).

These algorithms have different triggers, interventions, advantages, and disadvantages (Table 6.10), and some of them have been shown to result in a significant decrease in ventricular pacing [25,26]. These algorithms should be used with caution, especially in patients with AV block or when prolonged pause may increase the risk of ventricular arrhythmias.

Pacemaker-mediated tachycardia

Pacemaker-mediated tachycardia, commonly known as endless-loop tachycardia, is seen in patients with repetitive retrograde VA conduction. PMT can *only* occur in DDD or VDD pacing modes (P-synchronous ventricular pacing) and has also been referred to as pacemaker circus movement tachycardia, repetitive reentrant pacemaker VA synchrony, reentrant VA pacemaker tachycardia, or antidromic reentrant dual-chamber pacemaker tachycardia [27].

PMT is a "reentrant" arrhythmia that initiates only in those patients with intact VA conduction, where the device senses a retrograde P wave (after the PVARP expires) regardless of the trigger. Thus, a retrograde P wave initiating PMT can be triggered by (i) PVC; (ii) failure of atrial capture during AV sequential pacing (Figure 6.42); and (iii) at the end of ventricular threshold testing in VVI mode, where the device switches immediately to DDD pacing mode sensing retrograde P wave (Figure 6.43).

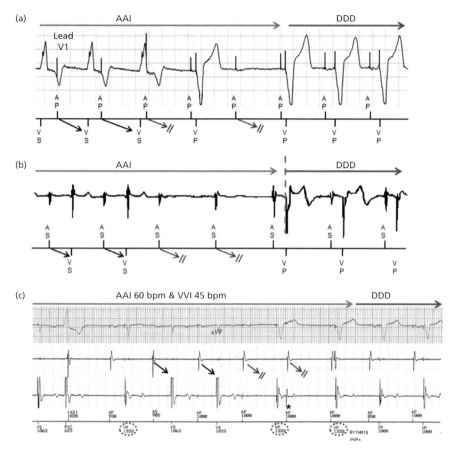

Figure 6.41 Algorithms to promote intrinsic atrioventricular (AV) conduction: Part II. (a) Managed ventricular pacing (MVP): AAI switches to DDD pacing mode due to AV nodal Wenckebach (Mobitz I AV block) after two of four P waves do not demonstrate intrinsic AV conduction. Back-up P-synchronous ventricular pacing is delivered after transient loss of AV conduction with an AVI of 80 ms. (b) Sorin SafeR: AAI changes to DDD mode after two consecutive P waves lack intrinsic AV conduction (high-degree AV block). (c) RythmIQ: simultaneous AAI 60 bpm and VVI 45 bpm (15 bpm below the AAI lower rate limit). The criterion of three slow ventricular beats (dashed ovals: event markers) in an 11 rolling window is met, changing to a DDD pacing mode at 60 bpm. A premature ventricular contraction (PVC, event marker) resets AA timing, resulting in atrial pacing (AP) 1000 ms after the PVC (PVC–AP interval of 1000 ms). Note that PVC also resets the VV interval and ventricular pacing (VP: slow ventricular beat) occurs at the programmed VVI 45 bpm (1333 ms) even though intrinsic AV conduction is noted (fusion beat) on the aVF lead. Source: modified from Huizar JF, Kaszala K, Ellenbogen KA. Cardiac pacing modes and terminology. In: Sakena S, Camm AJ, eds. *Electrophysiological Disorders of the Heart*, 2nd edn. Philadelphia, PA: Elsevier Saunders, 2012: 441–456. Reproduced with permission of Elsevier.

Once a retrograde P wave is sensed, AVI is initiated. Upon completion of the AVI and MTR interval, ventricular pacing is delivered (anterograde limb) and this can once again result in VA conduction (retrograde limb), with retrograde P wave perpetuating this reentry. Once established, this reentrant mechanism continues until it is interrupted or until the retrograde limb of the circuit is exhausted. The ventricular pacing rate cannot violate the programmed MTR or URL; thus, PMT often occurs at the MTR. The cycle length of the PMT is the sum of the VA conduction time and the programmed sensed AV delay. If the VA conduction time is sufficiently long, PMT could occur below the MTR. PMT may be asymptomatic if the programmed MTR is low; however, symptoms

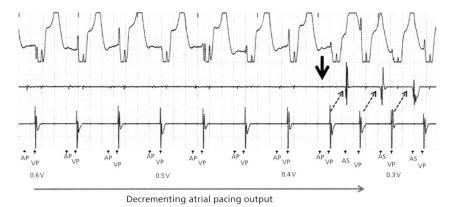

Decrementing atrial pacing output

Figure 6.42 Pacemaker-mediated tachycardia (PMT) initiated during an atrial threshold test in DDD pacing mode. This test induced PMT due to loss of atrial capture (solid arrow) followed by ventricular pacing with retrograde VA conduction (dashed arrows). Retrograde atrial signal outside the post-ventricular atrial refractory period (PVARP) [terminates the ventriculoatrial interval (VAI) and initiates an atrioventricular interval (AVI)] is tracked by ventricular pacing (maximum tracking rate 120 bpm), which will perpetuate itself as long as the retrograde atrial signal does not occur within the PVARP.

may be significant if the MTR is programmed relatively high.

Algorithms to prevent, identify, and terminate pacemaker-mediated tachycardia

Many mechanisms have been adopted to prevent, identify, and terminate PMT (Table 6.11). Among the early preventive algorithms is *PVARP extension after PVC*, since they are the most common triggers. Extension of the PVARP after a PVC prevents tracking of retrograde P wave (PMT initiation) as this will force it to fall within the PVARP. However, PMT could also initiate despite PVARP extension after a PVC, due to ineffective atrial pacing soon after retrograde P wave (during the ARP), followed by ventricular pacing with retrograde VA conduction, initiating PMT (Figure 6.43a).

Commonly, PMT is prevented by programming the PVARP longer than VA conduction during ventricular pacing, as it will no longer track P waves falling within the PVARP. Nevertheless, VA conduction can change based on ventricular rate (decremental conduction), as well as vagal and adrenergic tone. Thus, the PVARP should be programmed based on VA conduction at the MTR in order to assess the longest VA conduction time.

Paradoxically, a similar form of VA dyssynchrony (distinct from PMT) may occur when PVARP is significantly extended. After a PVC with retrograde P wave (VA conduction), a long PVARP avoids initiation of PMT. Since resetting of the VAI does not occur, ineffective or non-capture atrial pacing (due to atrial refractoriness) is followed by ventricular pacing (AV sequential pacing) and retrograde atrial conduction. Thus, repetitive atrial pacing during refractoriness followed by ventricular pacing will perpetuate this cycle [27]. This phenomenon is called repetitive non-reentrant VA synchrony (RNRVAS), also known as AV desynchronization arrhythmia or VA synchrony nonreentrant arrhythmia (Figure 6.43b,c).

The basic requirements, predisposing factors, and programing changes to prevent RNRVAS are detailed in Table 6.12 [28]. Under certain circumstances, RNRVAS may convert spontaneously to PMT and vice versa. As noted in Table 6.12, RNRVAS is more common with high LRL or rate-modulated pacing mode (DDDR) since the sensor-driven increase in VAI will increase the probability of a non-captured atrial-paced event allowing retrograde VA conduction after ventricular pacing. PVARP shortening could prevent RNRVAS at the expense of an increasing probability of PMT. Thus, decreasing sensor-driven response or MSR and shortening the AVI could decrease the probability of recurrence of this undesired rhythm and yet still prevent PMT. The main differences between PMT and RNRVAS are summarized in Table 6.13.

(a)

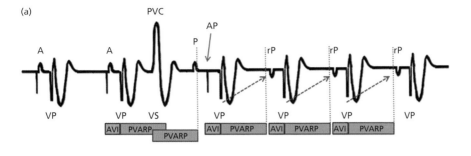

(b)

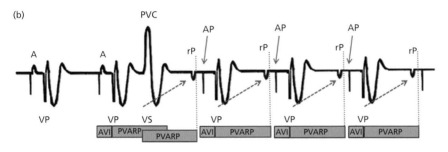

(c)

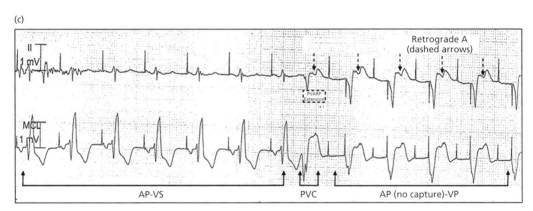

Figure 6.43 (a) Paradoxical mechanism of pacemaker-mediated tachycardia (PMT) initiation by an inappropriately long post-ventricular atrial refractory period (PVARP). Early premature ventricular contraction (PVC) reinitiates PVARP and VA interval (VAI). A sinus P wave falls within the PVARP (without resetting VAI), followed by ineffective atrial pacing (AP) due to atrial refractoriness. Ventricular pacing (VP) occurs after the atrioventricular interval (AVI) is completed, causing a retrograde P wave (rP) due to unopposed ventriculoatrial (VA) conduction (dashed red arrows) with subsequent initiation of PMT. (b) Repetitive non-reentrant VA synchrony. To avoid PMT, a long PVARP is programmed. An rP after an early PVC falls within the PVARP, followed by an ineffective AP (after the VAI is completed), initiating an AVI. VP occurs after completion of the AVI, and finds unopposed VA conduction (retrograde P wave), falling again within the PVARP, causing repetitive ineffective AP and VP with VA conduction. (c) Representative case of repetitive non-reentrant VA synchrony (RNRVAS) documented in telemetry. Source: Sharma *et al.* [28]. Reproduced with permission of Elsevier.

While various algorithms are available to prevent, diagnose and terminate PMT (Table 6.11), only Abbott devices (previously St. Jude Medical) frequently store RNRVAS mislabeled as an atrial high rate episode. The simplest PMT algorithm assumes that atrial-sensed ventricular pacing occurring close to MTR is a PMT and, after a preset number of cycles, either withholds ventricular pacing or extends the PVARP. Withholding ventricular pacing will terminate retrograde VA conduction, whereas extending the PVARP will render the retrograde P wave "refractory" and terminate

Table 6.11 Different algorithms for pacemaker-mediated tachycardia (PMT)

Algorithm	Trigger	Intervention	Prevent PMT	Diagnose and treat PMT
PVC response (BS, MDT, SJM, BTK)	"PVC" beat (R without a preceding P wave)	Programmed PVARP is extended immediately after sensed PVC beat	Yes	No
PMT termination (BS)	16 successive VP at MTR following AS events. VA interval stability: PMT is declared if all the 15 VA intervals are <32 ms longer or shorter than first VA interval	Extend PVARP to fixed 500 ms for one cardiac cycle to break PMT	No	Yes
PMT intervention (MDT)	Nine consecutive VP events of <400 ms that end with an AS event. On eighth consecutive VA interval, activity sensor is checked (assess exercise-related tachycardia); PMT is declared if SIR < pacing rate and intervention will occur	Forces a 400-ms PVARP extension after the ninth VP event	No	Yes
PMT protection (BTK)	Eight consecutive VP events in which atrial events lie within a programmed PMT VA criterion (default 350 ms). PMT is confirmed by stable VA interval after decreasing MTR by 10 bpm or shortening AVI to next programmable length by 10 bpm	PVARP extension by measured V–V interval plus 50 ms	No	Yes
PMT response (SJM) (Figure 6.44)	Eight consecutive VP–AS events above PMT detection rate. PMT is confirmed if VP–AS interval remains stable (within 16 ms of prior eight VP–AS intervals) despite shortening or increasing AVI by 31 ms if AS–VP interval is greater or shorter than 100 ms, respectively	Suspends VP event and delivers atrial pulse at 330 ms after detected retrograde P wave	No	Yes

AS, atrial-sensed event; AV, atrioventricular; AVI, AV interval; BS, Boston Scientific; BTK, Biotronik; GDT, Guidant; SJM, St. Jude Medical; PVC, premature ventricular contraction; SIR, sensor-indicated rate; VIP, ventricular intrinsic preference; VP, ventricular paced event; for other acronyms, see Table 6.3.

inappropriate tracking. Thus, true PMT will terminate after one of these interventions, whereas atrial arrhythmias will continue. A further refinement to these algorithms allows the clinician to select a PMT rate that is below the MTR, in an attempt to adjust for PMT at slower rates based on slow retrograde VA conduction. The limitation of these algorithms is that they are activated regardless of whether the rhythm is PMT or an intrinsic atrial rhythm with appropriate ventricular tracking. For a native atrial rhythm, repeated pauses are caused by the activation of the PMT termination algorithm, which may be symptomatic or could result in intermittent loss of tracking in biventricular devices.

More sophisticated algorithms attempt to confirm PMT before PMT intervention is deployed.

These algorithms suspect PMT if retrograde VAI is stable within a predetermined number of cycles. Furthermore, PMT is confirmed if stability of retrograde VA conduction is preserved despite changing AVI or decreasing MTR. If the mechanism is *not dependent* on the ventricular-paced event (atrial or sinus tachycardia), the VP interval (VA conduction) on the next cycle is either lengthened or shortened by the same degree by which the AVI was changed. If atrial arrhythmia is confirmed, the pacemaker will continue to track atrial-sensed events. If PMT is confirmed, the device will intervene by withholding ventricular pacing, followed by atrial pacing at 330 ms if no intrinsic P wave is sensed. Successful atrial capture breaks the cycle and prevents retrograde conduction after the next ventricular-paced complex.

Table 6.12 Predisposing factors and programming to avoid repetitive non-reentrant VA synchrony (RNRVAS)

Factors predisposing to RNRVAS
Minimum requirements
Dual-chamber devices with AV sequential pacing mode (DDD, DDI, DDDR, DDIR)
Retrograde VA conduction
Other factors
High pacing rate, e.g. SIR, high LRL, rate drop response, overdrive pacing algorithms (e.g. AOP algorithm SJM)
Long AV delay
Long PVARP
Programming changes to avoid RNRVAS
Key management
Lower pacing rate (e.g. LRL, SIR including reaction sensor time, activity sensor threshold, intervention rate of rate drop algorithms, disable overdrive pacing algorithms)
Shorten AV delays, disable search AV algorithm (VIP, Search AV+)
Extend NCAP (Medtronic)
MVP, AAI-SafeR, RythmIQ

SJM, St. Jude Medical; for definition of other acronyms, see Table 6.3.
Source: Sharma *et al.* [28]. Reproduced with permission of Elsevier.

This algorithm also prevents pauses occurring with some of the earlier generation PMT algorithms (Figure 6.44).

Biventricular pacing

Cardiac resynchronization therapy (CRT) has been shown to improve heart failure symptoms and LV function by restoring ventricular coordination (biventricular pacing) primarily in patients with wide QRS (>150 ms) and left bundle branch block [2,3]. In order to achieve this effect, biventricular pacing must be maintained and intrinsic conduction limited. In patients with chronic AF, the VVIR mode is frequently used. Although initial clinical trials utilized the VDDOV pacing mode, most patients in sinus rhythm are programmed to DDDOV or DDDRV pacing mode.

Timing cycles

Overall, the timing cycles for biventricular pacing are similar to those in dual-chamber pacemakers. However, timing cycles in CRT can have numerous potential variations based on LV sensing (not all companies use LV sensing for timing purposes) [29]. Most of contemporary CRT devices use RV sensing for timing cycles, including base-rate behavior (Figure 6.45). One important distinction

Table 6.13 Main differences between pacemaker-mediated tachycardia (PMT) and repetitive non-reentrant VA synchrony (RNRVAS)

Feature	RNRVAS	PMT
Retrograde P wave	Occurs within PVARP	Occurs outside PVARP
Promoted by	Long PVARP Long AV delay Features that allow rapid AV sequential pacing: rate drop response, rate-adaptive response, AOP algorithm	Short PVARP
Ventricular pacing (pacing mode)	AV sequential pacing (DDD, DDDR, DDI, DDIR)	P-synchronous ventricular pacing (DDD, DDDR)
Detection	No algorithms are developed to prevent or identify these events. Some are stored as atrial high-rate episodes in SJM devices	Special algorithms are present in all manufacturers to prevent and recognize these events
Treatment	Algorithms are non-existent to terminate RNRVAS. Recommend to (i) decrease LRL or disable features that allow rapid AV sequential pacing, and (ii) shorten AV delay, both of which will result in extension of VA interval	Automatic extension of PVARP or withhold a single P-synchronous VP

SJM, St. Jude Medical; for definition of other acronyms, see Table 6.3.
Source: Sharma *et al.* [28]. Reproduced with permission of Elsevier.

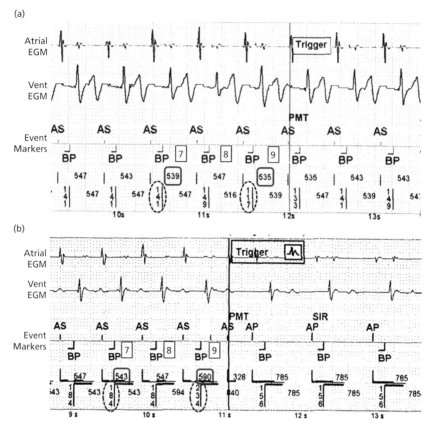

Figure 6.44 Pacemaker-mediated tachycardia (PMT) algorithm in a cardiac resynchronization therapy (CRT) device. (a) PMT response algorithm suspects PMT after eight consecutive VP–AS events. PMT is excluded since the ventriculoatrial interval (VAI) in beat 9 (VAI or BP–AS interval, 535 – 117 = 418 ms) changes more than 16 ms when compared to beat 7 (VAI, 539 – 141 = 398 ms) after decreasing the atrioventricular interval (AVI) from 141 to 117 ms (dashed oval). Thus, P-synchronous pacing continues as atrial arrhythmia was confirmed. (b) PMT is confirmed since the VAI (BP–AS interval) remains stable (<16 ms) between beat 9 (VAI, 590 – 234 = 356 ms) and beat 7 (VAI 547 – 184 = 363 ms) despite increasing AVI from 184 to 234 ms. PMT is terminated after ventricular pacing (VP) is withheld, restoring AV synchrony with atrial pacing (AP) 330 ms after the last atrial-sensed event (AS). Source: St. Jude Medical, Inc. Reproduced with permission of St. Jude Medical, Inc.

of CRT devices is the presence of two distinct PAVBs in some devices, one in the RV-sensing channel (PAVB$_{RV}$; similar to dual-chamber pacemakers) and one in the LV-sensing channel (PAVB$_{LV}$), in order to prevent inappropriate inhibition of LV pacing due to far-field atrial pace oversensing (Figure 6.46). The PVAB on CRT devices will also inhibit atrial sensing after an RV- or LV-paced event, which can be particularly important if a significant interventricular delay is programmed between LV and RV pacing (see section Interventricular delay or left ventricular offset).

It is particularly important to understand some unique timing cycles present in CRT devices (see Table 6.3) as these optimize appropriate biventricular pacing.

Left ventricular refractory period

Left ventricular refractory period (LVRP) is a programmable interval in which an LV-sensed event after an LV-paced (LVP) or LV-sensed (LVS) event will not affect or reset timing cycles. This period is intended to prevent oversensing of QRS or T wave following a sensed or paced event, preventing inappropriate loss of CRT (seen more commonly with unipolar LV leads). A long LVRP shortens the LV-sensing window that could affect timing cycles.

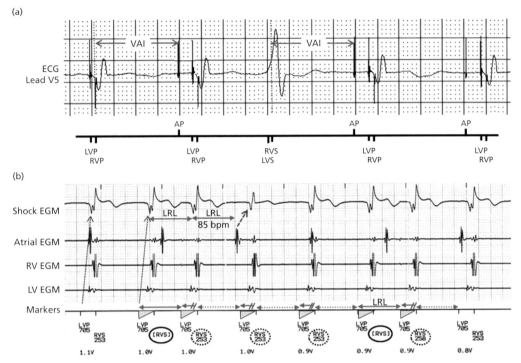

Figure 6.45 Role of right ventricular (RV) sensing for cardiac resynchronization therapy (CRT) timing cycles. (a) The device is programmed with an interventricular delay of 40 ms [left ventricular pacing (LVP) precedes RV pacing (RVP) by 40 ms]. During a premature ventricular contraction (LVS–RVS), the pacemaker uses RV sensing (RVS) as its reference to initiate a ventriculoatrial interval (VAI) even though this extrasystole was originated from the left ventricle (LVS occurs prior to RVS). (b) Intermittent RV sensing beyond the RV refractory period (RVRP) causes resetting of the lower rate limit (LRL) with subsequent variability on LV pacing rate during LV threshold testing. Arrows on left side of the panel demonstrate LV capture after LVP. Despite LV threshold testing programmed with an LRL of 85 bpm (VVI 795 ms), variability on LV pacing rate (RR interval 958 and 705 ms or 63 and 85 bpm, respectively) is noted due to intermittent sensing of right ventricle (RVS) within (solid circles) and beyond (dotted circles) the RVRP (designated by blue triangles), resetting the LRL (bold dashed arrow, RR 958 ms). Note that RV sensing occurs way beyond RVRP due to a significant latency (160 ms) between the LVP stimulus and deflection of QRS in the shock ECG, which could be explained by a scar.

Left ventricular protection period

Even though biventricular pacing should be delivered continuously to maximize CRT benefits, there are some circumstances in which it is appropriate to inhibit therapy (e.g. left-sided PVCs). The left ventricular protection period (LVPP) prevents the pulse generator from inadvertently delivering a pacing stimulus during the LV vulnerable period after an LVS event, such as when a left-sided PVC occurs. However, if the LVPP inhibits LV pacing, the device will still deliver RV pacing. Proper programming of this feature will help maximize CRT delivery while reducing the risk of accelerating the patient's rhythm to a ventricular tachyarrhythmia. However, programming a long LVPP will reduce the MTR and inhibit biventricular pacing at higher rates.

Interventricular delay or left ventricular offset

Nowadays, biventricular pacemakers allow programming of different timing between the RV- and LV-paced events, referred to as interventricular delay or LV offset (RV–LV delay). For the most part, RV–LV delay can be programmed positive, negative, or zero in an attempt to optimize biventricular pacing and maximize clinical response. However, programming an interventricular delay can affect the programmed AVI depending on the CRT manufacturer. For instance, a programmed sensed or

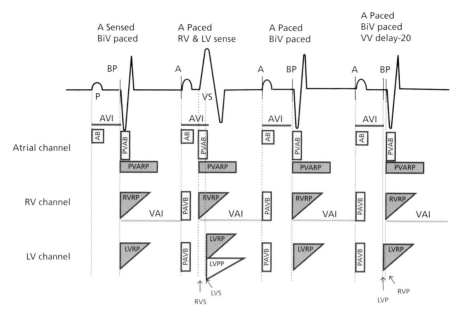

Figure 6.46 Blanking (red) and refractory (blue) periods in a biventricular pacemaker. The different blanking and refractory periods are demonstrated for different possible scenarios: atrial sense–BiV paced, atrial paced–RV&LV sensed, atrial paced–BiV paced, and atrial paced–BiV paced with LV offset of –20 ms. A, atrial; AB, atrial blanking; AVI, atrioventricular interval; BiV, biventricular; LVRP, left ventricular refractory period; LVP, LV-paced event; LVPP, LV protection period; LVS, LV-sensed event; PAVB, post-atrial ventricular blanking period; PVAB, post-ventricular atrial blanking period; PVARP, post-ventricular atrial refractory period; RVP, RV-paced event; RVRP, right ventricular refractory period; RVS, RV-sensed event; VAI, ventriculoatrial interval; VV delay, interventricular delay.

paced AVI of 180 ms and 160 ms, respectively, will demonstrate a true AVI of 140 ms and 120 ms if LV pacing is programmed to occur 40 ms earlier than RV pacing (LV offset –40 ms; Figure 6.47).

Most contemporary biventricular pacemaker models are available with the IS4 header to accept a quadripolar LV lead. This allows not only modification of pacing location in order to minimize phrenic nerve stimulation or optimize capture, but has also allowed for multisite or multipoint pacing within the LV lead. That has expanded the programming options of the interventricular delay as they allow for separate pacing timing of the RV and two LV sites. Multipoint pacing in the left ventricle has required the introduction of atrial blanking after LV1 or LV2 pacing to prevent far-field R-wave oversensing. Any events falling within this multipoint PVAB will not reset atrial timing, be used in SVT discriminators, or be used for the mode switch counter.

Loss of biventricular pacing

There are a number of circumstances that may cause loss of biventricular pacing (inhibition or fusion), with the possible negative hemodynamic consequences. Fusion of biventricular pacing with intrinsic conduction can be easily overlooked if we only depend on device interrogation, since the counters may show a high biventricular pacing percentage. Thus, true biventricular pacing capture may need to be confirmed by a 12-lead ECG or Holter monitor [30].

Common examples of loss of biventricular pacing include (i) rapid sinus or atrial rates above the MTR; (ii) short and dynamic PR intervals; (iii) PACs; (iv) frequent PVCs; (v) AF with ventricular response above the LRL or SIR; and (vi) setting inadequate pacing output. Fortunately, several device features and alternatives are available to assist in improving biventricular pacing.

Rapid sinus or atrial rates above the MTR

If an atrial rhythm including sinus tachycardia occurs above the MTR, biventricular pacing will not occur even with a short programmed AVI. Furthermore, Wenckebach-pacemaker behavior

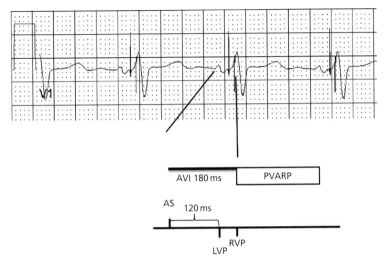

Figure 6.47 Left ventricular (LV) offset affecting atrioventricular interval (AVI) (Boston Scientific Corporation). Cardiac resynchronization therapy (CRT) has a programmed paced and sensed AV interval of 180 ms and 160 ms, respectively, with an LV offset of –40 ms. While right ventricular (RV) pacing will occur at a programmed AVI, LV pacing will occur at 140 and 120 ms after a paced or sensed P wave, respectively. AS, atrial-sensed event; AVI, AV interval; LVP, LV-paced event; PVARP, post-ventricular atrial refractory period; RVP, RV-paced event.

will not be seen unless the patient is pacemaker dependent. In this circumstance, it is important to consider reprogramming the MTR (if appropriate) or to treat the atrial dysrhythmia in order to allow resumption of biventricular pacing.

Short and dynamic PR intervals

The basic timing cycle for biventricular pacing is based on RV-based timing with a sensed or paced ventricular event initiating a VAI (Figures 6.45 and 6.46). The AVI must be sufficiently short to result in constant ventricular capture rather than intrinsic conduction. AV hysteresis (see section Atrioventricular interval hysteresis) may be used to promote ventricular capture in biventricular pacing. Furthermore, a rate-adaptive or dynamic AVI may be programmed in order to decrease the AVI during exercise or elevated heart rates. Finally, a feature called *ventricular-sensed response* or *biventricular trigger* allows LV pacing immediately after an intrinsic conduction or RV-sensed event occurs. This feature promotes synchronized RV and LV contractions (fusion between intrinsic activation and LV pacing) only if an RV-sensed event occurs between the LRL and MTR, although some devices will allow a distinct programmable maximum biventricular trigger rate (Figure 6.48). The clinical efficacy of this algorithm is questionable as triggered pacing occurs late in the depolarization cycle.

Premature atrial contractions

A common phenomenon is an atrial event occurring during the PVARP, resulting in failure to track the atrial event with subsequent intrinsic AV conduction and biventricular pacing inhibition. Because the PR interval may be relatively long compared with the sinus cycle length, the P wave may fall in the PVARP of the preceding R-wave interval. With a specific set of relationships between the AVI, PR interval, and PVARP, biventricular pacing may continue to be inhibited. As the atrial rhythm reaches rates faster than the total ARP (PVARP + AVI), biventricular pacing will stop. When the atrial rate falls, biventricular pacing will continue to be inhibited until the atrial rate is below the total intrinsic ARP (PVARP + PR interval). For instance, if the PR interval is 240 ms, the AVI is 150 ms and the PVARP is 300 ms (TARP 450 ms), at a sinus cycle length of 450 ms or 133 bpm, biventricular pacing will cease. As the rate slows, biventricular pacing will continue to be inhibited until the sinus cycle length increases to 540 ms (PVARP + PR interval) or 111 bpm.

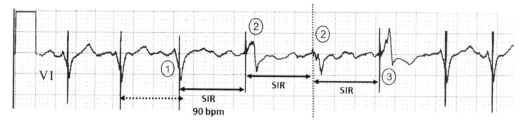

Figure 6.48 Biventricular trigger feature. Atrial fibrillation with a rapid ventricular response of 110 bpm (VVIR pacing mode) prevents appropriate biventricular pacing (first three beats, labeled "1") since the sensor indicator rate (SIR) is 90 bpm. However, the biventricular trigger delivers left ventricular (LV) pacing immediately after right ventricular (RV) sensing in an attempt to maintain LV pacing even when rates are higher than the SIR. The tracing also demonstrates fusion beats (labeled "2") and full biventricular paced beats (labeled "3") when the heart rate is close to or below 90 bpm, respectively.

Premature ventricular contractions

Frequent PVCs are commonly responsible for loss of biventricular pacing due to inhibition. A PVC trigger algorithm is frequently available in CRT devices (biventricular trigger or ventricular-sensed response, as already described), by which the device will immediately deliver LV pacing after an RV-sensed event (Figure 6.48). However, this response will commonly result in a fusion beat rather than true biventricular pacing with unclear hemodynamic effects. Even occasional PVCs can result in loss of biventricular pacing, since they will reset the VAI and create a new PVARP. Biventricular pacing is inhibited after a PVC if the following sinus P wave falls within the PVARP (lack of ventricular tracking). It is important to understand that PVC response algorithms (PVARP extension) will likely exacerbate loss of biventricular pacing and should be disabled if it is thought to be the main cause of loss of biventricular pacing. Because the PVARP may be markedly extended (e.g. to 600 ms), perpetuation of loss of biventricular pacing can occur even at slower rates. For example, a PVARP extended to 600 ms combined with an AVI of 140 ms would result in continued loss of pacing until the sinus cycle length dropped to 740 ms or 81 bpm. Algorithms that reduce the PVARP when a sensed ventricular event occurs may prevent perpetuation of loss of biventricular pacing. Finally, elimination of PVCs with either medical treatment (e.g. amiodarone) or invasive therapies (e.g. radiofrequency catheter ablation) should be considered in order to optimize biventricular pacing.

Atrial fibrillation with ventricular response above the LRL or SIR

Biventricular pacing in patients with chronic AF with rapid ventricular response is a common challenge. However, even subjects with relatively good rate control may have fusion or lack of biventricular pacing (mode switch to non-tracking pacing mode) if ventricular response occurs above LRL or SIR. This can be dealt with by increasing LRL or sensor response, enabling ventricular rate regularization (see section Rate enhancements) or ventricular sense response (biventricular trigger), or medical therapy or ablation (AF ablation or AV nodal ablation).

Noise reversion

All manufacturers have a noise reversion algorithm to prevent asystole or inappropriate bradycardia if a patient is exposed to an external source that can generate inappropriate sensing, such as electromagnetic interference (EMI). A ventricular-sensed event initiates a ventricular refractory period (nonprogrammable "noise window" in some devices), which will be reset if a ventricular-sensed event is noted within this period. Most algorithms will label these signals as electrical "noise" if they exceed physiological rates (400–600 bpm). Once the counter of the noise reversion algorithm is met, the device will adopt an asynchronous pacing mode, termed noise mode response, noise reversion mode, bradycardia noise mode, or noise rejection, depending on the device manufacturer (Figure 6.49).

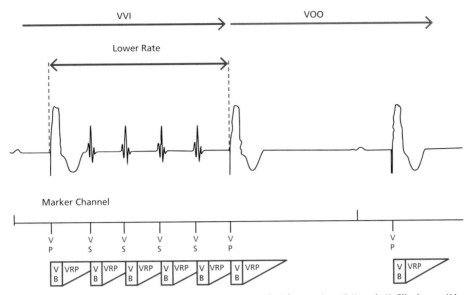

Figure 6.49 Noise reversion response. After a ventricular-sensed (VS) event occurs during the ventricular refractory period (VRP), this period will be reinitiated. Recurrent VS at non-physiological rates will be labeled as "noise" and switch to an asynchronous (VOO) pacing mode. Source: modified from Huizar JF, Kaszala K, Ellenbogen KA. Cardiac pacing modes and terminology. In: Sakena S, Camm AJ, eds. *Electrophysiological Disorders of the Heart*, 2nd edn. Philadelphia, PA: Elsevier Saunders, 2012: 441–456. Reproduced with permission of Elsevier.

Magnet response

Traditionally, magnet application has been used in special circumstances, such as (i) temporary asynchronous pacing (such as in a pacemaker-dependent individual who will undergo a procedure where pacing inhibition is likely due to EMI) and (ii) assessment of pacing and battery status (latter determined by base pacing rate).

The response of a pacemaker to magnet application depends on the manufacturer as well as the device programming. Overall, single- and dual-chamber pacemakers will *almost* always result in asynchronous pacing (AOO, VOO, DOO). Some pacemakers continue to pace asynchronously for a number of beats after magnet removal and most have a variable pacing rate with magnet application, determined by battery status. In "reset mode," some devices do not exhibit asynchronous pacing. Some pacemakers have a programmable "off" magnet response, while others may be programmed to store electrogram diagnostics when the magnet is applied. In contrast to pacemakers, defibrillators will *not* display asynchronous pacing mode, but will inhibit detection of ventricular arrhythmia (disabling therapies) and therefore patients should be monitored until the magnet is removed.

Summary

A clear understanding of pacing modes, timing cycles, and special pacemaker features is crucial for differentiating between appropriate and inappropriate pacemaker function, particularly when elucidating an ECG with an unusual pacing behavior.

Overall, all pacemakers follow the basic principles of timing cycles reviewed in this chapter. However, different pacemaker manufacturers and models have significant differences in their special pacemaker features, even when the goal is the same. When troubleshooting these cardiac devices, it is paramount to (i) interrogate the device to understand baseline programmed pacemaker settings; (ii) understand in depth the different algorithms or pacing features; and (iii) attempt to reproduce these episodes if possible, since both atrial and ventricular event markers (a pacemaker's interpretation of cardiac events) can assist us to further differentiate between appropriate and inappropriate pacemaker behavior response. Pacemaker manufacturers provide manuals and technical service experts around the clock to corroborate appropriate or inappropriate device function.

References

1 Bernstein AD, Daubert JC, Fletcher RD, *et al*. The revised NASPE/BPEG generic code for antibradycardia, adaptive-rate, and multisite pacing. *North American Society of Pacing and Electrophysiology/British Pacing and Electrophysiology Group. Pacing Clin Electrophysiol* 2002;25(2):260–264.

2 Ellenbogen KA, Kay GN, Lau C-P. *Clinical Cardiac Pacing, Defibrillation, and Resynchronization Therapy*, 3rd edn. Philadelphia: Saunders Elsevier, 2007.

3 Kaszala K, Huizar JF, Ellenbogen KA. Contemporary pacemakers: what the primary care physician needs to know. *Mayo Clin Proc* 2008;83(10):1170–1186.

4 Cleland JG, Coletta AP, Abdellah AT, *et al*. Clinical trials update from Heart Rhythm 2007 and Heart Failure 2007: CARISMA, PREPARE, DAVID II, SAVE-PACE, PROTECT and AREA-IN-CHF. *Eur J Heart Fail* 2007;9(8):850–853.

5 Biotronik. *Cyclos Pacemaker Feature Handbook*. Lake Oswego, OR: Biotronik Inc., 2006.

6 Higano ST, Hayes DL. P wave tracking above the maximum tracking rate in a DDDR pacemaker. *Pacing Clin Electrophysiol* 1989;12(7 Pt 1):1044–1048.

7 Boston Scientific Corporation. *Cognis™ 100-D System Guide*. St. Paul, MN: Boston Scientific Corp., 2008.

8 Boston Scientific Corporation. *Altrua 20 and Altrua 40 Multiprogrammable Pacemakers*. St. Paul, MN: Boston Scientific Corp., 2008.

9 St. Jude Medical, *Inc. Bradycardia Devices: Help Manual*. Sylmar, CA: St. Jude Medical, Inc., 2008.

10 Medtronic, Inc. *Adapta/Versa/Sensia Pacemaker Reference Guide*. Minneapolis, MN: Medtronic, Inc., 2006.

11 Connolly SJ, Sheldon R, Roberts RS, Gent M. The North American Vasovagal Pacemaker Study (VPS). A randomized trial of permanent cardiac pacing for the prevention of vasovagal syncope. *J Am Coll Cardiol* 1999;33(1):16–20.

12 Palmisano P, Zaccaria M, Luzzi G, *et al*. Closed-loop cardiac pacing vs. conventional dual-chamber pacing with specialized sensing and pacing algorithms for syncope prevention in patients with refractory vasovagal syncope: results of a long-term follow-up. *Europace* 2012;14(7):1038–1043.

13 Connolly SJ, Sheldon R, Thorpe KE, *et al*. Pacemaker therapy for prevention of syncope in patients with recurrent severe vasovagal syncope: Second Vasovagal Pacemaker Study (VPS II): a randomized trial. *JAMA* 2003;289(17):2224–2229.

14 Lau CP, Leung SK, Tse HF, Barold SS. Automatic mode switching of implantable pacemakers: II. Clinical performance of current algorithms and their programming. *Pacing Clin Electrophysiol* 2002;25(7):1094–1113.

15 Lau CP, Leung SK, Tse HF, Barold SS. Automatic mode switching of implantable pacemakers: I. Principles of instrumentation, clinical, and hemodynamic considerations. *Pacing Clin Electrophysiol* 2002;25(6):967–983.

16 Medtronic, Inc. *Entrust Implantable Cardioverter Defibrillator systems: Reference Manual*. Minneapolis, MN: Medtronic, Inc., 2005.

17 Mitchell AR, Sulke N. How do atrial pacing algorithms prevent atrial arrhythmias? *Europace* 2004;6(4):351–362.

18 Carlson MD, Ip J, Messenger J, *et al*. A new pacemaker algorithm for the treatment of atrial fibrillation: results of the Atrial Dynamic Overdrive Pacing Trial (ADOPT). *J Am Coll Cardiol* 2003;42(4):627–633.

19 Israel CW, Lawo T, Lemke B, Gronefeld G, Hohnloser SH. Atrial pacing in the prevention of paroxysmal atrial fibrillation: first results of a new combined algorithm. *Pacing Clin Electrophysiol* 2000;23(11 Pt 2):1888–1890.

20 Ellenbogen KA. Pacing therapy for prevention of atrial fibrillation. *Heart Rhythm* 2007;4(3 Suppl):S84–S87.

21 Israel CW, Hugl B, Unterberg C, *et al*. Pace-termination and pacing for prevention of atrial tachyarrhythmias: results from a multicenter study with an implantable device for atrial therapy. *J Cardiovasc Electrophysiol* 2001;12(10):1121–1128.

22 Lee MA, Weachter R, Pollak S, *et al*. The effect of atrial pacing therapies on atrial tachyarrhythmia burden and frequency: *results of a randomized trial in patients with bradycardia and atrial tachyarrhythmias. J Am Coll Cardiol* 2003;41(11):1926–1932.

23 Padeletti L, Purerfellner H, Adler SW, *et al*. Combined efficacy of atrial septal lead placement and atrial pacing algorithms for prevention of paroxysmal atrial tachyarrhythmia. *J Cardiovasc Electrophysiol* 2003;14(11):1189–1195.

24 Gold MR, Adler S, Fauchier L, *et al*. Impact of atrial prevention pacing on atrial fibrillation burden: primary results of the Study of Atrial Fibrillation Reduction (SAFARI) trial. *Heart Rhythm* 2009;6(3):295–301.

25 Savoure A, Frohlig G, Galley D, *et al*. A new dual-chamber pacing mode to minimize ventricular pacing. *Pacing Clin Electrophysiol* 2005;28(Suppl 1):S43–S46.

26 Sweeney MO, Bank AJ, Nsah E, *et al*. Minimizing ventricular pacing to reduce atrial fibrillation in sinus-node disease. *N Engl J Med* 2007;357(10):1000–1008.

27 Barold SS. Repetitive reentrant and non-reentrant ventriculoatrial synchrony in dual chamber pacing. *Clin Cardiol* 1991;14(9):754–763.

28 Sharma PS, Kaszala K, Tan AY, *et al*. Repetitive nonreentrant ventriculoatrial synchrony: an underrecognized cause of pacemaker-related arrhythmia. *Heart Rhythm* 2016;13(8):1739–1747.

29 Wang P, Kramer A, Estes NA III, Hayes DL. Timing cycles for biventricular pacing. *Pacing Clin Electrophysiol* 2002;25(1):62–75.

30 Kamath GS, Cotiga D, Koneru JN, *et al*. The utility of 12-lead Holter monitoring in patients with permanent atrial fibrillation for the identification of nonresponders after cardiac resynchronization therapy. *J Am Coll Cardiol* 2009;53(12):1050–1055.

31 Sweeney MO, Hellkamp AS, Ellenbogen KA, *et al*. Adverse effect of ventricular pacing on heart failure and atrial fibrillation among patients with normal baseline QRS duration in a clinical trial of pacemaker therapy for sinus node dysfunction. *Circulation* 2003;107(23):2932–2937.

CHAPTER 7

Evaluation, troubleshooting, and management of pacing system malfunctions

Karoly Kaszala

Cardiac Electrophysiology Laboratory, Hunter Holmes McGuire VA Medical Center, VCU School of Medicine, Richmond, VA, USA

Introduction

Advanced functionality and programmability of modern pacemaker systems allow specific options to manage cardiac arrhythmias. Increasing complexity of both the mechanical (as in dual- and multichamber devices) and software features (such as complex algorithms and pacemaker behaviors) create the potential for increased component or software malfunction and appearance of unusual device behavior (pseudo-malfunction) that may challenge the providers. Over the last two decades, while challenges continue, technological advances have also improved the reliability and diagnostic capabilities of cardiac pacemakers and implantable cardioverter–defibrillators (ICDs). Miniaturization has allowed incorporation of increasing memory function and automatization that support simpler device follow-up and advanced troubleshooting. In this chapter, commonly encountered problems relating to pacing in pacemakers and ICDs will be discussed.

General considerations: approach to evaluation of pacemaker function and malfunction

Proper device evaluation and troubleshooting requires a review of clinical and device history, a comprehensive and systematic clinical assessment of the patient, and interrogation of the device and review of the ancillary data. Intraoperative evaluation for diagnostic purposes is very rarely required, but is important for final confirmation of hardware abnormalities. The order of the diagnostic steps should be directed by the clinical circumstances and urgency of the problem but, in general, evaluation should start with non-invasive assessment and tests. During initial clinical encounters some of the historical information may not be readily available and in these cases the ancillary data become even more important. Obtaining a focused medical history may help to clarify the indication of device therapy and identify prior system problems until other records become available. Comorbidities may have significant implications regarding pacemaker programming, appropriate device selection, and risk of complications. The surgical implantation note should be carefully reviewed. The operative report should describe the indication for device therapy, vascular access site, lead type and position, device position, as well as any procedural difficulties. Device and lead parameters, including lead polarity, lead connection type, lead fixation mechanism, product manufacturer, and serial numbers should also be listed. Baseline programming parameters as well as post-implant electrocardiogram (ECG) and chest

Cardiac Pacing and ICDs, Seventh Edition. Edited by Kenneth A. Ellenbogen and Karoly Kaszala.
© 2020 John Wiley & Sons Ltd. Published 2020 by John Wiley & Sons Ltd.

X-ray are also important references. Any advisories related to the leads and device should be noted (Table 7.1). The next step is evaluation for the presence of any symptoms. While certain symptoms, such as syncope, are commonly linked to pacemaker malfunction, other less common signs may also indicate malfunction and should be looked for under appropriate clinical circumstances (Table 7.2). A focused physical examination may identify signs of heart failure and valvular abnormalities. Inspection of the jugular venous pressure may reveal the presence of cannon A waves, suggesting loss of atrioventricular (AV) synchrony as atrial contraction takes place against a closed tricuspid valve. Presence of pectoral or intercostal muscle stimulation or diaphragmatic capture may point to mechanical malfunction. If lead integrity failure or skeletal muscle oversensing is suspected, provocative maneuvers, such as isometric arm exercise, hyperventilation or Valsalva maneuver, may be useful for triggering abnormal function.

Inspection should also extend to the device pocket to assure proper healing and look for postoperative complications such as infection or erosion. A current ECG is important to confirm the heart rhythm and presence or absence of pacing. The ECG may identify atrial and ventricular sensing or pacing abnormality and the morphology of paced atrial and ventricular complexes provides rough information of the pacing site. Review of a baseline ECG before device implantation may also be useful. Pacemaker lead position and gross lead integrity may be further evaluated by anteroposterior and lateral chest X-ray images. While analysis of the ancillary information rarely reveals all details of an abnormality, it is helpful with triaging until a device-specific programmer becomes available for further analysis. The programmer is required to retrieve information from the device memory and test the pacing system. It is therefore essential to

Table 7.1 Baseline data needed for pacemaker troubleshooting

Pacemaker system	Pacemaker generator
	Manufacturer
	Model and serial numbers
	Current programming
	Date of implant
	Alert or recalls
	Header type
	Special features
Lead system	Manufacturer
	Model and serial numbers
	Polarity and fixation mechanism
	Pin type
	Insulation material
	Date of implant
	Alert or recalls
Patient	Indication for pacemaker
	Implant operative report
	Medical and cardiac diagnosis
	Medications
	History of recent medical procedures (e.g. cardioversion, defibrillation, MRI, electrocautery)
	History of electrical current exposure, trauma

Table 7.2 Symptoms suggestive of pacemaker abnormality

Symptom[a]	Cause
Fatigue	Pacemaker syndrome:
Confusion	hemodynamic and neurohormonal
Dyspnea	abnormality related to ventricular
Orthopnea	pacing and/or loss of AV synchrony
Chest pain	Loss of capture or pacing output
Palpitations	Sensing abnormality
Presyncope	Special algorithms
Syncope	Suboptimal rate-modulated pacing
	Arrhythmias: with or without suboptimal pacemaker programming
Hiccups (due to diaphragmatic stimulation)	LV pacing close to phrenic nerve
	RA pacing close to phrenic nerve
	RA lead dislodgement to SVC
	Lead perforation
Chest wall/pectoral muscle contractions (due to pectoral muscle or intercostal muscle capture)	Unipolar pacing
	Loose set-screw
	Lead insulation damage
	Lead perforation

[a] Many of the symptoms are not specific for a pacemaker abnormality. Correlation with additional clinical and ancillary data is required to make the diagnosis.
AV, atrioventricular; LV, left ventricular; RA, right atrial; SVC, superior vena cava.

(a)

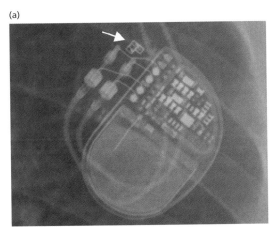

(b)

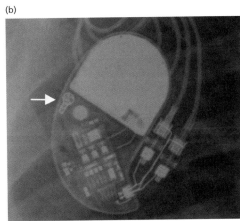

Figure 7.1 Examples of radiographic device identifiers. (a) EnRhythm device with Medtronic logo and PNP device identifier (white arrow). (b) Logo of a St. Jude Medical Identity pacemaker (white arrow). Bipolar leads are identified based on two pin electrodes for each lead.

know the manufacturer of the device in order to perform a full evaluation. Manufacturer's information may be retrieved from the operative report or from the device identification card that is mailed to the patient following an implant. If these are not available, the radiographic identifier of the pulse generator (Figure 7.1) on a chest radiograph or pacing response to magnet application over the pacemaker (magnet response) may help to narrow down the device manufacturer. The X-ray image showing the profile of the device may also provide additional clues [1]. If all these efforts fail, a technical service representative of the device companies (current major device manufacturers in the United States include Biotronik, Boston Scientific, Medtronic, LivaNova and St. Jude Medical) may be able to retrieve the patient information from their implant database. Technical services may also assist with interpretation of the device interrogation and provide additional information about the leads, pulse generator, and certain device- and manufacturer-specific algorithms.

Differential diagnosis of device malfunction

Pacing system malfunctions may be categorized according to electrocardiographic manifestations including abnormal sensing, lack of pacing or lack of capture, and abnormal or unexpected rate of pacing. In broader terms, pacemaker malfunction also includes symptoms associated with the pacing or pacemaker programming or complications from the pacemaker system. Malfunctions may also be categorized according to the particular cause, including mechanical abnormalities, programming abnormalities, and extrinsic/external causes. In clinical practice, malfunction is usually suspected based on abnormal ECG or symptoms. Latent abnormalities may also be diagnosed from stored device data and proper action may halt an impending clinical problem. Ultimately, the particular cause is determined following correlation of all ancillary information with the interrogated device data.

Abnormalities of the mechanical components of a pacing system

A pacing system comprises a pulse generator and the pacemaker lead(s). The pulse generator, which houses the battery and electrical circuitry, is hermetically sealed and connected to the pacemaker leads through the header. The pacemaker lead pins are secured in the header with one or two setscrews during the implant procedure. The leads maintain a connection to the cardiac tissue by either an active screw mechanism or passive fixation. The pacemaker leads consist of one or more conductors surrounded by insulation material. In a bipolar lead, the conductors connect the tip and ring electrodes to the terminal pin, whereas in a unipolar lead only a tip electrode is present and the can serves as the anode (Figures 7.1 and 7.2). The ICD leads are more complex structures incorporating, in addition, one or two coils for high-voltage defibrillation. These additional components make lead engineering more difficult and are likely major contributors to a poorer long-term lead survival compared to pacemaker leads. The electrical circuit of a pacer system is completed by the tissue between the anode and cathode. The distance between the anode and cathode is the major difference between a unipolar and bipolar system in terms of sensing characteristics and current and energy requirement to capture the myocardium. A larger distance in a unipolar system predisposes to sensing far-field signals from cardiac or noncardiac sources. Pacing impedance is lower during

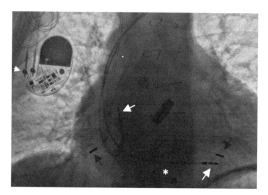

Figure 7.2 Posteroanterior radiographic image of a unipolar pacemaker system. Note the single pin electrode on each lead and header (small white arrow). Lead integrity failure occurred in the system and the patient underwent implantation of two new bipolar leads. Due to venous occlusion, a completely new system was implanted from the left subclavian system. Black arrows point to the passive fixation unipolar lead tips and large white arrows to the new bipolar active fixation pacemaker leads. A mechanical aortic valve is also present. A broken old epicardial pacer wire is marked with an asterisk. This system is over 30 years old and it required a special header to accommodate 5-mm lead pins. Special consideration is required when plans are made for pulse generator change in such a patient as a standard header would not accommodate the lead. In addition, the pacemaker generator serves an active part in the pacing circuit and capture would not take place once the device is removed from the body (in contrast to a bipolar pacing system). Another implication of a unipolar system is that there is an increased chance of noise oversensing, and special attention is required especially in the hospital environment. Note that the electrodes of the second set of leads (large white arrows, new implant) are more than 1 cm away from other lead components.

unipolar pacing compared to bipolar pacing in the same system. Any defect in the integrity of the lead and pacemaker header assembly may result in introduction of noise and cause sensing abnormality or divert pacing current away from the myocardium with resultant capture failure.

Pulse generator hardware and software

A predictable failure of any current pacer or ICD system is related to battery depletion, and this is the most common reason for device explantation [2]. One of the goals of regular device follow-up is to ascertain that there is adequate battery capacity to maintain appropriate device function. Among the several challenges of battery engineering are the constant efforts to minimize device (and battery) size yet maximize longevity in a very reliable manner. In addition, in order to allow adequate time to diagnose battery depletion and schedule generator replacement, battery depletion has to follow a very predictable pattern. For the purpose of cardiac pacing, the characteristics of lithium/iodine batteries have been optimal and have been utilized for decades with great reliability. Battery voltage remains relatively flat during much of the device's lifetime, with decline only close to end of service. Battery impedance on the other hand increases continuously, with a very rapid rise as battery depletion approaches. Impedance is therefore a better overall predictor of battery longevity at any given time point. Manufacturers differ in whether they express battery parameters in numerical or graphical fashion, but battery status is one of the key parameters followed in the clinic. Application of a magnetic field over a pacemaker (clinically by placing a special donut-shaped magnet) results in a device-specific magnet response. This response may be observed during clinic follow-up or during transtelephonic monitoring (TTM). In most pacemakers, magnet application results in asynchronous pacing at a certain rate (except for rare circumstances when different special magnet function is programmed "on"). As the battery approaches end of service, the magnet-activated pacing rate gradually decreases or remains stable in some generators until the battery reaches elective replacement indicator (ERI) status. At this point a specific model or company-specific magnet rate indicates that the device is nearing end of service (Figure 7.3). An additional 3 months' battery support is available at ERI until the

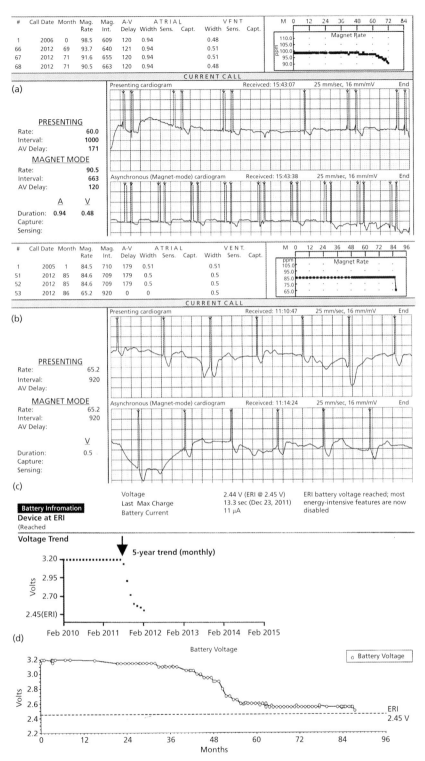

Figure 7.3 Pacemaker transtelephonic transmission (TTM) summaries: (a) St. Jude Medical and (b) Medtronic. A typical, gradual decline in magnet response rate is seen in the St. Jude device (model: Identity Adx), whereas there is a sudden drop to VVI 65 bpm in the Medtronic pacemaker (model: EnRhythm). Electrogram strips show current presenting rhythm as well as current magnet rate. (c) Battery voltage trend from an ICD. This device was found with an abnormal, sudden battery depletion (arrow) 2 years after implant. The abnormality was recognized during remote device monitoring. This was a random component failure and no specific cause was identified. (d) Normal ICD battery depletion curve of a St. Jude Atlas device with two plateau phases, one at the beginning of life and one before elective replacement indicator (ERI).

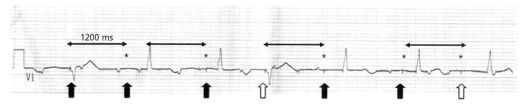

Figure 7.4 Pacemaker battery depletion. The rhythm strip (lead V1) from a patient who had undergone VVI pacemaker implantation 14 years earlier and had subsequently not obtained any further pacemaker follow-up. Pacing stimuli are denoted by the vertical closed arrows; pacing is occurring at a cycle length of 1200 ms (horizontal arrows). There is both intermittent failure to capture (*) and failure to sense (vertical open arrows). The combination of sensing and capture problems suggested a problem intrinsic to the lead; however, at pacemaker generator change, the lead demonstrated no abnormality. The erratic pacing behavior is best explained by near-complete depletion of the pacemaker's battery.

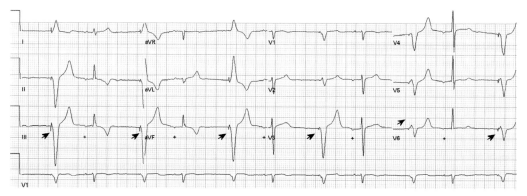

Figure 7.5 A patient with sinus node dysfunction presented with shortness of breath. The Medtronic device had reached elective replacement indicator (ERI) and current ECG shows VVI pacing at 65 bpm with appropriate sensing and capture [pacing artifact (arrows) is followed by ventricular depolarization]. There is slow retrograde conduction with echo beats (+). The ninth beat is a fusion beat between a ventricular ectopic beat and paced beat. This presentation with acute loss of atrioventricular synchrony due to pacing mode change is consistent with pacemaker syndrome. His symptoms resolved after pacemaker generator change.

device reaches end of life (EOL). At EOL, device reliability is not guaranteed and erratic behavior may be observed (Figure 7.4). As ERI may also trigger a change in pacing mode (rate response turned "off," switch to single-chamber VVI mode), in rare patients clinical decompensation may occur as ERI is reached (Figure 7.5). Increasing availability of web-based remote home monitoring has revolutionized patient follow-up and this technology has nearly completely replaced TTM [3].

ICD batteries are designed differently in order to support standard pacing requirements (1–20 µJ per pacing pulse) and deliver rapid charge to high-voltage capacitors (up to 30–40 J) for defibrillation or cardioversion therapy of tachyarrhythmias. These tasks are achieved more efficiently with currently used lithium/silver/vanadium oxide or lithium/manganese dioxide based batteries; indeed some of these battery technologies are also applied in pacemakers to support additional energy requirements, such as wireless monitoring and extended diagnostics. The discharge curves of these batteries vary based on the composition material and also differ from the discharge curves of traditional pacemaker batteries. It is important to understand the individual variations in order to make informed decisions during follow-up. Assistance from the technical service at the device company may be helpful in unclear situations. In ICD generators, battery voltage and capacitor charge time is used most commonly to follow the battery status.

While the reliability of pacemaker and ICD generators continues to improve, random system failure or mechanical (e.g. battery, circuitry, header, wiring) or software design flaws continue to occur, as has been seen in recent advisories [4]. Depending on which particular component is affected, inappropriate pacing behavior, battery or wiring short with lack of pacing or defibrillation, or accelerated battery depletion may result (Figure 7.3c). Early battery depletion may be caused by suboptimal device programming or lead/patient-related events (exit block, high pacing threshold, frequent ICD therapy in ICDs). Other causes of generator failure or malfunction may be suspected based on clinical circumstances, such as recent mechanical trauma to the device site; exposure to significant electromagnetic interference (EMI), especially in the hospital setting, such as electrocautery, MRI scan, TENS; or radiation (mainly therapeutic). While EMI has caused system failures in early devices, these types of serious events are much less common with modern pacemakers and ICDs due to advanced filtering and shielding and increased awareness of these potential interactions [5]. EMI may cause temporary changes in pacemaker or ICD behavior and trigger a reset or a partial reset of the device. These are fallback safety settings that are activated in an event of suspected software or hardware malfunction. Most commonly, a change in bradycardia programming (and/or tachycardia programming in ICDs) or loss of stored data occurs. The programming changes are usually reversible, but generator change may be required in rare instances when changes are non-programmable (Figure 7.6). Direct or scattered radiation may affect the device circuitry and cause various levels of reset. Direct radiation over the device may cause permanent damage to the circuitry if the radiation dose exceeds a device-specific safety level. Radiation exposure for the device needs to be calculated, especially when therapeutic radiation is applied close to the device site. The maximum tolerated radiation dose for a particular device is available from the manufacturer. If the safety dose is exceeded, the reliability of the device may be impaired and the generator has to be replaced. If the planned radiation path is close to or over the device, the generator may need to be repositioned before treatment, especially in pacemaker-dependent patients. The mechanism of radiation-induced changes is multifactorial. Modern devices utilize complementary metal oxide semiconductor (CMOS) circuitry. Radiation may induce ionization in CMOS with build-up of a charge [6]. The time course of these changes and possible consequences

Boston Scientific	ZOOM ® View™	Report Created
	Safety Mode Report	Last Office Interrogation
	Date of Birth	
	Device	Implant Date

Warning: Pulse Generator is in Safety Mode.

For patient protection the device has been switched to Safety Mode. Device function is permanently limited to ventricular tachy single zone operation with ventricular paced support.

Please contact Boston Scientific Technical Services at 1.800.CARDIAC (North America) or contact your local Boston Scientific representative.

Tachy Mode	Monitor + Therapy
VF Threshold	165 ppm
Duration	1 sec
Energy	Max X 5
Brady Mode	VVI
Pacing Rate	72 ppm
Amplitude	5.0 V
Pulse Width	1.0 ms

Figure 7.6 Biventricular ICD generator switched to non-programmable safety mode due to exposure to electromagnetic interference in the hospital environment. The patient underwent open heart surgery and electrocautery was used very close to or over the coronary sinus lead and this was the likely cause of the problem. A new generator was implanted after the patient recuperated from surgery.

are variable, and include increased current drain and shortened battery life or changes in sensing. Scattered radiation may also affect the random access memory (RAM) and result in errors in device function or data storage. RAM is increasingly used in more complex ICDs, but also in newer generation pacemakers.

Software abnormalities had been common reasons for device advisories in the past. Increasing sophistication of the device circuitry and memory have increasingly allowed non-invasive postoperative software upgrades via the programmer and the clinical consequences of software anomalies in recent years have been less significant. An example of software upload includes the update of Medtronic ICDs with the Lead Integrity Alert™ algorithm in order to minimize risk of inappropriate ICD therapies in the event of a lead fracture. This software was retrofitted to several earlier classes of Medtronic devices [7]. As software-specific information is proprietary, providers need to rely on information from the manufacturers about any updates or to confirm abnormalities.

Failure of pacemaker circuitry or complete depletion of the battery results in system failure and inability to interrogate the device. In clinical situations when communication with the device cannot be established, several possible confounders need to be ruled out before a generator change is contemplated. First, an environmental factor that may affect communication with the device, such as EMI (as may be seen in a patient with left ventricular assist device), or a malfunctioning programmer has to be excluded. As part of the evaluation process, the manufacturer of the device has to be ascertained, as already discussed, to ensure that the proper programmer is used for interrogation. This is critical for assessing a new patient, but may also be an embarrassing oversight in a patient who is normally followed in the device clinic and had a device exchange or upgrade performed in another facility between visits.

Leads

Pacemaker and ICD leads are commonly referred to as the Achilles heel of the pacer/ICD system as they remain the main source of mechanical failure. Starting at the implantation procedure and over the lifetime of the system, leads are exposed to significant chemical and mechanical stress in the hostile intravascular environment. The restricted space at the intersection of the first rib and clavicle may cause additional stress and this is the site where subclavian crush injuries develop. Lead-to-lead and lead-to-can interaction as well as tight anchoring sutures are other common mechanical points for potential lead failure. Lead-to-lead interactions may also occur between the leads as they make their way to the heart in the vascular system. Repetitive stress due to friction, pressure, and cyclical repetitive movement may result in lead insulation defect or fracture of the conductors. Certain pacemaker or ICD leads are more prone to develop structural failure for various reasons, such as defects in the design or manufacturing of insulation material, type of insulation material, or other parts of the lead assembly. Long-term survival data of individual leads are available from the performance report of the manufacturers. Lead failures are notoriously underreported and it is difficult to know the true incidence of this problem. In case there are concerns about lead reliability, advisories are initiated by the manufacturer or Food and Drug Administration (FDA) to inform clinicians and assist with clinical decision-making. While the reliability of pacemaker leads has improved over the past decades, two major advisories drew attention to design failures and the risk of premature lead degradation in certain ICD leads, affecting tens of thousands of patients (Sprint Fidelis™, Medtronic in 2007 and Riata™, St. Jude Medical ICD leads as well as left ventricular leads from St. Jude Medical, 2011) [8]. Review of recommendations about the management of these advisories is beyond the scope of this chapter but, in general, an individualized approach is recommended with enhanced surveillance. Routine invasive interventions are rarely beneficial or advised for prophylactic purposes.

In general, abnormalities in lead insulation manifest as decreased lead impedance, whereas conductor fracture is associated with increased lead impedance (Figures 7.7 and 7.8). Insulation or conductor failure may cause noise, oversensing, or failure to capture. The normal lead impedance values usually vary between 300 and 1800 Ω depending on the particular lead characteristics but remain relatively stable following the lead maturation period. Out-of-range values would not

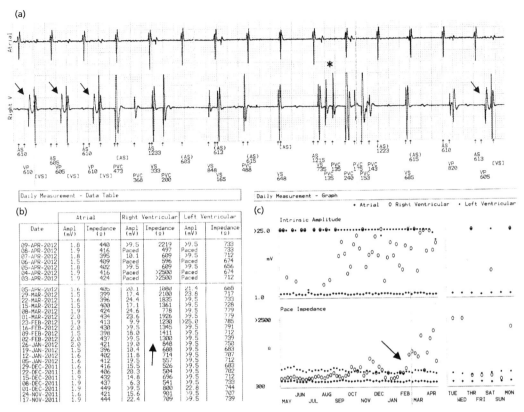

Figure 7.7 (a) Atrial and right ventricular (RV) electrogram recording from a biventricular pacemaker. At the beginning of the tracing, there is atrial-synchronous biventricular pacing but only the left ventricular lead captures (arrows). A subsequently delayed RV signal (marked as VS) represents loss of capture at the RV pacing site. There are make-or-break signals consistent with noise (*) and suggestive of lead integrity failure. Lead fracture was confirmed by sudden increase and erratic changes in RV lead impedance (b, c, arrows). This example shows that while the biventricular pacemaker provides some safety advantage in case of a lead fracture, significant noise in the RV lead would result in inhibition of pacing (a, *) and cause asystole.

necessarily mean abnormal lead function (Figure 7.9). On the other hand, significant variation in lead impedance, even if within the range of "normal" values, should raise concerns about possible lead failure [9]. Subclinical mechanical abnormality may present with sudden erratic change in lead impedance in the lead trend data or non-physiological noise may be recorded as an arrhythmia event (Figure 7.7). Lead failure in a pacemaker system may result in oversensing and lack of, or inappropriate, pacing or lack of capture. In certain pacemakers, automatic polarity switch (from bipolar to unipolar) takes place if lead impedance values reach an out-of-range value. This safety feature may help to reestablish pacing if only the ring electrode circuit is damaged (Figure 7.10).

In ICD patients, noise and oversensing may present with inappropriate ICD therapies or dizziness and syncope due to oversensing and pauses. In some newer generation ICDs, a near-field or sensed intracardiac electrogram (EGM) is correlated with a far-field EGM to rule out oversensing of non-physiological signals (Securesense™, St. Jude Medical; Smartshock™, Medtronic). A special algorithm, developed by Medtronic, monitors lead impedance change, ventricular tachycardia episodes in non-physiological range, and non-physiological ventricular sensing events (VV intervals in the range of 120–130 ms that are too closely coupled to represent physiological ventricular depolarization) and this technology has been helpful in identifying impending lead integrity failure before any clinical event and reducing the risk of inappropriate

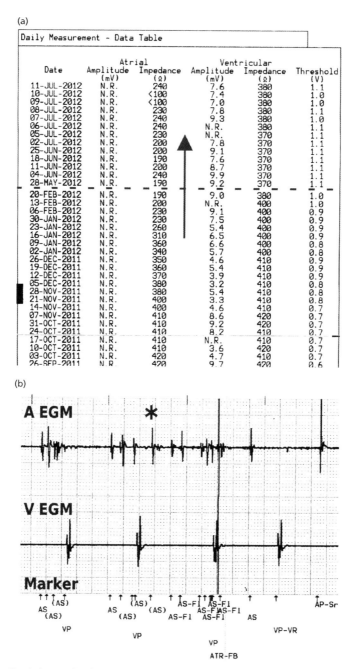

Figure 7.8 Example of lead abnormality due to insulation failure. (a) Long-term lead trends. There is gradual decline in lead impedance and subsequent variability (arrow) with minimum impedance recorded as <100 Ω. (b) Noise with oversensing was recorded in the device memory as mode switch episode. Following mode switch (ATR-FB), DDI pacing is initiated with ventricular rate regularization (VP–VR).

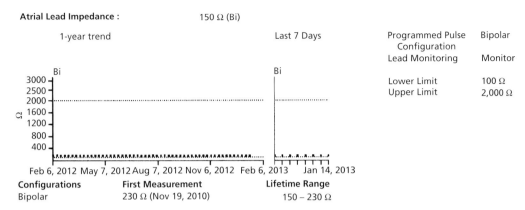

Atrial Lead Impedance :   150 Ω (Bi)

1-year trend   Last 7 Days

Programmed Pulse   Bipolar
Configuration
Lead Monitoring   Monitor

Lower Limit   100 Ω
Upper Limit   2,000 Ω

Configurations   First Measurement   Lifetime Range
Bipolar   230 Ω (Nov 19, 2010)   150 – 230 Ω

Figure 7.9 Chronic low impedance trend of a bipolar atrial lead. Note long-term stable impedance value in this lead with normal function.

Ventricular Impedance Trend - Chronic Report   Page 1

Ventricular Impedance Trend - Chronic Report

○ Initial	■ min/max vs. time
✕ At Interrogation	— Lifetime min/max

Initial Interrogation

Pace Polarity	Unipolar
Sense Polarity	Unipolar
Lead Monitor	Monitor Only
Lead Trend	On

Measured Impedances

Initial	674 ohms
At Interrogation	53,526 ohms
Lifetime Min	596 ohms
Lifetime Max	34,018 ohms

Notable Data

High Impedance	16,777,222
Low Impedance	0
Polarity Switch	

Figure 7.10 Polarity change from bipolar to unipolar pacing due to sudden marked elevation in lead impedance. In this case, the impedance remained abnormal even in unipolar mode, suggesting that the lead fracture involved both electrodes.

ICD therapies [7]. Any suggestion of lead integrity failure has to be taken very seriously, especially in ICD leads or in pacemaker-dependent patients, as the functionality of the lead may change very rapidly and failure to act on it in a timely manner may have catastrophic consequences.

In broader terms, lead failure may be seen with mechanically intact leads when fixation to the heart is suboptimal, such as in the case of micro- and macro-dislodgement or lead perforation. Macro- dislodgement is suspected based on alterations in pacing parameters and change in lead position based on imaging studies (mainly chest X-ray). A change in the paced ECG morphology may also be evident following significant ventricular lead migration. Atrial lead dislodgement to the ventricle may mimic switched lead pins in the header. Micro-dislodgement is suspected when pacing parameters change (decreased sensing, increased pacing threshold, change in lead impedance, or the combination of these) within the first days to weeks following implantation without a noticeable change in lead position based on X-ray appearance. It is important to remember that during normal lead maturation an inflammatory reaction takes place in the myocardium near the lead tip. This may result in an increased capture threshold and decrease in sensing and can be expected to resolve within several weeks. Almost all contemporary transvenous leads now have steroid-eluting tips and these have markedly reduced the incidence of significant tissue reaction. Once the healing process is complete, some degree of fibrosis develops at the lead tip contact site and when this process is excessive, permanent exit block and sensing abnormality may develop. Micro-perforation may also present in a similar way. Exit block usually develops in the chronic stage, weeks to months after implant, whereas perforation may occur at any time. Differentiation between exit block and micro-dislodgement is difficult, especially if the abnormality is identified weeks to months after implant. Lead dislodgement may be due to inadequate fixation to the cardiac tissue, inadequate lead redundancy, loose fixation of the lead in the suture sleeves, or patient-related causes (such as non-compliance with activity or twiddler's syndrome). It is important to identify the mechanism of failure (if possible) in order to minimize the chance of the same problem occurring again. Lead repositioning would resolve the problem with dislodgement, but exit block is related to tissue reaction and a similar response may develop again at the new implant site. The decision to manage lead abnormalities invasively or non-invasively is dependent on the clinical circumstances, such as the lead affected, urgency of need for pacing, and degree of change in parameters.

Acute lead perforation usually presents as a hemodynamic catastrophe in the perioperative period and usually requires emergency pericardiocentesis and lead repositioning. Subacute and chronic lead perforation may cause pericarditis, pericardial effusion, pneumothorax (may be seen with right atrial lead perforation), and pectoral muscle stimulation, and are associated with changes in pacing, sensing and impedance values. In the case of gross lead perforation, chest X-ray is very helpful (Figure 7.11). In these cases complete loss of capture and sensing may be seen. Microperforation may be suspected if the unipolar tip pacing threshold is significantly higher than the ring threshold in the appropriate clinical settings. If high-output pacing causes pectoral muscle stimulation, the possibility of perforation should be considered. Advanced imaging studies with CT scan or

echocardiography to evaluate microperforation are limited due to streaming artifact from the lead tip, but may be of diagnostic value [10]. In most cases lead revision is required to correct the problem.

Lead-to-lead interaction may cause chatter and oversensing when the tip or ring electrode collides with other intracardiac leads during the cardiac cycle. This is best avoided by paying meticulous attention to lead positioning when more than one lead is present in the cardiac chamber. X-rays in two orthogonal views should document that the lead tips and electrodes are ideally at least 1 cm apart (Figure 7.2).

Inadequate connection of the lead pins (using devices with non-compatible headers, connecting to the wrong pinhole, or improper tightening of the set-screw) is a cause of a completely avoidable mechanical malfunction. Another, usually reversible, abnormality may be seen when an air bubble remains entrapped around the lead pin following securing of the lead in the header during implantation. Once the air evaporates from the chamber (generally within a few hours to days), the noise usually subsides. Rarely, reoperation may become necessary if sensing or pacing abnormality persists [11]. Careful implantation techniques may help to reduce the risk of future mechanical problems.

Radiographic imaging of pacer systems

Radiographic imaging is a routine part of the clinical assessment following device implant and in chronic settings when clinical questions arise. Two perpendicular X-ray projections are required to adequately assess the pacing system structure and position. In general, posteroanterior and lateral projections are used during outpatient follow-up and right and left anterior oblique views during implant. As the left cardiac chambers are positioned in a posterolateral orientation relative to the right chambers, posteroanterior projection alone is not sufficient to adequately assess lead position (Figure 7.12). Inadvertent lead placement in the left chambers may easily be missed unless lateral projections are included in the evaluation. Besides providing information on lead position, chest X-ray also helps to identify the number and type of leads present (such as unipolar or bipolar, active or

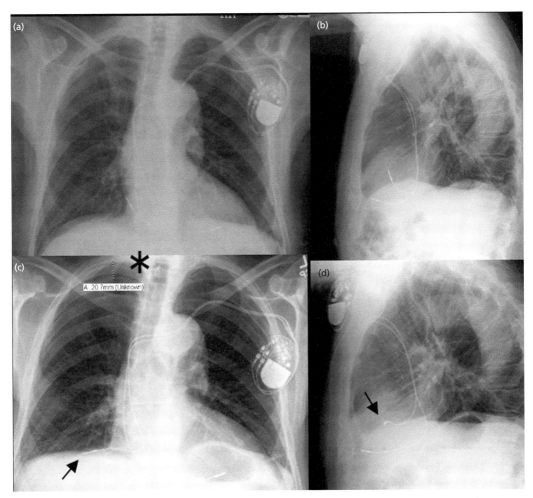

Figure 7.11 (a) Posteroanterior and (b) lateral chest X-ray 24 hours after a pacemaker implantation using active fixation leads. The atrial lead is located in an anterolateral position in the right atrial appendage. The right ventricular lead is placed in the anterior free wall/apical area. The patient presented 3 weeks later with right-sided diaphragmatic stimulation. There was no sensing or pacing with the right atrial lead but diaphragmatic capture was reproduced with high pacing output. This symptom commonly occurs when the right atrial lead pulls back to the superior vena cava and pacing results in phrenic nerve capture. In this case the cause for diaphragmatic stimulation was right atrial perforation (c, d). Note the migration of the right atrial lead tip (arrows). The lead was found in the pleural space and there was evidence of a small asymptomatic pneumothorax (*). The patient was receiving chronic high-dose oral steroid therapy at the time of the implant, which is a significant risk factor for lead perforation.

passive fixation, pacemaker or ICD lead; Figure 7.2). Company-specific radiographic markers of the pacemaker may be identified and adequate connection of the lead pins confirmed (Figure 7.1). Certain lead abnormalities, such as integrity failure or fracture, may also become apparent on an X-ray and X-rays are primary screening tools for certain complications related to the pacing system (Figure 7.13).

Electrocardiographic manifestations of pacer malfunction

Interpretation of electrocardiogram

Abnormal pacer function may be suggested by a telemetry strip or a 12-lead ECG and consultations to pacemaker clinics are common for this reason. When one faces a challenge in analyzing

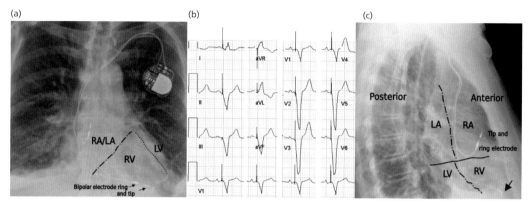

Figure 7.12 Chest X-ray and ECG features of a typical dual-chamber pacing system. (a) Posteroanterior projection of a chest X-ray. The dash–dot line delineates the approximate location of the atrioventricular (AV) groove and the dotted line approximates the septum between the right ventricle (RV) and left ventricle (LV). The right atrial lead is an active fixation bipolar lead (screw visible at the tip), whereas the RV lead is a passive fixation bipolar lead. There is significant overlap between the RV and LV in this view. (b) ECG features of typical RV apical pacing. There is left axis deviation with purely negative, left bundle branch block-like QRS morphology in V1. (c) Lateral X-ray projection in the same patient. The dash–dot line illustrates the septum between the left and right chambers and the solid line indicates the AV groove. The arrow marks the RV lead tip. LA, left atrium; RA, right atrium.

an ECG strip, the first task is to identify the intrinsic cardiac complexes, the underlying atrial rhythm, and the presence of P waves and QRS complexes. The presence of P waves, but occasionally even QRS complexes, may not be evident, especially from a single-lead ECG. Multiple ECG leads should be examined if there are uncertainties. It is important to look for clues such as presence of a T wave despite a "missing" QRS complex. This may be the case when the QRS vector is small or relatively isoelectric in a particular lead (Figure 7.14). The isoelectric QRS vector is occasionally seen in TTM strips. The next step is to search for pacing artifacts and establish their relationship and timing to intrinsic complexes (P wave, QRS). Once pacing artifacts are identified, electrical capture of the related cardiac chamber has to be evaluated (i.e. pacing artifact consistently followed by P wave or QRS complex; Figure 7.15). Based on timing of the pacing spikes, the base rate, AV interval, ventriculoatrial (VA) interval and AA interval should be determined if possible. Measurements of these basic pacing intervals on a 12-lead ECG and their correlation with intrinsic cardiac events often clarify device behavior without further need of device testing. It is important to note that digital ECG recording systems may

reduce or eliminate pacing artifacts due to filtering or assign pacing artifacts spuriously. Electrical artifacts may also be recorded as signals from non-cardiac devices; therefore, just like any other test, ECGs should be interpreted in the clinical context (Figure 7.16).

A standard 12-lead ECG with pacing is helpful for identifying the pacing site by analyzing the QRS vector and morphology. This is even more important with the advent of increased use of His and left bundle branch pacing. An ECG with pacing should ideally be collected following every device implant as a subsequent change in pacing morphology may indicate lead migration. In general, right ventricular (RV) apical pacing gives a left bundle branch block-type appearance and left superior axis (Figure 7.9). As the pacing site is moved up on the septum, the QRS axis gradually rotates to the right, reaching an inferior axis with pacing in the RV outflow tract. Typically, selective His pacing would show a pacing spike followed by a short isoelectric interval and subsequent QRS complex mimicking intrinsic activation (Figure 7.9). Parahisian pacing would show fusion between RV septal pacing and pure His capture. If there is right bundle branch block appearance in the precordial leads, then inadvertent left ventricular (LV) placement (via the arterial system or a

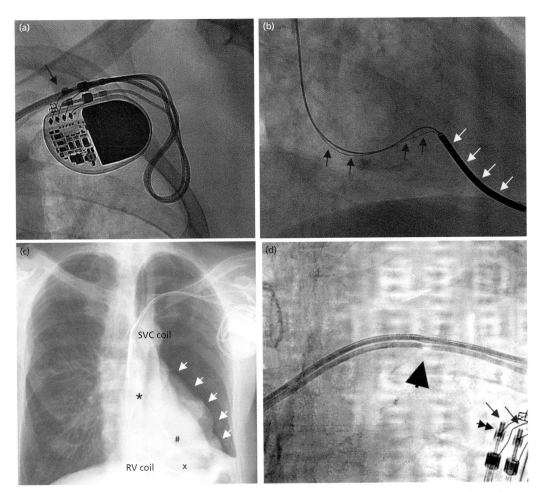

Figure 7.13 Examples of pacing system abnormalities on chest X-ray. (a) Loose pacemaker lead pin. Arrow points to a withdrawn lead pin, which now hardly reaches the distal screw location (atrial lead). Compare this to the correctly positioned ventricular lead pin. This patient was referred for lead revision due to noise, inappropriate mode switches, and pocket stimulation during pacing. During operative evaluation, lead was easily pulled out of the header without loosening the screw and diagnosis confirmed. The lead was functioning properly. (b) Typical fluoroscopy appearance of "inside-out" insulation failure of a St. Jude Medical Riata ICD lead. The black arrows point to the separation of high voltage (HV) cable from the remainder of the lead. Due to additional insulation around the HV cable, this finding is usually not associated with immediate electrical malfunction and currently the best long-term management for this lead abnormality is unclear. White arrows point to the HV coil. This lead component is only present in ICD leads. (c) Chest X-ray 24 hours following a biventricular ICD implant in a patient with severe chronic obstructive pulmonary disease. There is complete collapse of the left lung (white arrows). This patient was asymptomatic. There was tympany and complete loss of air movement in the left lung during auscultation. The patient fully recovered following chest tube placement. The superior vena cava (SVC) and right ventricular (RV) coils of ICD lead are marked. Bipolar active fixation atrial lead tip (*); left ventricular bipolar pacing lead tip (#); ICD lead tip (x). (d) Magnified X-ray image of lead fracture at the first rib/clavicle junction (large arrow). This is the typical site for subclavian crush injury. Small arrows point to the lead pins in the header. Both pins pass well beyond distal header posts (double arrowhead).

patent foramen ovale), perforation with LV pacing, deep septal LV pacing, or biventricular/coronary sinus pacing has to be considered. Mechanical lead complications may be further assessed with echo-cardiography, chest X-ray or CT. During biventricular pacing, there is fusion between RV and LV pacing and the QRS axis is mainly determined by the LV and RV lead locations and presence and

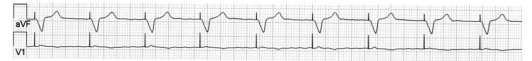

Figure 7.14 While pacer spikes are very well seen, assessment of proper capture in an ECG lead with isoelectric QRS complex is very difficult (V1). Analysis of a different ECG lead (aVF) reveals clear capture with each pacing stimulus.

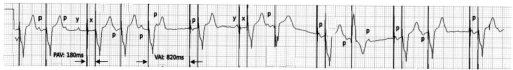

Figure 7.15 Example of how to analyze a paced ECG. The underlying rhythm is atrial pacing with frequent premature atrial complexes. All P waves are marked as P. There is consistent ventricular capture and two premature ventricular contractions (#8 and #10 beats). Dual-chamber pacemaker is present as evidenced by short coupled (180-ms) pairs of pacing artifacts and tracking of P waves. This latter fact is confirmed by the presence of irregularity in ventricular pacing which correlates with the P waves. Paced atrioventricular delay (PAV = 180 ms) and ventriculoatrial (VA) interval may be measured in the middle of the tracing (VAI = 820 ms). Pacemaker lower rate may be calculated as 1000 ms or 60 bpm. The last three atrial pacing spikes result in atrial capture. There are at least two P waves that are not sensed properly (marked as y). These are followed by close-coupled atrial pacing and functional non-capture (marked as x). The post-ventricular atrial refractory period (PVARP) is not known but P waves in a range of 400–440 ms following V pacing are tracked, suggesting that PVARP is shorter. The second P wave may be in the refractory period or below the sensing threshold. There is no evidence of atrial or ventricular capture abnormality. Pacemaker was interrogated and P-wave undersensing was confirmed and sensitivity adjusted.

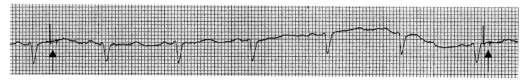

Figure 7.16 ECG recorded from a patient who received a gastric stimulator for gastric hypomotility. Pacing impulses (arrows) are unrelated to the cardiac cycle for obvious reasons.

extent of scar. In typical cases, the axis is rightward with a prominent R wave in V1 and Q wave in lead I [12]. A multilead ECG may help to identify intermittent loss of His or LV capture in a biventricular device that may otherwise be unnoticed in a single lead tracing (Figure 7.17). Occasionally, right bundle branch morphology may be seen with RV pacing. Repeating the ECG with repositioning of leads V1 and V2 one intercostal space below the standard position usually eliminates the right bundle branch pattern and confirms RV pacing [13]. In terms of atrial pacing localization, ECG has a limited role. A negative P-wave morphology in lead I suggests left atrial pacing and negative inferior P waves point to a pacing site near the coronary sinus. The duration of the paced P wave reflects intra-atrial conduction time and a shorter P-wave duration is expected with septal lead position.

Interpretation of intracardiac electrograms

Current pacemakers and ICDs provide a wealth of information both real-time as well as in stored data summaries, statistics. and stored EGMs. Real-time EGMs of the atrial and ventricular channel, surface ECG and marker channel is usually included in dual-chamber pacemakers. Additional EGM configurations may be available in ICDs or biventricular pacemakers. Connection of a surface ECG during interrogation should be encouraged especially in complex cases, when a far-field EGM is not available or in pacemaker-dependent patients (Figure 7.18). The first step during interpretation is analysis of the surface ECG and correlation with intracardiac EGMs. After distinguishing the atrial and ventricular signals, their relationship has to be determined

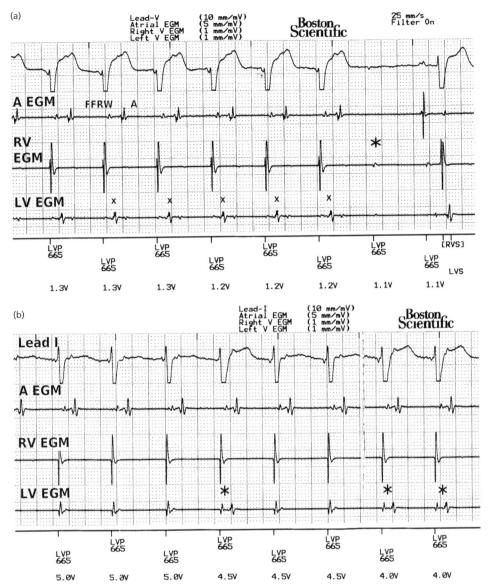

Figure 7.17 Left ventricular (LV) threshold assessment in a biventricular pacemaker. The first threshold test (a) showed LV threshold 1.2V, loss of capture at 1.1V (*). The last beat of the tracing is sinus at loss of capture with A–RV–LV activation. A closer look at the tracing reveals that the LV electrogram (EGM) (marked as x) follows the right ventricular (RV) EGM. This should not be the case during LV capture. These findings are most consistent with anodal capture at the RV ring electrode and loss of LV capture. When pacing takes place between the LV electrode (cathode) and a relatively small-sized RV ring electrode (anode), occasionally capture threshold may be lower at the anodal site, which results in RV capture. (b) Anodal capture was proven by pacing at a higher output. There is now RV/LV capture at 5V with intermittent LV capture at 4.5V and loss of capture at 4V (*). Also note a subtle change in QRS morphology in lead I with the RV-only beats. Multiple ECG leads or other ECG lead configuration would be helpful in this case. Anodal capture may be associated with arrhythmias. Commonly available configurations in biventricular pacemakers include LV tip–LV ring, LV tip–RV ring, and LV ring–RV ring. Other configurations may be available depending on the particular device and manufacturer. A different configuration was chosen for this patient (LV tip to can) for chronic pacing which eliminated anodal capture.

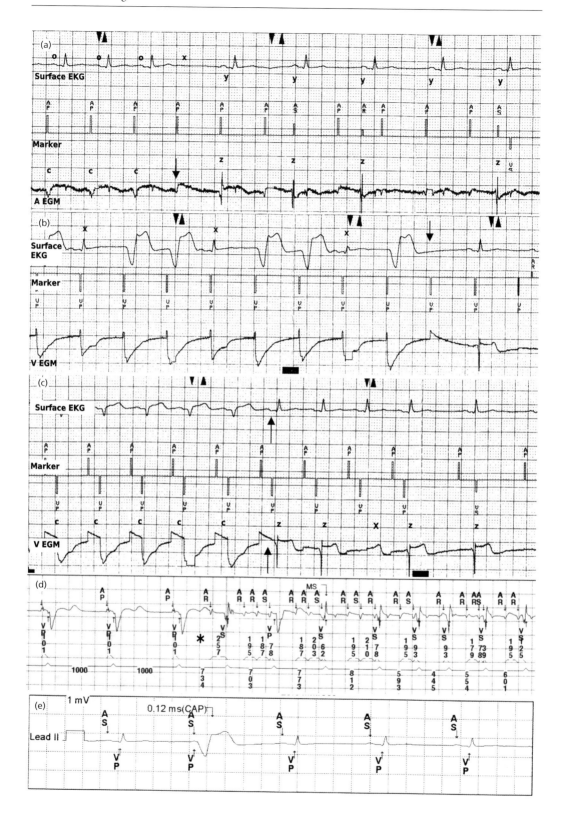

(i.e. presence of pacing and capture, driving chamber of an arrhythmia). The next step is to correlate the intracardiac EGMs to the marker channel signals. The marker channel reading is helpful because it signifies when the device senses events or paces, and correlating these to the intracardiac EGM components is key to evaluating proper function (Figure 7.18). Occasionally only a marker channel recording is available in stored event data, which is often helpful but in and of itself does not provide absolute diagnostic information as appropriate sensing or capture cannot be confirmed from the marker channel alone (Figure 7.19).

Problems with sensing

Undersensing or failure to sense

Pacing artifacts appearing at an unexpected interval often incite questions relating to sensing abnormalities. Sensing of intrinsic electrical activity is indeed of key importance as this is closely linked to pacemaker timing intervals. In most pacemakers there is a (programmable) fixed sensing level. If the amplitude of an intrinsic complex is less than the programmed sensitivity level, it will not be recognized by the device and the event will be disregarded in the timing cycle (Figure 7.15). There is occasionally confusion regarding the concept and relationship of sensitivity level to sensing. Only signals that measure above the programmed sensitivity are counted. Device sensitivity is increased (i.e. smaller signals will be detected by the device) when the programmed sensitivity level is decreased (e.g. sensitivity level programmed from 2.5 mV to 0.6 mV) and vice versa.

Sensing algorithms that automatically readjust the sensing level have been increasingly introduced into newer generation devices [14]. In ICDs, fixed sensing in the ventricle cannot be used as it would risk undersensing of ventricular fibrillation (if the sensing level is set too high) or cause oversensing (if the sensing level is set too low). For this reason variable sensitivity adjustment (or variable signal gain; Boston Scientific) is used in all defibrillators. In these algorithms, sensitivity is adjusted in a beat-to-beat fashion after each sensed or paced signal. Variable sensitivity is increasingly being applied in the atrial channel. Following a sensed

Figure 7.18 Interpretation of intracardiac electrograms. (a) Real-time atrial electrogram (A EGM) in addition to marker channel and surface ECG during atrial threshold testing. Atrial output is automatically decremented by the pacemaker (double arrowheads). Initially, there is atrial capture based on the presence of surface-paced P wave (o) with each stimulus and consecutive activation of the ventricle. Capture is lost (arrow) with only minor change in paced A EGM signal. There is no surface-paced P wave present (x) as capture is lost and sinus P waves (y) and local atrial EGMs (z) are dissociated from the pacing stimulus. Note the subtle difference between P-wave morphology of the paced (o) and intrinsic (y) P waves. (b) Ventricular threshold test in VVI mode in the same patient. As ventricular output is decremented (double arrowheads) there is variation of wide and narrow QRS complexes (x). This occurs because there is no ventriculoatrial (VA) conduction and every third beat is a capture beat from intrinsic sinus activation and not due to loss of capture. The clue is that on each occasion the narrow beat is simultaneous with the pacing spike. Once threshold is reached, true loss of capture is indicated (arrow) by the fact that no QRS complex follows the pacing spike and there is change in V EGM morphology. If intrinsic beats confuse the situation, pacing rate may be increased or, as shown in (c), DDD mode may be used.

Loss of capture is easily recognized with change in surface QRS morphology (arrow). The paced intracardiac EGM also changes: the deep negative component is absent (arrow) and subsequent conducted intrinsic activation appears (z). While there is no depolarization component present with beat x, there is a clear T wave indicating that local depolarization did occur (this may be confirmed with surface ECG). (d) Stored EGM strip from a Medtronic pacemaker. Some devices are capable of storing only one EGM, so either the atrial or ventricular signal has to be chosen. Availability of a summed EGM, as illustrated here, may be helpful in differentiating between certain arrhythmias. The EGM is recorded between the atrial and ventricular lead and provides the composite of the atrial and ventricular activation. Sequential AV pacing takes place at the first part of the strip until atrial fibrillation develops (*) and mode switch takes place (MS). Atrial depolarization is correctly marked as AS and AR; the larger ventricular signals are marked as VS. The strip confirms appropriate mode switch. (e) An example of automatic threshold testing in a Medtronic device. Note the markedly shortened PR interval with the beat during capture testing (CAP). As the device tests daily threshold (mainly at night), this finding during telemetry monitoring may cause some confusion regarding pacemaker function.

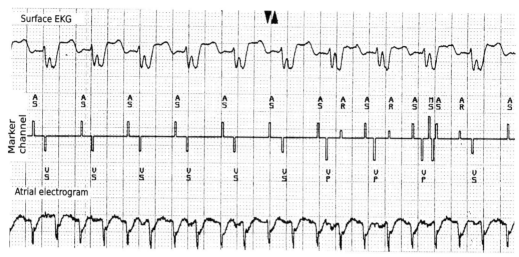

Figure 7.19 Tracing showing atrial undersensing during atrial flutter due to long post-ventricular atrial blanking period (PVAB). Only every other atrial electrogram (EGM) is identified as AS event, whereas the other atrial EGMs are blanked. PVAB was changed from 200 ms to 140 ms (double arrowheads), which resulted in unblanking of the flutter EGMs (AR) and appropriate mode switching (MS). If only the marker channel on the left of the strip had been examined without access to the atrial EGM, normal device function would have been indicated.

event, sensitivity is set to a percentage of the signal and after a brief blanking period sensitivity gradually increases until maximum programmed sensitivity is reached or a new signal is sensed. In some ICDs, specific aspects of sensitivity adjustments are programmable, which is a very useful feature for the management of sensing problems, such as T-wave oversensing. Algorithms for sensitivity adjustment in the atrial channel are similar but specific adjustments are made following a ventricular depolarization in order to minimize far-field R-wave oversensing. In newer generation pacemakers, ICD-type beat-to-beat adjustable sensitivity is increasingly used. Traditional pacemaker sensitivity level (especially in the ventricular channel) is generally programmed at 30–60% of the measured parameters. When choosing sensitivity settings for the ventricle, the polarity of the pacemaker system and clinical characteristics of the patient, such as pacemaker dependence and presence of variable amplitude signals [e.g. frequent premature ventricular complexes (PVCs)], have to be considered. Unipolar sensing (used uncommonly) predisposes to oversensing of non-cardiac signals and in pacemaker-dependent patients especially, avoiding it or programming a less sensitive setting is advised (Figure 7.20). Attention should

also be directed to excluding sensing abnormalities with oversensing PVCs, T waves, or myopotentials. Programming sensitivity in the atrial channel may be challenging. If there are intermittent atrial arrhythmias, measured EGM amplitude may change significantly between sinus rhythm and an atrial arrhythmia. If atrial arrhythmias are not sensed properly, intermittent palpitations may develop due to tracking and lack of mode switching (Figure 7.21). In contrast, if atrial sensitivity is set too low, non-atrial signals may be oversensed (such as far-field R wave) and result in inappropriate mode switching and loss of AV synchrony. In these cases, careful adjustment of atrial sensitivity and post-ventricular atrial blanking period (PVAB) is required (Figure 7.22). Optimization of PVAB and atrial sensitivity setting allows adequate monitoring of atrial arrhythmias and appropriate mode switching in most clinical situations [15].

In general, undersensing results in pacing at higher than expected rates (intrinsic signal would not inhibit pacing or modify pacing behavior due to lack of sensing). Undersensing may be caused by inadequate programming of sensitivity settings or refractory periods, lead or device failure, micro- or macro-dislodgement of leads, or a change in signal amplitude due to change in tissue characteristics.

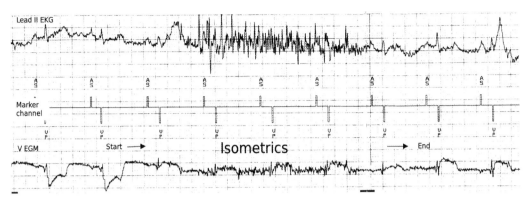

Figure 7.20 Noise on the right ventricular (RV) lead due to myopotential signals in a unipolar pacemaker. Following the initiation of isometric exercise, high-frequency noise is noted on the RV lead (isometrics). Sensitivity programming is adequate as there is no oversensing of the noise and atrial synchronous ventricular pacing takes place during the event.

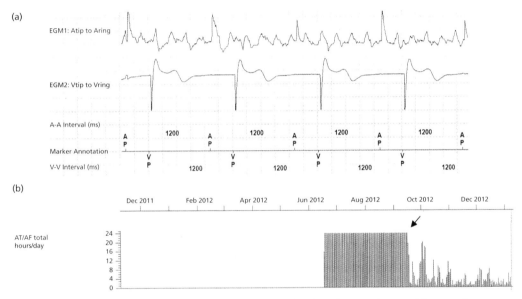

Figure 7.21 (a) An episode of atrial fibrillation (AF) with atrioventricular (AV) sequential pacing and undersensing of the atrial arrhythmia due to low-amplitude signals. AF is present while sequential AV pacing takes place. (b) Summary of daily AF episode burden. The patient developed persistent AF in June with appropriate detection of AF (AF present 24 hours/day). Starting in September (arrow), the measured AF burden is reduced due to decreased P-wave size and undersensing.

If the lead is otherwise functional and the position is stable, increasing the sensitivity is the first step. If programming options fail, lead repositioning may be required. Undersensing may occur even when sensitivity settings are programmed appropriately. Functional undersensing is an undersensing event that is due to an interaction between paced and sensed events and pacemaker refractory periods. As discussed in Chapter 6 in detail, blanking and refractory periods are designed to minimize oversensing of undesirable cardiac signals and to eliminate interactions between atrial and ventricular pacing and tracking. A blanking period is initiated in all chambers after each pacing stimulus to minimize the chance of oversensing of a polarization artifact or a far-field chamber signal. If an intrinsic cardiac depolarization occurs during the blanking period (i.e. PVC occurs at the time of atrial pacing), the signal may not be sensed (Figure 7.23). If a signal falls into the refractory

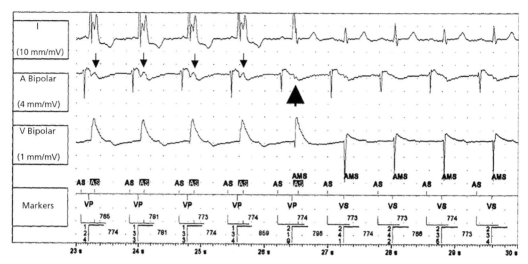

Figure 7.22 A method for testing far-field R-wave oversensing in order to assist with programming of the post-ventricular atrial blanking period (PVAB). For test purposes, atrial sensing is maximized (0.1 mV) and PVAB shortened to 60 ms. During ventricular pacing, far-field R-wave signals are oversensed. They fall in the post-ventricular atrial refractory period (PVARP) and are marked as AS refractory (white AS in black box; small arrows). Events in PVARP count toward mode switch counter and in this case inappropriate mode switch takes place (AMS; large arrow). Setting PVAB 25–30 ms longer than the VP–AS refractory interval would prevent future far-field R-wave oversensing. Alternatively, P-wave sensitivity may be decreased.

period, it will be sensed and added to the counters, but in most cases it will not reset or affect the pacing timing cycle. Clinically common examples are seen in the atrial channel during dual-chamber pacing. The post-ventricular atrial refractory period (PVARP) is designed to eliminate tracking of a retrograde P wave in order to prevent pacemaker-mediated tachycardia (PMT). If the P wave falls in the PVARP it causes functional undersensing. Clinical examples of this type of undersensing is seen following a PVC with retrograde conduction, upper rate behavior with pacemaker Wenckebach periodicity (during atrial tachycardia), or repetitive non-reentrant ventriculoatrial synchrony (see section Pacemaker-mediated tachycardia and repetitive non-reentrant ventriculo-atrial synchrony; Figures 7.24 and 7.25). Another common example is when PVAB covers every other flutter wave and results in undersensing of atrial flutter (Figure 7.23). Rapid pacing may also result in undersensing of ventricular tachycardia and delay or prohibit tachycardia therapy [16]. Functional undersensing is not a mechanical problem but rather a programming problem and invasive management is very rarely required. It is also important to recognize that under certain circumstances the pacemaker operates in asynchronous mode and intrinsic events are disregarded. A typical example of asynchronous pacing is seen when a magnet is placed over the device (magnet rate pacing) or when a device is programmed in asynchronous mode (for example, during a procedure that may result in EMI or oversensing of non-cardiac signals). Pacemakers may temporarily switch to asynchronous mode automatically if noise is sensed. This safety feature is designed to minimize the risk of asystole due to oversensing of non-physiological signals. R waves during rapid ventricular rate may fall in ventricular refractory period and cause asynchronous pacing (Figure 7.26).

Oversensing

Oversensing is an event when signals other than the local cardiac activation at the lead electrode site are counted as cardiac signal. These may include other signals from the heart (far-field signals from P and R wave or near-field T wave), myopotentials (from the diaphragm or pectoral muscle), or electrical artifact (noise) related to structural abnormalities in the lead/pacemaker system (fracture, insulation defect, header connection problem) or environmental effects (EMI). In general, ventricular oversensing

(a)

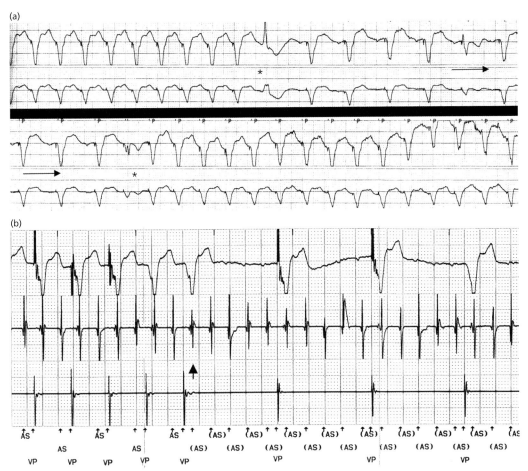

Figure 7.23 (a) An electrogram from a patient who complained of intermittent palpitations. The telemetry recording showed intermittent rapid ventricular pacing. The tachycardia is initiated and terminated with a premature ventricular contraction (PVC). The rhythm strip is a continuous recording. (b) Pacemaker interrogation confirmed atrial flutter and intermittent 2 : 1 ventricular pacing. In the first part of the tracing only every other atrial signal (AS) is sensed due to atrial blanking [every other atrial electrogram falls in the post-ventricular atrial blanking period (PVAB)]. The atrial flutter response was turned "on," which allows uncovering of atrial activity by extending the post-ventricular atrial refractory period (PVARP). The first AS falls outside the PVAB, and the second AS is refractory and not tracked due to the extended PVARP. This allows appropriate mode switching. The PVC in (a, *) changed the timing of the PVAB relative to the atrial depolarization and allowed uncovering of the flutter waves, whereas another PVC (*) had the opposite effect and 2 : 1 tracking recurred.

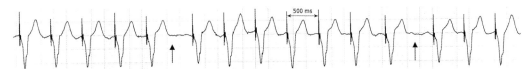

Figure 7.24 Rhythm strip from a patient with a dual-chamber pacemaker who developed atrial tachycardia. The tachycardia was tracked with ventricular pacing (pacing stimulus precedes each QRS) until upper tracking rate was reached at 120 bpm. Intermittent pauses are due to upper rate behavior as P wave falls in the post-ventricular atrial refractory period (PVARP) and is not tracked.

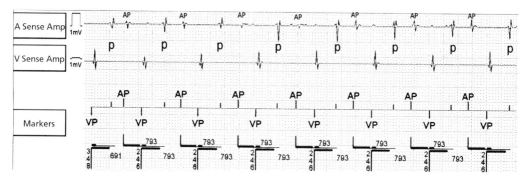

Figure 7.25 Repetitive non-reentrant ventriculoatrial synchronous rhythm. The arrhythmia is perpetuated by ventricular pacing with retrograde atrial conduction. Atrial activation falls in the post-ventricular atrial refractory period (PVARP) and is therefore not tracked (p). If it had fallen outside the PVARP, the result would be pacemaker-mediated tachycardia. Close-coupled atrial pacing (AP) likely does not capture the atrium (functional loss of capture) and is followed by ventricular pacing (VP), which starts the cycle again.

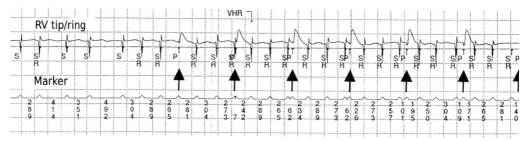

Figure 7.26 Ventricular high-rate episode recorded in a single-chamber Medtronic pacemaker. There is atrial fibrillation with rapid, irregular ventricular response. Ventricular cycle length exceeds the ventricular refractory period (VRP; set at 320 ms) and sensed events are counted as SR (sensed refractory). These events are disregarded for pacing timing purposes and pacing is initiated at 857 ms/70 bpm after two consecutive R waves fall in the VRP (first arrow). Asynchronous pacing continues, as indicated by the subsequent arrows (marked as P on the marker channel), as long as R waves fall in the VRP. VRP is reset after each refractory event. While SR events are not counted in pacemaker timing, they count toward the high-rate V counter in addition to asynchronous pacing.

manifests as pacing below the programmed rate. Atrial oversensing in dual-chamber devices may present with tracking and rapid ventricular pacing or mode switching to a non-tracking mode (if oversensing is recorded as atrial arrhythmia) (Figure 7.27). It is important to categorize these episodes appropriately as they may be sources of symptoms or may be precursors of a more serious problem. Furthermore, oversensing episodes may be recorded in the device memory as tachyarrhythmias and failure to recognize the correct diagnosis may trigger recommendations for otherwise unnecessary or inappropriate therapies (Figure 7.28).

Specific types and characteristics of oversensing and management are discussed in the following sections. In general, especially in an emergency situation when oversensing is suspected, magnet application over a pacemaker will initiate asynchronous pacing and prevent asystole (as long as there is a working pacemaker circuit and intact lead) until a programmer is available for reprogramming of the device. It is important to note that magnet application will not change the pacing mode in most ICDs, but will result in temporary suspension of ICD tachycardia therapy.

Cross-talk

An important and rare complication of dual-chamber pacing is AV cross-talk. A particularly dangerous situation may occur during dual-chamber pacing if, following atrial pacing, the electrical polarization from atrial pacing is sensed at the ventricular electrode and recorded as a sensed ventricular event. The result is inhibition of ventricular

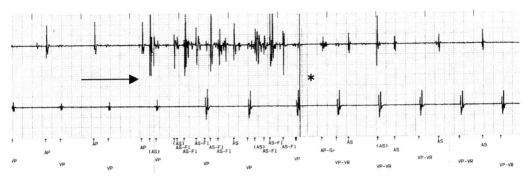

Figure 7.27 Atrioventricular (AV) sequential pacing with noise (arrow) due to lead integrity failure. Oversensing of electrical artifact results in tracking and subsequent mode switching to DDI mode (*). VP-VR, ventricular pacing with ventricular rate regularization.

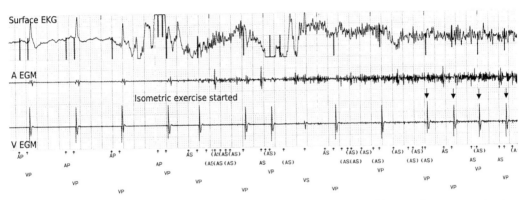

Figure 7.28 This patient with a dual-chamber unipolar system presented to routine follow-up with palpitations and over 2000 episodes of mode switches. Mode switch episodes due to pectoral muscle potential oversensing were reproduced with isometric exercise. Oversensing resulted in loss of AV synchrony and occasional rapid ventricular tracking (arrows).

pacing (Figure 7.29) and possible asystole. The post-atrial ventricular blanking period (PAVB) is used in the ventricular sensing algorithm to cover the immediate interval that follows an atrial pacing output signal in order to eliminate post-pacing signal oversensing. If the blanking period is not long enough, there is another programmable safety feature that may be used to minimize consequences of cross-talk, called safety pacing. This algorithm is applied to minimize the risk of asystole. There is a cross-talk window following the PAVB. If sensing occurs in this time interval, a ventricular pacing stimulus is initiated (at the programmed AV delay or shorter AV delay, depending on the specific device). This safety feature allows ventricular pacing even if there is oversensing in the cross-talk window (Figure 7.30). The best programming option to eliminate cross-talk is extension of the

PAVB. Other options include changing to VVI/VDD mode or reducing atrial pacing output and pulse width. Reducing the lower rate limit to allow intrinsic atrial activation may also help but it is not a safe long-term solution as lack of atrial pacing in the future is not guaranteed. Because of possible severe consequences of these events, in pacemaker-dependent patients it is prudent to check for cross-talk at the time of original or new implant.

Oversensing cardiac signals

These events include double counting of T, R, or P waves (Figure 7.31). Prolonged bradycardia may result from oversensing of intrinsic T wave (Figure 7.32). Electrolyte abnormalities, hyperkalemia and severe hyperglycemia or severe ventricular hypertrophy has been associated with permanent or temporary T-wave oversensing.

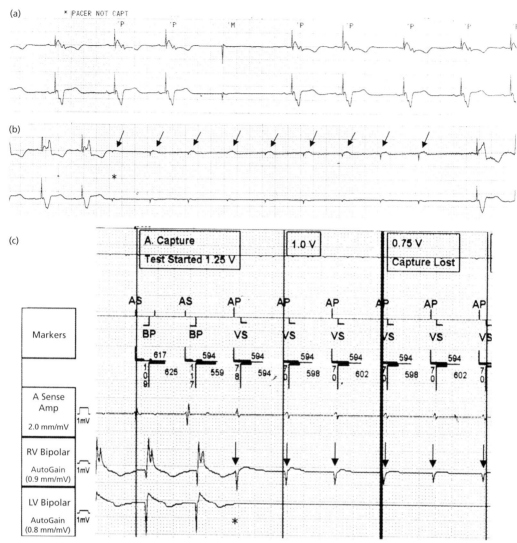

Figure 7.29 (a) Telemetry strip in a pacemaker-dependent patient following upgrade to a biventricular defibrillator. There is a pacing spike (M) followed by atrial capture but no ventricular conduction or pacing. This finding raises the possibility of cross-talk. There is no loss of capture here, contrary to the automatic alert at the top of the tracing. (b) Device interrogation reproduced asystole with atrial threshold testing in DDD mode (starting at the asterisk). The other possible explanation would be AAI pacing in a pacemaker-dependent patient. (c) Real-time electrogram during device interrogation confirmed cross-talk during atrial pacing. As the atrial threshold test started, a large signal became apparent on the right ventricular (RV) channel, corresponding to the atrial-paced event (arrows). This signal is sensed and the event is consistent with ventricular oversensing (AP followed by VS) and cross-talk. While there is no surface ECG, asystole is confirmed by the left ventricular (LV) lead electrogram (*). No safety pacing occurred in this case despite adequate programming.

T-wave oversensing may be eliminated by extending the ventricular refractory period in pacemakers. T-wave oversensing is a more common problem in ICDs because ventricular refractory periods are kept short to minimize the risk of undersensing ventricular fibrillation. In order to maximize sensing of small signals and without double counting cardiac signals or oversensing non-cardiac signals, either signal gain is modified (automatic gain control) or various sensitivity

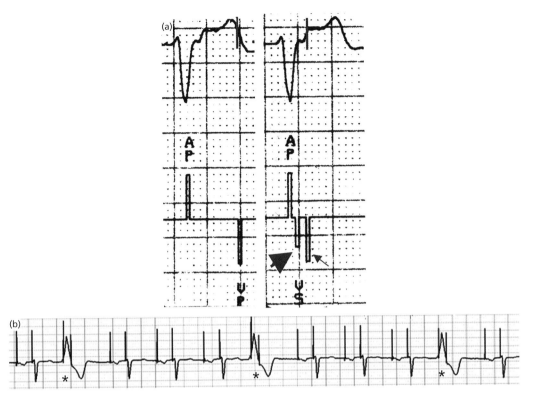

Figure 7.30 (a) Premature ventricular contraction (PVC) and simultaneous timing with atrial pacing. The first PVC falls in the post-atrial ventricular blanking period (PAVB) and is not sensed. Ventricular pacing occurs after atrioventricular (AV) delay times out, but is not captured as the ventricle is not fully repolarized. In the same patient, the second PVC occurs slightly later and now falls in the cross-talk window (large arrow) and initiates safety pacing (small arrow). Note that AV delay is now shorter. (b) ECG strip showing AV sequential pacing and capture. There are three PVCs marked with asterisks. PVC occurs at the time of atrial pacing and during the AV interval. A PVC is sensed in the cross-talk window (interval following PAVB). As this event, from the device-sensing prospective, may represent cross-talk, a ventricular pacing stimulus is delivered at a shorter paced AV delay to minimize the risk of asystole. Shorter AV delay reduces the chance of pacing in the vulnerable area of the T wave in case an intrinsic beat triggers safety pacing, as seen in this example. The beats marked (*) are pseudo-pseudofusion beats (see text for details).

adjustments are made with each sensed event (discussed in more detail in Chapter 8). T-wave oversensing may be eliminated in ICDs by decreasing sensitivity if R-wave sensing is adequate. In some ICDs, post-sensing or post-pacing sensitivity settings are programmable and may be tailored to the specific clinical problem (adjustment of initial sensing level and decay delay timing in St. Jude Medical and Biotronik devices). In some ICDs (St. Jude Medical) there is also a programmable option for setting different sensitivities for pacing and tachycardia detection purposes.

Although less common with modern bipolar pacemaker leads with closely spaced electrodes, oversensing of the far-field R wave is still the most common cause of atrial oversensing. The best way to eliminate this problem is to pay meticulous attention to lead placement and assure a minimized far-field R-wave recording during the implant procedure. However, complete elimination during implant may not be feasible or the problem may surface later with a change in P-wave signal amplitude or change in relative position of the lead and development of larger far-field signal. There are several programming options to eliminate far-field R-wave oversensing, such as decreasing atrial sensitivity (programming higher sensitivity cutoff if P-wave sensing allows), increasing PVAB, or minimizing RV pacing (Figure 7.22). In some Medtronic ICDs, atrial blanking is minimized and instead an algorithm

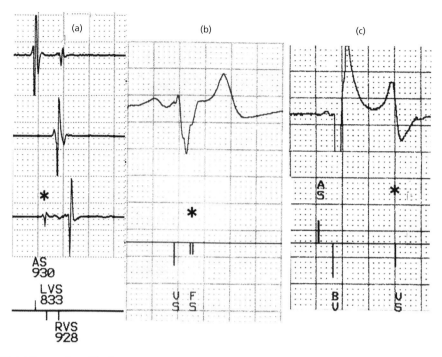

Figure 7.31 (a) Oversensing of far-field P wave on the left ventricular (LV) lead (*, marked as LVS in marker channel) in a biventricular device resulted in inhibition of pacing. Oversensing resolved after reprogramming the LV pacing configuration. (b) R-wave double counting in an ICD. The late component of the R wave is counted as an FS event (VF sensed; marked with an asterisk), which follows the VS marker at a non-physiological interval (120 ms). Oversensing occurred only with a particular premature ventricular contraction (PVC) morphology. Decreasing right ventricular (RV) sensitivity eliminated the problem. (c) Example of T-wave oversensing. VS marker times out with T wave on the electrogram (*). Adjustment in ventricular sensitivity mitigated the problem.

is used to differentiate between far-field signal oversensing and arrhythmias. As blanking is very short in these devices, atrial arrhythmia detection is markedly improved. If far-field signal is intermittent or the algorithm fails, traditional blanking periods may be activated in the most current devices.

Oversensing non-cardiac signals

Other sources of oversensing are related to myopotential oversensing, EMI, or intermittent noise due to lead chatter and lead or connection integrity failure (Figures 7.33 and 7.34). In many cases, the typical appearance of these artifacts establishes the diagnosis, but in atypical presentations it may be more complex to make the diagnosis. It is very helpful to identify the circumstances of the event. Artifacts during straining or coughing may point to diaphragmatic oversensing. Significant arm or upper body isometric exercise would be a typical trigger for pectoral muscle oversensing, especially in a unipolar system or lead insulation failure in the device pocket. On the other hand, noise with structural abnormalities has a probabilistic appearance, although certain events may trigger intermittent malfunction. For example, if noise is brought on by pocket manipulation, a faulty lead pin connection or lead integrity failure in the pocket has to be considered. Lead integrity abnormality usually results in changes in lead impedance, but alterations may be subtle and intermittent. Stable impedance does not completely rule out a structural abnormality. Other, non-structural causes of noise do not affect the lead impedance. As mentioned earlier, looking at the signal characteristics of noise is helpful. A myopotential oversensing signal is continuous and of sudden onset, high frequency, and relatively low amplitude. EMI is commonly sudden in onset, but EMG appearance may be different depending on the specific source. It is generally a high-frequency

(a)

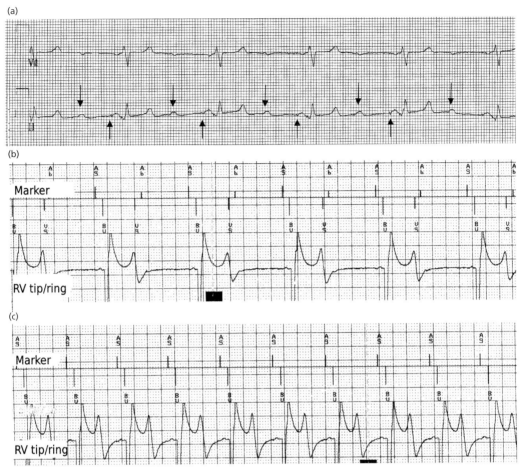

(b)

(c)

Figure 7.32 A pacemaker-dependent patient with biventricular pacing presented with new-onset heart failure symptoms. The pulse rate was in the 40s and the ECG strip (a) shows the presenting rhythm. There is alternating atrial pacing and sequential biventricular pacing (up arrows) and sinus without ventricular tracking (down arrows). (b) Device interrogation showed sinus rhythm with biventricular pacing (AS, BV). Every paced beat is followed by a VS marker which corresponds to the timing of the T wave. This represents T-wave oversensing. Usually T-wave oversensing results in a delay of the paced RR interval equal to the QT interval (350–500 ms). Here, as the T-wave signal is oversensed as an R wave, a blanking period is initiated. The sinus beat falls in the blanking period and is not tracked. (c) Once ventricular sensitivity was decreased, appropriate tracking resumed. This patient has a biventricular ICD and therefore programming options are limited (see text for further discussion).

continuous signal. Occasionally, a typical 60-Hz noise is seen. While the trigger for EMI commonly goes unrecognized unless there are symptoms, the time stamp from the event may help to correlate the activity or circumstances at the time of the event. Signal abnormalities related to structural hardware abnormalities usually cause make-or-break type EGM changes. Differentiation between conductor fracture and lead insulation failure is made primarily based on change in impedance (low with insulation failure, high with fracture).

It is important to remember that impedance changes may vary and temporarily revert to normal. Insulation abnormality on the ring electrode may be suspected when pacing impedance during unipolar (tip to can) pacing is higher than during bipolar pacing. Chest X-ray has low yield in finding lead fracture but it still should be obtained. Lead failure requires lead revision if clinically indicated. If lead integrity is intact, avoidance of the trigger or decreasing the sensitivity level is the best next step in management.

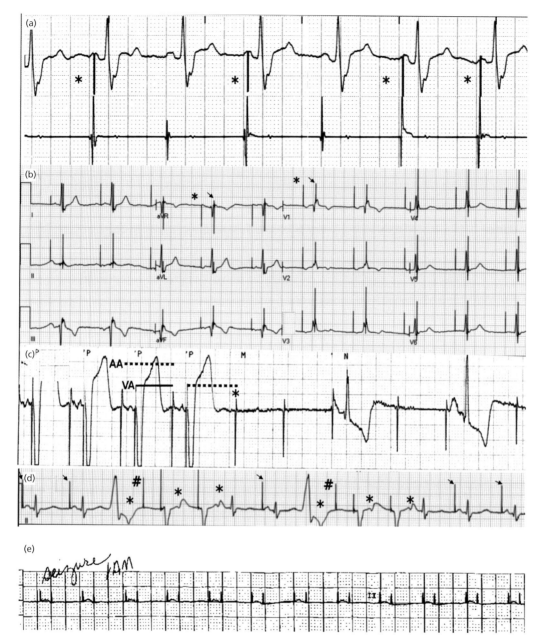

Figure 7.33 (a) Sinus rhythm at a rate close to the lower rate limit. Occasional atrial pacing occurs (*) and a pacing spike appears in the middle of the P wave. There is adequate sensing as the intrinsic P wave of <800 ms cycle length resets atrial pacing. Atrial capture is confirmed by subtle degree of fusion in the intracardiac atrial electrogram (EGM). (b) Example of atrioventricular (AV) sequential pacing. There is atrial capture (*) and conduction to the ventricle (arrows) with right bundle branch block (RBBB) in 1 : 1 fashion. Ventricular pacing stimulus is delayed and appears late in the QRS. This phenomenon is more common in the setting of RBBB due to delayed activation at the site of the right ventricular (RV) lead. RV capture cannot be ascertained from this ECG alone as fusion is not proven. (c) AV sequential pacing and capture during the first three beats, which is then followed by pacing artifacts without capture (pacing spike is not followed by depolarization). The measured paced AV delay is 200 ms. The VA time and AA time are indicated by the solid line and dashed line, respectively. The first non-captured beat (*) times out with the AA interval after the last paced ventricular beat. This pacing spike is most likely of ventricular origin. An atrial spike would time out with a shorter VA interval. Further investigations revealed evidence of lead fracture. (d) ECG example of dual-chamber pacing and premature ventricular contractions (PVCs). Atrial pacing is followed by atrial capture and normal intrinsic conduction (arrows). PVC causes retrograde P-wave activation (first asterisk). The retrograde P wave falls in the post-ventricular atrial refractory period (PVARP) and atrial pacing follows at a time when the atrium is still refractory (#) and causes (functional) loss of atrial capture (atrial pacing without capture). The next two P waves (*) are retrograde and the

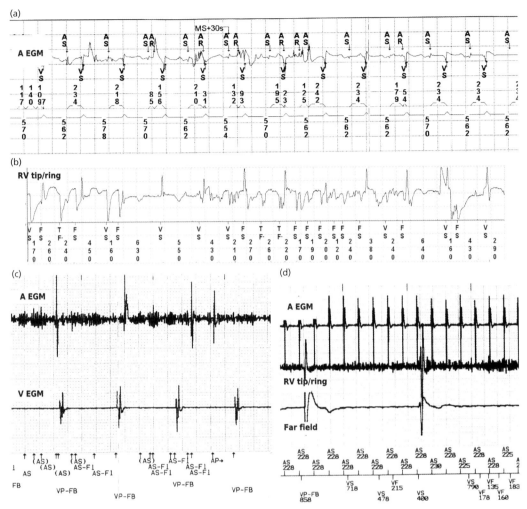

Figure 7.34 (a) Noise, recorded as mode switch episode, appearing in the right atrial lead electrogram following a pacemaker generator change. There was fluctuation in lead impedance and the patient complained of pectoral muscle stimulation during atrial pacing. Pectoral stimulation was worse with bipolar pacing and improved with unipolar pacing. The patient was referred for lead replacement with suspected fracture. Fluoroscopy showed inappropriate lead pin position and the diagnosis of loose set-screw was made during intraoperative testing (see corresponding Figure 7.13a). The lead was functioning normally. (b) Fracture of the pace/sense portion of a Spring Fidelis lead (Medtronic). There is evidence of make-or-break signals, occasional saturation of the amplifier, and non-physiological RR intervals. (c) Electromagnetic interference and noise on the atrial lead recorded as a mode switch episode. The origin of this noise could not be determined. (d) Diaphragmatic muscle potential oversensing in an ICD lead during straining. There is bradycardia due to inhibition of pacing and tachycardia detection is initiated. Oversensing resolved once ventricular sensitivity was decreased.

Figure 7.33 (*Continued*) result of ventricular pacing. The sequence is terminated with an echo beat (third and sixth asterisks). The same sequence is repeated with the subsequent PVC. (e) Rhythm strip from a pacemaker-dependent patient who developed seizure-like activity and syncope while in the hospital. His pacemaker was upgraded to an ICD 8 months before the admission. He suffered a myocardial infarction and was diagnosed with intermittent loss of ventricular capture due to exit block. The telemetry strip shows an episode of dual-chamber pacing with prolonged loss of ventricular capture. Exit block was likely due to recent myocardial infarction. Cross-talk is ruled out by the presence of ventricular pacing. He remained stable after RV pacing output was increased. This unusual event would have been prevented if the autocapture feature had been available in the device.

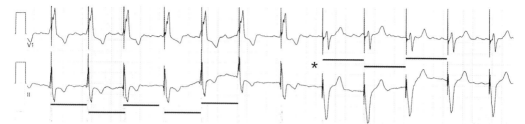

Figure 7.35 Example of atrial fibrillation in a patient with a pacemaker. The first part of the tracing shows atrial fibrillation and a right bundle branch QRS morphology. Pacing artifacts are apparent with each QRS complex but pacing spikes are timed *after* the initiation of the QRS. The RR intervals are irregular (marked with solid lines, which are of equal length) but the R wave always precedes the pacing spike. This is consistent with triggered pacing. Triggered pacing algorithms are commonly used in biventricular devices to maximize biventricular pacing during rapid atrial arrhythmias or premature ventricular contraction (PVCs). The upper rate of triggering is programmable and is usually set well above the base rate (see text for further details). Once the ventricular response slows (*), biventricular pacing ensues. Note that pacing rate has slowed and is regular. There is a change in QRS morphology and pacing spikes now precede each QRS. This is normal behavior. If rate control and/or rhythm control fails, AV node ablation may be considered in some patients.

Problems with capture

Pacing capture is confirmed by documenting a stable relationship between the pacing stimulus and depolarization of the cardiac chamber (Figure 7.15). If lack of capture is suspected (pacing artifact present without a corresponding cardiac depolarization), change in capture threshold, pacing during the cardiac refractory period, lead dislodgement, lead fracture, pacemaker generator failure, or metabolic factors have to be considered (Figures 7.30 and 7.33). Pacing artifact may appear within a P wave or QRS complex and occasionally considered a device malfunction. It is important to understand that a bipolar pacing electrode records summed electrical activity from a relatively small cardiac area and the local activation in these regions may be delayed compared to the earliest electrical activity of the corresponding chamber. In these situations a pacing artifact may be delayed compared to the surface ECG-onset of the signal (P wave or QRS complex) and result in fusion or pseudofusion. Fusion means that the surface EGM has a morphology "in-between" that of the intrinsic and purely paced complex, and evidence of fusion confirms capture from the pacing site. Pseudofusion occurs when the pacing artifact appears after the initiation of the P wave or QRS complex but the morphology is identical to the intrinsic complex. In this case, capture cannot be evaluated. An example of ventricular pseudofusion is illustrated in Figure 7.33. In biventricular devices, the goal is to provide maximum percentage ventricular pacing. All major manufacturers offer some sort of algorithm that allows triggered pacing in the left and/or right ventricle if a ventricular signal is sensed. The trigger for pacing is a sensed signal in either the RV or LV chamber (such as PVC or conducted atrial arrhythmia). Consequently, the resultant triggered pacing will occur at the time of earliest intracardiac sensing, which is commonly timed after the initial part of the QRS complex. Characteristically, a pacing spike is seen after the initiation of an R wave, mimicking loss of sensing or capture (Figure 7.35). The rationale for these algorithms is to provide at least some ventricular resynchronization to conducted complexes (or PVC) when ventricular response exceeds the programmed lower pacing rate. The effectiveness of these algorithms to change clinical response to biventricular pacing is moderate at best [17].

Pseudo-pseudofusion occurs when timing of an atrial pacing spike coincides with the early part of the QRS complex, commonly with a PVC. Due to summation of the atrial and ventricular EGMs on the ECG, these spikes appear to cause the QRS complex but in fact they are independent.

When there is loss of capture at a time when the myocardium is expected to be excitable, a broad differential diagnosis has to be considered. If loss of capture occurs within a few weeks of a new implant, once appropriate programming of output is confirmed, a search should be made for lead dislodgement, lead perforation, loose set-screw, air bubble

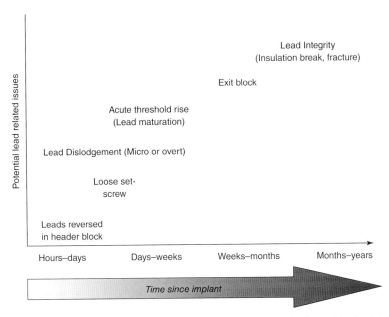

Figure 7.36 The relationship between time since device implantation and commonly observed lead-related complications.

in the header, or exit block at the lead tip due to maturation (Figure 7.36). Air in the pacemaker pocket in a unipolar pacing system may also result in change in pacing threshold. Under more chronic circumstances, every component of the pacing system has to be scrutinized (Table 7.3 and Figure 7.37). It is important to be methodical and systematic, starting with the generator (Is the battery status OK? Was pacing output programmed appropriately? Is there a change in threshold?) and the lead (Is there a change or fluctuation in lead impedance? Is it gradual or sudden change?). If the basic system parameters are stable, provocative arm exercise or pocket manipulation may result in noise and suggest lead integrity failure or myopotential oversensing. A chest X-ray helps to distinguish lead dislodgement and may identify lead fracture. Clinical history may reveal initiation of new medication (most typical examples are Vaughan Williams class I antiarrhythmic agents) or presence of renal failure. Abnormalities in serum electrolytes, such as acidosis or hyperkalemia, should always be considered (Figure 7.38). A history of recent procedures such as surgery, radiofrequency ablation, cardioversion, MRI scan, or radiation therapy may point toward secondary lead or device abnormality. Immediate manage-

ment should include increasing pacing output and treating the underlying cause(s) if possible. If an appropriate safety margin cannot be programmed, placement of a temporary pacemaker may be considered for select patients until final resolution of the problem (Figure 7.6).

Programming adequate pacing output is an important part of safe pacing therapy. Temporarily, an increased pacing output is required following a new lead implant to cover occasional threshold changes in the first weeks to months during the lead maturation period. Chronic output parameters are usually programmed 8–12 weeks after implant. Expert opinion may differ on programming chronic output but in general twice the voltage threshold at or close to chronaxie (pulse width 0.3–0.5 ms) gives an ideal safety margin with the least energy consumption. Determining the capture strength–duration curve may help to clarify the relationship of output programming to true safety margin. When choosing the final pacing output, the chance and consequences of loss of pacing have to be considered, bearing in mind the effects of programming on battery life (Figure 7.39). Obviously, safety of pacing should override concerns about battery longevity. For example in a pacemaker-dependent, end-stage

Table 7.3 Causes and management of sensing and pacing abnormalities

Cause	Treatment
Pulse generator hardware/software abnormality	Change device/load new software if possible
Suboptimal device programming	Reprogram device:
Subthreshold programming for capture	Increase pacing output (consider temporary increased pacing threshold during lead maturation period
Undersensing/oversensing	Adjust sensitivity
Inadequate mode selection	Change pacing mode
Inadequate rate-modulated pacing	Adjust rate-modulated pacing settings
Suboptimal programming of specific algorithms	Readjust algorithm
Functional abnormality	
Functional undersensing	Change blanking period or adjust refractory interval
Functional loss of capture	Optimize sensing parameters
Loose set-screw	Tighten set-screw
Lead insulation failure/fracture	Revise lead. Consider temporary unipolar mode
Lead dislodgement	Reposition lead and:
Loose suture sleeve	Tighten lead sutures
Inadequate lead redundancy during implant	Readjust lead redundancy
Twiddler's syndrome	Tighten device to pectoral muscle/consider subpectoral implant
Inadequate fixation to the myocardium	Reposition lead; consider different fixation mechanism
Change in lead–myocardium interface	
Exit block due to fibrosis/myocardial infarction; micro-dislodgement	Increase output/reposition lead or implant new lead
Electrolyte abnormality	Treat underlying problem, readjust pacing output or sensitivity if needed
New medication effect	Change medication or increase pacing output
Oversensing	If urgent intervention needed, apply magnet
Cross-talk	Change PAVB or eliminate atrial pacing
P, R, T wave oversensing	Adjust sensitivity or refractory period
Myopotential oversensing	Adjust sensitivity, use bipolar sensing
Electromagnetic interference (EMI)	Avoid triggers. Adjust pacing mode or use magnet during hospital procedures with EMI

PAVB, post-ventricular atrial blanking period.

renal disease patient, who may frequently have fluctuations in serum electrolyte levels, programming a borderline ventricular safety margin would be dangerous and many providers would consider programming output above twice the voltage safety margin. On the other hand, in a patient with sinus node disease who has chronotropic incompetence and occasional pauses with dizziness, most providers would be more aggressive in programming toward improving battery longevity. Current state-of-the-art devices now provide extensive options for management of changes in capture threshold. Daily automatic capture threshold measurements (Biotronik, Medtronic) or beat-to-beat capture management (Boston Scientific, St. Jude Medical) allow automatic testing and adjustment of pacing threshold to achieve adequate safety margin or consistent capture, respectively.

Pacing at an unexpected rate or sudden change in pacing rate

A sudden change in pacing rate often raises concerns about adequate pacemaker function. In some cases these represent normal pacemaker behavior, but symptoms may be associated with these events and proper understanding of the cause is important in order to provide reassurance or initiate proper programming changes. The main differential diagnoses for sudden rate changes include atrial arrhythmias or noise with tracking, initiation of PMT, a special algorithm

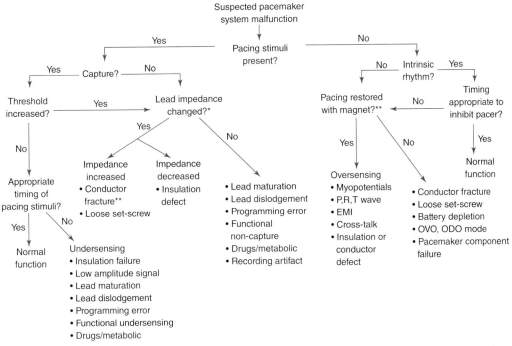

Figure 7.37 Simplified schematic for pacemaker trouble-shooting. EMI, electromagnetic interference. *, >300-Ω change in impedance as measured at the time of malfunction; **, or programmed to asynchronous mode; there can be no change in impedance with concomitant insulation failure.

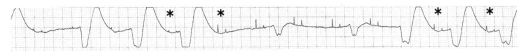

Figure 7.38 This tracing was recorded during severe hyperkalemia. Atrioventricular sequential pacing is present with loss of atrial and ventricular capture. Intermittent sensing is present following some of the wide QRS complexes, as evidenced by intermittent resetting of the pacing timing cycle (*).

(Table 7.4), sensor-based pacing, runaway pacemaker, and antitachycardia pacing. Specific details of these behaviors are discussed in the following section.

Special algorithms

Questions may occasionally arise when an ECG in a pacemaker patient shows no pacing artifacts or when the rate of pacing appears to be slower or faster than expected. The programmed base rate and sensor rate are the main determinants of minimum pacing rate in a single-chamber device. Exceptions to this rule may be seen when special algorithms are operational that are designed to minimize pacing near the intrinsic heart rate (e.g. rate hysteresis or sleep mode).

These algorithms allow the heart rate to decrease below the base rate, and pacing will only ensue again at the base rate if intrinsic heart rate reaches the lower hysteresis rate.

Most manufacturers provide algorithms to promote overdrive pacing over the intrinsic sinus rate in an attempt to regularize the rate, minimize short–long cycles, and reduce the occurrence of atrial arrhythmias. These algorithms manifest as accelerated atrial pacing rate (i.e. post mode switch response, atrial preference pacing, post mode switch overdrive pacing). Some of these algorithms are now less commonly used as their overall clinical benefit has been shown to be minimal. Rate regularization, especially during atrial fibrillation (AF), may help with rate control or reduce symptoms related to irregular

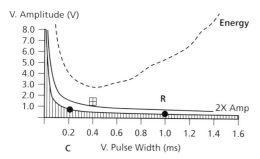

Figure 7.39 Print-out of calculated strength–duration curve in a Medtronic pacemaker. The device measures voltage threshold at 1 ms (R, rheobase) followed by pulse width threshold at twice rheobase voltage (C, chronaxie). The safety margin setting for 2× amplitude is indicated. For illustration purposes, a dotted line of relative energy expenditure per pacing stimulus has been manually added. Increasing the voltage at the extreme left part of the strength–duration curve or multiplying the pulse width above 0.4 ms would result in a rapid increment in energy without providing an appropriate safety margin in capture. In the current example, a 2× amplitude safety margin at a pulse width of 0.1 ms would require about a 4-V amplitude output and result in similar safety as programming 2 V at 0.2-ms pulse width. Similarly, increasing the pulse width above 0.6 ms (without changing the amplitude) would not meaningfully improve the safety margin but would increase energy expenditure significantly.

ventricular rate. Accelerated pacing rate may be seen when these algorithms are operational (e.g. ventricular rate regularization, conducted AF response). More recent data point to adverse effects from unnecessary pacing, especially in the right ventricle. Increased RV pacing has been shown to promote systolic dysfunction and AF [18,19]. Algorithms are now increasingly used to allow intrinsic ventricular activation, employing either AV search hysteresis or special hybrid pacing modes. These hybrid pacing modes (RythmIQ™, Boston Scientific; Managed Ventricular Pacing™, Medtronic; SafeR™, LivaNova) may cause unusual ECG presentations, such as very prolonged PR interval, occasional AV block, and sudden changes in AV timing (Figure 7.40). Temporary changes in AV timing may also be seen during automatic threshold testing in certain devices. As capture is determined by measuring the evoked response, fusion with intrinsic rhythm has to be minimized. Ventricular capture test algorithms achieve this by temporary shortening of the AV interval (or acceleration of the pacing rate in single-chamber devices) for the duration of the threshold test (Figure 7.18e).

Sudden accelerated pacing may be seen when pacing treatment is programmed "on" for management of cardioinhibitory autonomic syndromes. Algorithms may initiate accelerated pacing rate for 1–2 min (or longer if desired) if the intrinsic rate suddenly decreases significantly (e.g. rate drop response, sudden brady response; Figure 7.41).

In certain advanced pacemakers, programmable antitachycardia pacing (ATP) therapy is available for the treatment of atrial arrhythmias. After the tachycardia is detected, bursts of rapid overdrive pacing are initiated in an attempt to terminate the arrhythmia. Multiple rounds of pacing may be programmed for these episodes and present as cycles of rapid atrial pacing. Ventricular ATPs are frequently used in ICDs for treatment of ventricular tachycardia.

Triggered pacing

In dual-chamber devices, complex interactions between atrial- and ventricular-sensed events and pacing may be encountered depending on the programmed pacing mode (discussed in Chapter 6). In the commonly used DDD mode, lower rate pacing is determined by the base rate whereas faster rate may be due to atrial tracking or sensor-based pacing rate (Figure 7.23). On the other hand, if the intrinsic rate exceeds the base rate and sensor-modulated rate, pacing will be inhibited and this is normal pacemaker behavior. Depending on the clinical circumstances, these episodes may be asymptomatic or may be associated with palpitations or, rarely, with more severe hemodynamic compromise.

In DDD mode, at the initiation of an atrial tachycardia or AF, tracking will take place if mode switch is not programmed "on" or until the algorithm is initiated (Figure 7.42). If noise occurs in the atrial channel and tracking is programmed "on," pacemaker behavior is often similar to what is seen during an atrial arrhythmia, such as tracking or mode switching. Maximum ventricular tracking or sensor rate will determine the peak paced heart rate. Intermittent palpitations and rate changes may also develop if there is periodical undersensing during an atrial arrhythmia. A common problem is seen with atrial flutter when tracking occurs at a 2 : 1 rate. In these cases, every other atrial signal falls in the PVAB while the other events are sensed and tracked up to the maximum tracking rate. Algorithms have been designed and used by all manufacturers that temporarily extend the PVARP,

Table 7.4 Pacemaker functions that may be interpreted as malfunction (pseudo-malfunctions)

	Diagnostic clue
Pacing when not expected	
Rate smoothing	Graded rate slowing toward lower rate limit
Rate drop response	Abrupt pacing 90–110 bpm after sudden slowing
Dynamic atrial overdrive	Atrial pacing after atrial ectopy
Ventricular rate regularization	Pacing after shorter VV intervals in atrial fibrillation or after PVC
Ventricular-based timing	Faster ventricular rate during A_pV_s–A_pV_p cycle
Safety pacing	Ventricular pacing with shortened AV delay
Separate mode switch rate or post-mode switch overdrive rate	Pacing during or after atrial tachyarrhythmia or oversensing
Atrial pace for AV resynchronization	Pacing simultaneous with PVC or delayed after atrial ectopy
Atrial pacing preference	Atrial pacing after atrial-sensed events
Automated capture determinations	Closely coupled stimuli for P wave or QRS, sudden increase in paced rates
No pacing when expected	
Hysteresis	Pause after sensed events
Rate smoothing	Graded rate acceleration toward upper rate limit
PMT intervention	Ventricular output absent after V_pA_s near upper rate limit
Mode switching	Failure to track atrial activity
Separate mode switch rate	Lower pacing rate during mode switch
Intrinsic AV conduction search	Periodic extension of AV delay
Non-competitive atrial pacing	Delay in atrial output following atrial sense in PVARP
Separate sleep rate	Reduced lower rate limit at rest
Atrial-based timing	Prolongation of VV interval during A_pV_s–A_pV_p cycle
Automatic sensing check	Periodic delay in pacing after prolonged pacing
MVP/RythmIQ/SafeR algorithms	AAI pacing behavior and allowed AV block (with pause) before switching to DDD mode
Apparent undersensing	
Mode switching	Failure to track atrial activity
PMT intervention	Failure to track single P wave during prolonged A_sV_p at upper rate limit
Rate-adaptive AV delay	Evidence of shorter AV delays at faster rates
Non-tracking modes (DDI, DVI, etc.)	Typical non-tracking behavior
Blanked flutter search	Failure to track P wave when atrial tracking at rate <2× TARP
Noise mode	Evidence of EMI
PVARP extension post PVC	Failure to sense P wave after PVC
MVP/RythmIQ/SafeR algorithms	Single ventricular events in AA interval do not reset atrial pacing

AV, atrioventricular; EMI, electromagnetic interference; MVP™, Managed ventricular pacing, Medtronic; PMT, pacemaker-mediated tachycardia; PVARP, post-ventricular atrial refractory period; PVC, premature ventricular contraction; RythmIQ™, AAI(R) with VVI back-up, Boston Scientific; SafeR™, AAI/DDD mode pacing, Sorin Group; TARP, total atrial refractory period.

which allows functionally undersensed atrial events to be uncovered and promotes proper mode switching (Figure 7.23). At the termination of an arrhythmia, reversal of these rate changes may be seen, going from tachycardia to sudden bradycardia. Different algorithms have been designed to minimize symptoms due to irregular ventricular rate by reducing sudden heart rate changes (rate smoothing up and down; ventricular rate regularization, Boston Scientific; conducted AF response,

Medtronic). These algorithms may be operational during an irregular rhythm and cause pacing at an unexpected rate. An example of these algorithms is illustrated in Figure 7.42.

Pacemaker-mediated tachycardia and repetitive non-reentrant ventriculoatrial synchrony

PMT remains a relatively common problem, although sustained episodes are less common with

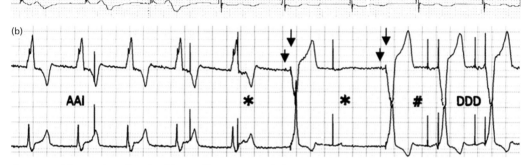

Figure 7.40 (a) Operation of an algorithm to allow intrinsic activation and minimization of ventricular pacing. The ventricular intrinsic preference (VIP™) algorithm extends the atrioventricular (AV) delay (in this example from 145 ms to 245 ms, marked by * and #, respectively) and allows intrinsic ventricular activation to take place. Note the change from VP to VS on the marker channel and wide to narrow QRS on surface ECG as the AV delay is extended and intrinsic conduction returns. (b) ECG showing managed ventricular pacing (MVP™) mode behavior. AAI pacing takes place at the beginning of the tracing with a very long AV interval. When AV block develops (first asterisk), AV pacing takes place with short (80 ms) AV interval (first double arrow). If AV block occurs in two of four beats (second asterisk), the device switches to DDD mode (#). The second AV block event (second asterisk) is also followed by AV pacing with a short AV delay. This is a typical response and represents normal pacemaker behavior.

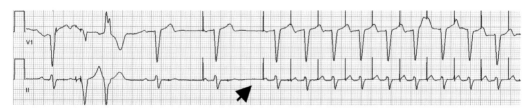

Figure 7.41 Rate drop response in a patient with carotid sinus hypersensitivity. There is a sudden drop in heart rate (following tracked premature atrial and ventricular contraction) to 50 bpm for two beats, which initiates dual-chamber pacing at 115 bpm for 2 min (arrow).

the advent of contemporary algorithms that are designed to prevent or identify and terminate them. The basic mechanism of the arrhythmia is persistent retrograde atrial conduction following ventricular pacing while the retrograde, non-refractory atrial signal is continuously tracked with ventricular pacing. Therefore beat-to-beat ventricular pacing and atrial sensing is necessary to

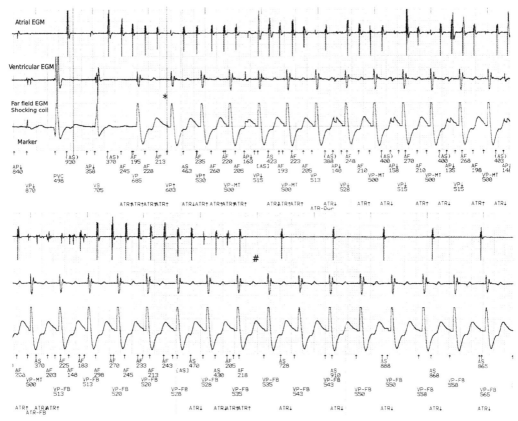

Figure 7.42 Continuous tracing retrieved from a dual-chamber ICD memory. Atrial fibrillation starts following a premature ventricular contraction (PVC) and retrograde conducted P wave. Atrial depolarization falls in the post-ventricular atrial refractory period (PVARP) and subsequent atrial pacing results in initiation of the arrhythmia. There is an immediate change in pacing rate due to tracking. Subsequent pacing occurs at a slower rate due to rate smoothing down (*; VP↓). There are also examples in the tracing when rate smoothing causes accelerated pacing (VP↑) in order to reduce irregularity in the ventricular rate. Once appropriate mode switching occurs, ventricular-based timing slowly decreases the pacing rate (fallback rate, marked as VP-FB) until the programmed mode switch lower rate is reached (note the slowing of pacing rate in the bottom tracing). At the termination of the arrhythmia (#), VVI pacing continues with ventriculoatrial (VA) dissociation until the mode switch episode terminates (not shown in the tracing). Symptoms in this patient may occur due to rapid pacing or loss of AV synchrony.

maintain the circuit. Pacing mode has to be dual chamber with tracking (PMT cannot be present with AAI, DDI or VVI pacing or ventricular sensing). The most common initiating trigger is a PVC with retrograde atrial conduction that falls outside of the atrial refractory period (PVARP). Other common situations include loss of atrial sensing and failed capture of the subsequent atrial paced beat due to tissue refractoriness. Subsequent ventricular pacing would cause retrograde atrial activation and initiate PMT. Other possibilities are long programmed AV delays with ventricular pacing, loss of atrial capture (spontaneously or during atrial threshold test), or termination of VVI pacing to DDD mode (i.e. ventricular threshold test in VVI mode, end of mode switching). Symptoms may be absent or include palpitations or pacemaker syndrome. The tachycardia rate is variable, depending on VA conduction time and programmed AV delay but typically the heart rate is close to the upper tracking rate. PMT may be terminated by applying a magnet over the device. This will initiate a temporary, asynchronous, non-tracking pacing mode. Alternatively, non-tracking pacing modes may be programmed "on" with a programmer. For long-term management, first reversible causes

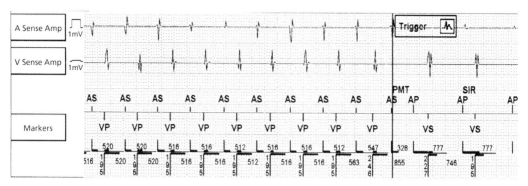

Figure 7.43 Treatment of pacemaker-mediated tachycardia (PMT) in a St. Jude Medical device. Once the PMT algorithm is satisfied, sensed atrial signal (AS) is not tracked but is followed by atrial pacing. This breaks the tachycardia and atrial pacing at sensor-indicated rate (SIR) resumes.

need to be treated, such as adjusting sensing or pacing output. The next step is to test for retrograde conduction and measure retrograde VA conduction time. Based on this information, PVARP has to be extended beyond the timing of the retrograde atrial signal. If indicated, special PMT prevention algorithms may be used, such as atrial pacing on PVC or PVARP extension on PVC. If PMT is detected and the PMT termination algorithm is programmed "on," most commonly the PVARP is extended for one beat and this usually breaks the tachycardia (Figure 7.43). Occasionally, upper rate behavior is misclassified by the device as PMT. In this case, there will be no change in tachycardia rate when extended PVARP is applied, but one beat that falls in the PVARP would not be tracked.

Elimination of PMT may result in another, relatively common arrhythmia, called repetitive non-reentrant ventriculoatrial synchrony. The initiating triggers are the same as for PMT. In this case, the retrograde P wave falls in the atrial refractory period (PVARP) and therefore in this case it is not tracked. As the event is recorded in PVARP, it is not counted for timing purposes in most devices. Thus, if the next V–AP interval is short enough to find the atrium inexcitable, there will be functional loss of capture. Atrial pacing will be followed by ventricular pacing, which causes retrograde atrial conduction and the rhythm perpetuates. Algorithms are available to limit this problem. For example, the non-competitive atrial pacing algorithm (in Medtronic devices) takes into consideration the atrial event in PVARP (normally disregarded for timing purposes) and delays the

next atrial pacing event beyond the refractory period of the atrium (nominally 300 ms). Programming features that decrease the atrial escape interval (long AV delay, high atrial pacing rate) promote the development of this rhythm and vice versa. Symptoms are usually consistent with pacemaker syndrome and a high level of suspicion is required to make the diagnosis. In certain devices the event may trigger mode switching or cause arrhythmia and these episodes may be recorded in the device memory (Figure 7.44).

Sensor-driven pacing
Rate-modulated pacing is an important programing feature for patients with chronotropic incompetence. Sensors are used to obtain simulated information regarding activity level in order to mimic a physiological heart rate response that is appropriate for that level of activity. While there have been significant efforts to develop pacemaker algorithms for automatic adjustments in sensor-driven pacing rate, programming and fine tuning rate-modulating sensors, especially in an active and young person, may be challenging. Depending on the specific sensor or combination of sensors, there may be many instances in which inappropriate rate acceleration occurs. Some of the examples are detailed in this section. Activity sensors, such as accelerometers, monitor the movement and vibrations of the body. These sensors may activate during a bumpy car ride, air travel or helicopter ride, or in the hospital environment while moving the patient or tapping on the patient's chest. Other types of activities, such as cycling or swimming, may be undersensed.

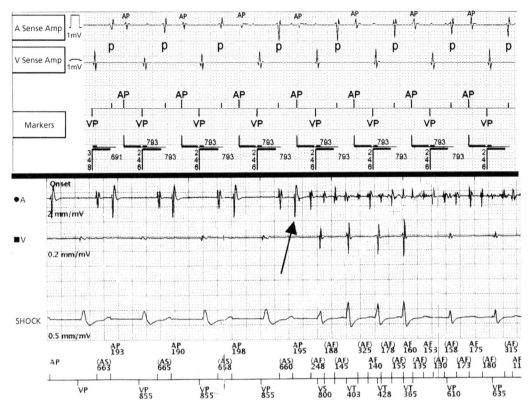

Figure 7.44 (*Top*) A recorded event that resulted in inappropriate mode switching. Ventricular pacing (VP) is followed by retrograde atrial conduction that falls in the post-ventricular atrial refractory period (p). When the ventriculoatrial (VA) interval times out (disregarding AS in the refractory period), atrial pacing (AP) takes place, which is closely coupled at the time that the atrium is refractory and there is functional loss of capture. Atrial pacing (AP) is followed by ventricular pacing (VP), which results in a retrograde P wave and the cycle continues. This arrhythmia is called repetitive non-reentrant ventriculo-atrial synchronous rhythm (RNRVAS). It may result in symptoms of pacemaker syndrome or arrhythmias. (*Bottom*) Another example of RNRVAS. The fouth ventricular pacing beat is followed by retrograde atrial conduction and early-coupled atrial pacing (arrow), which induces atrial fibrillation.

Minute ventilation sensors estimate exertion by measuring transthoracic impedance changes related to ventilation. Interference may occur in the hospital environment due to erroneous signals related to monitoring equipment, or during mechanical ventilation or an echocardiography examination. Hyperventilation or excessive arm movement may also promote sensor-driven pacing. QT sensor-based pacemakers are prone to false activation due to medication or ischemia-induced QT changes.

Runaway pacemaker

Runaway pacing, an uncontrolled rapid pacing above the programmed upper rate, is a serious medical emergency. Pacing rates from 150 to 1000 bpm have been reported, but most cases were described decades ago. The number of these rare abnormalities has dramatically declined with hermetic sealing of the devices, improvements in battery technology, and development of central processing unit (CPU)-controlled circuitry. A runaway pacemaker, in contrast to PMT, is not affected by magnet application, and pacing rate with PMT will not exceed the programmed upper pacing or tracking rate. If emergency VVI pacing through the programmer fails to override the tachycardia, emergency device replacement is required.

Analysis of stored device data

Storage and diagnostic capabilities in modern pacemakers and ICDs continue to improve. Automatic sensing and pacing capabilities and auto-adjustment and increasing compatibility with telephone or internet-based remote monitoring has revolutionized the follow-up of device patients. Summaries of basic device information, in addition to lead trends, extensive counter information and stored EGMs, allow the providers to obtain a more complex picture of the clinical events and device information.

Basic device data

The basic device data provide the backbone information regarding the device function. This includes information about battery status, which may be expressed as measured battery voltage, battery impedance, or graphic expression as "gas-gauge." In most contemporary devices there is also a reference regarding predicted battery longevity. Lead parameters include the measured impedance, lead polarity, and previous threshold measurements. Longitudinal recording of lead impedance and threshold information are invaluable during long-term follow-up and serve as a reference to identify lead abnormalities. Programming parameters summarize the pacing mode and basic intervals (Figure 7.45).

Event counters and histograms

There are different counters and statistical data that provide a rough overview of pacing and rhythm characteristics. These measured parameters include percentage of pacing and sensing in each chamber, and frequently subgroups are also identified, such as the relationship of sensing and pacing between the chambers. Counters often show the number of premature atrial contractions or PVCs and percentage of atrial arrhythmias or mode switches. The validity of the data summary depends on the characteristics of the patient and also the sensing accuracy of the pacemaker (Figure 7.21). For example, a high percentage of ventricular pacing may be present in the device counter yet this finding in the presence of pseudofusion may not indicate a true clinical ventricular pacing percentage. Critical review of the histograms (graphical or numerical) is helpful in screening for chronotropic incompetence or identifying possible clusters of tachyarrhythmias based on bimodal distribution of heart rate. This information may be useful in patients who have unexplained palpitations and helps to direct further investigations (Figure 7.46).

(a)

Figure 7.45 (a, b) Basic device data and programming parameters from a print-out of a Boston Scientific pacemaker. Battery and lead status, lead parameters, and atrial arrhythmia burden are shown in graphical fashion (b). These graphs suggest that there are episodes of atrial arrhythmias and also variable P-wave amplitude. Decreased P-wave amplitude is seen during atrial arrhythmias. Appropriate diagnosis cannot be made based on these data unless intracardiac tracings are available to confirm these findings. The discontinuities in the right ventricular (RV) amplitude recordings are the result of frequent RV pacing and periodic inability to record R-wave measurement. There is some variation in lead impedances in this patient without any lead abnormality.

(b)

Settings

Ventricular Tachy Settings

Ventricular Tachy EGM Storage	On
Detection Rate	160 bpm

Atrial Tachy Settings

ATR Mode Switch   170 bpm   DDIR

Brady Settings

Mode	DDDR	Pacing Output	
Lower Rate Limit	60 ppm	Atrial	3.5 V @ 0.5 ms
Maximum Tracking Rate	120 ppm	Ventricular	Auto 1.6 V @ 0.4 ms
Maximum Sensor Rate	130 ppm	Sensitivity	
Paced AV Delay	130 - 180 ms	Atrial	Fixed 0.25 mV
Sensed AV Delay	110 - 150 ms	Ventricular	Fixed 2.5 mV
A-Refractory (PVARP)	370 ms	Leads Configuration (Pace/Sense)	
V-Refractory (VRP)	230 - 250 ms	Atrial	Bipolar
		Ventricular	Bipolar
		Rate Adaptive Pacing	
		Minute Ventilation	On
		Accelerometer	Passive

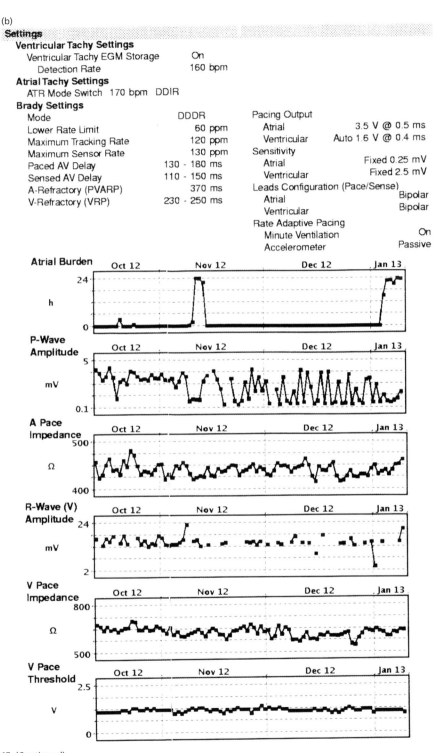

Figure 7.45 (Continued)

Brady Counters	Reset Before Last 2012	Since Last Reset 2012
Counters		
% A Paced	77	58
% V Paced	95	95
Intrinsic promotion		
AV Search +		
% Successful	0	0
Rate Hysteresis		
% Successful	0	0
Atrial Burden		
Episodes by Duration		
< 1 minute	0	175
1 min - < 1 hr	0	236*
1 hr - < 24 hr	0	51
24 hr - < 48 hr	0	0
> 48 hr	0	0
Total PACs	39.7K	126.8*
Ventricular Counters		
Total PVCs	3.4K	21.5K
Three or More PVCs	7	3

Histograms Reset Before Last (2012) (Continued)

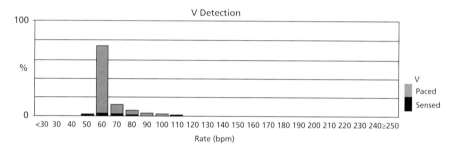

Histograms Since Last Reset (2012) (Continued)

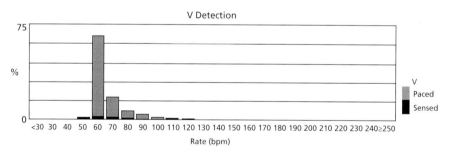

All Events Since last Reset (11 Oct 2012)

2013 14:07	ATR at 308 bpm, Avg V Rate in ATR: 0 bpm
2013 14:03	ATR at 209 bpm, Avg V Rate in ATR: 72 bpm
2013 14:02	ATR at 182 bpm, Avg V Rate in ATR: 74 bpm
2013 14:00	ATR at 181 bpm, Avg V Rate in ATR: 75 bpm

Figure 7.46 Summary page of counters and histogram information from a Boston Scientific pacemaker. A significantly increased number of premature atrial contractions and high rate atrial events are seen compared to the previous device check (*).

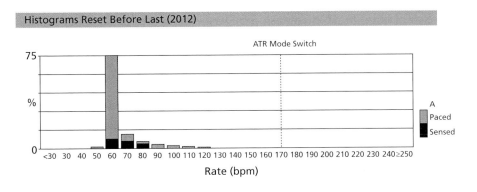

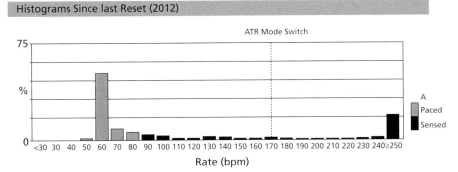

All Events Since Last Reset (Continued) (2012)

2013 13:56	ATR at 185 bpm, Avg V Rate in ATR: 72 bpm
2013 13:46	ATR at 279 bpm, Avg V Rate in ATR: 90 bpm
2013 13:43	ATR at 220 bpm, Avg V Rate in ATR: 105 bpm
2013 13:31	RV Auto
2013 11:52	ATR at 216 bpm, Avg V Rate in ATR: 71 bpm
2013 11:47	ATR at 225 bpm, Avg V Rate in ATR: 104 bpm
2013 11:32	ATR at 217 bpm, Avg V Rate in ATR: 78 bpm
2013 11:30	ATR at 181 bpm, Avg V Rate in ATR: 81 bpm
2013 11:17	ATR at 198 bpm, Avg V Rate in ATR: 77 bpm
2013 09:58	ATR at 296 bpm, Avg V Rate in ATR: 75 bpm
2013 09:47	ATR at 168 bpm, Avg V Rate in ATR: 81 bpm
2013 09:44	ATR at 194 bpm, Avg V Rate in ATR: 85 bpm
2013 15:32	NonSustV at 163 bpm
2012 17:40	NonSustV at 153 bpm
2012 13:29	NonSustV at 144 bpm
2012 20:14	NonSustV at 174 bpm
2012 17:21	NonSustV at 163 bpm
2012 19:58	PMT at 120 bpm
2012 16:30	NonSustV at 168 bpm
2012 14:26	NonSustV at 163 bpm
2012 23:25	NonSustV at 163 bpm
2012 23:25	NonSustV at 162 bpm

Figure 7.46 (Continued)

Arrhythmia logbook and stored electrograms

EGM recording capability is a very important component of the diagnostic armamentarium in pacemakers and ICDs. In most pacemakers, a memory segment is reserved for storing EGMs. Based on the clinical circumstances and the type of problem investigated, or perhaps for general screening purposes, programming may be adjusted to focus EGM recording on certain types of arrhythmias or abnormalities, such as atrial or ventricular tachyarrhythmias, PMT episodes, mode switches, or noise reversion recording (may be helpful when there are questions about environmental effects or a

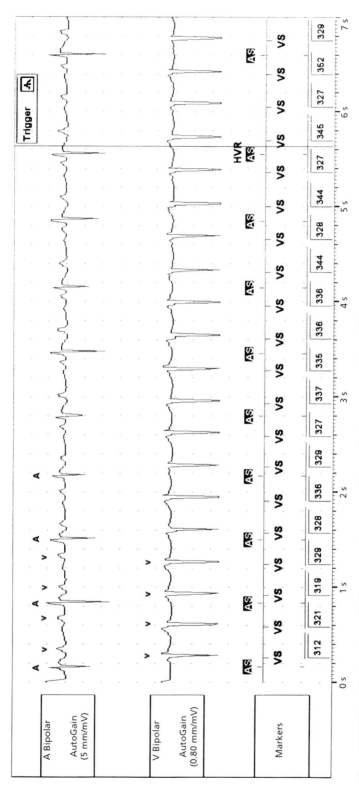

Figure 7.47 High ventricular rate recorded in a pacemaker memory. The ventricular channel (V Bipolar) records a tachycardia (VS, ventricular sensed) with dissociation from the atrial signals (A Bipolar; AS, atrial sensed). The first four ventricular events are marked with (v). The corresponding (v) signals on the atrial channel represent far-field R-wave signals. Large electrograms (A) are dissociated atrial signals. The presence of VA/AV dissociation indicates that the episode is ventricular tachycardia.

Table 7.5 Pacemaker mode selection.

Clinical problem	Optimal	Acceptable	Avoid
Sinus node dysfunction with intact AV node	DDD(R) long AV delay AAI(R) with special mode-switch algorithm	Single-chamber AAI (age <70 years) Single-chamber VVI (significant comorbidities, rare pacing expected) Single-chamber leadless pacemaker (rare pacing is expected)	
Moderate AV nodal disease	DDD(R) long AV delay AAI(R) with special algorithm	Single-chamber VVI (significant comorbidities, rare pacing expected) Single-chamber leadless pacemaker (rare pacing is expected)	Single-chamber AAI
Third-degree AV block	DDD(R) or VDD mode	Single-chamber VVI (significant comorbidities, rare pacing expected)	Single-chamber AAI
Permanent AF	Single-chamber VVI(R) Leadless pacemaker		Single-chamber AAI Dual-chamber pacemaker

AF, atrial fibrillation; AV, atrioventricular.
Source: modified from Gillis AM, Russo AM, Ellenbogen KA, *et al.* HRS/ACCF expert consensus statement on pacemaker device and mode selection. *J Am Coll Cardiol* 2012;60:682–703.

subclinical lead integrity problem). While these logbooks and EGMs are very helpful for clarifying symptoms or identifying arrhythmias, the EGMs have to be carefully reviewed and adjudicated as misclassification may frequently occur (Figures 7.2d, 7.26, 7.34, 7.44, and 7.47).

Pacemaker programming

Pacing mode and pacing rate

The detrimental effects of pacing have been increasingly recognized and the importance of selecting the appropriate mode and rate of pacing may mitigate these risks. Before any device implantation, a thoughtful evaluation of the clinical circumstances and expected disease progression should be taken into consideration in order to choose the most appropriate type of device, such as single, dual, biventricular, His or leadless pacemaker, or ICD (see Chapter 3). Device selection will also significantly

influence (and may limit) future programming options. The availability and need of special device features or algorithms, such as high ventricular sensitivity (for His pacemaker), rate drop response, or availability of atrial ATP, may be important and should also be considered. The first step in device programming is the selection of pacing mode. A general approach is summarized in Table 7.5 and also discussed extensively in Chapter 3. Next, basic pacing parameters are programmed, such as rate, output, AV delay, and refractory periods. While nominal settings work most of the time, individualized programming of rest rate, upper tracking and sensor rate, and AV delay may prevent future problems (Table 7.6). Finally, after an initial 1–3 months' acute maturation phase, chronic pacing output settings may be programmed and special pacing algorithms may be activated. Examples of common clinical scenarios that may require special programming are detailed in Table 7.7.

...

Table 7.6 Basic pacemaker programming

Clinical problem	Program rate response "on" Rationale: To treat chronotropic incompetence	Program AV delay (AVD) Rationale: Extend to minimize RV pacing if possible. Consider hemodynamic consequences of short or long AV delay. Use dynamic AV interval with higher pacing rates to avoid 2 : 1 tracking or pacemaker Wenckebach	Program PVARP, PVAB and other considerations Rationale: Decrease chance of PMT, minimize VA cross-talk. Nominal settings are usually acceptable. Check VA conduction and extend PVARP beyond timing of retrograde P wave. Check atrial signal during ventricular pacing and adjust PVAB to cover far-field R wave if oversensing present
Sick sinus syndrome with normal AV node function	If CI present: yes If no CI: no	Extend AVD; use special algorithms (MVP, RhythmIQ, VIP)	Consider hemodynamic consequences of long AV delay
Intermittent AV block	If CI present: yes If no CI: no	Extend AVD; use special algorithms (MVP, RhythmIQ, VIP)	Consider hemodynamic consequences of long AV delay
Third-degree AV block	If CI present: yes If no CI: no	Fixed AVD at rest, use dynamic AV delay for higher rates	Avoid atrial-only pacing modes Avoid algorithms to minimize RV pacing

AV, atrioventricular; CI, chronotropic incompetence; MVP™, Managed ventricular pacing, Medtronic; PMT, pacemaker-mediated tachycardia; PVAB, post-ventricular atrial blanking period; PVARP, post-ventricular atrial refractory period; RV, right ventricular; RythmIQ™, AAI(R) with VVI back-up, Boston Scientific; VIP™, Ventricular intrinsic preference, St. Jude Medical; VA, ventriculoatrial.

Table 7.7 Programming considerations in special clinical situations

Special situation	Problem	Solution
Atrial flutter	2 : 1 functional undersensing, rapid tracking due to lack of mode switching	Apply algorithm to uncover flutter wave Perform flutter ablation Consider atrial ATP
Atrial fibrillation (AF)	Undersensing, intermittent mode switching and tracking with rapid pacing	Increase atrial sensitivity Use DDI(R) mode Treat AF
Drug-refractory atrial tachycardia	Symptomatic tachycardia Inappropriate tracking due to slow atrial tachycardia rate	Adjust medical therapy; program atrial ATP therapy; perform ablation Use lower atrial tracking rate setting and higher rate response pacing rate if chronotropic incompetence is present Consider atrial ATP therapy
Post AV node ablation	Sudden bradycardia, risk of TdP	Use temporary increased base rate (80–90 bpm) for 30–90 days
Hypertrophic cardiomyopathy with dynamic outflow obstruction	Heart failure	Use short AV delay to force RV apical pacing Use negative AV hysteresis
Cardioinhibitory vasovagal syncope, carotid sinus hypersensitivity	Occasional sudden bradycardia but no pacing needs otherwise	Use low base pacing rate and program rate drop algorithm "on"

ATP, antitachycardia pacing; AV, atrioventricular; RV, right ventricular; TdP, torsade de pointes.

References

1 Jacob S, Shahzad MA, Maheshwari R, Panaich SS, Aravindhakshan R. Cardiac rhythm device identification algorithm using X-rays: CaRDIA-X. *Heart Rhythm* 2011;8(6):915–922.

2 Hauser RG, Hayes DL, Kallinen LM, *et al*. Clinical experience with pacemaker pulse generators and transvenous leads: an 8-year prospective multicenter study. *Heart Rhythm* 2007;4(2):154–160.

3 Burri H, Senouf D. Remote monitoring and follow-up of pacemakers and implantable cardioverter defibrillators. *Europace* 2009;11(6):701–709.

4 Maisel WH, Moynahan M, Zuckerman BD, *et al*. Pacemaker and ICD generator malfunctions: analysis of Food and Drug Administration annual reports. *JAMA* 2006;295(16):1901–1906.

5 Manegold JC, Israel CW, Ehrlich JR, *et al*. External cardioversion of atrial fibrillation in patients with implanted pacemaker or cardioverter-defibrillator systems: a randomized comparison of monophasic and biphasic shock energy application. *Eur Heart J* 2007;28(14):1731–1738.

6 Last A. Radiotherapy in patients with cardiac pacemakers. *Br J Radiol* 1998;71(841):4–10.

7 Swerdlow CD, Gunderson BD, Ousdigian KT, *et al*. Downloadable software algorithm reduces inappropriate shocks caused by implantable cardioverter-defibrillator lead fractures: a prospective study. *Circulation* 2010;122(15):1449–1455.

8 Liu J, Brumberg G, Rattan R, Jain S, Saba S. Class I recall of defibrillator leads: a comparison of the Sprint Fidelis and Riata families. *Heart Rhythm* 2012;9(8):1251–1255.

9 Sharif MN, Wyse DG, Rothschild JM, Gillis AM. Changes in pacing lead impedance over time predict lead failure. *Am J Cardiol* 1998;82(5):600–603.

10 Hirschl DA, Jain VR, Spindola-Franco H, Gross JN, Haramati LB. Prevalence and characterization of asymptomatic pacemaker and ICD lead perforation on CT. *Pacing Clin Electrophysiol* 2007;30(1):28–32.

11 Essebag V, Champagne J, Birnie DH, *et al*. Nonphysiologic noise early after defibrillator implantation in Canada: incidence and implications. A report from the Canadian Heart Rhythm Society Device Committee. *Heart Rhythm* 2012;9(3):378–382.

12 Ammann P, Sticherling C, Kalusche D, *et al*. An electrocardiogram-based algorithm to detect loss of left ventricular capture during cardiac resynchronization therapy. *Ann Intern Med* 2005;142(12 Pt 1):968–973.

13 Coman JA, Trohman RG. Incidence and electrocardiographic localization of safe right bundle branch block configurations during permanent ventricular pacing. *Am J Cardiol* 1995;76(11):781–784.

14 Alings M, Vireca E, Bastian D, *et al*. Clinical use of automatic pacemaker algorithms: results of the AUTOMATICITY registry. *Europace* 2011;13(7):976–983.

15 Kolb C, Wille B, Maurer D, *et al*. Management of far-field R wave sensing for the avoidance of inappropriate mode switch in dual chamber pacemakers: results of the FFS-test study. *J Cardiovasc Electrophysiol* 2006;17(9):992–997.

16 Wood MA, Ellenbogen KA, Shepard RK, Clemo HS. Atrioventricular sequential pacing by an implantable cardioverter defibrillator during sustained ventricular tachycardia: what is the mechanism? *J Cardiovasc Electrophysiol* 2002;13(12):1309–1310.

17 Kamath GS, Cotiga D, Koneru JN, *et al*. The utility of 12-lead Holter monitoring in patients with permanent atrial fibrillation for the identification of nonresponders after cardiac resynchronization therapy. *J Am Coll Cardiol* 2009;53(12):1050–1055.

18 Tse HF, Lau CP. Long-term effect of right ventricular pacing on myocardial perfusion and function. *J Am Coll Cardiol* 1997;29(4):744–749.

19 Sweeney MO, Hellkamp AS, Ellenbogen KA, *et al*. Adverse effect of ventricular pacing on heart failure and atrial fibrillation among patients with normal baseline QRS duration in a clinical trial of pacemaker therapy for sinus node dysfunction. *Circulation* 2003;107(23):2932–2937.

CHAPTER 8

The implantable cardioverter–defibrillator

Michael E. Field and Michael R. Gold
Medical University of South Carolina, Charleston, SC, USA

Introduction

The implantable cardioverter–defibrillator (ICD) was developed by Mirowski and colleagues about 40 years ago and the Food and Drug Administration (FDA) approved its use in 1985 [1]. The early pulse generators were large, requiring thoracotomy for epicardial patch placement, and were implanted in the abdomen. This complex surgery resulted in postoperative hospitalization averaging approximately 1 week. The pulse generators had a longevity of less than 2 years and almost no diagnostic or pacing capabilities. These early devices were approved by the FDA for use only in patients who had survived multiple cardiac arrests. Over the ensuing decades, ICD technology has evolved to provide detailed information on the morphology and rates of arrhythmias, stored electrograms (EGMs) before, during, and after therapy, as well as diagnostic information to assess lead integrity and physiological states such as activity and heart failure. The miniaturization of components, including processors, has allowed the downsizing of pulse generators so that the implantation procedure approaches those of pacemakers, with outpatient placement now routine. Despite the marked reduction in size and increase in diagnostic capabilities, device longevity is now greater than 10 years even for complex multilead systems. While the fundamental role of ICDs is still the treatment and prevention of sudden cardiac death (SCD), these devices have the capabilities to treat multiple problems, including bradyarrhythmias, atrial arrhythmias, and heart failure with cardiac resynchronization therapy (CRT). Most recently, subcutaneous lead systems have been developed for ICDs that have no transvenous components [2]. In this chapter, the contemporary indications, device selection, and programming are reviewed.

Indications

ICD implantation is now indicated for both secondary prevention of SCD among patients who have experienced life-threatening arrhythmias (i.e. ventricular tachycardia or fibrillation) and a wide variety of cohorts at increased risk for SCD (i.e. primary prevention). A summary of the current indications for ICD therapy is given in Table 8.1 and a flow chart summarizing the indications for ICD implant in Figure 8.1.

Secondary prevention

Three major multicenter randomized trials (AVID, CIDS, CASH) involving patients who had suffered a cardiac arrest or life-threatening ventricular arrhythmia compared ICD with antiarrhythmic

Cardiac Pacing and ICDs, Seventh Edition. Edited by Kenneth A. Ellenbogen and Karoly Kaszala.
© 2020 John Wiley & Sons Ltd. Published 2020 by John Wiley & Sons Ltd.

Table 8.1 Summary of indications for ICD therapy in patients with ischemic and non-ischemic cardiomyopathy

Secondary prevention	
Class I ICD is recommended	• Survivors of sudden cardiac arrest due to VT/VF or those with hemodynamically unstable VT (LOE: B-R) or stable sustained VT (LOE: B-NR) not due to reversible causes • Unexplained syncope in a patient with ischemic cardiomyopathy with inducible sustained monomorphic VT on EP study (LOE: B-NR)
Class IIa ICD is reasonable	• Syncope presumed to be due to VA in an NICM patient who does not meet ejection fraction criteria for a primary prevention ICD (LOE: B-NR)
Primary prevention[a]	
Class I ICD is recommended	• Ischemic cardiomyopathy or NICM with LVEF ≤35% and NYHA class II or III heart failure despite GDMT[b] (LOE: A) • LVEF ≤30% ischemic cardiomyopathy, NYHA class I heart failure despite GDMT[b] (LOE: A) • Ischemic cardiomyopathy with NSVT and LVEF ≤40% with inducible sustained VT or VF at EP study[b] (LOE: B-R)
Class IIa ICD is reasonable	• Non-hospitalized patients with NYHA class IV who are also candidates for cardiac transplantation or an LVAD[b]
Class IIb ICD may be considered	• NICM with LVEF ≤35% despite GDMT and NYHA class I heart failure (LOE: B-R)

[a] Primary prevention patients with ischemic cardiomyopathy should be at least 40 days post myocardial infarction and at least 90 days post revascularization prior to ICD placement unless another urgent indication for pacing present.
[b] All ICD indications apply to patients if meaningful survival of greater than 1 year is expected.
EP, electrophysiology; ICD, implantable cardioverter–defibrillator; GDMT, guideline-directed management and therapy; LOE, level of evidence; LVAD, left ventricular assist device; LVEF, left ventricular ejection fraction; NICM, non-ischemic cardiomyopathy; NYHA, New York Heart Association; NSVT, non-sustained VT; VA, ventricular arrhythmia; VT, ventricular tachycardia.
Source: Al-Khatib *et al.* [19]. Reproduced with permission of American Heart Association.

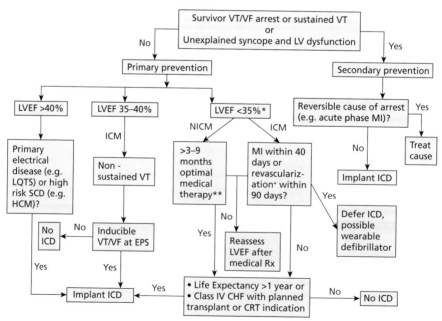

Figure 8.1 Flow chart summarizing indications for ICD implant. CHF, congestive heart failure; CRT, cardiac resynchronization therapy; EPS, electrophysiological study; HCM, hypertrophic cardiomyopathy; ICM, ischemic cardiomyopathy; LQTS, long QT syndrome; LVEF, left ventricular ejection fraction; MI, myocardial infarction; NICM, non-ischemic cardiomyopathy; Rx, therapy; VF, ventricular fibrillation; VT, ventricular tachycardia; *, LVEF <35% with class II or III heart failure or <30% with class I heart failure; **, period of 3–9 months on medical therapy after new diagnosis of NICM not part of scientific guidelines but required for reimbursement in the USA; +, surgical or percutaneous procedures.

drug therapy, predominantly amiodarone [3–5]. Although only one of these trials was sufficiently powered to be statistically significant for a reduction in total mortality, the results of all three are consistent and a meta-analysis demonstrated that ICD therapy was associated with a 28% reduction in the relative risk of death and a 50% reduction in arrhythmic death [6]. An analysis of the AVID trial results demonstrated that the benefit was confined primarily to patients with a left ventricular ejection fraction (LVEF) below 35% [7]. These studies established the benefit of ICD therapy as first-line treatment among patients with a history of life-threatening arrhythmias, particularly those with left ventricular (LV) dysfunction. In clinical practice, this therapy is used routinely in all secondary prevention patients other than those with significant comorbidities limiting longevity; thus, antiarrhythmic drugs have been relegated to adjunctive therapy to reduce arrhythmia recurrence rates.

Primary prevention of cardiomyopathy

Evidence supporting ICD therapy for primary prevention in ischemic cardiomyopathy

A primary prevention ICD is placed to prevent SCD in a patient who has not had sustained ventricular tachycardia (VT) or sudden cardiac arrest (SCA), but who is at increased risk for these events. The Multicenter Automatic Defibrillator Implantation Trial (MADIT) and Multicenter Unsustained Tachycardia Trial (MUSTT) were the first large multicenter studies of ICD use in primary prevention of SCD. These trials evaluated patients with coronary artery disease, LV systolic dysfunction, non-sustained VT, and inducible sustained monomorphic VT. In the MADIT trial, patients were randomized to receive either an ICD or "conventional" medical therapy, which was most commonly amiodarone [8]. In the MUSTT study, patients were randomized to either no antiarrhythmic therapy or drug therapy guided by electrophysiological study. In 46% of the latter group, ICD implantation was performed because of the failure of antiarrhythmic drugs to suppress inducible arrhythmias [9]. Despite these differences in study design, the results of the two trials were remarkably similar. ICD use decreased mortality by greater than 50% in these cohorts with ischemic cardiomyopathy [10]. Despite these results,

the impact of these studies was limited in part by the requirement for electrophysiological studies, documentation of non-sustained VT, restriction to patients with ischemic cardiomyopathy, and suboptimal medical therapy in both arms of the trials.

A further analysis of MUSTT indicated limited prognostic value of the electrophysiological study for risk stratification [11]. For this reason, as well as those already noted, subsequent primary prevention trials were designed to simplify and broaden the identification of patients who would benefit from ICD placement. The MADIT II study was a prospective randomized trial of 1232 subjects with previous myocardial infarction (MI) and LVEF of 30% or less [12]. Spontaneous non-sustained VT or electrophysiological testing were not required for enrollment in this trial. The ICD and control groups had similar clinical characteristics, with 67% with congestive heart failure (CHF) [New York Heart Association (NYHA) class II–IV], a mean age of approximately 65 years, and mean LVEF of 23%. During a mean follow-up of 20 months, the mortality rates were 14.2% in the ICD group and 19.8% in the control group. The long-term 8-year follow-up of this trial showed persistence of the benefit, with a remarkably low number needed to treat of six patients to reduce one mortality.

The Sudden Cardiac Death in Heart Failure Trial (SCD-HeFT) was the first large multicenter primary prevention study to eliminate the inclusion criteria of coronary artery disease. In this trial, 2521 subjects with CHF (NYHA class II and III) and LV systolic dysfunction (LVEF ≤35%) were randomized, irrespective of etiology (i.e. ischemic or non-ischemic cardiomyopathies) [13]. ICD implantation was associated with a 23% reduction in all-cause mortality, but amiodarone showed no benefit. The benefit of ICDs was only observed among patients with mild (NYHA class II) CHF. Table 8.2 provides a summary of trials for the primary prevention of SCD with ICDs.

ICD therapy for primary prevention in patients with non-ischemic cardiomyopathy

Although patients with heart failure due to non-ischemic cardiomyopathy have an increased risk of SCD, the strength of the evidence supporting the use of ICD therapy in this population is weaker than that supporting ICD use in ischemic cardiomyopathy.

Table 8.2 Selected ICD trials for primary prevention of sudden cardiac death

Trial	No. of patients	Etiology	Major inclusion criteria	HR mortality (ICD)	P value
MADIT	196	ICM	EF ≤35%, NSVT, inducible VT	0.46	0.009
MUSTT[a]	704	ICM	EF ≤40%, NSVT, inducible VT	0.45[a]	<0.001
MADIT II	1232	ICM	EF ≤30%, prior MI	0.69	0.016
SCD-HeFT	2521	ICM and NICM	EF ≤35%, CHF NYHA class II or III	0.77[b]	0.007
DEFINITE	458	NICM	EF ≤35%, PVCs or NSVT	0.65	0.08
COMPANION[c]	1520	ICM and NICM	EF ≤35%, CHF NYHA class II or III, QRS >120	0.64[c]	0.003
DINAMIT	676	ICM	EF ≤35%, HRV, recent MI (<40 days)	1.08	0.66
CABG Patch	900	ICM	EF ≤35%, CABG, abnormal SAECG	1.07	0.64
DANISH	556	NICM	NYHA class II, III or IV (if CRT), EF ≤35%, increased NT-proBNP	0.87	0.28

[a] The MUSTT results listed are the adjusted relative risk for overall mortality for patients receiving electrophysiologically guided therapy with an ICD compared with no antiarrhythmic therapy.
[b] SCD-HeFT mortality is compared with guideline-directed medical therapy and not amiodarone.
[c] The COMPANION results listed are for CRT + ICD versus medical therapy alone. The hazard ratio for overall mortality for CRT alone versus medical therapy was 0.76 (P = 0.059).
CABG Patch, Coronary Artery Bypass Graft Patch; CHF, congestive heart failure; COMPANION, Comparison of Medical Therapy, Pacing, and Defibrillation in Heart Failure Trial; DANISH, Danish Study to Assess the Efficacy of ICDs in Patients with Non-ischemic Systolic Heart Failure on Mortality; DEFINITE, Defibrillators in Non-Ischemic Cardiomyopathy Treatment Evaluation; DINAMIT, Defibrillator in Acute Myocardial Infarction Trial; EF, ejection fraction; HR, hazard ratio; HRV, heart rate variability; ICM, ischemic cardiomyopathy; MADIT, Multicenter Automatic Defibrillator Implantation Trial; MI, myocardial infarction; NICM, non-ischemic cardiomyopathy; MUSTT, Multicenter Unsustained Tachycardia Trial; NSVT, non-sustained VT; NT-proBNP, N-terminal pro-B-type natriuretic peptide; NYHA, New York Heart Association; PVC, premature ventricular contraction; SAECG, signal-averaged ECG; SCD-HeFT, Sudden Cardiac Death in Heart Failure Trial; VT, ventricular tachycardia.
Source: Sroubek and Buxton [22]. Reproduced with permission of Elsevier.

SCD-HeFT included patients with both ischemic and non-ischemic cardiomyopathy and showed similar relative mortality reductions among the subgroups, with ischemic as well as the 792 non-ischemic cardiomyopathy patients enrolled, although absolute mortality was lower in the non-ischemic subgroup as expected. Additionally, the Defibrillators in Non-Ischemic Cardiomyopathy Treatment Evaluation (DEFINITE) trial enrolled only patients with non-ischemic cardiomyopathy. This smaller study failed to show a statistically significant reduction in overall mortality in the ICD cohort but there was a significant reduction in the incidence of SCD [14]. Interestingly, this trial showed a greater benefit of ICD implantation among patients with heart failure treated for less than 3 months compared with those treated for longer

periods. Patients with such short-duration heart failure were not included in SCD-HeFT, but current guidelines recommend ICD implantation only if heart failure has been treated medically for at least 3 months in patients with non-ischemic cardiomyopathy. This is based on studies showing a high probability of improving LV function with medical therapy in this cohort [15].

A more contemporary trial, the Danish Study to Assess the Efficacy of ICDs in Patients with Nonischemic Systolic Heart Failure on Mortality (DANISH trial) enrolled patients with a non-ischemic cardiomyopathy [NYHA class II or III heart failure symptoms, LVEF ≤35%, and elevated serum N-terminal pro-B-type natriuretic peptide (NT-proBNP)] to receive either an ICD (intervention) or usual clinical care (control group).

The DANISH trial showed a reduction in SCD but not in all-cause mortality with use of an ICD [16]. The subgroup of younger patients in the trial appeared to benefit from ICD therapy.

There were a number of important differences between the DANISH trial and the previous trials evaluating the non-ischemic population (SCD-HeFT and DEFINITE). More than half of patients in the DANISH trial received CRT (either CRT pacemakers in the control group or CRT defibrillators in the intervention group). CRT is a therapy that reduces all-cause mortality and SCD [17]. The observed mortality rate in the control arm of the DANISH trial was 3–4%, substantially lower than previous studies evaluating medical therapy in similar patients, and there was a very high rate of guideline-directed medical therapy used. The SCD rate was also lower than seen in other trials of pharmacological or device therapies in heart failure. The high use of CRT and medical therapy in the DANISH trial likely reduced their statistical power to show a significant difference in the primary outcome. It remains unclear if patient selection, medical therapy, or a decline in SCD rates in general was responsible for the observed results.

Several different meta-analyses have shown survival benefit with ICD in the non-ischemic cardiomyopathy population and support the current guideline recommendations for primary prevention ICD in patients with LVEF ≤35% (Table 8.1) [18–20]. Despite the controversy associated with the DANISH trial, it demonstrated that improvements in medical therapy and appropriate use of CRT have contributed to a decline in mortality rate, decreasing the potential benefit of ICD therapy. More specific predictors for SCD beyond LVEF, such as late gadolinium enhancement on cardiac MRI, may be helpful for identifying patients with non-ischemic cardiomyopathy who might derive the greatest benefit from ICD therapy [21].

Practical decisions regarding primary prevention ICD implantation
One of the more challenging cohorts of patients to manage are those with unexplained syncope and underlying structural heart disease. There is a paucity of data to guide therapy, as syncope was an exclusion criterion for primary prevention tri-als and these patients were rarely included in secondary prevention studies. Programmed ventricular stimulation may help risk-stratify patients with syncope and ischemic heart disease, again with less severe LV dysfunction (LVEF >35%). In addition, electrophysiological studies may be useful for identifying the risk of heart block in patients with moderate reductions of LV function (LVEF >35%) in the presence of conduction system disease. However, among patients with marked LV dysfunction and syncope, ICD therapy is generally the preferred treatment in the absence of contraindications.

Under current guidelines issued by CMS (Centers for Medicare and Medicaid Services), important exclusions to primary prevention ICD implantation include coronary artery bypass graft (CABG) or percutaneous coronary intervention within the past 3 months, MI within the past 40 days, treatment of heart failure for less than 3 months in patients with non-ischemic cardiomyopathy, and clinical symptoms and findings that make the patient a candidate for coronary revascularization. Another group of patients in whom an ICD is not indicated are those with NYHA class IV heart failure, where rates of deaths from non-arrhythmic causes are exceedingly high and an ICD is not expected to meaningfully prolong survival, unless the patient is also a candidate for CRT or advanced therapies such as left ventricular assist device (LVAD) or heart transplantation.

Shared decision-making (SDM) is now required by CMS for primary prevention ICDs. The 2017 guidelines recommend that "clinicians should adopt a shared decision-making approach in which treatment decisions are based not only on the best available evidence but also on the patients' health goals, preferences, and values" [19]. The SDM interaction must occur prior to ICD implantation. The effectiveness of SDM tools for ICDs is under evaluation in a multicenter randomized clinical trial.

Rare, arrhythmogenic disorders
Several genetic or acquired conditions are associated with increased risk of sudden death and may benefit from ICD implantation. These include genetic conditions resulting in channelopathies (long and short QT syndrome, Brugada syndrome,

and catecholaminergic polymorphic VT) or cardio-myopathy (arrhythmogenic right ventricular cardiomyopathy and hypertrophic cardiomyopathy), and infiltrative disorders such as cardiac sarcoidosis and amyloidosis. Unlike the more common conditions of ischemic and non-ischemic dilated cardiomyopathies, where the effectiveness of ICDs has been evaluated in several large randomized controlled trials, the evidence supporting the benefit of ICD in these less common arrhythmogenic disorders is limited and often based on expert consensus and case series. Prospective randomized trials are currently unavailable because of ethical reasons and practical limitations, predominantly linked to relatively low disease prevalence and low event rate.

In addition, inherited cardiac diseases often present in younger patients in whom the consequences of lifelong ICD implantation are more significant due to increased risks of lead dysfunction, need for multiple generator changes, and psychological consequences. Furthermore, these disorders are sometimes characterized by variable expressivity and incomplete penetrance, presenting challenges in the interpretation of genetic results in patients and family members and difficult decisions about placement of an ICD. Several guideline documents, expert consensus statements, and review articles summarize the important and often nuanced considerations in these populations [23–28]. Table 8.3 presents a summary of the guideline indications for ICD therapy in patients with rare arrhythmogenic conditions [19].

Contraindications and neutral trials: high-risk patients who do not benefit from ICDs

Not all high-risk groups benefit from ICD implantation. The current guidelines mandate a 40-day waiting period following MI or 3 months after coronary revascularization before a primary prevention ICD can be implanted based on data from three randomized controlled trials. In the Coronary Artery Bypass Graft (CABG) Patch trial, patients with ischemic cardiomyopathy and an abnormal signal-averaged electrocardiogram (ECG) were randomized to receive an ICD or no antiarrhythmic treatment at the time of CABG surgery. No effect on mortality was observed with ICD use in this cohort [29]. The Defibrillator in Acute

Myocardial Infarction Trial (DINAMIT) evaluated patients with acute MI, LV systolic dysfunction, and reduced heart rate variability. No mortality benefit was observed with ICD implantation [30]. The Immediate Risk Stratification Improves Survival (IRIS) trial had a very similar design with similar outcomes [31]. The reasons for the failure of these studies to show a benefit of ICD therapy are unclear. The use of non-invasive risk stratification, such as signal-averaged ECG or heart rate variability, may be insufficient to identify a high-risk cohort. Also, the competing mortality risks early post MI may offset any benefit of ICD therapy. This concept was supported by a subsequent analysis of DINAMIT showing that increased non-arrhythmic death offset the benefit of a reduction in arrhythmic death in the ICD arm [32].

One major challenge is to develop better methods to risk-stratify patients for SCD, allowing clinicians to implant devices only in those patients who will be likely to use them. The major trials for primary prevention already mentioned have shown that only approximately one-third of patients who receive ICDs for primary prevention will receive an appropriate shock for a ventricular tachyarrhythmia over 4–5 years. The results of retrospective analyses of clinical predictors of ICD shocks or mortality generally show that the incidence of shocks or mortality increases with the severity of heart failure, the lower the ejection fraction, QRS prolongation, atrial fibrillation, renal failure, and age. Clinical scores were developed to help identify subgroups of patients most likely and least likely to benefit from ICDs for primary prevention of SCD [33]. These tools demonstrate the competing factors of risk of arrhythmic events versus non-arrhythmic risk of death associated with comorbidities.

Finally, perhaps the most important challenge for prevention of SCD is that most deaths occur in victims without a guideline indication for ICD implantation. Population-based studies from both the Netherlands and Oregon have shown that only about half of SCD victims had an LVEF less than 50% prior to their event, and only 20–30% of these patients had severe LV dysfunction that meet criteria for ICD implantation according to current guidelines [34,35]. The challenge of such studies is that while the number of patients who experience sudden death in such groups is increased, the

Table 8.3 Summary of indications for ICD therapy in patients with rare conditions[a]

Class I ICD is recommended	• ARVC and an additional marker of increased risk of SCD (resuscitated SCA, sustained VT, significant ventricular dysfunction with RVEF or LVEF 35% or less) (LOE: B-NR) • HCM with SCA or spontaneous sustained VT causing syncope or hemodynamic compromise (LOE: B-NR) • Cardiac channelopathy with SCA (LOE: B-NR) • CPVT and recurrent sustained VT or syncope, while receiving adequate or maximally tolerated beta-blocker (alternatives to ICD include treatment intensification with either combination medication therapy such as combined beta-blocker and flecainide or left cardiac sympathetic denervation) (LOE: B-NR) • Brugada syndrome with spontaneous type 1 Brugada ECG pattern and SCA, sustained VA or a recent history of syncope presumed due to VA (LOE: B-NR) • Cardiac sarcoidosis with sustained VT or SCA or LVEF ≤35% (LOE: B-NR) • High-risk symptomatic long-QT syndrome patients in whom a beta-blocker is ineffective or not tolerated (alternatives to ICD include intensification of therapy with additional medications guided by consideration of the particular long-QT syndrome type or left cardiac sympathetic denervation) (LOE: B-NR)

Class IIa
ICD is reasonable
	• ARVC and syncope presumed due to VA (LOE: B-NR)
	• HCM and one or more of the following risk factors:
	  a Maximum LV wall thickness ≥30 mm (LOE: B-NR)
	  b SCD in one or more first-degree relatives presumably caused by HCM (LOE: C-LD)
	  c One or more episodes of unexplained syncope within the preceding 6 months (LOE: C-LD)
	• HCM with spontaneous NSVT (LOE: C-LD) or an abnormal blood pressure response with exercise (LOE: B-NR) who also have additional SCD risk modifiers or high-risk features
	• Cardiac sarcoidosis and LVEF >35% who have syncope and/or evidence of myocardial scar by cardiac MRI or PET scan, and/or have an indication for permanent pacing (LOE: B-BR)
	• Cardiac sarcoidosis and LVEF >35% with sustained VA is inducible at EP study (LOE: C-LD)
	• Emery–Dreifuss or limb-girdle type IB muscular dystrophies with progressive cardiac involvement (LOE: B-NR)
	• NICM due to a lamin A/C mutation who have two or more risk factors (NSVT, LVEF <45%, non-missense mutation, and male sex)

Class IIb ICD may be considered	• Asymptomatic patients with long-QT syndrome and a resting QTc >500 ms while receiving a beta-blocker (alternatives include intensification of therapy with medications guided by consideration of the particular long-QT syndrome type or left cardiac sympathetic denervation) (LOE: B-NR) • Myotonic dystrophy type 1 with an indication for a permanent pacemaker (LOE: B-NR)

[a] All ICD indications apply to patients if meaningful survival of greater than 1 year is expected.

ARVC, arrhythmogenic right ventricular cardiomyopathy; CPVT, catecholaminergic polymorphic ventricular tachycardia; EP, electrophysiology; HCM, hypertrophic cardiomyopathy; ICD, implantable cardioverter–defibrillator; LOE, level of evidence; LVEF, left ventricular ejection fraction; NICM, non-ischemic cardiomyopathy; NSVT, non-sustained VT; PET, positron emission tomography; RVEF, right ventricular ejection fraction; SCA, sudden cardiac arrest; SCD, sudden cardiac death; VA, ventricular arrhythmia; VT, ventricular tachycardia.

Source: Al-Khatib et al. [19]. Reproduced with permission of American Heart Association.

overall pool of patients is much larger, so that the relative risk of SCD is lower.

Management of patients with temporary SCD risk

Survivors of SCA that may be due to transient or reversible factors (acute MI, proarrhythmic medication effects, or marked electrolyte disturbances) generally should not receive an ICD. However, as observed in the AVID registry, this is a subgroup that still has a high mortality rate and still requires thorough evaluation, treatment, and close follow-up and many clinical scenarios can be borderline [36]. For example, for a cardiac arrest clearly temporally related to an acute ST-elevation MI (within 48 hours), revascularization would be the treatment without need for ICD. However, a cardiac arrest, even in the absence of an acute coronary syndrome, is often associated with small increases in troponin. For a patient presenting with successful resuscitation from VT/ventricular fibrillation (VF), it may be difficult to determine whether a troponin elevation is indicative of a primary acute ischemic event, in which revascularization would be the treatment, or secondary ischemia from the cardiac arrest and resuscitation, in which case an ICD is likely warranted. It is also worth considering whether the arrest was due to VF or monomorphic VT. Monomorphic VT more likely indicates the presence of scar-related reentry and revascularization alone is unlikely to reduce the recurrence.

An alternative to ICD is a wearable cardioverter–defibrillator (WCD), which may be prescribed for patients perceived to be at high risk of SCD in the short term but ineligible for ICD at the time of evaluation, such as those with a reduced LVEF but recent MI and/or revascularization, myocarditis or secondary cardiomyopathy, systemic infection, or a newly diagnosed non-ischemic cardiomyopathy in which recovery in ventricular function is anticipated. The WCD is capable of rapid external defibrillation for ventricular tachyarrhythmias.

The evidence supporting use of the WCD is limited and based primarily on registry data that demonstrate the ability of the device to provide successful defibrillation. The Vest Prevention of Early Death Trial (VEST) is the only randomized controlled trial that has examined whether a WCD could reduce SCD early after acute MI in patients with LVEF ≤35%. There was no benefit demonstrated in this trial for the primary end point of reduction of arrhythmic death, with some notable limitations including low rates of device adherence [37]. There are a number of limitations of the WCD, including lack of pacing capability and risk of inappropriate shocks. From a practical standpoint, the WCD remains a useful option for patients perceived to be at short-term risk of SCD but should not receive a permanent device, particularly in the well-informed and motivated patient. Formal recommendations for use are provided in a clinical practice guideline and a scientific advisory (summarized in Table 8.4) [19,38].

Device selection

Single- versus dual-chamber ICD

Among patients receiving a primary prevention transvenous ICD without a bradycardia pacing indication, a choice must be made between implanting a single-chamber versus dual-chamber ICD. Advantages of a single-chamber ICD include reduced rates of complications related to placement of an atrial lead, such as dislodgement or lead perforation leading to need for reoperation and increased risk of infection. Advantages of a dual-chamber system include the potential benefit of improved discrimination between atrial and

Table 8.4 Guideline recommendation for the use of wearable cardioverter–defibrillator

Guideline recommendation	LOE	Clinical scenario
Class IIa (WCD is reasonable)	B-NR	Temporary removal of an ICD is needed and History of SCD or sustained VA present
Class IIb (WCD may be considered)	B-NR	Increased risk of SCD but ineligible for ICD 1 ICD indicated but acute infection present 2 Potentially reversible cardiomyopathy: a MI <40 days b New NICM c Recent revascularization d Acute myocarditis

LOE, level of evidence; MI, myocardial infarction; NICM, non-ischemic cardiomyopathy; NR, non-randomized; SCD, sudden cardiac death; VA, ventricular arrhythmia; WCD, wearable cardioverter–defibrillator;
Source: modified from Al-Khatib *et al.* [19].

ventricular arrhythmias to avoid inappropriate therapy and the ability to provide atrial pacing and sensing should the patient develop a pacing indication during follow-up. Practice patterns vary, as evidenced by data from US registries showing that about half of patients undergoing primary prevention ICD implantation without a bradycardia pacing indication received a dual-chamber device. However, a systematic review of trials evaluating the benefits of single- versus dual-chamber systems found no significant difference in rates of inappropriate therapies, mortality, pneumothorax, or lead dislodgement. Given the lack of clear benefit of a dual-chamber device over single-chamber device in patients without pacing indications, an expert consensus document recommends that it is reasonable to choose single-chamber ICD therapy in preference to dual-chamber ICD therapy to reduce both lead-related complications and the cost of ICD therapy [39].

Transvenous versus subcutaneous ICDs

The risks associated with transvenous leads has led to the development of alternative implantation techniques and devices for ICDs [40]. Complications, both perioperative (pneumothorax, cardiac tamponade, and upper-extremity deep venous thrombosis) and long term (lead malfunction and infection), are a concern for endocardial leads. Studies have shown that more than 20% of patients will have failure of a lead due to mechanical problems or infection by 10 years, and advisory leads have much higher failure rates [41]. To address this problem, an entirely subcutaneous ICD (S-ICD) was developed to reduce or even eliminate many of the complications associated with transvenous ICDs [42]. Several multicenter registries have demonstrated that this device provides reliable and effective detection and termination of ventricular arrhythmias [43].

By avoiding vascular access, the S-ICD offers advantages over transvenous ICDs. Patients who may be considered appropriate candidates for an S-ICD are shown in Table 8.5. Notable limitations of the S-ICD include the lack of pacing capabilities, other than brief post-shock transthoracic pacing, a larger pulse generator size, and shorter battery life.

Patients for whom a transvenous system is preferred (poor candidates for S-ICD) include those

Table 8.5 Factors involved in considering appropriate candidates for S-ICD

S-ICD preferred
No or poor venous access (occluded veins or congenital anomalies)
High risk of complications from transvenous system (dialysis, pediatric, and immunocompromised)
Previous device infection
History of endocarditis

S-ICD considered
Young patients
Channelopathies (long-QT syndrome, Brugada, hypertrophic cardiomyopathy)
Primary prevention indicated patients with heart failure
Prosthetic heart valve(s)
Selected secondary prevention indicated patients (survivors of out-of-hospital VF, no evidence of monomorphic VT)

S-ICD should be avoided
Symptomatic bradycardia requiring pacing
Documented sustained monomorphic VT for whom ATP is deemed appropriate
Systolic heart failure and QRS prolongation with indication for CRT

ATP, antitachycardia pacing; CRT, cardiac resynchronization therapy; VF, ventricular fibrillation; VT, ventricular tachycardia.
Source: modified from Poole and Gold [47].

who require bradycardia pacing or CRT. Similarly, the S-ICD is not appropriate for patients with monomorphic VT that can be terminated by antitachycardia pacing (ATP). Compared with transvenous ICDs, the S-ICD has a higher incidence of inappropriate shocks from T-wave oversensing or myopotentials, but a lower risk from supraventricular arrhythmias [44].

Early studies of the S-ICD included many patients with "niche" indications, such as long QT syndrome, hypertrophic cardiomyopathy, and idiopathic VF. Thus these cohorts tended to be younger with less LV dysfunction and comorbidities. The more recent studies, including the US post-approval study and UNTOUCHED cohorts, have patient characteristics much more similar to transvenous ICD populations [45,46] (Table 8.6).

Table 8.6 S-ICD trial comparison of patient demographics

	EFFORTLESS[1]	S-ICD PAS[2]	UNTOUCHED[3]
Study region	Primarily EU	USA	USA + EU
Patients (number)	450	1637	1117
Age (years)	49 ± 18	53.2 ± 15.0	56 ± 12
Male (%)	72	68.6	73.8
Ejection fraction (%)	42 ± 19	32.0 ± 14.6	27 ± 7
Primary prevention (%)	63	77	100
Heart failure (%)	29	74	87
Hypertension (%)	24	62	68
Diabetes (%)	12	34	31.7
Kidney disease (%)	9	26	14

EU, European Union; PAS, post-approval study; S-ICD, subcutaneous ICD, USA.

Sources: 1, Burke *et al.* [43]; 2, Gold *et al.* [45]; 3, Boersma *et al.* [46].

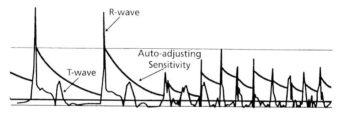

Figure 8.2 Schematic of automatic adjustment of sensitivity during sinus rhythm and ventricular fibrillation. In sinus rhythm, sensitivity increases slowly to avoid oversensing T waves. However, with the onset of ventricular fibrillation, high sensitivity is maintained to minimize undersensing. Source: Medtronic, Inc. Reproduced with permission of Medtronic, Inc.

Moreover, the safety and efficacy of the device is maintained in these populations, supporting an expanding role for subcutaneous devices [45].

Function

Sensing, detection, and arrhythmia discrimination

Rate sensing

Sensing of ventricular tachyarrhythmias is a critically important function of an ICD system [48,49]. The ability to detect small-amplitude signals rapidly during VF, while not oversensing T waves or noise in the absence of tachyarrhythmias, is mandatory for proper ICD function. Unlike pacemaker systems, which use fixed gain sensing, all ICD pulse generators use automatic adjustment of amplifier gain or sensing threshold to ensure appropriate detection of ventricular arrhythmias. ICDs increase the amplifier sensitivity over time between sensed or paced ventricular events to search for low-amplitude fibrillatory EGMs that may be undersensed at lower sensitivities, while retaining relatively insensitive settings shortly after the sensed ventricular EGM to prevent T-wave oversensing (Figure 8.2).

Undersensing of VF was rarely noted with early epicardial or bipolar transvenous leads after automatic gain or sensitivity was employed. Both true bipolar sensing, with a dedicated tip and ring, and integrated sensing, where the distal coil is used for both sensing and shocks, are available in commercial devices. Typically, sensed R-wave amplitude of greater than 5 mV in the baseline rhythm (i.e. sinus or atrial fibrillation) is sufficient to ensure adequate sensing of VF. In a retrospective analysis of induced and spontaneous VF episodes from two clinical trials with over 2000 patients, there was no significant relationship between sinus rhythm R-wave amplitude and either undersensing of induced VF or detection delay due to VF undersensing. These results did not support any recommended minimum sinus rhythm R wave to ensure reliable sensing of VF or the necessity of inducing VF to verify sensing for rectified sinus rhythm R waves with amplitude greater than or equal to 3 mV [50]. Uniformly excellent sensing of VF was demonstrated in a comparative study of multiple transvenous and subcutaneous ICD pulse generators, using both dedicated bipolar and integrated leads [51].

Although undersensing of ventricular tachyarrhythmias is very unusual with modern lead systems and pulse generators, oversensing of other biological signals is still problematic. The maximum sensitivity of transvenous pulse generators is increased (up to 0.15 mV) with contemporary low-noise amplifiers and these values are even lower for subcutaneous devices. This can lead to oversensing from electromagnetic interference or other external noise sources. Oversensing of T waves with double counting is another problem observed more frequently with modern pulse generators because of increased maximum sensitivity and aggressive sensing algorithms. Again, this can often be avoided with device programming, including use

of automated T-wave oversensing algorithms, reducing the maximum sensitivity, prolonging the refractory period, or reducing the aggressiveness of the autosensitivity algorithm. The frequency of T-wave oversensing varies among devices from different manufacturers, but is most often noted with the S-ICD. Recent advances in the detection algorithms of these devices should reduce the incidence of T-wave oversensing [52].

Extensive data logging capabilities are present in pulse generators. All systems provide beat-to-beat interval data for detected tachyarrhythmias. This is helpful for identifying the arrhythmias associated with shocks. For example, very irregular intervals are suggestive of atrial fibrillation (AF), whereas the sudden onset of a regular tachycardia is indicative of either monomorphic VT or paroxysmal supraventricular tachycardia (SVT). A very rapid rhythm with non-physiological intervals (<130 ms) is indicative of a sensing malfunction, typically due to either a lead defect or a loose set-screw in the pulse generator header.

Stored EGMs are used as a further diagnostic tool (Figure 8.3). This significantly improves the ability to interpret the appropriateness of defibrillation shocks. The electrodes used to record the EGM may or may not be the same electrodes used

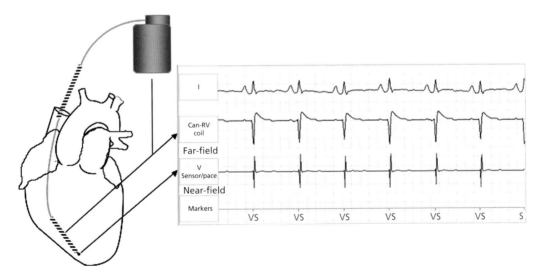

Figure 8.3 ICD electrograms. Near-field electrograms are true bipolar recordings between the tip and ring electrodes of the right ventricular (RV) lead. Far-field electrograms are recorded between the RV coil and the ICD can, which gives a more global representation of ventricular activity, not dissimilar from a precordial ECG lead. A surface ECG lead (top tracing) and a marker channel are also printed on this output, illustrating how the ICD interprets these signals. VS indicates sensed ventricular activity.

for the detection of arrhythmias. Near-field EGMs are recordings of the local bipolar ventricular EGM, which is also used for arrhythmia detection. This can either be true bipolar sensing, with recording from the electrode tip to a more proximal ring, or extended bipolar sensing, with recording from the tip to a right ventricular (RV) shocking coil. For far-field EGMs, recordings are made between shocking electrodes, which for a typical transvenous lead system includes an RV coil, a left pectoral active pulse generator, and sometimes a more proximal coil in the right atrium or superior vena cava. Far-field recordings potentially allow for the identification of atrial activity to aid in arrhythmia classification. In addition, the change in morphology of ventricular arrhythmias is often more obvious in the far-field EGMs. The source of stored EGMs is important for interpreting arrhythmia episodes, particularly inappropriate therapy. For example, if the far-field EGM recorded from the shocking electrodes is being monitored, then this is not the same signal that is being sensed by the amplifier for the determination of tachyarrhythmias. Thus, if no tachycardia is noted at the time of therapy for a rapid rate, then oversensing of the rate-sensing lead can be deduced, but extraneous noise may not be demonstrated. Examples of stored EGMs with a lead malfunction are shown in

Figure 8.4. With dual-chamber ICDs, atrial recordings further simplify the interpretation of arrhythmias (Figure 8.5). Table 8.7 summarizes other causes of rapid oversensing with normal impedance that may be considered in the differential diagnosis of lead failure.

Arrhythmia detection

Arrhythmia detection requires effective sensing of the intrinsic cardiac activity and fulfillment of the programmed detection algorithm. For VT, most ICDs require that a certain number of consecutive RR intervals be shorter than the tachycardia detection interval for the VT zone (Figure 8.6). Because the VF EGMs may transiently have low amplitude and be undersensed, the VF detection algorithms require that a certain percentage (typically 75%) of RR intervals in a rolling window of cardiac cycles be shorter than the VF detection interval (Figure 8.6). If the rate and duration criteria for detection of VF are met and shock therapy is programmed, the ICD charges the high-voltage capacitor, a process that typically takes 5–12 s. Before delivering the shock, the ICD confirms (reconfirms) that a tachyarrhythmia is still present by measuring a few intervals after the charging has completed. If VT or VF is no longer present, the shock is aborted (Figure 8.7). After each delivered

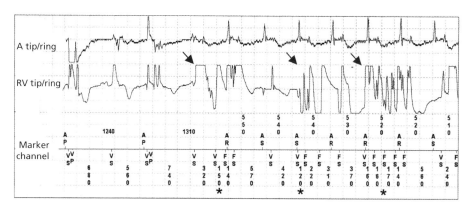

Figure 8.4 Stored electrograms from a dual-chamber ICD with a fracture of the pace/sense component of the right ventricular (RV) ICD lead. Note the oversensing of non-physiological electrical activity on the near-field (RV tip-to-ring) electrogram (*). This was interpreted by the device as ventricular fibrillation, as highlighted on the marker channel, and a shock was delivered (not shown). Also note the make-or-break type pattern of the noise with intermittent saturation of the amplifier (arrows). The patient received multiple inappropriate shocks for this noise, necessitating a lead revision procedure. A tip/ring, near-field atrial channel; AP, atrial-paced event; AS, atrial-sensed event; FS, ventricular-sensed event in VF rate zone; RV tip/ring, near-field RV bipolar signal; VP, ventricular-paced event; VS, ventricular-sensed event.

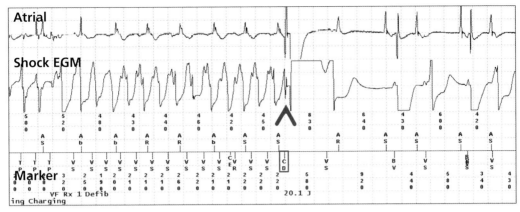

Figure 8.5 Dual-chamber electrograms from a cardiac resynchronization ICD showing polymorphic ventricular tachycardia (VT) with atrioventricular (AV) dissociation treated with shock. Atrial and high-voltage ("Shock") electrograms and the dual-chamber marker channel are shown. The arrowhead denotes shock, designated by CD (charge delivered) on the marker channel. After the shock, the atrial rhythm is sinus with premature atrial contractions; the ventricular rhythm is biventricular paced (BV) with premature ventricular contractions (PVCs) in the sinus rate zone (VS). The second BV beat (BV/VS) has a slightly shorter paced AV delay (110 vs. 130 ms) than the first BV beat because a PVC occurs during the AV delay, triggering "safety pacing," a feature that reduces cross-talk inhibition. Source: Swerdlow CD, Hayes DL, Zipes DP. Cardiac pacemakers and cardioverter-defibrillators. In: Bonow RO, Libby P, Mann DL, Zipes DP, Braunwald E, eds. *Braunwald's Heart Disease: A Textbook of Cardiovascular Medicine*, 9th edn. Philadelphia: Elsevier Saunders, 2013. Reproduced with permission of Elsevier.

Table 8.7 Rapid oversensing with normal pacing impedance: differential diagnosis of lead failure

	Sensing electrogram characteristics	Clues to diagnosis
Early or late after implant		
Conductor fracture	Typical non-physiological signals[a]	Postpacing oversensing
Insulation breach: in pocket	Pectoral myopotentials on dedicated bipolar electrogram	Pectoral muscle exercise reproduces oversensing
Insulation breach: inside out	Spikes	Simultaneous spikes on multiple electrogram channels
Connection problems	Indistinguishable from lead fracture	Radiography, pocket manipulation, repeat measurement of impedance
Electromagnetic interference	Reflects characteristics of source	More common in integrated bipolar than dedicated bipolar leads. History may suggest source. In dedicated bipolar leads, amplitude usually greater on shock channel than sensing channel
Diaphragmatic myopotentials	Uniformly low amplitude and relatively uniform morphology vs. lead failure signals, which vary in morphology, amplitude, or both	Usually occur in paced rhythm or bradycardia with integrated bipolar leads at right ventricular apex; may be reproduced by deep breath or Valsalva
Ventricular fibrillation	Variable	Present on both shock and sensing channels
Lead–lead mechanical interactions	Spiky electrogram	Presence of other leads by history; cinefluoroscopy with real-time electrogram recordings confirms diagnosis
Perioperative period only		
Air trapped in header	Uniform, medium-frequency signals	Postoperatively it is a diagnosis of exclusion

[a] Characteristics of non-physiological signals include (i) intermittent, high-dominant frequency; (ii) not cyclic; (iii) intervals in the ventricular fibrillation zone; (iv) in dedicated bipolar leads, not on shock channel; (v) variability of amplitude, morphology, or frequency; and (vi) may saturate sensing amplifier.
Source: adapted from Swerdlow et al. [48].

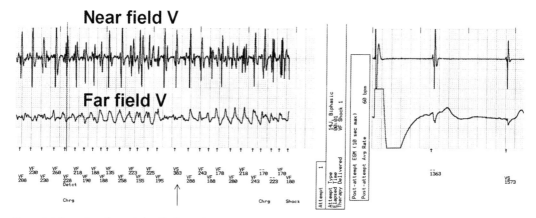

Figure 8.6 Detection of ventricular fibrillation (VF) with undersensing. Near-field and far-field electrograms and ventricular marker channel during induced VF. "VF" and "VS" markers indicate intervals sensed in the VF and sinus rate zones, respectively. VF is detected, and the ICD charges (Chrg) and delivers a shock at the break between the VF and baseline rhythm (shown on the right), despite the fact that not all intervals are classified as VF (arrow). Rapidly varying amplitude on near-field electrograms can contribute to undersensing but does not contribute in this episode.

therapy, the ICD must determine whether the tachycardia was terminated. The redetection criteria after therapy are usually less demanding than the initial detection criteria for each zone. The detection criteria in the VT zone may be modified by algorithms to prevent inappropriate therapy for SVTs. Multiple studies have demonstrated that significant prolongation of detection times and rate cutoffs are associated with better outcomes with ICD systems and fewer delivered inappropriate therapies as well as unnecessary appropriate therapies [53,54].

SVT–VT discrimination

The SVT–VT discrimination algorithm is a programmable sub-algorithm of the detection process for VT/VF. It withholds therapy if SVT is diagnosed. This sub-algorithm is applied after a sequence of sensed events meets the rate and duration criteria for VT or VF and, in some ICDs, after these sensed events are validated as representing true ventricular activations (versus oversensing). They apply over a range of cycle lengths, bounded on the slow end by the VT detection interval and on the fast end by a specific parameter, the SVT limit.

SVT–VT discrimination algorithms operate in a stepwise manner, using a series of logical discriminator "building blocks" (Table 8.8) based on the timing relationships of sensed events and morphology of sensed ventricular EGMs. Algorithms combine complementary discriminators to make a final rhythm classification of VT or SVT. Each discriminator building block has advantages and limitations. Some are redundant and some interact differently depending on the order in which they are applied. Rather than concentrating on the specifics of their implementation in each commercial ICD, the general principles of how these are assembled into a comprehensive algorithm is presented.

Blocks 1–4 in Table 8.8 apply to single-chamber ICDs or the ventricular component of dual-chamber ICDs. Blocks 5–9 combine atrial and ventricular information in dual-chamber algorithms. Block 10 incorporates atrial rate into dual-chamber algorithms. In contrast to the passive discriminators in blocks 1–10, block 11 is an active discriminator based on response to pacing.

Single-chamber ventricular building blocks

Ventricular electrogram morphology

The ventricular EGM morphology discriminator classifies tachycardia as SVT if the morphological characteristics of the EGM are similar to those of validated supraventricular beats and as VT if they are not. It is the only single-chamber building block that can classify all SVTs correctly, including sudden-onset regular SVT with a 1 : 1 atrioventricular (AV) relationship or atrial flutter. Thus, it is the cornerstone of modern single-chamber algorithms and the central single-chamber component of

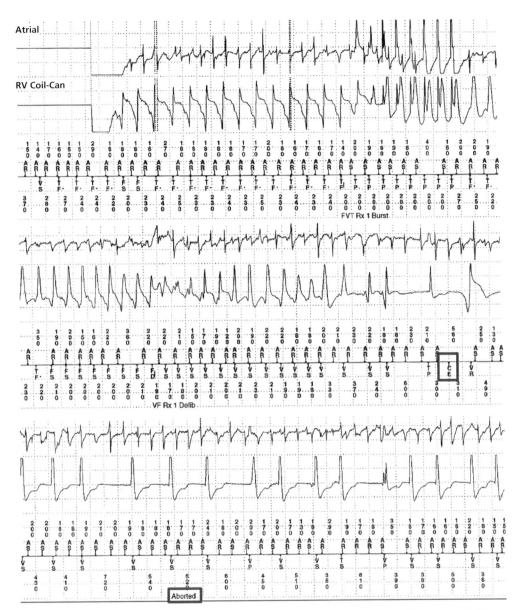

Figure 8.7 Aborted shock for ventricular tachycardia (VT) that terminates after capacitor charging. Continuous tracing of atrial and high-voltage (RV Coil–Can) electrograms and dual-chamber markers during an episode detected as fast VT (FVT; cycle length 200–250 ms) during ongoing atrial fibrillation (AF). Atrial markers indicate that the atrial rhythm is AF. Antitachycardia pacing is delivered at the end of the top panel (FVT Rx 1 Burst, TP markers). After antitachycardia pacing, the rhythm accelerates and becomes polymorphic. It is redetected as VF, and the high-voltage capacitor begins to charge (VF Rx 1 defib). Capacitor charging is complete near the end of the middle panel, as indicated by the CE marker in the red rectangle ("charge end"). After a sufficient number of intervals, the shock is aborted in the bottom panel (red rectangle). Antitachycardia pacing (ATP) accelerated the rhythm to VF, which then terminated. This would be classified as successful, but it is not known if the VT would have terminated spontaneously without ATP. Source: Swerdlow CD, Hayes DL, Zipes DP. Cardiac pacemakers and cardioverter-defibrillators. In: Bonow RO, Libby P, Mann DL, Zipes DP, Braunwald E, eds. *Braunwald's Heart Disease: A Textbook of Cardiovascular Medicine*, 9th edn. Philadelphia: Elsevier Saunders, 2013. Reproduced with permission of Elsevier.

Table 8.8 Discriminator building blocks for SVT–VT discrimination algorithms

Building block	Purpose	Limitation	Role in dual-chamber algorithms	
			V = A (rate)	V < A (rate)
Ventricular (single- or dual-chamber ICDs)				
1 VV regularity (stability)	Discriminates monomorphic VT (regular) from conducted AF (irregular)	Unreliable at ventricular rates of >170 bpm; underdetection of irregular VT		+
2 VV sudden onset	Discriminates abrupt onset of VT from gradual acceleration of sinus tachycardia	Detects abrupt onset of SVTs; misclassifies VT that starts in sinus zone and accelerates gradually into VT zone or starts in VT zone	+	
3 Ventricular EGM morphology	Discriminates VT based on EGM morphology change vs. baseline	Confounded by aberrant conduction; multiple technical issues; Cannot be used in redetection	+	+
4 Ventricular EGM width	Discriminates VT based on EGM width change vs. baseline	Measured EGM width may not be reproducible; patients with bundle branch block may not have width increase in VT	+	+
Atrioventricular (dual chamber ICDs)				
5 Comparison of atrial vs. ventricular rate	VT diagnosed if A rate < V rate; cornerstone of dual-chamber algorithms	Confounded by atrial undersensing or far-field R-wave oversensing	+	+
6 AV dissociation	AV dissociation usually indicates VT	VT with 1 : 1 retrograde conduction; rapidly conducted AF		+
7 Pattern of A/V events	Discriminates VT based on pattern of AV events	Unreliable for 1 : 1 tachycardias		+
8 Chamber of origin	Discriminates whether tachycardia initiates in atrium or ventricle	A single oversensed/undersensed event may cause misclassification		+
9 Dual-chamber sudden onset	Discriminates VT based on abrupt change in ventricular rate and AV interval	Unreliable if baseline rhythm is ventricular paced		+
Atrial (dual chamber ICDs)				
10 Atrial rate	Identifies AF to modify single-chamber ventricular discriminators	Atrial undersensing/oversensing causes measurement error. VT/VF may occur during AF	+	
Active discrimination				
11 A, V, or AV pacing during tachycardia	May terminate tachycardia; discriminates 1 : 1 tachycardia that persists based on pattern of AV intervals after pacing	Proarrhythmia		+

AF, atrial fibrillation; AV, atrioventricular; EGM, electrogram; SVT, supraventricular tachycardia; VF, ventricular fibrillation; VT, ventricular tachycardia.

dual-chamber algorithms. It is also the most complex building block.

All morphology discriminators designed for SVT–VT discrimination share common steps (Figure 8.8).
1 Record a template EGM of baseline rhythm.
2 Construct and store a quantitative representation of this template.
3 Record EGMs from an unknown tachycardia.
4 Time-align the template and tachycardia EGMs.
5 Construct a quantitative, normalized representation of each tachycardia EGM.
6 Compare the representation of each tachycardia EGM with that of the template to determine the degree of morphological similarity.
7 Classify each tachycardia EGM as a morphology match or non-match with the template.
8 Classify the tachycardia as VT or SVT based on the fraction of EGMs that match the template.
Steps 3–8 are performed in real time.

Morphology discriminators differ according to EGM source, methods of filtering and alignment, and details of quantitative representations. Figure 8.9 provides an example of one such discriminator. The source EGM should be recorded from widely spaced electrodes, such as the high-voltage electrodes of transvenous ICDs or the subcutaneous sensing electrodes of S-ICDs. All ICDs now apply the morphology discriminator to EGMs recorded from widely spaced electrodes. EGMs should be aligned using a robust method that is insensitive to minor changes in EGM morphology. Often, the EGM peak is used as a fiducial point. Alignment errors often result in complete failure of template matching. If a tachycardia EGM that is visually indistinguishable from the template has a match score of near 0%, then an alignment error has occurred.

Limitations of morphology discriminators. Morphology discriminators share common failure modes that are summarized in Table 8.9 and illustrated in Figure 8.10.
- *Inaccurate template.* The template may be inaccurate because the baseline EGM has changed (e.g. post-implantation lead maturation, new bundle branch block) or because the template was recorded during intermittent bundle branch block or from an abnormal rhythm (e.g. idioventricular or bigeminal premature ventricular contractions).

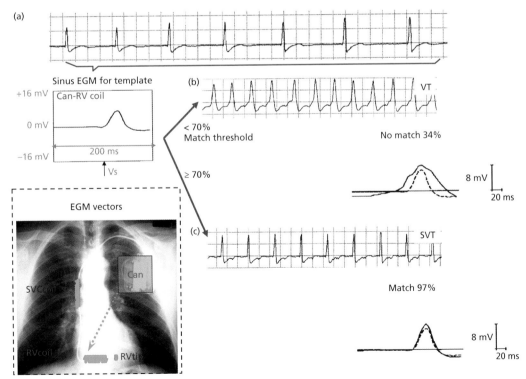

Figure 8.8 Structure of morphology algorithm. (a) The stored template representing the sinus rhythm coil-to-can electrogram (EGM) is stored and compared with real-time EGMs of tachycardia: (b) ventricular tachycardia (VT) and (c) supraventricular tachycardia (SVT). See text for details.

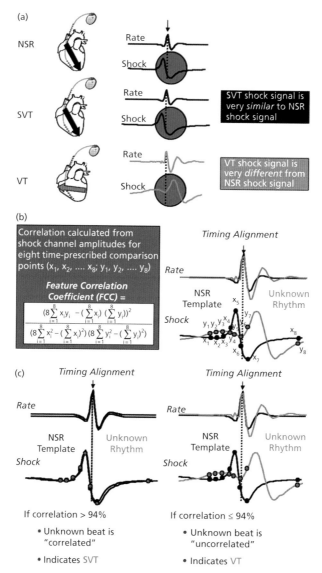

(a)

NSR

Rate

Shock

SVT

Rate

Shock

SVT shock signal is very *similar* to NSR shock signal

VT

Rate

Shock

VT shock signal is very *different* from NSR shock signal

(b)

Correlation calculated from shock channel amplitudes for eight time-prescribed comparison points (x_1, x_2, ... x_8; y_1, y_2, ... y_8)

Feature Correlation Coefficient (FCC) =

$$\frac{(8\sum_{i=1}^{8} x_i y_i - (\sum_{i=1}^{8} x_i)(\sum_{i=1}^{8} y_i))^2}{(8\sum_{i=1}^{8} x_i^2 - (\sum_{i=1}^{8} x_i)^2)(8\sum_{i=1}^{8} y_i^2 - (\sum_{i=1}^{8} y_i)^2)}$$

Timing Alignment

Rate

NSR Template

Unknown Rhythm

Shock

(c)

Timing Alignment

Rate

NSR Template   Unknown Rhythm

Shock

If correlation > 94%

- Unknown beat is "correlated"
- Indicates SVT

Timing Alignment

Rate

NSR Template   Unknown Rhythm

Shock

If correlation ≤ 94%

- Unknown beat is "uncorrelated"
- Indicates VT

Figure 8.9 A morphology discrimination algorithm. (a) The algorithm works by comparing shock electrogram (EGM) morphology during tachycardia with that obtained and stored during normal sinus rhythm (NSR), under the premise that the morphology and timing relationships between the two EGMs during supraventricular tachycardia (SVT) will be similar to that during NSR (barring any aberrant conduction), whereas the shock EGM will be markedly different during ventricular tachycardia (VT) compared with NSR. (b) The correlation between the shock channel morphologies during NSR and the unknown rhythm is calculated from amplitudes for eight time-prescribed comparison points. (c) If the correlation between the shock channel morphologies during NSR and the unknown rhythm is >94%, the algorithm identifies the beat as supraventricular, otherwise it indicates that it is VT. Source: Rhythm ID, Boston Scientific Corporation. Reproduced with permission of Boston Scientific.

- *Electrogram truncation.* EGM truncation ("clipping") occurs when the recorded EGM signal amplitude exceeds the range of the EGM amplifier, often due to postural changes. The maximum absolute peak of the EGM is clipped, removing EGM features for analysis and altering the timing of the tallest peak, which can cause alignment errors.

- *Alignment errors.* Alignment errors occur when one feature of the tachycardia EGM is aligned with a different feature of the template EGM. These prevent match between a tachycardia EGM and a morphologically similar template EGM. The mechanisms depend on the method used for EGM alignment. Usually,

Table 8.9 Failure modes of the electrogram morphology discriminator

Root cause		Solution or mitigation
Incorrect classification of VT as SVT		
Inaccurate template	Change in baseline EGM; automatic updating during bigeminy or bundle branch block	Automatic template updating after implant Operator confirmation of template in follow-up
EGM truncation	Inadequate amplifier range	Evaluate baseline EGM amplitude in various postures Adjust dynamic range of amplifier so that EGM amplitude is 50–75% of range
Alignment errors	Failure of alignment procedures	Algorithm specific (reference CDS)
Interfering signal in tachycardia	Superposition of extraneous signal such as pectoral myopotentials on true ventricular EGM degrades percentage match	Evaluate percentage match during pectoral muscle exercise Select alternative source EGM if interference is reproducible
Rate-related aberrancy	Alteration of interventricular conduction at rapid rate	Reduce fraction of EGMs (e.g. 5 of 8 to 3 of 8) required to exceed SVT match threshold, if programmable Disable automatic updating if template acquired at fast rate
SVT soon after shock	Post-shock EGM distortion	Program additional single-chamber discriminators in patients with repetitive VT
Incorrect classification of SVT as VT		
Analysis of morphology in single lead	Similar VT and SVT morphology in analyzed lead	Change lead if programmable Program other discriminators with "OR" logic for classification of VT Program high-rate timeout

EGM, electrogram; SVT, supraventricular tachycardia; VT, ventricular tachycardia.

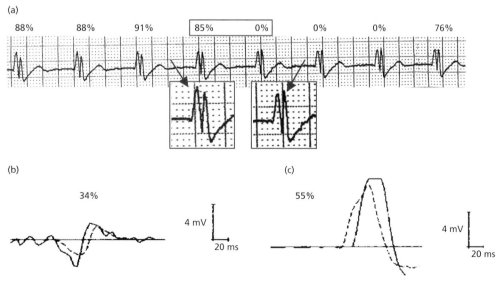

Figure 8.10 Failure modes of morphology algorithms. (a) Alignment error. (b) Interfering baseline myopotentials with low-amplitude coil-to-can electrogram (EGM). (c) Truncation of the EGM peak during tachycardia due to postural changes.

tachycardia EGMs are assigned morphology match scores of 0%.

- *Interfering signals during tachycardia.* All modern transvenous ICDs use morphology discriminators that include the pulse generator shell (i.e. "can") in the default EGM. Oversensing of pectoral myopotentials may prevent an SVT from matching the sinus template if the EGM amplitude is small.

- *Rate-related aberrancy.* If complete bundle branch aberrancy occurs reproducibly, the template may be recorded during rapid atrial pacing, but variable aberrancy in rapidly conducted AF is rarely reproducible. If a template is acquired at a fast rate, automatic template updating should be deactivated to prevent subsequent automatic acquisition of a slow baseline template without aberrancy.

- *SVT soon after a shock.* After a shock, ICD detection algorithms reclassify the rhythm as sinus and revert to their initial detection mode within a few seconds, but post-shock distortion of EGM morphology persists for 30 s to several minutes [57,58]. If a supraventricular tachyarrhythmia starts after the rhythm has been classified as sinus, but before post-shock EGM distortion dissipates, morphology discriminators misclassify SVT as VT [57].

Older discriminators

Interval stability. The *VV regularity* building block (VV interval stability or "Stability") discriminates between the regular ventricular intervals usually present in monomorphic VT and the irregular ventricular intervals usually present in rapidly conducted AF. Regularity criteria can reject AF with ventricular rates slower than 170 bpm in the absence of antiarrhythmic drugs. At faster rates, they cannot discriminate AF from VT reliably, because VV intervals in AF become more regular [59–61]. This discriminator may prevent detection of monomorphic VT that becomes irregular after therapy with amiodarone or type Ic antiarrhythmic drugs [60,61].

Sudden onset. The *RR onset* building block discriminates sudden-onset VT from gradual-onset sinus tachycardia. "Onset" has high specificity for rejecting sinus tachycardia [61], providing premature beats do not occur as the sinus rate accelerates across the sinus–VT boundary. However, when used in isolation, it prevents detection of VT that

originates during SVT or VT that starts abruptly with an initial rate below the VT detection limit. In the latter case, the ICD misclassifies the "onset" of the arrhythmia as the gradual acceleration of the VT rate across the VT rate boundary. Most single- and dual-chamber discriminators reevaluate classification of ongoing tachycardias, but Onset only classifies it once as it crosses the sinus–VT boundary. Both for this reason and because the morphology discriminator usually is highly accurate for rejection of sinus tachycardia, Onset should not be used as the only discriminator.

Dual-chamber ventricular building blocks
Atrial versus ventricular rate
Comparison of atrial and ventricular rates is the cornerstone and first step of most dual-chamber algorithms. The central role of this discriminator is predicated on accurate atrial sensing during high ventricular rates, which has proved to be the weakest link in performance of dual-chamber SVT–VT discrimination algorithms.

Discriminators that evaluate relative timing of atrial/ventricular events. The primary role of these building blocks is to discriminate VT with 1 : 1 ventriculoatrial (VA) conduction from SVT with 1 : 1 AV conduction. Their two secondary roles are to classify tachycardia with stable 2 : 1 AV relationships as atrial flutter and to classify dissociated isorhythmic tachycardias (similar atrial and ventricular rates) as VT. The *AV dissociation* building block detects VT during any SVT, but classifies conducted AF as dissociated. The *AV patterns* building block identifies stable associations of atrial and ventricular events. It also identifies tachycardias with stable 2 : 1 AV patterns as atrial flutter. The *chamber of origin* building block discriminates between VT and SVT with 1 : 1 AV association by identifying whether the tachycardia originates in the atrium or ventricle. In ICD patients, most AV nodal or AV reciprocating tachycardias are ablated. Abrupt-onset SVTs typically represent atrial tachycardia, which usually begins with an intrinsic atrial event in the interval between the last ventricular event in the sinus rate zone and the first ventricular event in the VT zone. Conversely, at the start of spontaneous VT, there is usually no atrial event in this interval. Dual-chamber sudden onset (Sinus Tachycardia Rule, Medtronic) is a substantial refinement of the single-chamber rule, applied only to tachycardias with a 1 : 1 AV association, and based on the observation that sinus tachycardia is characterized by gradual changes in both AV and V–V intervals [62]. Unlike single-chamber Onset, dual-chamber Onset identifies VT that begins during sinus tachycardia by the change in the expected AV relationship. However, it misclassifies rare VTs with 1 : 1 VA conduction that begin in the sinus rate zone and accelerate across the VT rate boundary. More problematically, if the baseline rhythm is ventricular paced (e.g. all cardiac resynchronization ICDs), it collapses to single-chamber Onset.

Single-chamber atrial building blocks in dual-chamber algorithms. Although atrial correlates of the single-chamber ventricular discriminators can be calculated, they are not employed in any current dual-chamber algorithm. However, *atrial rate* (A–A interval) is applied to determine the presence or absence of AF/flutter and to invoke or prioritize a single-chamber ventricular interval stability only if atrial tachyarrhythmia is present. This prevents underdetection of irregular VT in the absence of AF/flutter.

Importance of accurate atrial sensing. Atrial undersensing or oversensing invalidates comparison of atrial and ventricular rates. Atrial undersensing may be caused by either low-amplitude EGMs (especially during AF) or functional interactions with the post-ventricular atrial blanking period (PVAB) triggered by ventricular-sensed or -paced events (Figure 8.11). At high ventricular rates, long PVABs may comprise a sufficient fraction of the cardiac cycle that they blank enough atrial EGMs to prevent correct estimation of atrial rate.

Atrial oversensing is most commonly caused by far-field R waves (FFRWs; Figure 8.12) that are either high in amplitude, comparable in amplitude to small P waves, or sufficiently late relative to the sensed ventricular EGM that they time outside the PVAB. Consistent or inconsistent FFRW oversensing may result in incorrect classification of SVT as VT either by the AV dissociation, AV pattern, or chamber-of-origin discriminators. The best way to prevent atrial oversensing of FFRWs is to position the atrial lead where a large atrial EGM is recorded with no or minimal FFRWs.

Active discrimination: response to pacing. In the electrophysiology laboratory, the response of the opposite chamber to pacing is commonly used for diagnosing tachycardias with a 1 : 1 AV relationship. The *response to pacing* building block is conceptually different from others because it requires an active intervention that either terminates a 1 : 1 tachycardia or discriminates VT from SVT by the pattern of atrial and ventricular events at the end of pacing.

Operation of complete SVT–VT discrimination algorithms

Single-chamber algorithms

The morphology discriminator is the primary single-chamber discriminator. In transvenous ICDs it may be linked with Stability to withhold therapy unless both discriminators indicate VT. As noted, it is linked with ventricular EGM width in S-ICD (see section S-ICD sensing and discrimination).

Dual-chamber algorithms

Dual-chamber algorithms are more complex than single-chamber ones. Those that apply comparison of atrial and ventricular rates as a first step limit the fraction of VTs to which single-chamber discriminators are applied, since the ventricular rate exceeds the atrial rate in more than 80% of VTs in the VT zone of dual-chamber ICDs and a higher fraction of VTs in the VF zone [63,64]. Thus, these algorithms apply additional discriminators to fewer than 20% of VTs, reducing the risk of misclassifying VT as SVT by subsequently applied discriminators, provided that the atrial rate is measured accurately. However, they apply additional discriminators to all SVTs. The integration of building blocks into dual-chamber algorithms may be considered in terms of relative atrial and ventricular rates.

Operation for atrial rate less than ventricular rate (V > A). The rhythm is classified as VT.

Operation for atrial rate equal to ventricular rate (V = A). The vast majority of tachycardias with a 1 : 1 AV relationship are SVTs, primarily sinus tachycardias. The relevant building blocks are shown in Table 8.8.

Operation for atrial rate greater than ventricular rate (V < A). The building blocks that apply to these challenging rhythms are summarized in Table 8.8. Although various combinations successfully discriminate VT from SVT in VT zones, most VT during AF is sufficiently rapid to be detected in the VF zone, where some discriminators do not apply (e.g. Stability) and others lose specificity for

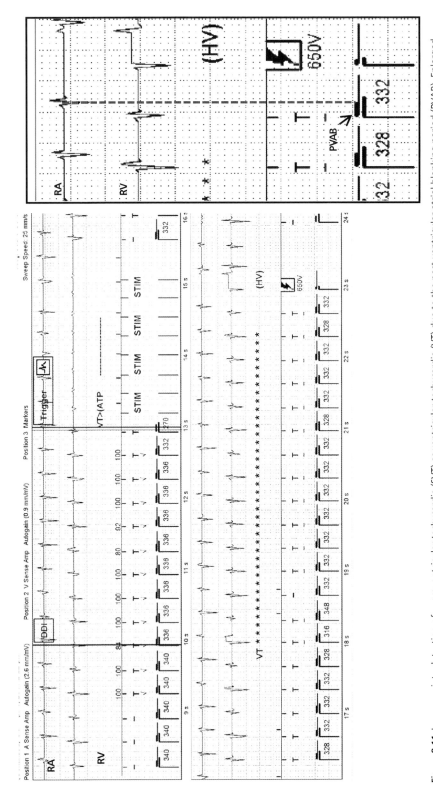

Figure 8.11 Inappropriate detection of supraventricular tachycardia (SVT) as ventricular tachycardia (VT) due to the post-ventricular atrial blanking period (PVAB). Enlarged panel at right shows that the peak of the atrial electrogram (EGM) times within the 90-ms PVAB after the ventricular EGM (top, dark short line on marker channel). At right of top panel, VT is detected in the V > A rate branch and antitachycardia pacing (ATP) is delivered (V > ATP). Note that there is a good morphology discriminator match (numerical values on marker channel > match threshold of 60%), but this is overridden by incorrect dual-chamber determination of V rate > A rate. In the lower panel, the asterisks indicate capacitor charging, and (HV) above the lightning symbol indicates an inappropriate 650-V shock.

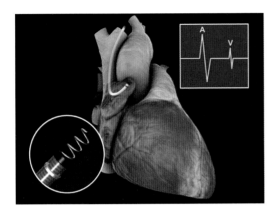

Figure 8.12 Far-field R-wave oversensing in a dual-chamber ICD. The close proximity between the atrial lead in the right atrial appendage and the right ventricle increases the likelihood of sensing far-field R waves on the atrial channel. Source: Seet RCS, Friedman PA, Rabinstein AA. Prolonged rhythm monitoring for the detection of occult paroxysmal atrial fibrillation in ischemic stroke of unknown cause. *Circulation* 2011;124:477–486. Reproduced with permission of Wolters Kluwer Health.

SVT (e.g. morphology templates may misclassify aberrantly conducted beats) [65].

Duration-based "Safety-Net" features to override discriminators

These programmable features deliver therapy if an arrhythmia satisfies the ventricular rate criterion for an extended duration even if discriminators indicate SVT. The premise is that VT will continue to satisfy the rate criterion, but the ventricular rate during transient sinus tachycardia or AF will decrease below the VT rate boundary before the duration is exceeded. The limitation is delivery of inappropriate therapy when SVT exceeds the programmed duration, which occurs commonly for durations of less than 1 min and in up to 10% of SVTs at 3 min, depending on the VT detection interval and AV conduction [59]. Durations of 5–10 min are required to minimize inappropriate therapy. The beneficial effects of these features are limited and we recommend programming them only in specific individualized indication.

SVT–VT discrimination algorithms: performance and clinical role

Measuring and comparing performance

Clinical comparisons of algorithm performance require the consideration of multiple factors,

including tachycardia episodes not stored in ICD memory and those faster than the SVT limit to which discriminators may not apply. Programmed parameters may influence algorithm performance. Not all algorithm failures have equivalent clinical significance. Inappropriate ATP is usually less significant than an inappropriate shock, and failure to detect asymptomatic self-terminating VT is less significant than failure to detect VT that requires resuscitation. Head-to-head comparisons of different SVT–VT discrimination algorithms show that there are substantive differences in performance, but it is difficult to be certain which of multiple differences among building blocks account for these findings [51].

Performance of single-chamber versus dual-chamber discriminators

When dual-chamber ICDs were developed before the advent of single-chamber morphology discriminators, there was great optimism that they would provide superior SVT–VT discrimination to single-chamber ICDs, both with respect to fewer inappropriate therapies and fewer underdetected VTs. Multiple studies have compared dual- versus single-chamber SVT–VT discrimination and a meta-analysis found no superiority of dual-chamber ICDs in terms of mortality or inappropriate therapies [66]. Despite some variation in results, a few conclusions can be drawn: (i) currently, unselected primary prevention patients do not benefit from dual-chamber SVT–VT discrimination; (ii) a randomized "bench test" comparison using prerecorded induced SVTs (mostly rapidly conducted AF) showed no benefit of dual-chamber discriminators with devices [51]; and (iii) currently recommended programming for primary prevention patients (Tables 8.10 and 8.11) reduces inappropriate therapy for SVT compared with traditional programming [53]. Additionally, current standard-of-care use of beta-blockers may reduce ventricular rates in SVT. The combination of these factors, combined with improved morphology discriminators, makes it unlikely that unselected primary prevention patients will ever benefit from dual-chamber SVT–VT discrimination. Dual-chamber algorithms have been reported to provide a modest performance improvement over single-chamber algorithms in secondary prevention patients who have SVT and slower VT at overlapping ventricular rates. Currently, experts

Table 8.10 ICD programming recommendations from 2015 Heart Rhythm Society consensus statement on optimal ICD programming and testing

Detection suggestions

- Program tachyarrhythmia detection duration to require the tachycardia to continue for at least 6–12 s or for 30 intervals before completing detection (primary or secondary prevention patients)
- Slowest tachycardia therapy zone limit between 185 and 200 bpm (primary prevention patients)
- Turn on SVT discrimination algorithms
- Program SVT discrimination algorithms to include rhythms with rates >200 bpm (potentially up to 230 bpm, unless contraindicated)
- For secondary prevention patients for whom the clinical VT rate is known, program the slowest tachycardia therapy zone at least 10 bpm below the documented tachycardia rate but not faster than 200 bpm
- Program more than one tachycardia detection zone to allow effective use of tiered therapy and/or SVT–VT discriminators and allow for a shorter delay in time-based detection programming for faster arrhythmias
- Choose single-chamber ICD therapy over dual-chamber ICD therapy if the sole reason for the atrial lead is SVT discrimination
- For the subcutaneous ICD, program two tachycardia detection zones:
- Zone with tachycardia discrimination algorithms at rate ≤200 bpm
- Second zone without tachycardia discrimination algorithms at rate ≥230 bpm
- Program tachycardia monitoring zone to alert clinicians to untreated arrhythmias
- Activate lead-failure alerts to detect potential lead problems
- Disable the SVT discriminator timeout function
- Activate lead "noise" algorithms
- Activate T-wave oversensing algorithms

Therapy suggestions

- Program ATP therapy "on" for all ventricular tachyarrhythmia detection zones to include arrhythmias up to 230 bpm in patients with structural heart disease[a]
- Program ATP to deliver at least one ATP attempt with a minimum of eight stimuli and a cycle length of 84–88% TCL[a]
- Use burst ATP therapy in preference to ramp ATP therapy
- Program the initial shock energy to the maximum available energy in the highest rate detection zone (unless specific defibrillation testing demonstrates efficacy at lower energies)

[a] Except when ATP is documented to be ineffective or proarrhythmic.
ATP, atrial tachycardia pacing; ICD, implantable cardioverter–defibrillator; SVT, supraventricular tachycardia; TCL, tachycardia cycle length; VT, ventricular tachycardia.
Sources: modified from Wilkoff *et al.* [56] and Stiles *et al.* [55].

disagree about whether or not dual-chamber ICDs benefit patients who are likely to have rapidly conducted SVT in the programmed VT detection zone. These conclusions are further complicated by head-to-head comparisons that show that the specificity of device-based algorithms differs among manufacturers, depending on programmed rate and whether single- or dual-chamber detection is employed [67].

Additionally, dual-chamber ICDs provide other features not available in single-chamber ICDs, including dual-chamber pacing algorithms that minimize RV pacing in patients with sinus node disease, diagnostics for AF, and stored EGMs that provide higher diagnostic accuracy than single-chamber ICDs. Dual-chamber ICDs may be considered if the benefits

of these features will outweigh the disadvantages of dual-chamber ICDs, which include higher cost, more implant complications, and decreased longevity. Figures 8.13–8.15 show representative examples.

Clinical role of SVT–VT discriminators
SVT–VT discriminators are only part of the solution to the problem of minimizing inappropriate therapy of SVT. Non-device elements include beta-blockers, antiarrhythmic drugs, and catheter ablation. Device elements include appropriate programming of rate and duration.

In clinical trials, approximately 25% of inappropriately treated SVTs are faster than the SVT limit [68]. The SVT limit must be programmed fast

Table 8.11 Manufacturer-specific ICD programming recommendations from 2015 Heart Rhythm Society consensus statement on optimal ICD programming and testing[a]

Manufacturer	Detection	Therapy (max. shocks energy)	Discriminators
Biotronik	VF: 30/40 intervals (if programmable, otherwise 24/30), 231 bpm VT2: 30 intervals, 188 bpm	VF: ATP One-Shot, one burst of 8 pulses at 88% CL VT2: ATP one or more bursts of 8 pulses at 88% CL, 10-ms scan decrement	Single: Morphology, Onset, Stability "on" Dual: SMART "on" Lead integrity check
Boston Scientific	*Option 1:* delayed therapy VF: 250 bpm; 5 s VT: 185 bpm; 12 s *Option 2:* high-rate therapy VF: 2.5-s duration, 200 bpm *Subcutaneous ICD* Shock Zone: ≥230 bpm Conditional Zone: ≥200 bpm	VF: QuickConvert "on" + shock VT: ATP-1: Scan, one or more bursts, 8 pulses at 84% coupling interval and cycle length (minimum 200 ms), 10-ms decrement	Single: Rhythm ID "on" Dual: Rhythm ID "on" or Onset/Stability "on" Sustained rate duration (SRD) "off" SVT discrimination zone <230 bpm
Medtronic	VF 188 bpm 30/40	VF: ATP before charge + shock ChargeSaver "on" VT (if "on"): Rx1: ATP, one or more bursts of 8 pulses at 88% VT CL, decrement 10 ms Rx2-6: All Shocks "on"	Single: Wavelet "on", Stability/Onset "off" Dual: PR logic "on", Wavelet "on", Stability/Onset "off" SVT discriminator: 230 bpm LIA and T-wave Oversensing "on" RV Lead Noise: "on" without timeout
Abbott (formerly St. Jude Medical)	VF: 240–250 bpm; 30 intervals VT: 187 bpm; 30 intervals	VF: ATP 8/85% + shock VT: ATP 8/85%/scan + shock	Single: Morphology 90% 3/10 Dual: Morphology + Onset + Stability SVT upper limit: 230 bpm SVT discrimination timeout "off" VT therapy timeout "off" Low Frequency Attenuation "on" SecureSense "on"

[a] Recommendations for empiric device programming for primary prevention patients. In patients where VT cycle length is known, VT zone is programmed to 10–20 bpm less than VT rate. Monitor zone can be added at user discretion. SVT Discriminators are not required in complete heart block.

CL, cycle length; RV, right ventricular; SVT, supraventricular tachycardia; VF, ventricular fibrillation; VT, ventricular tachycardia

Source: adapted from Wilkoff et al. [39] and Stiles et al. [55].

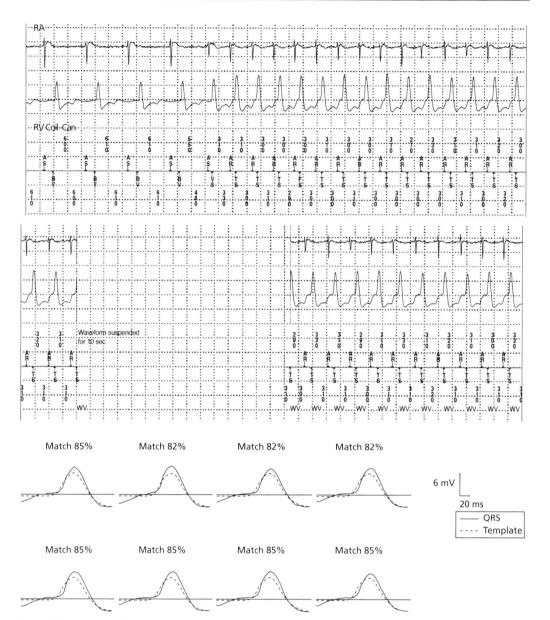

Figure 8.13 Correct classification of abrupt-onset supraventricular tachycardia (SVT) by morphology discriminator. Right atrial (RA) and shock (RV coil–can) electrograms (EGMs), and dual-chamber markers are shown. The fifth atrial EGM in the upper panel initiates SVT. VT detection based on rate alone would have occurred at the third (truncated) ventricular EGM in the lower panel, but the morphology discriminator (Wavelet, WV) classified the rhythm as SVT based on the match percentage being greater than the threshold value of 70% (bottom panel). Note the increase in shock EGM amplitude from sinus to SVT.

enough to apply to the most rapidly conducted SVT. An SVT–VT discrimination algorithm should be programmed in all patients with normal AV conduction. The algorithm should include a single-chamber ventricular morphology discriminator if available. A dual-chamber algorithm, usually including comparison of atrial and ventricular rates, should be programmed in patients with a stable functioning atrial lead. SVT–VT discriminators should be more specific in slower (VT) zones, in

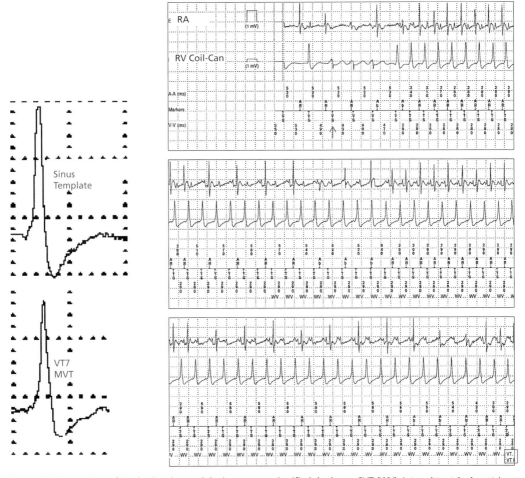

Figure 8.14 Interaction of single-chamber and dual-chamber algorithms. Right atrial (RA) and shock (RV coil–can) EGMs, and dual-chamber markers are shown. The left panel compares individual shock electrograms for the sinus template and seventh episode of monomorphic (M) ventricular tachycardia (VT), showing a close match. The red arrow shows onset of VT. The morphology algorithm classified rhythm as SVT (WV). Intermittent 1 : 1 ventriculoatrial (VA) conduction delays correct rhythm classification by comparison of atrial and ventricular rates, because classification is based on median value. After median ventricular rate exceeds median atrial rate, the algorithm delays for 10 beats before classifying rhythm as VT (bottom right).

which delay in detection of VT is well tolerated and underdetection of VT rarely causes collapse.

S-ICD sensing and discrimination

Although many principles of sensing and discrimination are similar to transvenous ICD systems, there are unique engineering challenges facing the S-ICD. Unlike the intracardiac EGM recorded by the transvenous system, the subcutaneous signal contains more morphological information that can be used for rhythm discrimination because it more closely resembles the surface ECG (Figure 8.16). S-ICD EGMs have smaller average R-wave amplitudes compared with transvenous ICD EGMs (from around 7 to 0.8 mV), as well as much smaller VF EGM amplitudes (from 5 to 0.5 mV). Moreover, the QRS complex can become quite broad, with a loss in slew rate differential [69]. When the R- to T-wave amplitude declines, the S-ICD signal is more vulnerable to cardiac oversensing, particularly T-wave oversensing, than the transvenous ICD (Figure 8.17). The R-wave to T-wave ratio becomes dependent on a number of factors, including patient's body habitus, posture, activity level, cardiac physiology, and

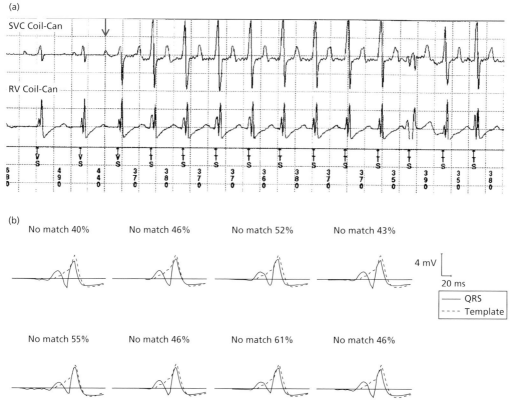

Figure 8.15 Inappropriate detection of abrupt-onset supraventricular tachycardia (SVT) as ventricular tachycardia (VT) in a single-chamber ICD that would have been prevented by the dual-chamber, chamber-of-onset discriminator. High-voltage electrograms (EGMs) recorded from the superior vena cava (SVC) and right ventricular (RV) coils are shown with single-chamber markers. Atrial EGMs are seen clearly on the SVC channel with the appearance of surface P waves. (a) Abrupt onset of SVT. Atrial tachycardia begins at third beat (arrow) with a premature atrial EGM wave that has a different morphology from the first two sinus atrial EGMs. (b) Moderate right bundle branch aberrancy results in match percentages between 40 and 60%, below the match threshold of 70%.

vector selection (Figure 8.16). This variability required the S-ICD to have a redesigned detection scheme that is primarily rhythm based rather than rate based like transvenous systems. A patient-specific morphology correlation analysis became the primary strategy for rate determination and rhythm discrimination algorithms [69]. To reduce T-wave oversensing, newer discrimination features were developed that helped recognize and reduce oversensing [52].

Prior to implant, the patient under consideration for S-ICD implant must be screened with a modified three-channel surface ECG that mimics the sensing vectors of the S-ICD system. The three different vectors are shown in Figure 8.16: the primary vector, which is programmed from the proximal ring to generator; the secondary vector, with the distal tip electrode to the generator; and the alternate vector, with the distal tip to the proximal ring electrode. For each vector, the R-wave to T-wave ratio is assessed for appropriate signal characteristics and relationships. The optimal sensing vector minimizes the likelihood of double counting of each cardiac event. If the screening is not satisfactory for at least one of the three vectors supine and standing, then implantation of an S-ICD is not recommended. After implant, the S-ICD automatically analyzes and selects the optimal vector from the three choices. If desired, the vector can be manually programmed. In general, the alternate vector is avoided if other vectors are acceptable because of a higher incidence of inappropriate shocks.

(a)

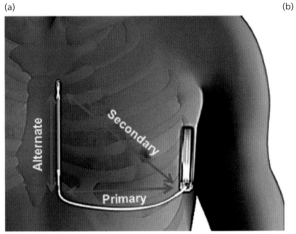

Anatomic location and sensing vectors of the subcutaneous implantable cardioverter-defibrillator system.

(b)

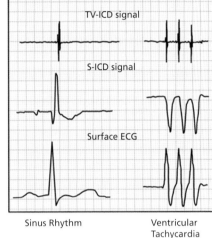

Sinus Rhythm   Ventricular Tachycardia

Figure 8.16 Subcutaneous-ICD (S-ICD) placement and sensing vectors. (a) The three available sensing vectors of S-ICD: primary (from proximal electrode ring to can), secondary (from distal electrode ring to can), and alternate (from distal to proximal electrode). During the implant procedure, the sense vector that provides the best sensing characteristics is evaluated and programmed, based on the signal quality of each vector evaluated by the device's programmer. (b) Examples of signals from transvenous (TV)-ICD, S-ICD, and surface ECG recordings. Note that the S-ICD signal, with the electrodes being some distance from the heart, more closely resembles the surface ECG and contains more morphological information than the near-field signal from the TV-ICD. Source: adapted from Brisben [70]. Reproduced with permission of Elsevier.

For tachycardia discrimination, the S-ICD utilizes automatic analysis in three stages: detection, certification, and therapy decision (Figure 8.18) [70].

- *Detection phase*: during the detection phase, the device uses a detection threshold to identify sensed events. The detection threshold is automatically adjusted continuously using amplitudes of recently detected electrical events. In addition, detection parameters are modified to increase sensitivity when rapid rates are detected (Figure 8.19). Events detected during the detection phase are passed on to the certification phase.
- *Certification phase*: this examines the detections and classifies them as certified cardiac events or as suspect events. Certified events are used to ensure that an accurate heart rate is passed to the decision phase. The device appraises waveforms to ensure detections are cardiac and not noise, and uses four algorithms that assess each detection to prevent oversensing. If the tachycardia EGM does not match the template ("static morphology" analysis), then a second "dynamic" morphology analysis is performed to discriminate VT from VF by a beat-to-beat comparison

of the morphology of tachycardia EGMs to determine their consistency. This step uses morphology to discriminate monomorphic VT from polymorphic VT or VF: a dynamic template match indicates monomorphic VT while a mismatch indicates polymorphic VT or VF. Morphology discriminators can also be used to reject T-wave oversensing reliably based on the poor match between the activation and repolarization components of the ventricular EGM.

- *Therapy decision phase*: this phase examines all certified events and continuously calculates a running four R–R interval average (four R–R average). The four R–R average is used throughout the analysis as an indicator of the heart rate.

In the shock-only zone, therapy decision is based solely on rate criteria. In addition, a second zone, termed the "conditional shock zone," uses a stepwise discrimination algorithm to distinguish shockable from non-shockable rhythms. The three discriminators used include the *static morphology analysis*, which identifies non-shockable rhythms, utilizing the normal sinus rhythm (NSR) template, a *dynamic morphology analysis*, which identifies shockable polymorphic rhythms by comparing each complex to the previous ones, and a *QRS width analysis*, which compares the QRS width to the baseline template QRS width (Figure 8.18).

Addition of a conditional shock zone reduces shocks due to both supraventricular arrhythmias and oversensing without prolonging detection times and with no increased incidence of syncope

[71]. In addition, when the S-ICD is programmed to have a conditional shock zone, the S-ICD VT detection algorithm has been demonstrated to be more effective than transvenous ICD systems programmed at nominal settings to prevent the detection of SVT [51]. Based on this, dual-zone programming is recommended for S-ICDs, with a conditional shock zone programmed at a rate of

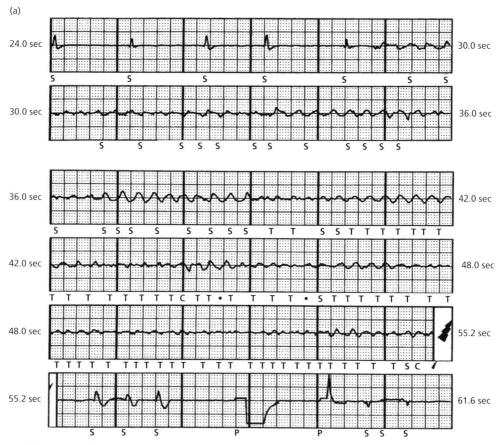

Figure 8.17 Examples of appropriate and inappropriate S-ICD shocks. (a) Electrogram of a spontaneously occurring ventricular fibrillation (VF) episode terminated with a single 80-J standard polarity shock by the S-ICD. On the early portion of the tracing, there is temporary undersensing due to signal amplitude variations. The device adjusts to higher sensitivity detection profiles as the VF continues, allowing identification and treatment with defibrillation therapy. (b) Inappropriate shock due to T-wave oversensing. Note that the low amplitude of the QRS complexes creates a challenge for the sensing algorithm to distinguish between QRS complexes and other physiological and non-physiological signals. The device annotates the "T" for tachy detection, tagging both the QRS complex and the T wave, in

some cases leading to double counting and inappropriate shock. The S-ICD has several options for reducing oversensing, including reprogramming of the sensing vector and gain setting and template optimization as well as newer filter-based algorithms. However, if the R-wave to T-wave ratio declines, which depends on final device position, patient activity and body habitus, posture, and changes in physiology, the S-ICD becomes more vulnerable to oversensing. Note that while low amplitude persists post shock, oversensing is not taking place. Some QRS complexes are undersensed, presumably due to the dissimilar detection profile. The dissimilar detection profile is invoked when the signal amplitude is found to differ by more than 20% between successive detections.

(b)

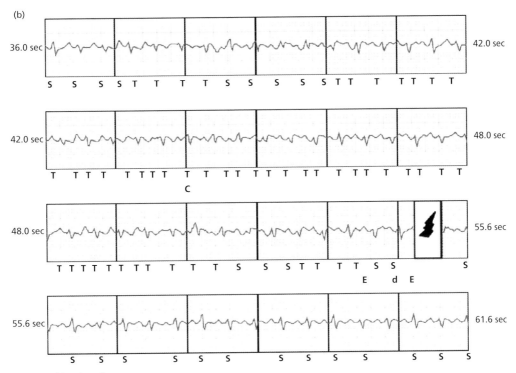

Figure 8.17 (Continued)

200 bpm or less and a shock zone programmed at 230 bpm or above [39]. Overall, the inappropriate shock rates are similar between transvenous ICDs and S-ICDs, although the distribution etiologies of such shocks differ. Specifically, inappropriate shocks for supraventricular arrhythmias are more common with transvenous devices, whereas shocks for T-wave oversensing and myopotentials are more common with the S-ICD.

Defibrillation

Basic physiology of defibrillation
An electrical stimulus interacts with cardiac cells via its resultant electrical field, which is proportional to the local rate of change of the applied voltage with respect to distance (spatial derivative). The cardiac response to the shock is determined by the passive and active (ion channel) properties of cell membranes, the properties of electrical connections between cells, and possibly by direct effects on intracellular events such as calcium release.

The electrophysiological requirement for defibrillation may be contrasted with the requirement for pacing. Pacemakers deliver a stimulus through closely spaced electrodes sufficient to depolarize local myocardium during diastole (phase 4 of the action potential) and initiate self-propagating depolarization. In contrast, initiation and termination of VF by shocks requires an electrophysiological effect throughout both ventricles during the plateau or repolarization phases of the action potential (phases 2 and 3, respectively). Shocks may have both direct effects related to the strength of the local electrical field and indirect effects related to the creation of *virtual electrodes*, secondary sources of electrical potential in tissue sites remote from the stimulating electrodes [72].

Defibrillation waveforms
The waveform of an electrical pulse is the temporal pattern of its amplitude, measured by voltage (or current). An ICD's shock waveform interacts with cardiac electrical activity via its electric field, which is the instantaneous spatial derivative of shock voltage. The response of the heart to the shock field is mediated by the passive and active (ionic channel) properties of cell membranes, the properties of

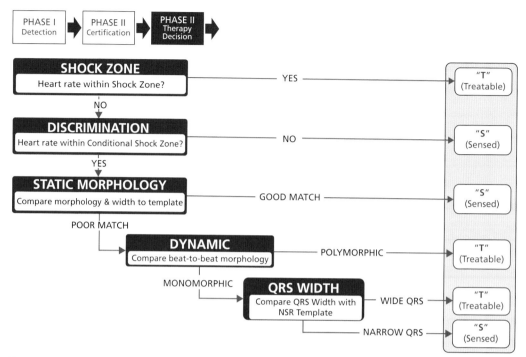

Figure 8.18 S-ICD algorithms during therapy decision phase: conditional zone discrimination. The S-ICD is programmed with two heart rate detection zones: a conditional shock zone and a shock zone. In this example, the conditional shock zone is programmed at 200–230 bpm and the shock zone at >230 bpm. The S-ICD annotates each certified detection with an "S" (sensed) or a "T" (treatable). First, detections in the shock heart rate zone (>230 bpm) are annotated with a "T" and then those in the "normal" heart rate zone (<200 bpm) are annotated with "S." When the heart rate is in the conditional zone (between 200 and 230 bpm), the rhythm discrimination algorithm is invoked, as shown. Detections are marked as "S" or "T" depending on the results of static and dynamic correlation waveform analysis (CWA). The static CWA score is calculated and, if the result is a match, the underlying rhythm is presumably an SVT, and the beat is marked "S." If the static CWA score indicates a poor match, then the dynamic CWA score is evaluated, where the morphology of the current detection is compared to the previous detection. If the dynamic CWA score is low, the rhythm is considered polymorphic and marked "T." On the other hand, if the dynamic CWA score is high, the rhythm is considered monomorphic. A last decision calculates the width of the current QRS complex and compares that width to the static template. If the detection's width is considerably wider than the static template, the rhythm is considered wide and ventricular in nature (marked "T"). Otherwise, the rhythm is considered supraventricular in nature and marked "S."

electrical connections between cardiac cells, and possibly the direct intracellular electrical effect.

The waveform parameters that most directly influence defibrillation are voltage and duration. Voltage is a critical parameter because its spatial derivative defines the electrical field that interacts with the heart. Similarly, waveform duration is critical because the shock interacts with the heart for the duration of the waveform. The electrical measure of defibrillation that is most relevant physiologically is voltage (or voltage gradient) as a function of time.

Shock energy is the most often cited metric of shock strength and an ICD's capacity to defibrillate, but it is not a direct measure of shock effectiveness. However, the maximum energy stored in an ICD's output capacitor is a major determinant of the size of the battery and capacitor, and thus the overall size of the pulse generator. Since minimizing pulse generator size is an important clinical goal, designing ICDs that defibrillate with minimum stored energy is an important engineering goal.

The plot of defibrillation threshold (DFT; usually leading-edge voltage) as a function of waveform duration is known as the defibrillation strength–duration curve, analogous to the strength–duration curve for pacing. Since there is

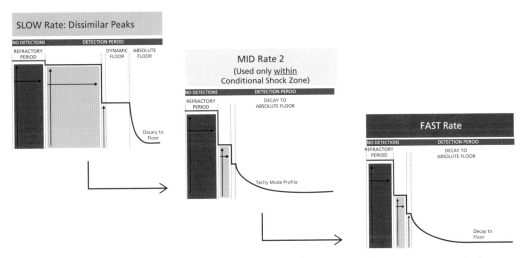

Figure 8.19 S-ICD system: detection profiles. As heart rate increases, the S-ICD system becomes more aggressive in detecting small or fast signals (ventricular tachycardia or ventricular fibrillation).

no true DFT, the plotted value may be considered as the shock strength required to achieve a given probability of defibrillation (e.g. 90%), but for simplicity we refer to it as the DFT. As shown in Figure 8.20, the effect on DFT of equivalent change in duration is much greater at short durations than long durations. The long-duration asymptote for DFT (the lowest value for an infinite pulse width) is referred to as the *rheobase*. The *chronaxie* is defined as the duration of a waveform that has a DFT of twice the rheobase amplitude. The chronaxie is close to the membrane time constant (τ_m).

Defibrillation testing

The goal of defibrillation testing is to ensure that the programmed shock strength has an extremely high probability of terminating VF in a given patient and that there is reliable sensing and detection of VF by the ICD. Multiple methods for calculating DFT have been developed [73], but the most commonly recommended programming of first shock strength is DFT + 10 J. When safety margin testing is used, the first shock for spontaneous arrhythmias is set to maximum output.

Defibrillation efficacy can be assessed directly by fibrillation–defibrillation ("defibrillation") testing or indirectly by vulnerability testing. Both methods can be used in either a patient-specific strategy or a safety margin strategy. DFT testing refers to a group of methods that assess defibrillation efficacy by

calculating a shock strength on the sloping portion of the curve based on successes and failures of a few shocks at different strengths. Thus, the DFT is based on a limited discrete sampling of a continuous statistical distribution. Clinical data show that conventional DFT testing has limited reproducibility [74].

In clinical practice, the usual goal is to identify those patients in whom ICD shocks are unreliable. *Safety margin strategies* limit testing to the minimum necessary to determine if there is a sufficient margin such that the maximum output of the ICD defibrillates reliably. Defibrillation efficacy is assessed one or more times, usually at only one shock strength chosen in relation to the maximum shock strength of the ICD. The outcome of each assessment is classified as either successful or unsuccessful, and the cumulative result is compared with the implant criterion. If defibrillation testing is performed, most commonly it is done using a safety margin strategy.

Early ICD systems using monophasic waveforms with epicardial patches or transvenous leads were associated with a substantial incidence of elevated DFTs, and DFT testing was an integral part of the ICD implantation procedure. However, contemporary ICD systems, with the pulse generator case (i.e. active can), biphasic waveforms, left pectoral pulse generators, and intravascular high-voltage leads, have considerably lowered the incidence of

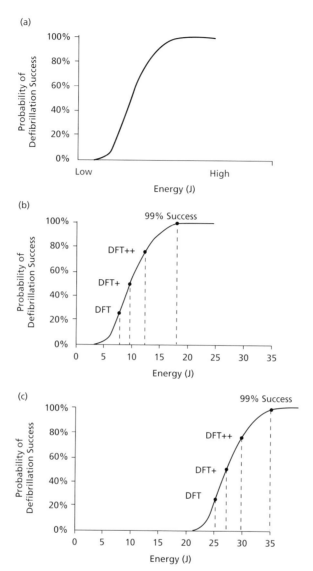

Figure 8.20 Graphical representation of the relationship between probability of successful defibrillation versus energy level of shock. (a) The generalized defibrillation success curve is sigmoidal in shape. (b) The defibrillation success curve for a hypothetical patient. If the defibrillation threshold (DFT) is measured as a single successful defibrillation at a given energy level, the confidence for repeated success is lower than if an energy level is tested that defibrillates twice (DFT+) or three times (DFT++) without failure. The safety margin for programming is the difference between the measured value of DFT and the energy needed for

>99% successful defibrillation. However, the energy level for 99% success is never really known for any patient. The safety margins for any measure of DFT are estimated empirically based on the assumption that the shape of the DFT curve is relatively consistent between patients. (c) In this hypothetical patient, all measures of DFT are high. Using a safety margin of 10 J added to the DFT+ or DFT++ would require a device with at least a 37-J output to ensure >99% successful defibrillation. This patient would require revision of the lead system to reduce the DFTs or the implantation of a high-output device.

elevated DFTs. Given the very low incidence of identifiable DFT issues and the potential serious complications, the safety of a primary implant approach without DFT testing was studied in a series of recent randomized controlled trials

assessing the effect of DFT on clinical outcomes. The Shockless Implant Evaluation (SIMPLE) trial was the largest [75]. Patients were randomized to DFT testing (1253 patients) or not (1247) at the time of ICD implantation and followed for a mean of 3.1 years. The primary outcome of arrhythmic death or failed appropriate shock was non-inferior in the no-testing group compared with patients undergoing DFT testing. DFT testing at the time of ICD implantation did not improve shock efficacy or reduce arrhythmic death but was also found to be generally well tolerated without a statistically significantly increased rate of complications. A second notable randomized trial, the No Regular Defibrillation Testing In Cardioverter Defibrillator Implantation (NORDIC-ICD) trial, patients were randomly assigned to first time ICD implantation with (540 patients) or without (537 patients) DFT testing [76]. All ICD shocks were programmed to 40 J irrespective of DFT testing results. The primary end point was average first-shock efficacy for all true VT and VF episodes occurring during follow-up. The secondary end points included serious adverse events and mortality. The primary end point was non-inferior with or without DFT testing and there was no difference in adverse events with either strategy. Altogether, the data support that DFT testing during left-sided transvenous ICD implantation is now optional and frequently not performed. However, testing is still recommended for right-sided implants.

Given the general practice of avoiding DFT testing at implant, the focus now is to identify patients who might be at higher risk of elevated DFTs (Table 8.12). It is worth emphasizing that the non-testing approach requires an anatomically well-positioned ICD lead with adequate sensing of intrinsic R waves, adequate pacing thresholds, and a thorough verification of proper lead connection. Clinical scenarios worth considering for DFT testing include patients with hypertrophic cardiomyopathy or channelopathies, those undergoing generator replacement, and procedures in the right pectoral location (Table 8.13). Additionally, DFT testing is reasonable when there is any question of the adequacy of lead integrity, sensing, or position. A suggested algorithm for management of the patient with an elevated DFT is shown in Figure 8.21.

Furthermore, there are several situations where DFT testing is contraindicated, such as the presence of a left atrial appendage thrombus, during inadequate anesthesia, suspected poor hemodynamic tolerance of testing, and unreliable external rescue shocks.

Table 8.12 Causes and corrections for high defibrillation thresholds (DFTs) at implant

Cause of elevated DFT	Diagnosis	Correction
Poor lead position	On fluoroscopy distal coil out of RV, proximal coil low in atrium	Reposition lead
Increased high-voltage impedance	Data from defibrillation attempt, commanded determination of impedance	Check header connections, reposition lead and/or coils, add SVC to single-coil system, add SQ array, relieve pneumothorax
Pneumothorax	High shock impedance, fluoroscopy, dyspnea	Relieve pneumothorax
Hypoxia	Low oxygen saturation	Lighten sedation, assist ventilation
Ischemia	Chest pain, ECG changes, hypotension	Anti-ischemic therapy
Multiple defibrillations	Numerous previous defibrillation attempts	Implant device in best configuration and retest
Antiarrhythmic drugs or anesthetics	Exclude other etiologies	Retest after stopping drugs, stop inhaled anesthetics
Poor current distributions	High or low shocking impedance, poor lead positions	Reposition coil, add SVC coil to single-coil system, add SQ array or azygous lead
Shunting current through guidewires or retained leads	Retained guidewires, temporary or permanent pacing leads	Retest after removing wires or leads
Poor myocardial substrate	Exclusion of other causes, failure of multiple lead configurations and polarity	Add coils, SQ array, azygous lead, epicardial patches to circuit, use high-output device, add class III antiarrhythmic drugs that reduce DFTs

RV, right ventricle; SQ, subcutaneous; SVC, superior vena cava.

ICD programming

Tachycardia detection programming

A series of clinical trials has helped determine programming parameters to optimize therapy and minimize unnecessary shocks, particularly in the primary prevention population. The PainFree trials showed that empiric programming of ATP was effective and reduced inappropriate shocks. Moreover, ATP for arrhythmias at rates as high as 250 bpm was shown to be safe [77]. The Comparison of Empiric to Physician-Tailored Programming of Implantable

Cardioverter-Defibrillators (EMPIRIC) study demonstrated that standard algorithms, including ATP for rapid arrhythmias, was preferable to individualized programming based on patient or arrhythmia characteristics [78]. An analysis of these early studies showed that many arrhythmias self-terminated, indicating that detection times were too short. This led to studies of both prolonged detection time and increased rate cutoff for therapy. The Primary Prevention Parameters Evaluation (PREPARE) study was one such study where arrhythmias at rates of less than 182 bpm were not treated and detection intervals were prolonged [79]. This programming strategy results in fewer appropriate as well as inappropriate shocks. It also reduces shocks for lead malfunctions and extraneous noise. An even more dramatic approach to ICD programming was employed in the MADIT-RIT trial, where separate arms of the study had devices programmed to withhold therapy for 60 s at rates of less than 200 bpm or to deliver no therapy for any arrhythmia of less than 200 bpm [53]. These arms were associated with fewer inappropriate therapies and lower mortality, without an increase in the rate of syncope. The link between inappropriate therapies and mortality is less clear from this study, as most therapies were ATP and not

Table 8.13 Scenarios where DFT testing is useful or might be considered

S-ICD
Right-sided ICD implantation
Antiarrhythmic drugs used (class I or amiodarone)
ICD replacement
Hypertrophic cardiomyopathy
Channelopathies
Concern regarding lead integrity, sensing or position
Significant programming change from default sensitivity or sensing

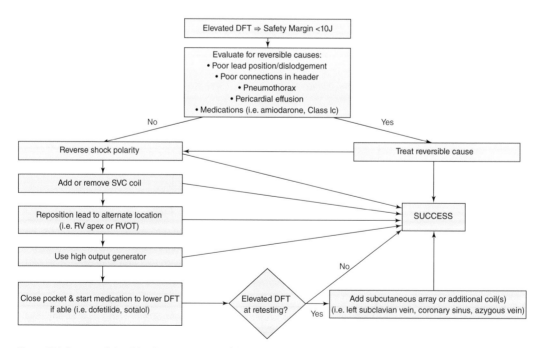

Figure 8.21 Suggested algorithm for management of the patient with an elevated defibrillation threshold (DFT), defined as a safety margin of <10 J below the maximal device output. The implanter should first rule out and treat reversible causes of elevated DFTs, and then attempt further modifications to the configurations and/or treatment regimen as illustrated. RV, right ventricular; RVOT, right ventricular outflow tract; SVC, superior vena cava.

shocks. Tables 8.10, 8.11 and 8.14 summarize the considerations and suggested ICD programming for primary and secondary prevention patients.

With increased awareness of the potential harm of inappropriate shocks, strategies to prolong detection times have been evaluated and shown to be beneficial. The benefit of delayed detection intervals was first reported in the PREPARE study and subsequently in several prospective randomized controlled trials including MADIT-RIT and ADVANCE-III [53,54,79]. A 2015 Heart Rhythm Society Consensus Statement on Optimal ICD Programming and Testing provides a detailed summary of the primary clinical evidence as well as expert recommendations regarding ICD programming [56] (Table 8.10). The document emphasizes the necessity to consider a long detection window setting as a "default" strategy for ICD programming.

High-rate overdrive pacing (known as ATP) is very effective for terminating VT. Adaptive algorithms are used in which the pacing rate is programmed based on the tachycardia cycle length of each episode of tachycardia (Figure 8.22). Randomized studies have shown similar efficacy of burst (constant cycle length in the train) and ramp (decremental cycle lengths in the train) pacing

Table 8.14 Considerations for ICD programming

Use of beta-blockers
Heart rate during exercise
Rate of prior documented clinical sustained ventricular tachycardia (VT)
Antiarrhythmic drugs that may slow VT rate
Rate and duration of prior documented non-sustained VTs
Rate of prior documented supraventricular tachycardias (SVTs) and likely effectiveness of SVT–VT discriminators in rejecting SVT

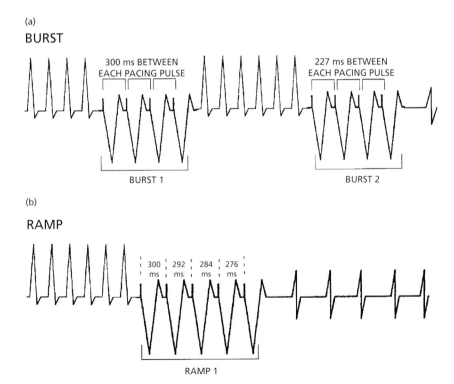

Figure 8.22 Schematic of burst and ramp antitachycardia pacing (ATP). (a) Four beats of ventricular tachycardia are followed by the first burst of ATP at 300 ms for four beats. The rate for this burst is determined as a programmable percentage of the tachycardia cycle length. Tachycardia continues after burst 1, so after redetection burst 2 is delivered at a programmable rate faster than burst 1 (227 ms in this example). The pacing interval for subsequent bursts will decrement further until a minimum pacing cycle length is reached, all ATP attempts are delivered, or the tachycardia terminates. (b) In ramp ATP there is a decrement in the pacing interval between consecutive stimuli. The initial pacing rate starts as a percentage of the tachycardia cycle length. Multiple ramp attempts can be programmed with shorter intervals in each subsequent attempt. Source: Boston Scientific Corporation. Reproduced with permission of Boston Scientific.

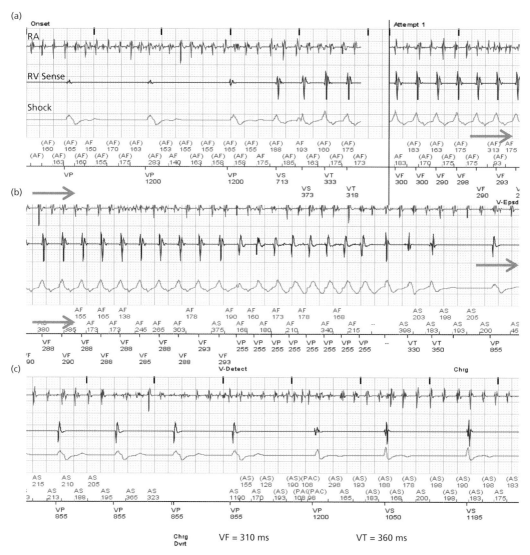

Figure 8.23 Example of successful antitachycardia pacing (ATP) for fast ventricular tachycardia (VT) in the ventricular fibrillation (VF) zone. The continuous stored electrogram (EGM) shows atrial (RA), near-field integrated-bipolar (RV Sense), and far-field (Shock) EGMs. The dual-chamber marker channel displays atrial intervals above and ventricular intervals below the line. The atrial rhythm throughout is atrial fibrillation (AF, marker channel). (a) The first three ventricular intervals are paced at 1200 ms (50 bpm). The fourth beat shows onset of regular tachycardia that accelerates to a cycle length of 300–290 ms. The vertical line denotes interruption of recording after onset of tachycardia and just before VF is detected initially (V-Epsd at end of panel). (b) Persistence of device-detected "VF" is confirmed in the middle of the panel (V-Detect), followed by ATP in the VF zone that terminates tachycardia. Because ATP was delivered in the VF zone, the ICD does not undergo a full redetection process, but rather a more limited reconfirmation process.

It begins to charge (Chrg) when two of three ventricular intervals after ATP are classified in the VT zone. ATP is followed by post-therapy pacing for five beats at 855 ms (70 bpm). (c) "Chrg Dvrt" indicates that the ICD classifies the tachycardia episode as completed so that the charge on the high-voltage capacitors is dissipated. Thus, the patient is spared a shock, but the battery loses the corresponding energy. The last two ventricular EGMs represent slowly conducted AF and differ markedly in morphology from tachycardia EGMs. The ICD's classification of this rhythm based on rate alone is "VF." It does not apply supraventricular tachycardia (SVT)–VT discriminators in the VF zone. The physician's classification is monomorphic VT during AF based on the abrupt onset of rapid, regular tachycardia with morphology different from the conducted beats during AF that terminates distinctly with ATP. The ICD may be reprogrammed so that this tachycardia is classified in a VT zone to increase the likelihood that ATP will be delivered without charging.

when applied to slower VTs, but greater efficacy for burst pacing when applied to VTs faster than 187 bpm. Figure 8.23 shows an example of ATP for fast VT in the VF zone. It also highlights several interpretive issues in analyzing ICD-stored EGMs. Early studies of ATP in ICDs reported high rates for pace termination of spontaneous episodes of relatively slow VT, typically approximately 90%, with low rates of arrhythmia acceleration (1–3%). More recent data indicate that many of these episodes would likely have terminated spontaneously. Success rates of 45–50% for episodes of VT faster than 182 bpm and lasting longer than 30 beats are observed. These observations support a strategy of empiric programming of ATP in patients with the underlying substrate for monomorphic VT. Older generation devices only allowed ATP in a VT detection zone. However, current devices typically allow one round of such pacing in the VF zone. This allows in some instances to program a single zone device while still allowing for ATP.

Summary

ICD therapy has undergone a remarkable transformation since the devices were first approved for human use. Modern devices provide detailed information about the rate and morphology of ECG signals, as well as physiological parameters that help manage patients remotely. The simplicity of defibrillator implantation now approaches that of pacemakers and more patients have been identified who can benefit from this therapy. However, the reliability of transvenous leads and the incidence and impact of unnecessary shocks are problems that have blunted full adoption of this therapy. Improvement in lead design, including subcutaneous systems, newer programming strategies, and better patient selection will hopefully contribute to improved outcomes and further reductions of SCD.

References

1 Mirowski M, Reid PR, Mower MM, *et al*. Termination of malignant ventricular arrhythmias with an implanted automatic defibrillator in human beings. *N Engl J Med* 1980;303(6):322–324.

2 Bardy GH, Smith WM, Hood MA, *et al*. An entirely subcutaneous implantable cardioverter-defibrillator. *N Engl J Med* 2010;363(1):36–44.

3 Antiarrhythmics versus Implantable Defibrillators Investigators. A comparison of antiarrhythmic-drug therapy with implantable defibrillators in patients resuscitated from near-fatal ventricular arrhythmias. *N Engl J Med* 1997;337(22):1576–1583.

4 Connolly SJ, Gent M, Roberts RS, *et al*. Canadian Implantable Defibrillator Study (CIDS): a randomized trial of the implantable cardioverter defibrillator against amiodarone. *Circulation* 2000;101(11):1297–1302.

5 Kuck KH, Cappato R, Siebels J, Ruppel R. Randomized comparison of antiarrhythmic drug therapy with implantable defibrillators in patients resuscitated from cardiac arrest: the Cardiac Arrest Study Hamburg (CASH). *Circulation* 2000;102(7):748–754.

6 Connolly SJ, Hallstrom AP, Cappato R, *et al*. Meta-analysis of the implantable cardioverter defibrillator secondary prevention trials. AVID, CASH and CIDS studies. Antiarrhythmics vs Implantable Defibrillator study. Cardiac Arrest Study Hamburg. Canadian Implantable Defibrillator Study. *Eur Heart J* 2000;21(24):2071–2078.

7 Sheldon R, Connolly S, Krahn A, *et al*. Identification of patients most likely to benefit from implantable cardioverter-defibrillator therapy: the Canadian Implantable Defibrillator Study. *Circulation* 2000;101(14):1660–1664.

8 Moss AJ, Hall WJ, Cannom DS, *et al*. Improved survival with an implanted defibrillator in patients with coronary disease at high risk for ventricular arrhythmia. Multicenter Automatic Defibrillator Implantation Trial Investigators. *N Engl J Med* 1996;335(26):1933–1940.

9 Buxton AE, Lee KL, Fisher JD, *et al*. A randomized study of the prevention of sudden death in patients with coronary artery disease. Multicenter Unsustained Tachycardia Trial Investigators. *N Engl J Med* 1999;341(25):1882–1890.

10 Gold MR, Nisam S. Primary prevention of sudden cardiac death with implantable cardioverter defibrillators: lessons learned from MADIT and MUSTT. *Pacing Clin Electrophysiol* 2000;23(11 Pt 2):1981–1985.

11 Buxton AE, Lee KL, DiCarlo L, *et al*. Electrophysiologic testing to identify patients with coronary artery disease who are at risk for sudden death. Multicenter Unsustained Tachycardia Trial Investigators. *N Engl J Med* 2000;342(26):1937–1945.

12 Moss AJ, Zareba W, Hall WJ, *et al*. Prophylactic implantation of a defibrillator in patients with myocardial infarction and reduced ejection fraction. *N Engl J Med* 2002;346(12):877–883.

13 Bardy GH, Lee KL, Mark DB, *et al*. Amiodarone or an implantable cardioverter-defibrillator for congestive heart failure. *N Engl J Med* 2005;352(3):225–237.

14 Kadish A, Dyer A, Daubert JP, *et al*. Prophylactic defibrillator implantation in patients with nonischemic dilated cardiomyopathy. *N Engl J Med* 2004;350(21):2151–2158.

15 McNamara DM, Starling RC, Cooper LT, *et al*. Clinical and demographic predictors of outcomes in recent onset

dilated cardiomyopathy: results of the IMAC (Intervention in Myocarditis and Acute Cardiomyopathy)-2 study. *J Am Coll Cardiol* 2011;58(11):1112–1118.

16 Kober L, Thune JJ, Nielsen JC, *et al*. Defibrillator implantation in patients with nonischemic systolic heart failure. *N Engl J Med* 2016;375(13):1221–1230.

17 Cleland JG, Daubert JC, Erdmann E, et al. The effect of cardiac resynchronization on morbidity and mortality in heart failure. *N Engl J Med* 2005;352(15):1539–1549.

18 Al-Khatib SM, Fonarow GC, Joglar JA, et al. Primary prevention implantable cardioverter defibrillators in patients with nonischemic cardiomyopathy: a meta-analysis. *JAMA Cardiol* 2017;2(6):685–688.

19 Al-Khatib SM, Stevenson WG, Ackerman MJ, *et al*. 2017 AHA/ACC/HRS guideline for management of patients with ventricular arrhythmias and the prevention of sudden cardiac death: a report of the American College of Cardiology/American Heart Association Task Force on Clinical Practice Guidelines and the Heart Rhythm Society. *J Am Coll Cardiol* 2018;72(14):e91–e220.

20 Anantha Narayanan M, Vakil K, Reddy YN, *et al*. Efficacy of implantable cardioverter-defibrillator therapy in patients with nonischemic cardiomyopathy: a systematic review and meta-analysis of randomized controlled trials. *JACC Clin Electrophysiol* 2017;3(9):962–970.

21 Kuruvilla S, Adenaw N, Katwal AB, *et al*. Late gadolinium enhancement on cardiac magnetic resonance predicts adverse cardiovascular outcomes in nonischemic cardiomyopathy: a systematic review and meta-analysis. *Circ Cardiovasc Imaging* 2014;7(2):250–258.

22 Sroubek J, Buxton AE. Primary prevention implantable cardiac defibrillator trials: what have we learned? *Card Electrophysiol Clin* 2017;9(4):761–773.

23 Birnie DH, Sauer WH, Bogun F, *et al*. HRS expert consensus statement on the diagnosis and management of arrhythmias associated with cardiac sarcoidosis. *Heart Rhythm* 2014;11(7):1305–1323.

24 Towbin JA, McKenna WJ, Abrams DJ, *et al*. 2019 HRS expert consensus statement on evaluation, risk stratification, and management of arrhythmogenic cardiomyopathy. *Heart Rhythm* 2019;16(11):e301–e372.

25 Gersh BJ, Maron BJ, Bonow RO, *et al*. 2011 ACCF/AHA guideline for the diagnosis and treatment of hypertrophic cardiomyopathy: a report of the American College of Cardiology Foundation/American Heart Association Task Force on Practice Guidelines. *J Am Coll Cardiol* 2011;58(25):e212–e260.

26 Schwartz PJ, Ackerman MJ, Wilde AAM. Channelopathies as causes of sudden cardiac death. *Card Electrophysiol Clin* 2017;9(4):537–549.

27 Priori SG, Wilde AA, Horie M, *et al*. HRS/EHRA/APHRS expert consensus statement on the diagnosis and management of patients with inherited primary arrhythmia syndromes: document endorsed by HRS, EHRA, and APHRS in May 2013 and by ACCF, AHA, PACES, and AEPC in June 2013. *Heart Rhythm* 2013;10(12): 1932–1963.

28 Maron BJ. Clinical course and management of hypertrophic cardiomyopathy. *N Engl J Med* 2018;379(7): 655–668.

29 Bigger JT. Prophylactic use of implanted cardiac defibrillators in patients at high risk for ventricular arrhythmias after coronary-artery bypass graft surgery. Coronary Artery Bypass Graft (CABG) Patch Trial Investigators. *N Engl J Med* 1997;337(22):1569–1575.

30 Hohnloser SH, Kuck KH, Dorian P, *et al*. Prophylactic use of an implantable cardioverter-defibrillator after acute myocardial infarction. *N Engl J Med* 2004;351(24): 2481–2488.

31 Steinbeck G, Andresen D, Seidl K, *et al*. Defibrillator implantation early after myocardial infarction. *N Engl J Med* 2009;361(15):1427–1436.

32 Dorian P, Hohnloser SH, Thorpe KE, *et al*. Mechanisms underlying the lack of effect of implantable cardioverter-defibrillator therapy on mortality in high-risk patients with recent myocardial infarction: insights from the Defibrillation in Acute Myocardial Infarction Trial (DINAMIT). *Circulation* 2010;122(25):2645–2652.

33 Goldenberg I, Vyas AK, Hall WJ, *et al*. Risk stratification for primary implantation of a cardioverter-defibrillator in patients with ischemic left ventricular dysfunction. *J Am Coll Cardiol* 2008;51(3):288–296.

34 de Vreede-Swagemakers JJ, Gorgels AP, Dubois-Arbouw WI, *et al*. Out-of-hospital cardiac arrest in the 1990s: a population-based study in the Maastricht area on incidence, characteristics and survival. *J Am Coll Cardiol* 1997;30(6):1500–1505.

35 Stecker EC, Vickers C, Waltz J, *et al*. Population-based analysis of sudden cardiac death with and without left ventricular systolic dysfunction: two-year findings from the Oregon Sudden Unexpected Death Study. *J Am Coll Cardiol* 2006;47(6):1161–1166.

36 Wyse DG, Friedman PL, Brodsky MA, *et al*. Life-threatening ventricular arrhythmias due to transient or correctable causes: high risk for death in follow-up. *J Am Coll Cardiol* 2001;38(6):1718–1724.

37 Olgin JE, Pletcher MJ, Vittinghoff E, *et al*. Wearable cardioverter-defibrillator after myocardial infarction. *N Engl J Med* 2018;379(13):1205–1215.

38 Piccini JP, Allen LA, Kudenchuk PJ, *et al*. Wearable cardioverter-defibrillator therapy for the prevention of sudden cardiac death: a science advisory from the American Heart Association. *Circulation* 2016;133(17):1715–1727.

39 Wilkoff BL, Fauchier L, Stiles MK, *et al*. 2015 HRS/EHRA/APHRS/SOLAECE expert consensus statement on optimal implantable cardioverter-defibrillator

programming and testing. *Heart Rhythm* 2016;13(2): e50–e86.

40 McLeod CJ, Boersma L, Okamura H, Friedman PA. The subcutaneous implantable cardioverter defibrillator: state-of-the-art review. *Eur Heart J* 2017;38(4):247–257.

41 Koneru JN, Jones PW, Hammill EF, Wold N, Ellenbogen KA. Risk factors and temporal trends of complications associated with transvenous implantable cardiac defibrillator leads. *J Am Heart Assoc* 2018;7(10):e007691.

42 Bardy GH, Smith WM, Hood MA, *et al.* An entirely subcutaneous implantable cardioverter-defibrillator. *N Engl J Med* 2010;363(1):36–44.

43 Burke MC, Gold MR, Knight BP, *et al.* Safety and efficacy of the totally subcutaneous implantable defibrillator: 2-year results from a pooled analysis of the IDE Study and EFFORTLESS Registry. *J Am Coll Cardiol* 2015;65(16):1605–1615.

44 Basu-Ray I, Liu J, Jia X, *et al.* Subcutaneous versus transvenous implantable defibrillator therapy: a meta-analysis of case-control studies. *JACC Clin Electrophysiol* 2017; 3(13):1475–1483.

45 Gold MR, Aasbo JD, El-Chami MF, *et al.* Subcutaneous implantable cardioverter-defibrillator post-approval study: clinical characteristics and perioperative results. *Heart Rhythm* 2017;14(10):1456–1463.

46 Boersma LV, El-Chami MF, Bongiorni MG, *et al.* Understanding Outcomes with the S-ICD in Primary Prevention Patients with Low EF Study (UNTOUCHED): clinical characteristics and perioperative results. *Heart Rhythm* 2019;16(11):1636–1644.

47 Poole JE, Gold MR. Who should receive the subcutaneous implanted defibrillator? The subcutaneous implantable cardioverter defibrillator (ICD) should be considered in all ICD patients who do not require pacing. *Circ Arrhythm Electrophysiol* 2013;6(6):1236–1244; discussion 1244–1245.

48 Swerdlow CD, Asirvatham SJ, Ellenbogen KA, Friedman PA. Troubleshooting implanted cardioverter defibrillator sensing problems I. *Circ Arrhythm Electrophysiol* 2014; 7(6):1237–1261.

49 Swerdlow CD, Asirvatham SJ, Ellenbogen KA, Friedman PA. Troubleshooting implantable cardioverter-defibrillator sensing problems II. *Circ Arrhythm Electrophysiol* 2015;8(1):212–220.

50 Ruetz LL, Koehler JL, Brown ML, *et al.* Sinus rhythm R-wave amplitude as a predictor of ventricular fibrillation undersensing in patients with implantable cardioverter-defibrillator. *Heart Rhythm* 2015;12(12):2411–2418.

51 Gold MR, Theuns DA, Knight BP, *et al.* Head-to-head comparison of arrhythmia discrimination performance of subcutaneous and transvenous ICD arrhythmia detection algorithms: the START study. *J Cardiovasc Electrophysiol* 2012;23(4):359–366.

52 Brisben AJ, Burke MC, Knight BP, *et al.* A new algorithm to reduce inappropriate therapy in the S-ICD system. *J Cardiovasc Electrophysiol* 2015;26(4):417–423.

53 Moss AJ, Schuger C, Beck CA, *et al.* Reduction in inappropriate therapy and mortality through ICD programming. *N Engl J Med* 2012;367(24):2275–2283.

54 Gasparini M, Proclemer A, Klersy C, *et al.* Effect of long-detection interval vs standard-detection interval for implantable cardioverter-defibrillators on antitachycardia pacing and shock delivery: the ADVANCE III randomized clinical trial. *JAMA* 2013;309(18):1903–1911.

55 Stiles MK, Fauchier L, Morillo CA, Wilkoff BL. 2019 HRS/EHRA/APHRS/LAHRS focused update to 2015 expert consensus statement on optimal implantable cardioverter-defibrillator programming and testing. *Heart Rhythm* 2020;17(1):e220–e228.

56 Wilkoff BL, Fauchier L, Stiles MK, *et al.*, editors. 2015 HRS/EHRA/APHRS/SOLAECE expert consensus statement on optimal implantable cardioverter-defibrillator programming and testing. *Heart Rhythm* 2016;13(2): e50–e86.

57 Swerdlow CD, Brown ML, Lurie K, *et al.* Discrimination of ventricular tachycardia from supraventricular tachycardia by a downloaded wavelet-transform morphology algorithm: a paradigm for development of implantable cardioverter defibrillator detection algorithms. *J Cardiovasc Electrophysiol* 2002;13(5):432–441.

58 Khalighi K, Florin TJ, Peters RW, Shorofsky SR, Gold MR. Distortion of intracardiac electrograms following defibrillator shocks for atrial tachyarrhythmias. *Pacing Clin Electrophysiol* 1997;20(6):1682–1685.

59 Brugada J, Mont L, Figueiredo M, *et al.* Enhanced detection criteria in implantable defibrillators. *J Cardiovasc Electrophysiol* 1998;9(3):261–268.

60 Le Franc P, Kus T, Vinet A, *et al.* Underdetection of ventricular tachycardia using a 40 ms stability criterion: effect of antiarrhythmic therapy. *Pacing Clin Electrophysiol* 1997;20(12 Pt 1):2882–2892.

61 Swerdlow CD, Chen PS, Kass RM, Allard JR, Peter CT. Discrimination of ventricular tachycardia from sinus tachycardia and atrial fibrillation in a tiered-therapy cardioverter-defibrillator. *J Am Coll Cardiol* 1994;23(6): 1342–1355.

62 Stadler RW, Gunderson BD, Gillberg JM. An adaptive interval-based algorithm for withholding ICD therapy during sinus tachycardia. *Pacing Clin Electrophysiol* 2003;26(5):1189–1201.

63 Wilkoff BL, Kuhlkamp V, Volosin K, *et al.* Critical analysis of dual-chamber implantable cardioverter-defibrillator arrhythmia detection: results and technical considerations. *Circulation* 2001;103(3):381–386.

64 Glikson M, Swerdlow CD, Gurevitz OT, *et al.* Optimal combination of discriminators for differentiating ventricular

from supraventricular tachycardia by dual-chamber defibrillators. *J Cardiovasc Electrophysiol* 2005;16(7):732–739.

65 Stein KM, Euler DE, Mehra R, *et al.* Do atrial tachyarrhythmias beget ventricular tachyarrhythmias in defibrillator recipients? *J Am Coll Cardiol* 2002;40(2):335–340.

66 Chen BW, Liu Q, Wang X, Dang AM. Are dual-chamber implantable cardioverter-defibrillators really better than single-chamber ones? A systematic review and meta-analysis. *J Interv Card Electrophysiol* 2014;39(3):273–280.

67 Gold MR, Ahmad S, Browne K, *et al.* Prospective comparison of discrimination algorithms to prevent inappropriate ICD therapy: primary results of the Rhythm ID Going Head to Head Trial. *Heart Rhythm* 2012;9(3):370–377.

68 Klein GJ, Gillberg JM, Tang A, *et al.* Improving SVT discrimination in single-chamber ICDs: a new electrogram morphology-based algorithm. *J Cardiovasc Electrophysiol* 2006;17(12):1310–1319.

69 Sanghera R, Sanders R, Husby M, Bentsen JG. Development of the subcutaneous implantable cardioverter-defibrillator for reducing sudden cardiac death. *Ann NY Acad Sci* 2014;1329(1):1–17.

70 Brisben A. How the S-ICD (subcutaneous implantable cardiac defibrillator) senses cardiac signals to minimize cardiac over-sensing and maximize rhythm discrimination. *J Electrocardiol* 2018;51(6 Suppl):S38–S43.

71 Gold MR, Weiss R, Theuns DAMJ, *et al.* Use of a discrimination algorithm to reduce inappropriate shocks with a subcutaneous implantable cardioverter-defibrillator. *Heart Rhythm* 2014;11(8):1352–1358.

72 Efimov IR, Cheng Y, Van Wagoner DR, Mazgalev T, Tchou PJ. Virtual electrode-induced phase singularity: a basic mechanism of defibrillation failure. *Circ Res* 1998;82(8):918–925.

73 Singer I, Lang D. Defibrillation threshold: clinical utility and therapeutic implications. *Pacing Clin Electrophysiol* 1992;15(6):932–949.

74 Swerdlow CD, Davie S, Ahern T, Chen PS. Comparative reproducibility of defibrillation threshold and upper limit of vulnerability. *Pacing Clin Electrophysiol* 1996;19(12 Pt 1):2103–2111.

75 Healey JS, Hohnloser SH, Glikson M, *et al.* Cardioverter defibrillator implantation without induction of ventricular fibrillation: a single-blind, non-inferiority, randomised controlled trial (SIMPLE). *Lancet* 2015;385(9970):785–791.

76 Bansch D, Bonnemeier H, Brandt J, *et al.* Intra-operative defibrillation testing and clinical shock efficacy in patients with implantable cardioverter-defibrillators: the NORDIC ICD randomized clinical trial. *Eur Heart J* 2015;36(37):2500–2507.

77 Wathen MS, Sweeney MO, DeGroot PJ, *et al.* Shock reduction using antitachycardia pacing for spontaneous rapid ventricular tachycardia in patients with coronary artery disease. *Circulation* 2001;104(7):796–801.

78 Wilkoff BL, Ousdigian KT, Sterns LD, *et al.* A comparison of empiric to physician-tailored programming of implantable cardioverter-defibrillators: results from the prospective randomized multicenter EMPIRIC trial. *J Am Coll Cardiol* 2006;48(2):330–339.

79 Wilkoff BL, Williamson BD, Stern RS, *et al.* Strategic programming of detection and therapy parameters in implantable cardioverter-defibrillators reduces shocks in primary prevention patients: results from the PREPARE (Primary Prevention Parameters Evaluation) study. *J Am Coll Cardiol* 2008;52(7):541–550.

CHAPTER 9

Cardiac resynchronization therapy

Yong-Mei Cha and Ammar M. Killu
Department of Cardiovascular Diseases, Division of Heart Rhythm Services, Mayo Clinic, Rochester, MN, USA

Heart failure and mechanisms of cardiac resynchronization therapy

Chronic heart failure (HF) is one of the leading epidemics in the USA, affecting 5 million patients overall and claiming nearly 300 000 lives annually. In the Framingham study, total mortality was 24% in women and 55% in men within 4 years of developing symptomatic HF [1]. Contemporary pharmacological therapies (beta-blockers, angiotensin-converting enzyme inhibitors, angiotensin receptor blockers with or without combined neprilysin inhibitors, mineralocorticoid receptor antagonists, and statins) have yielded substantial reductions in mortality from progressive HF. Despite these advances in medical therapy, HF still carries high morbidity and mortality. The estimated number of individuals with newly diagnosed HF has increased due to a rise in population size and age [2]. Each year, more than 1 million hospitalizations with a primary diagnosis of HF occur in the USA and contribute more than $34 billion to medical costs [3].

The fundamental pathophysiology is impaired myocardial contractility in systolic HF, leading to ventricular hypertrophy and dilation. Disordered electromechanical coupling at multiple levels contributes to reduced ventricular pump function.

Left bundle branch block (LBBB) is frequently accompanied by progression of left ventricular (LV) systolic dysfunction, with the consequence of delayed electrical conduction to the LV lateral wall. The loss of normal interventricular (VV) and intraventricular conduction via the His–Purkinje conduction system results in dyssynchronous ventricular excitation and contraction (Figure 9.1, left) [4]. This recognized ventricular dyssynchrony further reduces myocardial efficiency and cardiac output, worsening cardiac performance.

Cardiac resynchronization therapy (CRT), a non-pharmacological therapeutic approach developed more than two decades ago, resynchronizes electrical and mechanical coupling by placing leads to the right and left ventricles (via the coronary sinus [CS]) to excite the right ventricular (RV) and LV lateral wall simultaneously (Figure 9.1, right). The acute hemodynamic benefit is apparent, including improvement in ventricular contractility and cardiac output as well as reduction in mitral regurgitation and LV filling pressure. It has now been clearly proven that CRT can improve chronic LV systolic function with evidence of reverse LV remodeling [5–7]. These remodeling effects include reduction in LV volumes and chamber size [8] and improvement in LV ejection fraction (LVEF). At the cellular stage, CRT may upregulate β-adrenergic

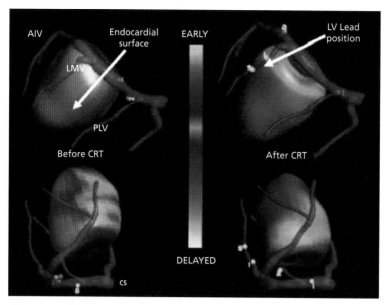

Figure 9.1 Image integration of functional (mechanical dyssynchrony) and anatomical (coronary venous anatomy) information before and after cardiac resynchronization therapy (CRT) at end systole. The branches of the coronary venous tree are displayed in the red reconstruction model. AIV, anterior interventricular vein; CS, coronary sinus; LMV, lateral marginal vein; PLV, posterolateral vein. Source: Tournoux *et al.* [4]. Reproduced with permission of John Wiley & Sons Ltd.

responses to signaling changes at receptor and post-receptor levels, improve ion-channel function, and promote mitochondrial energy production [9–11]. Furthermore, increased blood pressure with CRT may allow increased titration of neurohormonal antagonist medications that may further contribute to clinical improvement.

Indications and patient selection

CRT has been shown in numerous clinical trials to be an effective therapy for select HF patients. The American Heart Association, American College of Cardiology and Heart Rhythm Society (AHA/ACC/HRS) 2008 guidelines and focused updates in 2012 recommended CRT in patients with advanced HF [New York Heart Association (NYHA) class I–IV], evidence of severe LV systolic dysfunction (LVEF ≤35%), and evidence of ventricular conduction delay (QRS duration ≥120 ms but mainly LBBB) after failing optimal medical therapy [12,13]. Other societal guidelines that outline indications for CRT include the 2013 ACC/AHA heart failure guidelines and the 2016 European Society of Cardiology heart failure guidelines [14,15].

The Focused Update document further stratified the class indication by using QRS duration and morphology. Among those who meet the CRT criteria for the 2008 guidelines (NYHA class III or IV, LVEF ≤35%, QRS duration ≥120 ms), patients are considered class I with a QRS duration of ≥150 ms and LBBB; and class IIA with a QRS duration of 120–149 ms and LBBB or with a QRS duration of ≥150 ms and no LBBB (Table 9.1). This modification is based on evidence that CRT is most beneficial to those with a QRS duration ≥150 ms and LBBB morphology, in that up to 70% of these patients may have LV electrical and mechanical delay that can be corrected by the addition of LV pacing [5,7,16,17].

In patients with atrial fibrillation (AF) and LVEF of 35% or less, atrioventricular node (AVN) ablation or adequate drug suppression of the ventricular rate to achieve near 100% biventricular pacing is recommended. Anticipated ventricular pacing of 40% or more may be detrimental and could be amended by CRT [18,19].

The Focused Update of the guideline recommended CRT for those with NYHA functional class II HF, i.e. mild-to-moderate HF symptoms

Table 9.1 Recommendations for cardiac resynchronization therapy (CRT) in patients with systolic heart failure

Patient population	Class	Level
NYHA class II, III, or ambulatory NYHA class IV, LVEF ≤35%, sinus rhythm, QRS duration ≥150 ms, LBBB	I	A/B
NYHA class II, III, or ambulatory class IV, LVEF ≤35%, sinus rhythm, QRS duration 120–149 ms, LBBB	IIA	B
NYHA class III or ambulatory class IV, LVEF ≤35%, sinus rhythm, QRS duration ≥150 ms, non-LBBB	IIA	A

LVEF ≤35%, AF and:
  AVN ablation or medical rate control to allow 100% pacing or
  Anticipated device pacing >40%
	IIA	B/C

NYHA class I, ischemic cardiomyopathy, LVEF ≤30%, sinus rhythm, QRS duration ≥150 ms, LBBB	IIB	C
NYHA class III or ambulatory class IV, LVEF ≤35%, sinus rhythm, QRS duration 120–149 ms, non-LBBB NYHA class II, LVEF ≤35%, sinus rhythm, QRS duration ≥150 ms, non-LBBB	IIB	B
Mild-to-moderate reduced LVEF (36–50%) and LBBB (QRS ≥150 ms)	IIB	C
NYHA class I or II, QRS duration ≤150 ms, non-LBBB	III	B
Comorbidities and/or frailty limit survival to ≤1 year	III	C

AF, atrial fibrillation; AVN, atrioventricular node; CRT, cardiac resynchronization therapy; LBBB, left bundle branch block; LVEF, left ventricular ejection fraction; NYHA, New York Heart Association.

with LVEF ≤35%. Those with a QRS duration of ≥150 ms and LBBB are class I candidates for CRT. Patients with a QRS duration of 120–149 ms with LBBB (class IIA) or those with a QRS duration of ≥150 ms without LBBB (class IIB) are also potential candidates for CRT [6,7]. In the 2018 ACC/AHA/HRS Guideline on the Evaluation and Management of Patients With Bradycardia and Cardiac Conduction Delay, CRT can be considered (class IIB indication) in patients with HF, a mild to moderate reduced LVEF (36–50%), and LBBB (QRS ≥150 ms) [20].

In patients with asymptomatic LV systolic dysfunction (NYHA functional class I), LVEF of 30% or less, a QRS duration ≥150 ms, LBBB, and ischemic etiology of HF, CRT may be considered at the physician's discretion as a class IIB indication [7].

CRT has no benefit, and indeed is contraindicated, in those with mild HF symptoms (NYHA class I or II), with a QRS duration of less than 150 ms and no LBBB, and those with multiple comorbid conditions and/or expected survival of less than 1 year (Table 9.1) [4,6,7,21].

The Focused Update is essentially in agreement with the Heart Failure Society of America CRT Guideline Update published in 2012 [22]. The latter document states that to be candidates for CRT,

NYHA functional class IV patients should be ambulatory.

CRT implantation

There are currently a few approaches to achieving LV pacing. The most commonly used is the transvenous approach, which utilizes a specially designed delivery system for cannulating the CS to permit delivery of pacing leads into the branches of the epicardial venous trees. When the transvenous approach fails or is not available, an LV pacing lead can also be placed into the epicardial myocardium under direct visualization by using a left thoracotomy.

Coronary vein anatomy

Coronary venous blood returns to the CS, which opens to the posterior septum of the right atrium. The number of coronary veins and where these veins drain into the CS differ on an individual basis. From the proximal to the distal CS, the coronary veins are the middle cardiac, posterior, posterolateral, lateral, anterolateral, and antero-interventricular veins, as shown in Figure 9.2. These coronary venous trees serve as the vehicle and host for LV lead placement. Most coronary veins do not exclusively collect venous return from the LV region after which

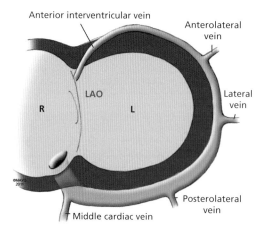

Figure 9.2 Coronary vein anatomy. The venous branches are named. LAO, left anterior oblique.

they are named. The anterolateral or lateral vein may have tributaries to the posterolateral, lateral, and anterolateral walls (Figure 9.3a,b). Approximately 60% of LV leads placed in the middle cardiac vein can be navigated to the posterolateral wall of the left ventricle (Figure 9.3c). Overall, lateral lead position can be accomplished through multiple venous tributaries, including anterolateral, lateral, posterolateral, and middle cardiac veins [23]. The LV free wall is the most common region of delayed electrical activation and mechanical contraction in HF. As such, it is critical to direct the LV lead to the lateral, anterolateral, or posterolateral position to achieve biventricular synchrony. Septal lead location has been considered an unfavorable location for resynchronization [7,23]. In some instances, target veins may be too small to host an LV lead or, paradoxically, may

be too large to achieve lead stability in the lateral location. In patients with complex congenital heart disease, coronary venous anatomy may significantly differ from "normal" and special expertise and planning is required.

Coronary sinus cannulation

The anatomical location of the CS overlaps the annular fat pad in the atrioventricular (AV) groove, where the CS is located (Figure 9.4). The fat pad appears more lucent than the myocardial tissue on fluoroscopy (Figure 9.4b). There are several ways to engage the CS.

- A 0.035-Fr guidewire, such as the SafeSheath® CSG® Worley guidewire (Pressure Products) or Radiofocus Angled Glidewire® (Terumo), can be used (Figure 9.4b). The wire with the angled tip (not J tip) can be successfully placed into the CS without difficulty in some cases.
- Often, a long sheath with a sub-selecting catheter is used to engage the CS. First, the delivery set (sheath and sub-selecting catheter) is placed in the right ventricle over the guidewire. After removing the guidewire, the delivery set is pulled back toward the CS with a counterclockwise rotation. The sub-selecting catheter often falls into the CS ostium where a small amount of contrast injection can confirm the anatomy (Figure 9.5a–c). The sheath is then advanced into the CS over the soft sub-selecting catheter. Contrast injection, with or without a balloon obstructing the CS backflow, helps to determine the options for selecting a target vein for LV lead placement.

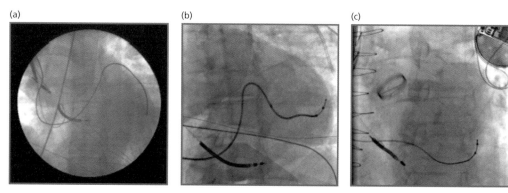

Figure 9.3 Fluoroscopy showing placement of the LV lead at the left ventricular lateral wall via (a) anterolateral, (b) lateral, and (c) middle cardiac veins in left anterior oblique review.

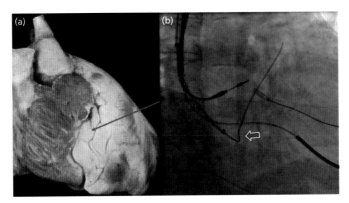

Figure 9.4 (a) Gross right anterior oblique heart anatomy showing the fat pad in the atrioventricular groove (arrow). (b) The fat pad is more lucent than the myocardium on fluoroscopy (arrow). The guidewire is placed into the coronary sinus as shown in this fluoroscopy RAO view.

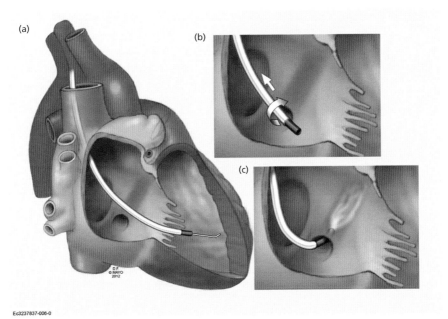

Figure 9.5 Engaging the coronary sinus using a long sheath and sub-selecting catheter. (a) The delivery set is first placed into the right ventricle over the wire. (b) The sheath and catheter are slowly pulled back with counterclockwise rotation, and fall into the coronary sinus ostium. (c) Contrast injection confirms the catheter location in the coronary sinus.

- In some instances, a steerable electrophysiology catheter can be used to engage the CS and support advancement of the long CS sheath (Figure 9.6). In this case, a straight Attain® sheath (Medtronic) or another preformed sheath may be used with the steerable catheter. This may be particularly useful when the guidewire or subselecting catheter does not provide sufficient support for advancing the CS sheath.

When the CS cannot be accessed despite these efforts, contrast hand injection into the right atrium or coronary angiography may be considered to facilitate visualization of the presence and location of the CS ostium in the contrast venous phase. The presence of a prominent Thebesian valve, a narrowed CS, or an obstructive valve of Vieussens may require coronary venoplasty to obtain venous access.

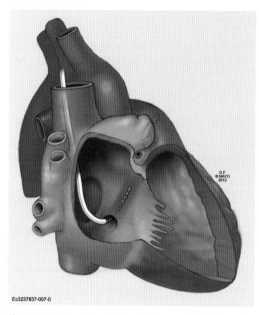

Figure 9.6 A mapping electrophysiology catheter is used to engage the coronary sinus. The sheath is advanced over the catheter.

Figure 9.7 shows the variety of commercially available LV lead delivery systems. The Attain® LV lead delivery set (Medtronic; Figure 9.7a) is 8 Fr in size and available in straight and curved shapes. Various sub-selecting 7-Fr catheters are available in different shapes and angles at the tip. The Rapido® (Boston Scientific; Figure 9.7b) LV lead delivery set comes with braided catheters of various shapes and lengths, with a breakable hub that allows for simplified cutting. The CPS Direct SL® slittable outer guide catheter (Abbott; Figure 9.7c) is designed for CS access and left heart lead delivery. It is compatible with CPS Aim® inner catheters (cannulators) and the CPS Luminary® bideflectable catheter with lumen. The soft tip, which is braid reinforced, provides torque transferability. Seven curve options meet the needs of various anatomies and different implanter techniques. The inner catheters have acute, 90°, and obtuse angles for selection. The SafeSheath CSG Worley (Pressure Product; Figure 9.7d) is designed specifically for

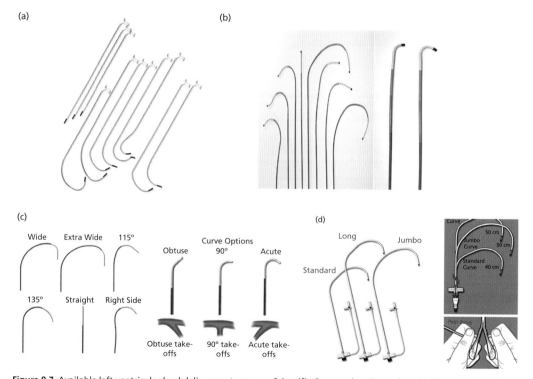

Figure 9.7 Available left ventricular lead delivery systems: outer sheath and sub-selecting catheter from (a) Medtronic; (b) Boston Scientific; (c) St. Jude Medical; and (d) Pressure Product. Sources: (a) Medtronic, Inc. Reproduced with permission of Medtronic, Inc. (b) Boston Scientific Corporation. Reproduced with permission of Boston Scientific. (c) St. Jude Medical, Inc. Reproduced with permission of St. Jude Medical, Inc. (d) Pressure Products Medical Supplies, Inc. Reproduced with permission of Pressure Products Medical Supplies, Inc.

ventricular resynchronization therapy where the right-sided chamber is considerably dilated. It has a larger lumen (9 Fr) and is available in standard, long, and jumbo sizes. The braided core provides improved torque control and its tip is radiopaque for better fluoroscopic visualization. The long gentle throw of the Worley causes its tip to virtually fall into the CS ostium while it is being pulled back from the right ventricle to the right atrium in counterclockwise rotation. The sheath can be peeled away easily after the LV lead is placed. When a right-sided CRT implant is planned, the appropriate choices are right-sided delivery systems available from the Attain, Rapido, CPS Direct SL, and Worley families.

Coronary vein navigation and left ventricular lead selection

Once the CS is successfully cannulated, coronary venography may be performed to delineate the coronary venous anatomy. This is done with a standard balloon occlusion catheter and hand injection of contrast. Care must be taken to achieve a good seal within the main body of the CS in order to obtain maximal opacification of the distal vasculature. Underfilling the coronary venous system is a common mistake that may result in failure to identify potentially suitable targets for LV pacing lead placement. Use of diluted contrast may be similarly suboptimal. Occasionally, the inflated balloon occludes the ostium of a suitable branch vessel for LV lead placement; therefore, occlusive venography at multiple levels within the main CS may be needed. If complete balloon occlusion of a large CS cannot be achieved, distal occlusion with prolonged imaging may help to identify more proximal vessels by filling via collaterals. Imaging in both right anterior oblique (RAO) and left anterior oblique (LAO) views may be helpful in complex cases.

Transvenous LV pacing leads may be either stylet driven or placed with the use of an over-the-wire delivery system, similar to that used for percutaneous coronary intervention. In general, the leads are delivered most commonly over a 0.014-Fr guidewire. Larger diameter leads may also accommodate a conventional stylet. With sheath support, the LV lead can be negotiated within the target vein, as it is advanced to more distal branches.

Overall, the success of LV lead placement is approximately 95% [24]. Lateral veins, including the posterolateral, lateral, and anterolateral veins, are prioritized to host the LV lead given that this generally correlates to the site of latest LV activation. The size and length of these venous branches are usually suitable for the available types of LV leads. Most commercially available LV leads are 2.6–6.0 Fr in size (tip or body) and shaped in straight, canted, spiral, or S-curve forms. A straight LV lead is usually universal, and is easily handled. It navigates curvature well and is suitable for torturous venous anatomy. It uses tines for fixation in the coronary veins. A canted-shape LV lead enables the lead to be wedged in a stable position. A spiral curved LV lead is often selected for a large, long venous branch. It increases the lead stability and provides good contact with the epicardium (Figure 9.8). The caveat is that the lead may retract and dislodge into the CS when the entire spiral segment is not well situated in the vein branch. The proximal end of the spiral curve should be anchored in the branch, not in the CS, as indicated by the arrow in Figure 9.8. Quadripolar LV leads provide over 16 or more configurations for LV pacing. These additional pacing poles provide options to minimize diaphragmatic stimulation and optimize pacing current output, thereby prolonging battery

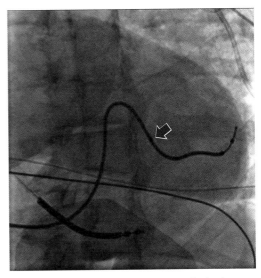

Figure 9.8 Spiral EASYTRAK® 3 left ventricular lead (Boston Scientific) is placed in the lateral vein. The arrow indicates the proximal end of the spiral curve.

longevity and improving CRT outcomes. Quadripolar leads also improve lead stability by allowing a more stable distal lead positioning and still providing options for more proximal pacing. It is worth mentioning that lead stability (wedging into the distal tributary of the vein) and non-apical pacing location need to be balanced during final lead positioning. Several studies have shown that an apical LV lead location has a higher non-responder rate and less favorable CRT outcome [7,23].

Figure 9.9a shows the Attain LV lead family from Medtronic. The Attain quadripolar lead family comprise canted, S-curve, and straight shapes to accommodate different venous anatomy. Figure 9.9b shows the LV leads from Boston Scientific. EASYTRAK® 3 is a bipolar lead with spiral fixation for larger vessels, while the EASYTRAK 2 lead with tined fixation is made for smaller vessels. ACUITY™ Spiral is a small (2.6-Fr tip, 4.5-Fr body) unipolar lead with three-dimensional helical bias designed for smaller tortuous vessels. ACUITY Steerable LV leads have a self-retaining cant at the tip that is able to unfold within the target vein, simultaneously compressing the distal segment of the lead against the outer wall of the vein, improving fixation and forcing the tip electrode against the epicardium, thus improving electrical contact for pacing. Figure 9.9c shows the St. Jude Medical QuickFlex Micro™ Model 1258 LV lead (4.3-Fr lead body, 4.0-Fr tip) and Quartet™ IS4 Quadripolar LV pacing lead (4.7-Fr lead body, 4.0-Fr tip, "S" curve fixation) with four electrodes, allowing multiple pacing configurations to overcome phrenic nerve stimulation and high pacing thresholds, potentially resulting in less need for lead repositioning and fewer surgical revisions, and providing multi-site LV pacing.

Multipoint left ventricular pacing

Quadripolar LV leads can provide multipoint pacing (MPP). Pacing impulses from two sites with adequate separation creates two pacing vectors that allow recruitment of more myocardium to contract simultaneously. A programmable delay (5–80 ms) can be introduced between the two LV pacing pulses, thereby delivering sequential pacing either before or after RV stimulation (Figure 9.10). The MPP IDE study has shown an 87% CRT response rate by programming two MPP vectors with wide two-cathode anatomical spacing ($\geq$30 mm, AS) and minimal timing delay (5 ms) [25,26]. Data from the MOre REsponse on Cardiac Resynchronization Therapy with MultiPoint Pacing phase I trial have shown that MPP-AS elicited a significantly higher non-responder conversion rate compared to MPP-Other (45.6% vs 26.2%, $P = 0.006$) and a trend in a higher conversion rate compared to biventricular pacing (45.6% vs 33.8%, $P = 0.10$) [27]. The MOre REsponse on Cardiac Resynchronization Therapy with MultiPoint Pacing phase II trial is currently underway. This is a prospective, randomized, multicenter study which plans to enroll 5000 patients who do not respond to 6 months of standard biventricular pacing (MPP off). These patients will be programed to MPP with wide LV electrode anatomical separation ($\geq$30 mm) to determine the benefit of MPP (MPP on) [28].

Assessment of optimal left ventricular lead position

The aim for empiric placement of LV leads is directed toward the lateral veins, including the posterolateral, lateral, or anterolateral veins, and the middle cardiac veins, which have tributary branches in the LV free wall, whereas the anterior interventricular vein in general is not optimal for LV pacing. At the time of lead placement, fluoroscopy is often used to assess the position of the LV lead tip, such as anterior or posterior, basal or apical location in the RAO view, or lateral versus septal location in the LAO view, as shown in Figure 9.11. A greater RV–LV lead tip separation is preferred. Improved clinical outcomes are associated with LV leads positioned at the basal or mid LV lateral wall instead of the apex. Figure 9.12 illustrates four examples of the final LV lead position at the anterolateral, lateral and posterolateral wall, and septum (interventricular groove via interventricular vein) in the LAO view, respectively. The septal lead location is considered an unfavorable pacing site under most circumstances.

Electrocardiography (ECG) is a useful tool for assessing whether LV free wall pacing is achieved. In RV pacing, ventricular depolarization propagates from right to left, commonly resulting in

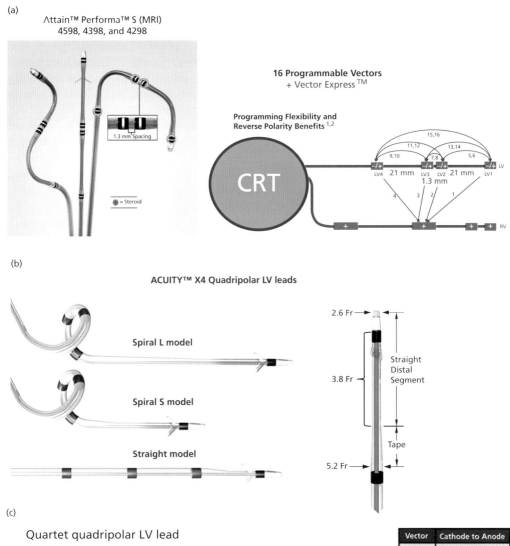

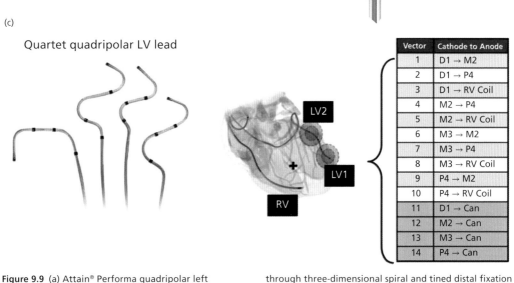

Figure 9.9 (a) Attain® Performa quadripolar left ventricular (LV) lead family from Medtronic. Leads are available in straight (S) and canted shapes. There are 16 programmable configurations available for programming flexibility in the Medtronic system. (b) Boston Scientific LV lead sections. The ACUITY™ X4 quadripolar LV leads for various sizes of vessels. The leads offer dual fixation through three-dimensional spiral and tined distal fixation mechanisms. (c) The Abbott Quartet™ quadripolar LV lead is available in four lead shapes, and features four pacing electrodes, multipoint pacing, and up to 14 pacing configurations. Source: (b) Boston Scientific Corporation. Reproduced with permission of Boston Scientific.

Multipoint Pacing

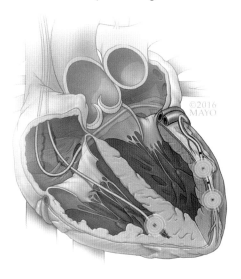

Figure 9.10 Diagram illustrating the concept of multipoint pacing (MPP) in which pacing impulses from two sites with adequate separation creates two pacing vectors. This allows recruitment of more myocardium to contract simultaneously.

positive forces in lead I. In LV free wall pacing, the depolarizing vector is in the opposite direction, resulting in a negative QS morphology in lead I (Figure 9.13) [29]. Lead III indicates whether the pacing vector is toward an inferior (pacing from the anterior wall) or anterior (pacing from the inferior wall) direction. The RV lead is often placed at the septal apex, resulting in QS in lead III, whereas the LV pacing vector usually directs inferiorly if the lead is situated at the anterolateral or lateral wall. Yet QS morphology in lead III may be seen when the LV lead is located posteriorly. Biventricular pacing (RV apex + LV lateral wall) produces a right superior axis as a result of fusion of RV and LV electrical axes. A qR or Qr complex in lead I is present in 90% of cases of biventricular pacing. In biventricular pacing, loss of the q or Q wave in lead I is predictive of loss of LV capture or exit delay. Figure 9.14a shows an example of ECG QRS morphologies during RV, LV, and biventricular pacing with the corresponding lead positions shown in Figure 9.14b (RAO and LAO views). The LV lead is located at the LV basal lateral wall. RV apical pacing alone has an LBBB-type and superior axis morphology (QRS duration 160 ms), whereas LV anterior free wall pacing gives rise to a right bundle branch block (RBBB)-type morphology (QRS 180 ms). Biventricular pacing (QRS 150 ms, VV delay 0 ms) has an appearance of RBBB and Qr in lead I.

Assessment of optimal LV lead position is summarized in Table 9.2.

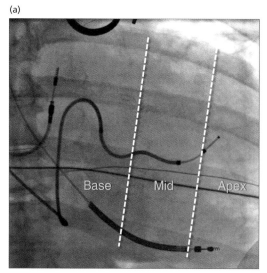

(a)

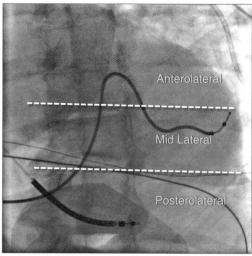

(b)

Figure 9.11 Assessment of left ventricular (LV) lead location using fluoroscopy. (a) The right anterior oblique view divides the left ventricle into three segments: basal, mid, and apical. (b) The left anterior oblique view separates the LV lateral wall from the septal position.

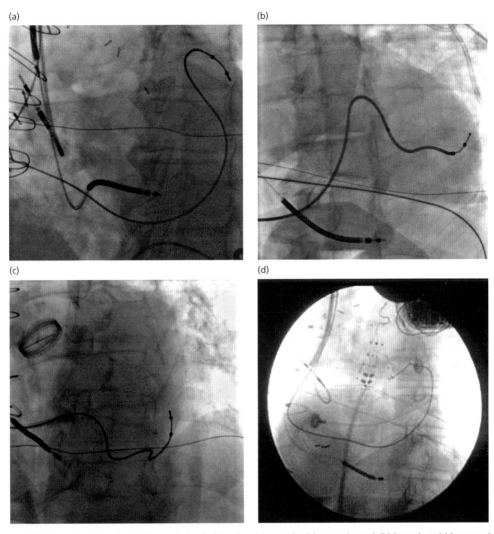

Figure 9.12 Examples of the final left ventricular (LV) lead position at the (a) anterolateral, (b) lateral, and (c) posterolateral wall, and (d) septum (interventricular groove) in the left anterior oblique view.

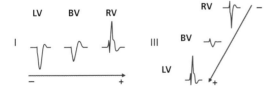

Figure 9.13 Mean QRS axis in the frontal plane during ventricular pacing. In right ventricular (RV) apical pacing, ventricular depolarization occurs from right to left; lead I is positive. In left ventricular (LV) free wall pacing, the depolarizing vector is in the opposite direction, resulting in a negative QS morphology in lead I. Lead III indicates the pacing vector is toward the inferior wall (pacing from the anterior wall) or anterior wall (pacing from the inferior wall). BV, biventricular.

Management of difficulties in placing left ventricular leads (Table 9.3)

Venous anatomy

The coronary venous circulation demonstrates considerably more variability than the parallel arterial circulation (Figure 9.15). Multiple factors may limit placement of LV leads at an ideal pacing location. The coronary venous target may be absent, inaccessible, or obstructed. Anterolateral, posterolateral, and lateral coronary veins serve the LV free wall, while none of the anterointerventricular and only some of the middle cardiac venous branches

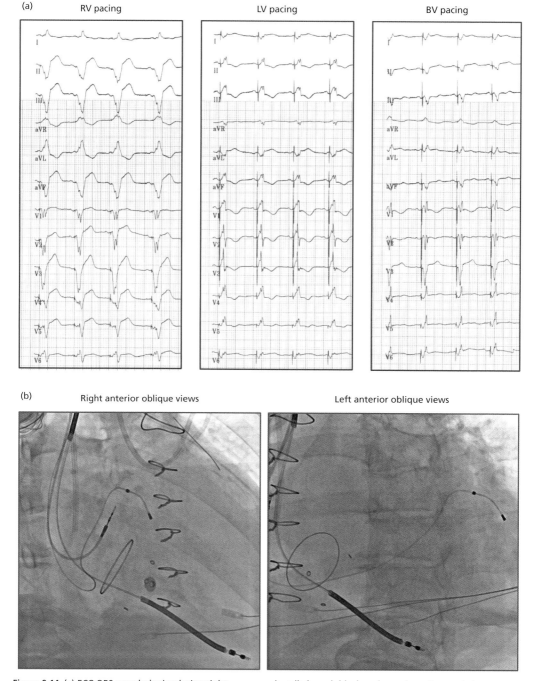

Figure 9.14 (a) ECG QRS morphologies during right ventricular (RV), left ventricular (LV), and biventricular (BV) pacing. (b) Corresponding lead positions in right and left anterior oblique views. The LV lead is located at the LV basal lateral wall. RV apical pacing alone gives rise to left bundle branch block and superior axis morphology, whereas LV anterior free wall pacing gives rise to a right bundle branch block (RBBB) morphology. Biventricular pacing has the appearance of RBBB and Qr in lead I.

Table 9.2 Assessment of optimal left ventricular (LV) lead position

• Occlusive coronary venography is helpful for selecting the optimal vein for LV lead placement
• LV lead placement in the lateral wall can be achieved via lateral, posterolateral, anterolateral, and even middle cardiac veins
• Fluoroscopy left anterior oblique view and QS morphology in lead I are quick ways to assess whether the LV lead is placed at a lateral location

Table 9.3 Management of difficulties when placing a left ventricular (LV) lead

• When a preferred LV lead location is not accessible, such as with a high pacing threshold or extracardiac pacing, venoplasty or repositioning the lead to an alternative lateral location should be considered
• Surgical placement of epicardial LV pacing leads or endocardial LV stimulation are options when the coronary venous anatomy precludes successful transvenous implant

contribute to the lateral wall [23]. Up to 20% of patients may not have a vein that reaches the optimal LV free wall site for delivery of CRT. In some instances, target veins are present but too small for cannulation with existing lead systems or, paradoxically, too large to achieve mechanical fixation. Currently available leads may navigate small tortuosities impassable to larger leads.

Another commonly encountered difficulty in transvenous LV lead placement is tortuosity of the target vessel take-off or main segment. These anatomical constraints can be extremely difficult to overcome and often require the use of multiple LV lead designs and delivery systems (Figure 9.16a,b). Tortuous take-offs may be overcome with the use of firm guidewires or double guidewires to straighten the vessel. Another technique is to use a sub-selecting catheter with the guide sheath, such as Renal Telescopic Braided Series (Pressure Product). The guide sheath can be advanced into the branch over the sub-selecting catheter and is able to overcome acute-angle take-off and curvature (Figure 9.16c). Thereafter, the guide sheath supports the LV lead engagement (double sheaths provide support, with the outer sheath at the CS and the guide sheath at the proximal vein take-off).

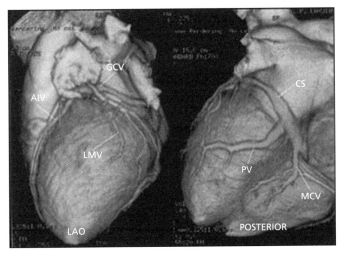

Figure 9.15 Three-dimensional reconstruction of epicardial coronary venous anatomy using computed tomography. AIV, anterior interventricular vein; CS, coronary sinus; GCV, great cardiac vein; LAO, left anterior oblique; LMV, lateral marginal vein; MCV, middle cardiac vein; PV, posterior vein. Source: Tada H. Three-dimensional computed tomography of the coronary venous system. *J Cardiovasc Electrophysiol* 2003;14:1385. Reproduced with permission of John Wiley & Sons Ltd.

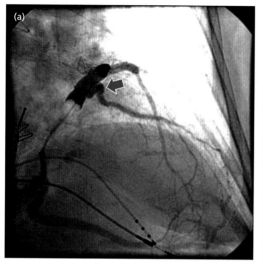

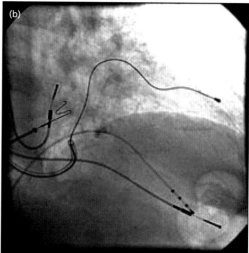

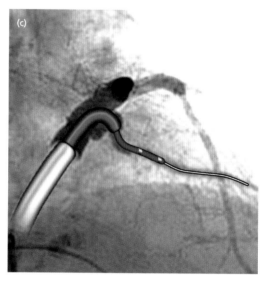

Figure 9.16 (a) "Shepherd's crook" take-off of the lateral marginal vein, with a kink just beyond the second bend (arrow). A 4-Fr over-the-wire left ventricular lead cannot navigate the venous kinking. (b) Same patient as shown in (a). Alternate 4-Fr over-the-wire lead successfully navigated the kinked portion of the vein. (c) Schematic illustrating the alternative approach using the Renal Telescopic Braided Series. The Worley outer sheath is in the coronary sinus, the telescoping guide sheath is advanced into the proximal vein branch to overcome the kink, and the lead can be delivered to the destination.

It is not uncommon that the target vein is found to be stenotic, preventing advancement of the LV lead. Venoplasty may be considered to open the area of stenosis. If an angioplasty wire can be advanced distally against the resistance of the stenosis, the wire may support a coronary angioplasty balloon to dilate the stenosis. The common balloons measure 3–4 mm in diameter and are relatively pliable [Maverick® Monorail Balloon Catheter (Boston Scientific) or VOYAGER™ RX Coronary Dilatation Catheter (Abbott Vascular)]. Figure 9.17 shows a venoplasty procedure performed in a patient with a left persistent superior vena cava (SVC). By means of a telescoping sheath system composed of a 5-Fr vein selector supported by a 7-Fr renal catheter and Worley sheath, a 0.014-Fr Whisper wire was advanced to a desirable location in the middle cardiac vein. The small target

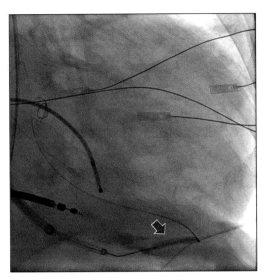

Figure 9.17 A venoplasty procedure performed in a patient with a persistent left superior vena cava (SVC). A telescoping sheath system composed of a 5-Fr vein selector supported by a 7-Fr renal catheter and Worley sheath, and 0.014-Fr Whisper wires was placed in the middle cardiac vein. The small target tributary would not accommodate the lead system. Venoplasty of the distal middle cardiac vein was performed using a 3.0 × 20 mm VOYAGER balloon to facilitate LV lead placement. The arrow shows the balloon inflation.

tributary would not accommodate the lead system. Venoplasty of the distal middle cardiac vein was performed using a 3.0 × 20 mm VOYAGER balloon to facilitate LV lead placement. Venoplasty should be performed by an experienced vascular interventionist teamed with a device implanter. Vein rupture or vein laceration may occur when the anchoring balloon exceeds the ability of the vein to expand. Choosing the optimal balloon size reduces the possibility of this complication. Although the CS has a low-pressure venous system, vein rupture may result in tamponade. Stand-by equipment for urgent echocardiography and pericardiocentesis should be available at the time of coronary venoplasty.

High left ventricular stimulation thresholds

The principal limitation of the transvenous approach is that the selection of sites for pacing is dictated entirely by navigable coronary venous anatomy. A commonly encountered problem is that an apparently suitable target vein overlaps a

site where ventricular capture threshold is high. The presence of scar or adipose tissue may prevent the electrical stimulation from capturing the myocardium. Alternative tributary branches in the same vein or in a different coronary vein may be approached when the pacing threshold is not acceptable. Fortunately, most myocardial scars, often from previous myocardial infarct, are located in the LV anterior, septal, or inferior wall or apex, sparing the free wall where the LV lead is the preferred target.

Phrenic nerve stimulation

The left and right sides of the diaphragm are innervated by the ipsilateral phrenic nerves, which derive from the third, fourth, and fifth cervical nerve roots [30]. The left phrenic nerve (Figure 9.18) passes over the pericardium of the LV free wall, supplying motor fibers to the diaphragm and sensory fibers to the fibrous pericardium, mediastinal pleura, and diaphragmatic peritoneum. The lead position may be near the left phrenic nerve, resulting in phrenic nerve capture. High-output pacing to provoke phrenic stimulation is a routine test during the procedure. A significant difference in the capture thresholds for phrenic nerve stimulation versus LV capture can be overcome by manipulation of LV voltage output. An increase in the chronic LV capture threshold may eliminate this safety gap and should be kept in mind during the implant procedure before final lead position is accepted at a site with phrenic nerve capture. Often, an alternative site for LV pacing is sought by repositioning the LV lead more proximally within the target vein or finding a different vein branch. A small change of lead position may eliminate the issue. Use of bipolar or quadripolar leads and/or pulse generators with multiple programmable LV pacing lead configurations may have advantages in overcoming phrenic stimulation. As there may be significant body positional changes in the anatomical proximity of the phrenic nerve and coronary veins, lack of phrenic nerve capture in the supine position during the implant procedure may not predict future lack of diaphragmatic capture even in the absence of lead dislodgement.

Most often, reprogramming of pacing output or pacing configurations corrects phrenic nerve stimulation. When the threshold causing

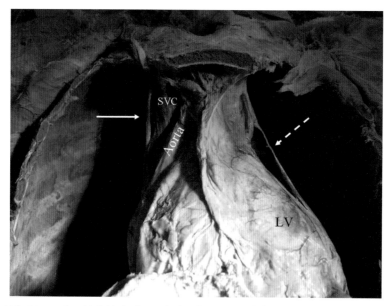

Figure 9.18 Right (solid arrow) and left (dashed arrow) phrenic nerves. LV, left ventricle; SVC, superior vena cava.

diaphragmatic stimulation is lower than the minimal LV capture, revision of the LV lead becomes necessary.

Complications related to left ventricular lead placement and management

Complications related to LV lead placement include coronary vein dissection, vein perforation, and lead dislodgement.

Coronary vein dissection/perforation

In a meta-analysis of randomized clinical trials, the event rates for coronary vein dissection and for perforation were both 1.3%, and tamponade occurred in 0.4% of CRT recipients (Table 9.4) [35]. Of note, more recent studies have reported lower incidences of coronary vein-related complications than earlier studies. The growing experience of implanters combined with the technical improvements in the LV lead and lead delivery tools may have contributed to this trend.

A coronary vein intimal tear with dissection can be associated with wire engagement or advancement of the sub-selecting catheter and sheath to the CS. The wire and sheath advancement must be gentle and stop when resistance is encountered. Contrast injection helps to assess the presence of

dissection. Pushing a delivery sheath alone without an accompanying guidewire, sub-selecting catheter, or lead poses the risk of vein dissection. Another common reason for CS dissection is related to the handling of the occlusion balloon. Advancement of the catheter without a guidewire, overinflation of the balloon, cannulation of the vein of Marshall, and inadvertent inflation in a side branch are common avoidable technical problems. Gentle contrast injection before inflation of the balloon is helpful to avoid these problems. Figure 9.19 shows an occlusive CS venogram that reveals a true CS lumen (red arrow) and a false lumen (blue arrow) with contrast staining. The guidewire or catheter may be trapped in the false lumen of the venous wall when dissection occurs. Coronary vein staining by contrast often resolves. A guidewire with a soft tip can be used to identify the true lumen of the coronary vein and the procedure can proceed. Coronary vein perforation may or may not cause tamponade. When it occurs, pericardiocentesis is required to restore hemodynamic stability. LV lead placement can be reattempted in a separate procedure. On occasion, an angioplasty guidewire may perforate distal venous branches into the pericardial space. Wire perforation rarely results in any hemodynamic consequences.

Table 9.4 Complications related to coronary sinus in recipients of a non-thoracotomy cardiac resynchronization therapy (CRT) device with or without defibrillation

Trial	Year	Number of patients undergoing implantation	Coronary vein dissection, perforation or tamponade [% (SD)]	Coronary vein dissection [% (SD)]	Coronary vein perforation [% (SD)]	Coronary vein tamponade [% (SD)]
MIRACLE [31]	2002	568	35 (6.2)	23 (4.0)	12 (2.0)	NR
COMPANION [32]	2004	1212	22 (1.8)	5 (0.4)	12 (1.0)	5 (0.4)
CARE-HF [17]	2005	404	6 (1.5)	5 (1.2)	NR	2 (0.5)
MIRACLE ICD [33]	2006	421	19 (4.5)	15 (3.6)	4 (1.0)	NR
RethinQ [34]	2007	176	1 (0.6)	1 (0.6)	NR	NR
REVERSE [5]	2008	642	3 (0.5)	3 (0.5)	NR	NR
MADIT-CRT [7]	2009	1089	5 (0.5)	5 (0.5)	NR	NR
Total		4512	91 (2.0)	57 (1.3)	28 (1.3)	7 (0.4)

RethinQ, Resynchronization Therapy in Narrow QRS. Other trial names are defined in the text.

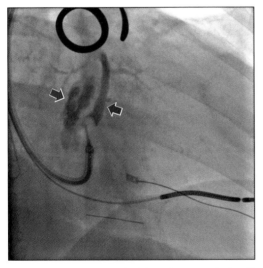

Figure 9.19 Coronary sinus (CS) dissection. An occlusive CS venogram that reveals a true CS lumen (red arrow) and a false lumen (blue arrow) with contrast staining.

Left ventricular lead dislodgement

The incidence of LV lead dislodgement is clearly higher than dislodgement of a right-sided lead, ranging from 2.8 to 10.6% in large clinical trials. The causes of LV lead dislodgement include not enough redundancy of the lead in the right atrium, unstable lead location, excessively proximal position of the lead in relation to the CS, placement of a spiral lead in a short vein branch, and others. The National Cardiovascular Data

Registry records indicate that among 79 909 patients who underwent CRT-D implantation, acute LV lead dislodgement occurred with a frequency of 1.8% [36]. As such, device interrogation and reviewing chest X-ray films within 24 hours of implant are recommended. Macro-dislodgement with loss of lead capture prompts lead revision. During LV lead revision, alternative vein branches and/or leads with different features are often used. In some instances, an acceptable pacing threshold may be achieved by device reprogramming to adjust the pacing output, pacing configurations, or both.

Clinical outcomes

The aggregate experience with CRT in more than 10 clinical trials involving more than 8000 patients has demonstrated undisputable proof that CRT is an effective therapy for select patients with HF, regardless of the severity of HF symptoms (Figure 9.20). The magnitude of the benefit is concordant, although the effects are heterogeneously distributed among different patient subtypes. These include improvement in NYHA class, quality-of-life measures, peak Vo_2, 6-min hall walk distance, HF hospitalization, and death. The favorable outcome may, in part, be attributable to improved volumetric remodeling and function of the failing LV.

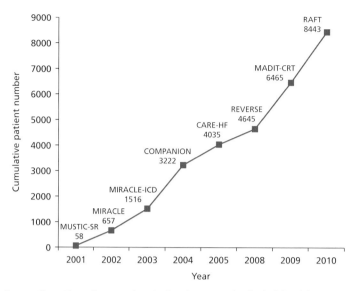

Figure 9.20 Cumulative enrollment in cardiac resynchronization therapy randomized trials. Trial names are defined in the text.

Severe heart failure

In the first decade of the twenty-first century, the application of CRT was aimed at those patients with severe symptoms and an advanced stage of HF. The Multisite Stimulation in Cardiomyopathies (MUSTIC), Multicenter InSync Randomized Clinical Evaluation (MIRACLE), Comparison of Medical Therapy, Pacing, and Defibrillation in Heart Failure (COMPANION), and Cardiac Resynchronization in Heart Failure (CARE-HF) studies were prominent stepping-stone trials of CRT use (Table 9.5).

The MUSTIC trial was one of the first studies. This single-blind, randomized, crossover study compared a 3-month trial of active CRT with inactive CRT in 58 subjects with severe HF and a QRS duration of longer than 150 ms. Biventricular pacing improved exercise tolerance and quality of life, and reduced hospitalizations for HF [37].

The MIRACLE study was the first randomized controlled trial without crossover. It randomized 453 subjects with an LVEF of 35% or less and a QRS duration of 130 ms or longer to CRT with pacemaker capability (CRT-P) or control arms. The CRT-P arm showed significant symptomatic and functional (6-min walk distance) improvement [31]. These improvements translated into a 40% reduction in death and HF hospitalization, a composite end point.

The COMPANION trial enrolled 1520 subjects with either ischemic or non-ischemic cardiomyopathy, NYHA class III or IV, LVEF of 35% or less, and QRS duration of 120 ms or longer. Patients were randomly assigned to one of three arms: optimal medical therapy alone, CRT-P, or CRT with defibrillation capability (CRT-D). Both CRT-P and CRT-D significantly reduced hospitalizations for HF, while mortality reduction was seen only in the CRT-D group [32].

The CARE-HF trial was the next landmark study that randomized 813 patients with LVEF 35% or less, NYHA class III or IV, QRS duration 150 ms or longer or QRS of 120–150 ms plus echocardiographic evidence of dyssynchrony to optimal medical therapy or CRT-P. The device therapy reduced the composite end point of hospitalization for HF and all-cause mortality by 37% [17]. This was the first trial showing that stand-alone CRT, without an ICD, improves survival in subjects with severe HF.

These clinical trials have consistently shown clear and continuous improvement in LVEF in both short-term and longer-term follow-up, as shown in Figure 9.21 [38]. Of note, extended improvement was observed even at 12 months after CRT implant. Concomitant reduction of LV volumetrics, an index of reverse structural remodeling, was seen in the MIRACLE-ICD, Resynchronization Reverses Remodeling in Systolic Left Ventricular

(95% CI) |

Parallel open | 490 | CRT-ICD vs. ICD | II–IV | 21.5 (7) | 158 (26) | Peak Vo_2
6MWT
NYHA
QOL
LVEF
LV volume | 32/245 39/245
0.82 (0.53–1.26) | 11/245 16/245
0.69 (0.33–1.45) |

Parallel double blind | 453 | CRT vs. OMT | III–IV | 22 (6) | 166 (20) | 6MWT
NYHA
QOL
LVEF
LVEDD
MR | 18/228 34/225
0.52 (0.3–0.9) | 12/228 16/225
0.73 (0.34–1.54) |

Parallel double blind | 369 | CRT-ICD vs. ICD | III–IV | 24 (6.2) | 163 (22) | NYHA
QOL | 85/187 78/182
1.06 (0.84–1.33) | 14/187 15/182
0.91 (0.45–1.83) |

2004 | Parallel double blind | 186 | CRT-ICD vs. ICD | I–II | 24.5 (6.7) | 165 (24) | NYHA
LVEF
LVEDV
LVESV | — | 2/85 2/101
1.19 (0.17–8.26) |

Parallel open | 1520 | CRT-ICD vs. CRT vs. OMT | III–IV | 22 | 160 | 6MWT
QOL
NYHA | — | 131/617 77/308
0.76 (0.58–1.01) |

(Continued)*

Table 9.5 (Continued)

Study	Year	Design	Total number	Group	NYHA class	EF [% (SD)]	QRS interval [ms, mean (SD)]	HF improvement	HF admission CRT (n/n) vs. control (n/n): RR (95% CI)	All-cause death CRT (n/n) vs. control (n/n): RR (95% CI)
CARE-HF	2005	Parallel open	813	CRT vs. OMT	III–IV	25	160	NYHA QOL LVEF LVESV	72/409 133/404 0.48 (0.36–0.64)	82/409 120/401 0.64 (0.48–0.85)
REVERSE [5]	2008	Parallel double blind	610	CRT vs. OMT	I–II	27 (7)	153 (21)	LVEF LVEDV LVESV	12/419 14/191 0.47 (0.18–0.83)	9/419 3/191 1.37 (0.37–4.99)
MADIT-CRT [7]	2009	Parallel blinded	1820	CRT-ICD vs. ICD	I–II	24 (5)	65% >150	LVEF LVEDV LVESV	151/1089 167/731 0.59 (0.47–0.74)	74/1089 53/731 1.00 (0.69–1.44)
RAFT [6]	2010	Parallel double blind	1798	CRT-ICD vs. ICD	II–III	23 (5)	158 (24)	—	174/894 236/904 0.68 (0.56–0.83)	186/894 236/904 0.75(0.62–0.91)

CI, confidence interval; EF, ejection fraction; HF, heart failure; ICD, implantable cardioverter–defibrillator; LVEDD, left ventricular end-diastolic diameter; LVEDV, left ventricular end-diastolic volume; LVEF, left ventricular ejection fraction; LVESV, left ventricular end-systolic volume; MR, mitral regurgitation; NYHA, New York Heart Association; OMT, optimal medical therapy; QOL, quality of life; RR, relative risk; SD, standard deviation; 6MWT, 6-min walk test. The study names are defined in the text.

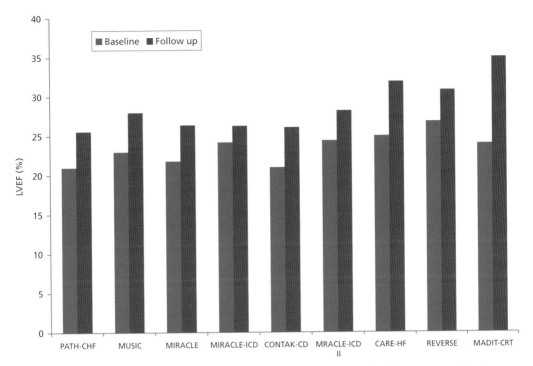

Figure 9.21 Change in left ventricular ejection fraction (LVEF) after cardiac resynchronization therapy (CRT) in heart failure patients with different New York Heart Association (NYHA) functional classes. In comparison to LVEF before CRT (blue bar), there was a statistically significant increase of LVEF in all studies after CRT (red bar). Trial names are defined in the text.

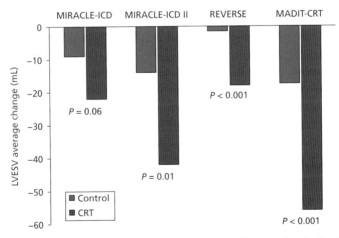

Figure 9.22 Changes in left ventricular end-systolic volume (LVESV) after cardiac resynchronization therapy (CRT) in control (blue bar) and CRT (red bar) groups from clinical trials. Trial names are defined in the text.

Dysfunction (REVERSE), and Multicenter Automatic Defibrillator Implantation Trial with Cardiac Resynchronization Therapy (MADIT-CRT) trials (Figure 9.22) [5,7,33]. The cardiac hemodynamic and structural benefit from CRT may have translated into the reduction of hospitalization for HF and cardiac mortality.

From a functional standpoint, CRT improves HF symptoms, NYHA class, overall wellness, exercise tolerance, and quality of life. Figure 9.23 summarizes

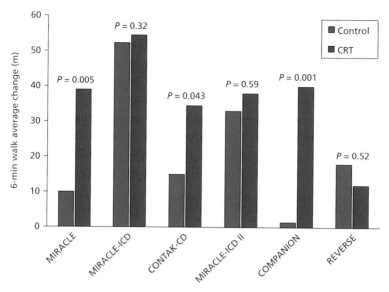

Figure 9.23 Changes in 6-min walk distance after cardiac resynchronization therapy (CRT) in control (blue bar) and CRT (red bar) groups from clinical trials. Trial names are defined in the text.

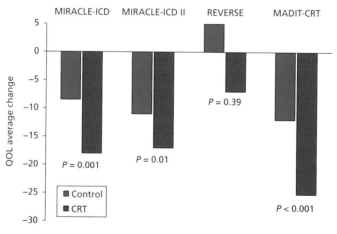

Figure 9.24 Changes in Minnesota Living With Heart Failure scores after cardiac resynchronization therapy (CRT) in control (blue bar) and CRT (red bar) groups from clinical trials. QOL, quality of life. Trial names are defined in the text.

the changes in 6-min walk distance in the control and CRT subjects after therapy from published clinical trials. Placebo effect was apparent in the two MIRACLE-ICD trials – there was a similar (30–50 m) gain in walking distance in both control and CRT subjects. However, a greater improvement in walking distance was found in the MIRACLE, CONTAK-CD, and COMPANION trials [31,32,39].

The quality of life was assessed in three MIRACLE and the CONTAK-CD trials. All three MIRACLE trials consistently showed greater changes in Minnesota Living With Heart Failure scores, whereas there was no improvement in quality of life in the CONTAK-CD trial (Figure 9.24).

Table 9.5 summarizes the outcomes in these clinical trials.

Mild-to-moderate heart failure
All the above-mentioned trials have investigated CRT outcomes in subjects with severe HF and ventricular conduction delay. The MADIT-CRT trial was expanded to enroll CRT candidates with

mild-to-moderate HF. The study enrolled 1820 subjects who had NYHA class I (20%) and II (80%), an LVEF of 30% or less, and QRS duration of 130 ms or longer (80% with QRS >150 ms). Subjects were randomly assigned to either CRT-D (the therapeutic group) or an ICD (the control group). The CRT-D group had a substantially lower combined end point of death and HF hospitalization than the ICD-alone group (17.2% vs. 25.3%; Figure 9.25) [7]. Furthermore, reverse LV remodeling with a reduction in LV end-systolic volume by 57 mL was seen in the CRT-D group compared with 18 mL in the ICD-alone group at 1-year follow-up (Figure 9.22).

In the future, CRT indications may expand to patients with LBBB and mild-to-moderate LVEF reduction (36–50%), which is currently a class IIB indication. A retrospective study demonstrated that patients with mildly to moderately reduced LVEF and LBBB have worse outcomes than those without conduction system disease [40]. A prospective, single center, randomized study is underway to evaluate the benefits of CRT in this group (clinicaltrials.gov, NCT03420833).

Results from the REVERSE-HF trial [5] concurred with those from the MADIT-CRT trial, observing a substantial reduction in the LV end-systolic volume in the CRT-on group compared with the CRT-off group (average 27.5 mL/m^2 vs. 2.7 mL/m^2) in 610 patients with NYHA class I or II, an LVEF of less than 40%, and QRS duration of 120 ms or longer.

Similarly, the Resynchronization–Defibrillation for Ambulatory Heart Failure Trial (RAFT) [6] randomly assigned 1798 patients with NYHA class II or III HF, LVEF of 30% or less, and an intrinsic QRS duration of 120 ms or more or a paced QRS duration of 200 ms or more to receive either an ICD alone (control) or an ICD plus CRT. The trial showed the relative risk reduction in HF and mortality from CRT to be comparable in patients with severe or mild-to-moderate HF.

These trials have consistently confirmed the benefit of CRT in patients with mild-to-moderate HF symptoms and LVEF of 30 or 40% or less. The vast majority of these patients were in NYHA class II. Reduction in LV volume, evidence of reverse LV structural remodeling, and improved LVEF are apparent, and this has been translated into a decrease in rates of hospitalization for HF. The mortality benefit has been shown in patients with NYHA class II and III (in RAFT study; ejection fraction <30%), but not in those with NYHA class I and II (in MADIT-CRT and REVERSE) within the studies' follow-up periods. A meta-analysis of five clinical trials showed that among mildly symptomatic patients (NYHA class II), CRT was associated with significantly lower all-cause mortality and HF hospitalization. In asymptomatic patients (NYHA class I), HF hospitalization risk was lower, although there was no difference in mortality (Table 9.6) [41].

QRS duration

To date, QRS duration determined from the surface ECG has been the most extensively evaluated selection criterion for CRT on the premise that ventricular electrical delay is a reliable marker for spatially dispersed mechanical activation. Numerous studies have reproducibly demonstrated that a baseline QRS duration of longer than 150 ms is predictive of acute and/or chronic hemodynamic improvement with CRT (Figure 9.26), whereas patients with a QRS duration shorter than 150 ms are less likely to respond [6,17,32]. Consistently, these observations appear to be corroborated by the COMPANION, CARE-HF, MADIT-CRT, RAFT, and REVERSE clinical trials across individuals with mild, moderate, and severe HF [5–7,17,32]: a significant clinical benefit from CRT was observed among patients with a QRS duration longer than 150 ms, whereas little or no benefit from CRT or CRT-D on death or HF hospitalization was observed among patients with a baseline QRS duration shorter than 150 ms. Subgroup analyses from several studies have suggested that a QRS duration shorter than 150 ms is a risk factor for failure to respond to CRT therapy [42].

Prolonged QRS duration may not always be accompanied by dyssynchronous mechanical activation. In this situation, despite electrically delayed ventricular activation, CRT would not be anticipated to modify mechanical performance. Conversely, patients with narrow QRS complexes can demonstrate echocardiographic evidence of dyssynchrony. CRT is likely to be of utility in only a minority of these patients [34].

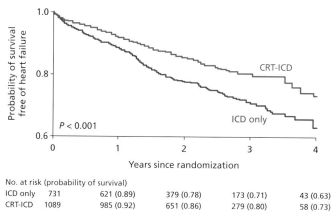

Figure 9.25 Kaplan–Meier estimates of the probability of survival free of heart failure from the MADIT-CRT trial. CRT, cardiac resynchronization therapy; ICD, implantable cardioverter–defibrillator. Trial name is defined in the text. Source: Moss *et al.* (7) Reproduced with permission of the Massachusetts Medical Society.

Table 9.6 Pooled mortality and heart failure (HF) events/hospitalizations with cardiac resynchronization therapy (CRT) among asymptomatic or mildly symptomatic patients with HF

Events/hospitalizations by NYHA class	CRT (%)	ICD (%)	RR	95% CI	P value	NNT
Class I–II						
Mortality	8.0	11.5	0.81	0.65–0.99	0.04	29
HF hospitalization	11.6	18.2	0.68	0.59–0.79	<0.001	15
Combined	17.5	26.4	0.72	0.65–0.81	<0.001	
Class II						
Mortality	9.6	13.1	0.78	0.65–0.95	0.01	28
HF hospitalization	14.6	21.5	0.67	0.57–0.79	<0.001	14
Combined	20.7	29.3	0.73	0.64–0.83	<0.001	
Class I						
Mortality	6.0	7.1	0.85	0.36–2.01	0.71	88
HF hospitalization	11.9	20.5	0.57	0.34–0.97	0.04	12
Combined	15.5	22.1	0.70	0.44–1.13	0.14	

CI, confidence interval; ICD, implantable cardioverter–defibrillator; NNT, number needed to treat; NYHA, New York Heart Association; RR, relative risk.
Source: Adabag *et al.* [41]. Reproduced with permission of Elsevier.

QRS morphology

The vast majority of candidates for CRT have either intrinsic LBBB or pacing-induced LBBB. The presence of LBBB confers a favorable response to CRT, independently and in addition to the QRS duration. Typically, LBBB is associated with delayed depolarization of the LV lateral wall, coupled with delayed mechanical activation in the same territory.

It is intuitive that preexcitation of the delayed LV lateral wall would result in improved synchronization of the left ventricle [44]. Patients with LBBB achieved more favorable survival and greater improvement in NYHA class and LVEF than those with RBBB. Similar survival outcomes may be achieved whether it is *de-novo* implantation or upgrade from an existing pacemaker or ICD [45].

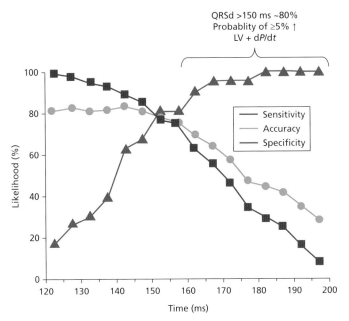

Figure 9.26 Sensitivity, specificity, and accuracy likelihoods are plotted for different QRS thresholds between 120 and 200 ms using acute hemodynamic data from PATH-CHF and PATH-CHF-II. The specificity curve indicates that there is an 80% chance of non-response in the presence of QRS duration of less than 150 ms. The sensitivity curve indicates there is an 80% chance of response if the QRS duration is more than 150 ms. Cardiac resynchronization therapy response is defined as more than a 5% acute increase in left ventricular (LV) dP/dt. Source: Stellbrink *et al.* [43].

A meta-analysis of four clinical trials showed that in patients with LBBB, CRT significantly reduced composite adverse clinical events [relative risk (RR) 0.64, 95% confidence interval (CI) 0.52–0.77; P <0.001]. No benefit was observed for patients with non-LBBB conduction abnormalities (RR 0.97, 95% CI 0.69–1.20; P = 0.49) [46]. An analysis of the benefit of CRT in subjects with RBBB from five randomized controlled trials (MIRACLE, CONTAK-CD, CARE-HF, MADIT-CRT, and RAFT) compared 259 patients randomly assigned to undergo CRT (4.3–12.5% of trial participants) with 226 randomly assigned to medical therapy. The data showed no favorable outcome with CRT in this subgroup [47]. However, the presence of RBBB does not preclude a coexisting LV conduction delay; rather it may represent a greater severity of right bundle or RV conduction abnormality than on the contralateral side. Three-dimensional mapping of both the left and right ventricle in patients with RBBB-type ECG shows that approximately one-quarter may have LV conduction delays comparable to LBBB; nearly 50%

Table 9.7 Key features of clinical outcomes

- A QRS duration of longer than 150 ms and/or left bundle branch block are favorable predictors of response to cardiac resynchronization therapy (CRT)
- CRT is an effective therapy across patients with mild-to-severe heart failure (HF)
- CRT improves HF symptoms, exercise effort, and quality of life
- CRT enhances LV systolic function and benefits structural remodeling
- CRT reduces hospitalization for HF
- CRT improves survival rate

have some delay that may be amenable to resynchronization [48].

The key clinical outcomes are summarized in Table 9.7.

Approach to CRT non-responders

The clinical measures for CRT response include improvement in NYHA class by one or more classes, 6-min walk distance by more than 10%

or 50 m, echocardiographic measures (e.g. change in ejection fraction or LV dimensions), or clinical scores. The agreement between various methods for defining response is inconsistent [49]. The most often used objective evidence of LV reverse remodeling in clinical studies is reduction in LV end-systolic volume by 10 or 15%. While the majority of eligible CRT recipients respond to CRT, there is an approximately 30% failure rate. These patients are so-called non-responders [21,50]. The non-response rate varies, depending on the criteria used for defining response. Clinical or echocardiographic response is typically assessed 3–6 months after CRT. Multiple factors may contribute to the failure of this therapy. Some factors are related to pre-implant clinical patient characteristics, including the nature of cardiomyopathy, width of the QRS complex, type of ventricular conduction delay, extent of LV scar burden, and presence of non-cardiac comorbidities. Other factors are related to post-implant elements that may be modifiable, such as LV lead position, percentage of biventricular pacing, and optimal AV and VV electrical coupling. The characteristics of CRT responders and non-responders are summarized in Table 9.8.

Etiology of underlying cardiomyopathy

In clinical practice, ischemic cardiomyopathy is more common than non-ischemic cardiomyopathy [7,51]. Conflicting data exist on the role of the underlying etiology of ventricular dysfunction and its impact on response [17,32,52,53]. Randomized clinical trials and cohort studies have shown CRT to be associated with a greater improvement in LVEF and reduced LV volume in patients who present with non-ischemic cardiomyopathy than in those with a predominant ischemic cardiomyopathy, despite similar LVEF in both groups before CRT (Figure 9.27) [7,17,51,54]. This preferential structural and hemodynamic response may be associated with the presence of more LBBB and less comorbidities in this entity. Higher mortality has been found among patients with an ischemic cause of HF than among patients with a non-ischemic cause [7,55,56]. In the MADIT-CRT trial, Kaplan–Meier event analysis demonstrated significantly higher rates of HF or death at 3 years in the ischemic cardiomyopathy group compared with rates of HF or death in the non-ischemic group (Figure 9.28), reflecting a poorer prognosis in the ischemic pathophysiological entity [54]. The interaction-term analysis did

Table 9.8 Factors affecting the outcomes of cardiac resynchronization therapy

Factor	Response more likely	Non-response more likely
Patient clinical characteristics		
Cardiomyopathy	Non-ischemic	Ischemic
Sex	Female	Male
QRS duration	>150 ms	<150 ms
QRS morphology	Left bundle branch block	Right bundle branch block, intraventricular conduction delay
LV end-diastolic volume	180–240 mL	>240 mL
Ventricular dyssynchrony	Present	Not present
Scar burden	Low, not transmural	High, transmural
Right ventricular enlargement, dysfunction	Not present	Present
Device-modifiable factors		
LV lead position	Lateral, base-mid LV	Anterior or inferior septum, apex
Percentage of biventricular pacing	99–100%	<99%, atrial fibrillation, PVCs
AV and VV optimization	Optimal	Not optimal

AV, atrioventricular; LV, left ventricular; PVC, premature ventricular contraction; VV, interventricular.

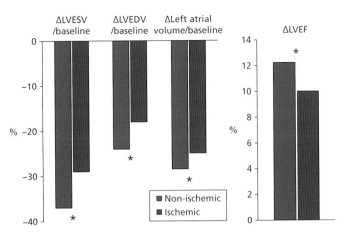

Figure 9.27 Effects of cardiac resynchronization therapy with defibrillation on echocardiographic measures in ischemic and non-ischemic cardiomyopathy patients in the MADIT-CRT trial. Asterisk indicate *P* <0.001. The bars represent median values. ΔLVEF indicates the 1-year LVEF (%) – baseline LVEF (%). ΔVolume/baseline indicates (1 year volume – baseline volume)/baseline volume. LVEDV, left ventricular end-diastolic volume; LVEF, left ventricular ejection fraction; LVESV, left ventricular end-systolic volume. Source: Barsheshet *et al.* [54]. Reproduced with permission of Oxford University Press.

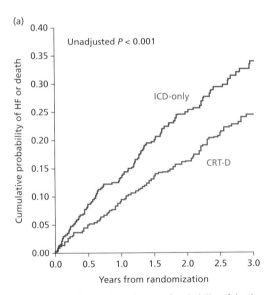
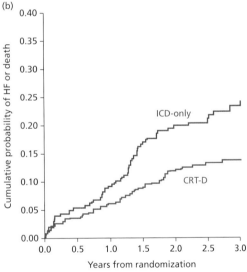

Figure 9.28 Kaplan–Meier estimates of probability of death or heart failure events in (a) all ischemic cardiomyopathy patients and (b) patients with non-ischemic cardiomyopathy. Unadjusted *P* = 0.537 for etiology-by-treatment interaction among all patients. CRT-D, cardiac resynchronization therapy with defibrillation; HF, heart failure; ICD, implantable cardioverter–defibrillator. Source: Barsheshet *et al.* [54]. Reproduced with permission of Oxford University Press.

not show a difference between ischemic and non-ischemic patients in the HF and death events with CRT-D therapy. It is difficult to be certain of the differential gain in terms of survival and HF events after CRT because ischemic heart disease has a worse natural course than non-ischemic disease.

Left ventricular structure and scar burden

The amount of scar tissue appears to be a predictor of response to CRT [57,58]. It is conceivable that a large scar burden, in some instances up to 50% of the LV mass, diminishes LV contractive force, irrespective of the pacing timing. Imaging

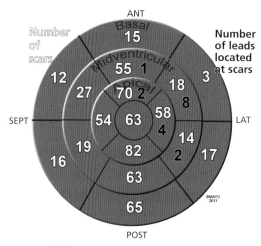

TOTAL NUMBER OF SCAR SEGMENTS: 651
TOTAL NUMBER OF LEADS LOCATED AT SCARS: 17
TOTAL NUMBER OF LEADS LOCATED AT NON-SCARS: 140

Figure 9.29 Distribution of scar sites and left ventricular (LV) leads located in a scar segment in the 17-segment polar map. In each location, the white number indicates the number of LV leads in a non-scar segment, and the black number indicates the number of LV leads located in a scar segment. Source: Xu *et al.* [57]. Reproduced with permission of the Society of Nuclear Medicine.

modalities, including echocardiography, nuclear imaging, and magnetic resonance imaging, can be used to quantify the scar burden and assess the scar locations prior to CRT. Most transmural scars are located in the anterior, septal, and inferior walls, and apex of the left ventricle. The LV lateral wall, a preferred LV lead location, is often spared from a large scar, especially in ischemic heart disease. A study has identified 651 scar segments using nuclear imaging assessment in 213 patients who received CRT devices [57]. Of these, only 11% of LV leads were positioned in scar segments, as shown in Figure 9.29. Patients may respond poorly to CRT when a posterolateral scar is present. In addition, a moderately dilated left ventricle, as opposed to a severely dilated one, predicts favorable reverse LV structural remodeling and response to CRT [59].

Optimal left ventricular lead position

The optimal LV pacing site varies between patients and is likely to be driven by multiple factors, such as regional and global LV mechanical function, myocardial substrate, characterization of electrical delay, and other factors. The success of resynchronization depends on pacing from a site that causes a change in the sequence of ventricular activation that translates to an improvement in cardiac performance. Presumably, this site corresponds to the site of maximal mechanical delay. Observed electrical dyssynchrony, as measured by the onset of QRS to LV delay (QLV), is strongly associated with CRT response, as seen in a substudy of the SMART-AV trial [60] (an example is shown in Figure 9.30). When separated by the median QLV value (95 ms in this study), LV dimension, ejection fraction, and quality-of-life responses were all significantly larger for patients with long as opposed to short QLV measurements. Ideally, the pacing site or sites that have the longest QLV would be selected for lead position [61]. This notion is supported by the fact that electrical and mechanical delays in the LV lateral wall frequently occur in patients with LBBB, often accompanied by HF [62–64]. Pacing free wall sites yields greater hemodynamic improvement than pacing anterior wall sites or any other LV region [61,65].

Comprehensive echocardiography has been used to assess the delayed activation of the LV lateral wall. The presence of ventricular dyssynchrony, determined by tissue Doppler, may predict CRT outcome. However, a large, prospective, randomized trial failed to demonstrate any meaningful utility for conventional and tissue Doppler-based echocardiographic methods of determining dyssynchrony (timing difference of peak contraction among all LV segments) in the prediction of CRT response [66].

The RethinQ multicenter study (patients with LVEF <35%, NYHA class III HF, and QRS interval <130 ms) failed to demonstrate improvements in peak oxygen consumption in patients with a QRS interval of <120 ms [34]. The larger EchoCRT study (patients with NYHA class III/IV HF, LVEF ≤35%, QRS duration <130 ms, *and* echocardiographic evidence of LV dyssynchrony) also failed to demonstrate any benefit of CRT in patients with a narrow QRS [67]. Newer echocardiographic parameters may overcome the limitations of dyssynchrony measurement. Speckle tracking permits analysis of motion by matching natural acoustic reflections from frame to frame to permit angle-independent assessment of tissue deformation and motion. Speckle tracking imaging with

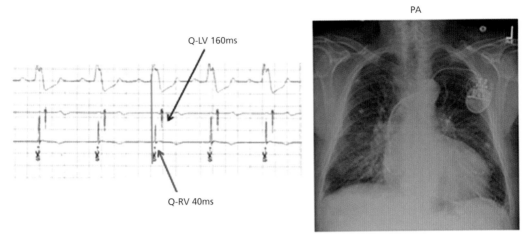

Figure 9.30 A 74-year-old male with dilated cardiomyopathy, left ventricular (LV) ejection fraction of 35%, NYHA class III and left bundle branch block who received a CRT-D. During the implant, the LV lead was placed in the posterior coronary vein (right panel: left anterior oblique view of LV lead position). The QLV time was 160 ms (left panel: light blue line indicates onset of QRS, red arrow RV bipolar electrogram, and blue arrow LV tip electrogram).

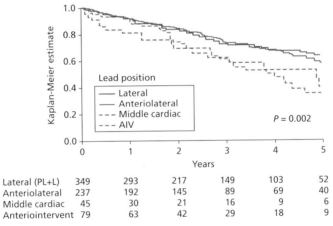

	0	1	2	3	4	5
Lateral (PL+L)	349	293	217	149	103	52
Anteriolateral	237	192	145	89	69	40
Middle cardiac	45	30	21	16	9	6
Anteriointervent	79	63	42	29	18	9

Figure 9.31 Kaplan–Meier estimates of survival among left ventricular lead positions. A greater survival outcome is seen when the leads are placed in the lateral and anterolateral coronary veins.
AIV: anterior interventricular vein

measurement of radial dyssynchrony and scar mass, combined with localization of the latest contracting segment, seems promising as a potential tool for improving response to CRT, although more studies are needed to confirm the utility of this imaging technology [68–70].

There is no consensus on the long-term outcomes of different lead locations and assessment of the tools to determine where a lead is best placed [71–73]. Improvement in NYHA class and LV systolic function may be seen for all lead position segments. The greater response to CRT derived from a lateral lead location may explain the greater survival outcome than that in patients with a non-lateral lead location [23] (Figure 9.31). However, sub-analysis of lead position on clinical outcome from clinical trials has not observed a survival difference with regard to the circumferential LV lead position [74,75]. Yet pacing at the LV basal and mid area has shown a greater response to CRT than pacing at the LV apex.

Attempts to move the LV lead to a more optimal location may improve CRT response. Figure 9.32 shows a 55-year-old female who received CRT-D

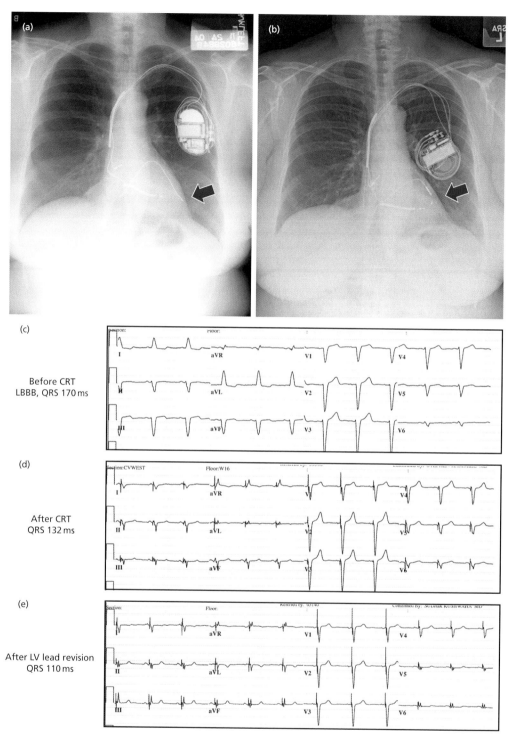

Figure 9.32 A patient received cardiac resynchronization therapy with defibrillation (CRT-D) for severe non-ischemic cardiomyopathy. (a) The left ventricular (LV) lead was initially placed in the anterolateral vein, more distally to the LV apex. (b) The LV lead was revised and moved toward the LV base in the same anterolateral vein. 12-lead ECG (c) before CRT (LBBB, QRS 170 ms), (d) after CRT (QRS 132 ms), and (e) after LV lead revision (QRS 110 ms). Note that lead I became more negative and lead III more positive with the change in the anatomical position of the LV lead.

for severe non-ischemic cardiomyopathy, NYHA class III, LVEF of 20%, and QRS duration of 170 ms with LBBB. The LV lead was initially placed in the anterolateral vein, more distally towards the LV apex (Figure 9.32a). She had minimal improvement in LVEF to 25%. During LV lead revision, the lead was moved toward the LV base in the same anterolateral vein (Figure 9.32b). Thereafter, the patient gradually achieved normalization of LVEF to 52% and LV chamber size was reduced from 71 to 49 mm. Her HF symptoms were resolved. Figure 9.32c–e shows her 12-lead ECG prior to CRT (LBBB, QRS 170 ms), after CRT (QRS 132 ms), and after LV lead revision (QRS 110 ms), respectively. Note that lead I became more negative and lead III more positive, corresponding to the anatomical change of LV lead position.

When deciding on lead revision, one should take precautions to balance the benefits and risks of the procedure in the individual patient. If the preferred location is not acceptable, owing to an anatomical barrier, high pacing threshold, or extracardiac pacing, venoplasty or a move to an alternative lateral location should be considered. Surgical placement of epicardial LV pacing leads or endocardial LV stimulation [76] are options when the coronary venous approach or lateral lead position fails. With the advent of quadripolar leads, transvenous pacing options have substantially improved due to the increase in available configurations.

Maximizing biventricular pacing

The percentage of biventricular pacing is an easily overlooked factor. The ideal target is 100% CRT, which is usually not difficult to attain in sinus rhythm. However, in AF, the adequacy of biventricular pacing depends on the competition between ventricular rate and pacing rate. Intermittent intrinsic ventricular conduction beats are often seen, diminishing the efficacy of CRT. There is no definitive percentage used as a biventricular pacing cutoff to separate non-responders from responders to CRT. The ALTITUDE study analyzed over 30 000 patients who were followed by the LATITUDE remote monitoring system. CRT-D survival by biventricular pacing quartiles showed a significant difference in survival. Patients who were paced 100% (Q4) had a 27% reduction in mortality compared to all other groups [hazard ratio (HR) 0.73; P <0.0001], while patients who were paced less than 95% (Q1) had a 35% increase in mortality (HR 1.35; P <0.0001). Thus, a small difference in missing biventricular pacing, such as 99% versus 97%, may show a substantial difference in survival benefit (Figure 9.33) [77]. Aggressive ventricular rate control is required to achieve the goal of CRT. Certain manufacturers have proprietary algorithms to maximize biventricular pacing in AF. These function by determining whether ventricular complexes over a certain period of time are sensed or paced and adjust the pacing rate

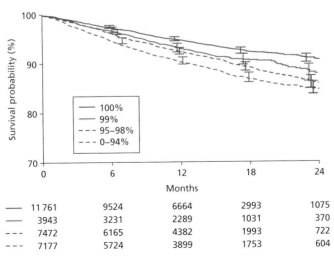

Figure 9.33 Cardiac resynchronization therapy (CRT-D) survival by biventricular pacing quartiles (time from first LATITUDE interrogation). Source: Hauser and Hayes [81]. Reproduced with permission of Elsevier.

accordingly to maximize biventricular pacing percentage. For example, the device will pace faster when ventricular-sensed events occur and slower when ventricular-paced events occur. Left ventricular triggered pacing (simultaneous LV pacing during RV sensing events) is commonly used but the effect is mostly pseudofusion and efficacy is limited. Unfortunately, in the majority of devices, the reported biventricular pacing percentage does not necessarily represent the accurate rate of effective biventricular pacing. Meanwhile, the device may still report this as biventricular pacing in the device counters. One manufacturer quantifies actual CRT delivery using beat-to-beat analysis of the paced morphology of the unipolar LV electrogram. The algorithm was shown to increase the percentage of effective CRT pacing during AF [78].

Often, permanent AVN ablation is advised to ensure 100% biventricular pacing and improve CRT outcome [77]. Meta-analysis has shown an association of AF with an increased risk of non-response to CRT when compared with responders (34.5% vs. 26.7%). Intriguingly, AVN ablation lowers the risk of clinical non-response (RR 0.40, 95% CI 0.28–0.58; P <0.001) and risk of death [79] (Figure 9.34). The benefit of AVN ablation in AF has been shown even in patients with narrow QRS. In the APAF-CRT trial, patients with symptomatic permanent AF, narrow QRS (≤110 ms), and at least one hospitalization for HF in the previous year were randomized to AVN ablation and CRT or to pharmacological rate control. Baseline average ejection fraction was 40%. Compared to pharma-

cological therapy, AVN ablation with CRT was superior in reducing HF hospitalization and improving quality of life.

Frequent premature ventricular contractions (PVCs) may impact on true biventricular pacing, despite the fact that modern devices can trigger biventricular pacing after sensing an intrinsic QRS. Targeted therapy of the PVCs is usually warranted. In a multicenter study, CRT non-responders with more than 10 000 PVCs in 24 hours underwent PVC ablation. In 88% of the cohort, the PVCs were successfully eliminated, which resulted in 7% improvement in LVEF [80]. The greater improvement in LVEF correlated with the greater frequency of PVCs (Figure 9.35). Whether reverse remodeling was the result of higher rate biventricular pacing or elimination of PVC-induced cardiomyopathy is unclear from the study.

AV and VV optimization

Optimization of programmed parameters is also considered important to maximize the therapeutic response. Both AV and VV timing intervals have demonstrated acute hemodynamic benefits. However, multicenter studies have not so far shown long-term clinical benefits. Echocardiography-guided methods have been used most commonly but have poor reproducibility. Hence, the role and efficacy of AV and VV optimization in improving clinical outcomes in CRT remain unclear. Currently, AV and VV optimization is used on an individualized basis (Table 9.9) (see also Chapter 3).

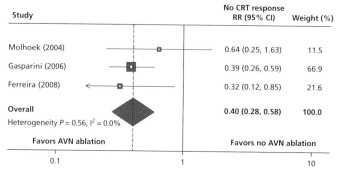

Figure 9.34 Meta-analysis of studies comparing the relative risk (RR) of clinical non-response to cardiac resynchronization therapy (CRT) among patients with atrial fibrillation who underwent concomitant atrioventricular nodal (AVN) ablation versus those who did not. P = 0.001 for the pooled RR. Source: Wilton et al. [79]. Reproduced with permission of Elsevier.

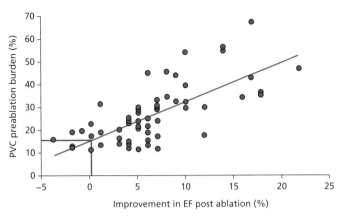

Figure 9.35 Correlation of premature ventricular contraction (PVC) frequency at baseline with improvement of left ventricular ejection fraction (EF) after PVC ablation.

Source: Lakkireddy *et al.* [80]. Reproduced with permission of Elsevier.

Table 9.9 Options for hemodynamic optimization in CRT devices

Parameter	Standard (current practice)	CRT optimization	Additional clinical benefit (compared to standard)
AV delay	Fixed empirical AV interval 120 ms (range 100–120 ms)	Echo-Doppler: shortest AV delay without truncation of the A wave (Ritter's method) or change in LV systolic function	Uncertain or mild (one small RCT and several observational positive)
		Device-based algorithms (SmartDelay, Quick-Opt)	Uncertain (two RCTs negative)
VV delay	Simultaneous BiV	Echo: residual LV dyssynchrony	Uncertain or mild (one RCT showed mild benefit)
		Echo-Doppler: largest stroke volume	Uncertain (one RCT negative, one controlled positive)
		ECG: narrowest LV-paced QRS; difference between BiV and preimplantation QRS	Unknown (no comparative study)
		Device-based algorithms (Expert-Ease, Quick-Opt, Peak endocardial acceleration)	Uncertain or mild (three RCTs)
LV pacing alone	Simultaneous BiV	NA	Non-inferior

AV, atrioventricular; BiV, biventricular; LV, left ventricular; RCT, randomized controlled trial; VV, interventricular.
Source: Brignole M, Auricchio A, Baron-Esquivias G, et al. (2013). 2013 ESC Guidelines on cardiac pacing and cardiac resynchronization therapy: the Task Force on cardiac pacing and resynchronization therapy of the European Society of Cardiology (ESC). Developed in collaboration with the European Heart Rhythm Association (EHRA). Eur Heart J; 34(29):2281–2329.

The key features of the approach to non-responders are summarized in Table 9.10.

Algorithm to approach non-responders

In all patients, heterogeneous factors may influence the outcome of CRT. Patient clinical characteristics, the anatomical limit for LV lead placement, and individualized device programming options have to be taken into consideration. Often, more than one factor may account for a poor response to CRT. Moreover, concomitant comorbidities, such as end-stage renal disease (cardiorenal syndrome), anemia, non-revascularizable coronary artery disease, and diabetes, can also dampen response to CRT [82].

Figure 9.36 shows an algorithm for approaching non-responders to CRT. The first step is to treat correctable factors or conditions, such as volume

Table 9.10 Key features to consider in the management of non-responders: the three Ps

Patient selection
No dyssynchrony (non-LBBB, narrow QRS)
Scar at the lead location
Right ventricular dysfunction, pulmonary hypertension
Arrhythmias (AF, PVC)
Severe mitral regurgitation
Suboptimal LV lead position
Too apical or anterior position
Lead malfunction
Non-optimal device programming
AV or VV optimization
Left ventricular-only pacing

AF, atrial fibrillation; LBBB, left bundle branch block; PVC, premature ventricular contraction.

overload, myocardial ischemia, new-onset AF, and suboptimal medical therapy. The second step is to confirm whether the patient is receiving 100% biventricular pacing. A 24-hour Holter monitoring may be required to determine *effective* CRT. The loss of LV capture or anodal stimulation of the right ventricle should be corrected. AF is the most common cause of low biventricular pacing rate. Definitive AVN ablation with complete AV block is recommended to attain 100% CRT. Frequent PVCs can be treated with either antiarrhythmic agents or catheter ablation. The third step is to consider individualized AV and/or VV optimization or multisite LV pacing, guided by echocardiography. The fourth step is to consider repositioning the LV lead if it is not located in the basal or mid LV lateral wall. The previous procedure note should be reviewed before considering LV lead revision.

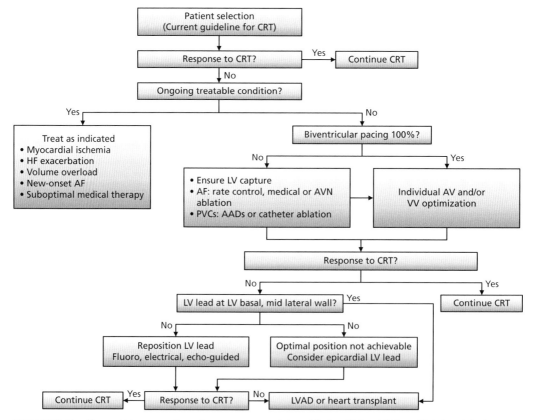

Figure 9.36 Algorithm used to approach cardiac resynchronization therapy (CRT) non-responders. AAD, antiarrhythmic drug; AF, atrial fibrillation; AV, atrioventricular; HF, heart failure; LV, left ventricular; LVAD, left ventricular assist device; PVC, premature ventricular contraction; VV, interventricular.

Repositioning of the LV lead can be guided under fluoroscopy. The local electrical activity identified by measuring the electrical conduction delay at the LV lead can be a useful reference. Placing the lead in the region of viable myocardium that is capable of contraction, measured by radial strain, has been shown to increase the CRT response rate [83]. In some cases, the optimal LV lead position may not be achievable due to anatomical or other constraints. An epicardial LV lead would be an alternative option. A new technology called WiSE LV endocardial pacing may benefit CRT non-responders who have anatomical limitation(s) to optimal LV lead placement. A prospective, randomized, double blind, multicenter study (SOLVE CRT, NCT02922036) has been initiated to test the benefit of "leadless" LV endocardial pacing in CRT. The study will use the WiSE (Wireless Stimulation of the Endocardium) system to provide LV endocardial pacing in conjunction with a co-implanted system that provides RV stimulation. The LV pacing is achieved by using an ultrasound transmitter that provides ultrasound energy to a receiver implanted on the inner surface of the left ventricle. When the receiver receives the ultrasound signal, it generates an electrical output and stimulates the left ventricle.

Summary

CRT has proven to be an effective non-pharmacological treatment for select patients with drug-refractory severe HF. Informed by recent clinical trials, updated CRT guidelines have recommended extension of resynchronization device therapy to patients with mild or moderate HF. A variable proportion of eligible patients fail to benefit from this treatment. Part of the complexity in the management of HF is related to the fact that the evolution of HF is unpredictable in the individual patient. Efforts to improve patient selection before implant and to optimize device management following implant are required to achieve optimal CRT outcomes.

References

1 Kannel WB, Plehn JF, Cupples LA. Cardiac failure and sudden death in the Framingham Study. *Am Heart J* 1988;115(4):869–875.

2 Conrad N, Judge A, Tran J, *et al.* Temporal trends and patterns in heart failure incidence: a population-based study of 4 million individuals. *Lancet* 2018;391(10120):572–580.

3 Gheorghiade M, Pang PS. Acute heart failure syndromes. *J Am Coll Cardiol* 2009;53(7):557–573.

4 Tournoux FB, Manzke R, Chan RC, *et al.* Integrating functional and anatomical information to facilitate cardiac resynchronization therapy. *Pacing Clin Electrophysiol* 2007;30(8):1021–1022.

5 Linde C, Abraham WT, Gold MR, *et al.* Randomized trial of cardiac resynchronization in mildly symptomatic heart failure patients and in asymptomatic patients with left ventricular dysfunction and previous heart failure symptoms. *J Am Coll Cardiol* 2008;52(23):1834–1843.

6 Tang ASL, Wells GA, Talajic M, *et al.* Cardiac-resynchronization therapy for mild-to-moderate heart failure. *N Engl J Med* 2010;363(25):2385–2395.

7 Moss AJ, Hall WJ, Cannom DS, *et al.* Cardiac-resynchronization therapy for the prevention of heart-failure events. *N Engl J Med* 2009;361(14):1329–1338.

8 Yu CM, Chau E, Sanderson JE, *et al.* Tissue Doppler echocardiographic evidence of reverse remodeling and improved synchronicity by simultaneously delaying regional contraction after biventricular pacing therapy in heart failure. *Circulation* 2002;105(4):438–445.

9 Chakir K, Depry C, Dimaano VL, *et al.* Gαs-biased β$_2$-adrenergic receptor signaling from restoring synchronous contraction in the failing heart. *Sci Transl Med* 2011;3(100):100ra88.

10 Wang S-B, Foster DB, Rucker J, *et al.* Redox regulation of mitochondrial ATP synthase: novelty and significance. *Circ Res* 2011;109(7):750–757.

11 Aiba T, Hesketh GG, Barth AS, *et al.* Electrophysiological consequences of dyssynchronous heart failure and its restoration by resynchronization therapy. *Circulation* 2009;119(9):1220–1230.

12 Epstein AE, DiMarco JP, Ellenbogen KA, *et al.* ACC/AHA/HRS 2008 guidelines for device-based therapy of cardiac rhythm abnormalities. *Circulation* 2008;117(21):e350–e408.

13 Tracy CM, Epstein AE, Darbar D, *et al.* 2012 ACCF/AHA/HRS focused update of the 2008 guidelines for device-based therapy of cardiac rhythm abnormalities: a report of the American College of Cardiology Foundation/American Heart Association Task Force on Practice Guidelines. *J Am Coll Cardiol* 2012;60(14):1297–1313.

14 Yancy CW, Jessup M, Bozkurt B, *et al.* 2013 ACCF/AHA guideline for the management of heart failure: a report of the American College of Cardiology Foundation/American Heart Association Task Force on practice guidelines. *Circulation* 2013;128(16):e240–e327.

15 Ponikowski P, Voors AA, Anker SD, *et al.* 2016 ESC guidelines for the diagnosis and treatment of acute and

chronic heart failure: The Task Force for the diagnosis and treatment of acute and chronic heart failure of the European Society of Cardiology (ESC). *Eur Heart J* 2016;37(27):2129–2200.

16 Abraham WT, Young JB, León AR, *et al.* Effects of cardiac resynchronization on disease progression in patients with left ventricular systolic dysfunction, an indication for an implantable cardioverter–defibrillator, and mildly symptomatic chronic heart failure. *Circulation* 2004;110(18):2864–2868.

17 Cleland JGF, Daubert J-C, Erdmann E, *et al.* The effect of cardiac resynchronization on morbidity and mortality in heart failure. *N Engl J Med* 2005;352(15):1539–1549.

18 Wilkoff BL, Cook JR, Epstein AE, *et al.* Dual-chamber pacing or ventricular backup pacing in patients with an implantable defibrillator: the Dual Chamber and VVI Implantable Defibrillator (DAVID) Trial. *JAMA* 2002;288(24):3115–3123.

19 Doshi RN, Daoud EG, Fellows C, *et al.* Left ventricular-based cardiac stimulation post AV nodal ablation evaluation (the PAVE study). *J Cardiovasc Electrophysiol* 2005;16(11):1160–1165.

20 Kusumoto FM, Schoenfeld MH, Barrett C, *et al.* 2018 ACC/AHA/HRS guideline on the evaluation and management of patients with bradycardia and cardiac conduction delay. *Circulation* 2019;140(8):e382–e482.

21 Bax JJ, Marwick TH, Molhoek SG, *et al.* Left ventricular dyssynchrony predicts benefit of cardiac resynchronization therapy in patients with end-stage heart failure before pacemaker implantation. *Am J Cardiol* 2003;92(10):1238–1240.

22 Stevenson WG, Hernandez AF, Carson PE, *et al.* Indications for cardiac resynchronization therapy: 2011 update from the Heart Failure Society of America Guideline Committee. *J Card Fail* 2012;18(2):94–106.

23 Dong YX, Powell BD, Asirvatham SJ, *et al.* Left ventricular lead position for cardiac resynchronization: a comprehensive cinegraphic, echocardiographic, clinical, and survival analysis. *Europace* 2012;14(8):1139–1147.

24 Gras D, Bocker D, Lunati M, *et al.* Implantation of cardiac resynchronization therapy systems in the CARE-HF trial: procedural success rate and safety. *Europace* 2007;9(7):516–522.

25 Niazi I, Baker J II, Corbisiero R, *et al.* Safety and efficacy of multipoint pacing in cardiac resynchronization therapy: the MultiPoint Pacing Trial. *JACC Clin Electrophysiol* 2017;3(13):1510–1518.

26 Tomassoni G, Baker J II, Corbisiero R, *et al.* Rationale and design of a randomized trial to assess the safety and efficacy of multipoint pacing (MPP) in cardiac resynchronization therapy: the MPP Trial. *Ann Noninvasive Electrocardiol* 2017;22(6):e12448.

27 Leclercq C, Burri H, Curnis A, *et al.* Cardiac resynchronization therapy non-responder to responder conversion rate in the MOre REsponse to cardiac resynchronization therapy with MultiPoint Pacing (MORE-CRT MPP) study: results from Phase I. *Eur Heart J* 2019;40(35):2979–2987.

28 Leclercq C, Burri H, Curnis A, *et al.* Rationale and design of a randomized clinical trial to assess the safety and efficacy of multipoint pacing therapy: MOre REsponse on Cardiac Resynchronization Therapy with MultiPoint Pacing (MORE-CRT MPP-PHASE II). *Am Heart J* 2019;209:1–8.

29 Barold SS, Stroobandt RX, Sinnaeve AF. *Cardiac Pacemakers Step-by-Step: An Illustrated Guide.* Oxford: Blackwell Publishing, 2004.

30 Maish MS. The diaphragm. *Surg Clin North Am* 2010;90(5):955–968.

31 Abraham WT, Fisher WG, Smith AL, *et al.* Cardiac resynchronization in chronic heart failure. *N Engl J Med* 2002;346(24):1845–1853.

32 Bristow MR, Saxon LA, Boehmer J, *et al.* Cardiac-resynchronization therapy with or without an implantable defibrillator in advanced chronic heart failure. *N Engl J Med* 2004;350(21):2140–2150.

33 Young JB, Abraham WT, Smith AL, *et al.* Combined cardiac resynchronization and implantable cardioversion defibrillation in advanced chronic heart failure: the MIRACLE ICD Trial. *JAMA* 2003;289(20):2685–2694.

34 Beshai JF, Grimm RA, Nagueh SF, *et al.* Cardiac-resynchronization therapy in heart failure with narrow QRS complexes. *N Engl J Med* 2007;357(24):2461–2471.

35 van Rees JB, de Bie MK, Thijssen J, *et al.* Implantation-related complications of implantable cardioverter-defibrillators and cardiac resynchronization therapy devices: a systematic review of randomized clinical trials. *J Am Coll Cardiol* 2011;58(10):995–1000.

36 Cheng A, Wang Y, Curtis JP, Varosy PD. Acute lead dislodgements and in-hospital mortality in patients enrolled in the National Cardiovascular Data Registry Implantable Cardioverter Defibrillator Registry. *J Am Coll Cardiol* 2010;56(20):1651–1656.

37 Cazeau S, Leclercq C, Lavergne T, *et al.* Effects of multisite biventricular pacing in patients with heart failure and intraventricular conduction delay. *N Engl J Med* 2001;344(12):873–880.

38 Auricchio A, Prinzen FW. Non-responders to cardiac resynchronization therapy. *Circ J* 2011;75(3):521–527.

39 Lozano I, Bocchiardo M, Achtelik M, *et al.* Impact of biventricular pacing on mortality in a randomized crossover study of patients with heart failure and ventricular arrhythmias. *Pacing Clin Electrophysiol* 2000;23(11 Pt 2):1711–1712.

40 Witt CM, Wu G, Yang D, *et al.* Outcomes with left bundle branch block and mildly to moderately reduced left ventricular function. *JACC Heart Fail* 2016;4(11):897–903.

41 Adabag S, Roukoz H, Anand IS, Moss AJ. Cardiac resynchronization therapy in patients with minimal heart failure: a systematic review and meta-analysis. *J Am Coll Cardiol* 2011;58(9):935–941.

42 Saxon LA, Ellenbogen KA. Resynchronization therapy for the treatment of heart failure. *Circulation* 2003;108(9):1044–1048.

43 Stellbrink C, Auricchio A, Butter C, *et al.* Pacing Therapies in Congestive Heart Failure II study. *Am J Cardiol* 2000;86(9A):138K–143K.

44 Auricchio A, Fantoni C, Regoli F, *et al.* Characterization of left ventricular activation in patients with heart failure and left bundle-branch block. *Circulation* 2004;109(9):1133–1139.

45 Wokhlu A, Rea RF, Asirvatham SJ, *et al.* Upgrade and de novo cardiac resynchronization therapy: impact of paced or intrinsic QRS morphology on outcomes and survival. *Heart Rhythm* 2009;6(10):1439–1447.

46 Sipahi I, Carrigan TP, Rowland DY, Stambler BS, Fang JC. Impact of QRS duration on clinical event reduction with cardiac resynchronization therapy: meta-analysis of randomized controlled trials. *Arch Intern Med* 2011;171(16):1454–1462.

47 Nery PB, Ha AC, Keren A, Birnie DH. Cardiac resynchronization therapy in patients with left ventricular systolic dysfunction and right bundle branch block: a systematic review. *Heart Rhythm* 2011;8(7):1083–1087.

48 Fantoni C, Kawabata M, Massaro R, *et al.* Right and left ventricular activation sequence in patients with heart failure and right bundle branch block: a detailed analysis using three-dimensional non-fluoroscopic electroanatomic mapping system. *J Cardiovasc Electrophysiol* 2005;16(2):112–119; discussion 120–121.

49 Fornwalt BK, Sprague WW, BeDell P, *et al.* Agreement is poor among current criteria used to define response to cardiac resynchronization therapy. *Circulation* 2010;121(18):1985–1991.

50 Auricchio A, Stellbrink C, Butter C, *et al.* Clinical efficacy of cardiac resynchronization therapy using left ventricular pacing in heart failure patients stratified by severity of ventricular conduction delay. *J Am Coll Cardiol* 2003;42(12):2109–2116.

51 McLeod CJ, Shen W-K, Rea RF, *et al.* Differential outcome of cardiac resynchronization therapy in ischemic cardiomyopathy and idiopathic dilated cardiomyopathy. *Heart Rhythm* 2011;8(3):377–382.

52 Diaz-Infante E, Mont L, Leal J, *et al.* Predictors of lack of response to resynchronization therapy. *Am J Cardiol* 2005;95(12):1436–1440.

53 Molhoek SG, Bax JJ, van Erven L, *et al.* Comparison of benefits from cardiac resynchronization therapy in patients with ischemic cardiomyopathy versus idiopathic dilated cardiomyopathy. *Am J Cardiol* 2004;93(7):860–863.

54 Barsheshet A, Goldenberg I, Moss AJ, *et al.* Response to preventive cardiac resynchronization therapy in patients with ischaemic and nonischaemic cardiomyopathy in MADIT-CRT. *Eur Heart J* 2011;32(13):1622–1630.

55 Likoff MJ, Chandler SL, Kay HR. Clinical determinants of mortality in chronic congestive heart failure secondary to idiopathic dilated or to ischemic cardiomyopathy. *Am J Cardiol* 1987;59(6):634–638.

56 Franciosa JA, Wilen M, Ziesche S, Cohn JN. Survival in men with severe chronic left ventricular failure due to either coronary heart disease or idiopathic dilated cardiomyopathy. *Am J Cardiol* 1983;51(5):831–836.

57 Xu YZ, Cha YM, Feng D, *et al.* Impact of myocardial scarring on outcomes of cardiac resynchronization therapy: extent or location? *J Nucl Med* 2012;53(1):47–54.

58 Bleeker GB, Kaandorp TA, Lamb HJ, *et al.* Effect of posterolateral scar tissue on clinical and echocardiographic improvement after cardiac resynchronization therapy. *Circulation* 2006;113(7):969–976.

59 Gasparini M, Regoli F, Ceriotti C, *et al.* Remission of left ventricular systolic dysfunction and of heart failure symptoms after cardiac resynchronization therapy: temporal pattern and clinical predictors. *Am Heart J* 2008;155(3):507–514.

60 Gold MR, Birgersdotter-Green U, Singh JP, *et al.* The relationship between ventricular electrical delay and left ventricular remodelling with cardiac resynchronization therapy. *Eur Heart J* 2011;32(20):2516–2524.

61 Butter C, Auricchio A, Stellbrink C, *et al.* Effect of resynchronization therapy stimulation site on the systolic function of heart failure patients. *Circulation* 2001;104(25):3026–3029.

62 Gold MR, Auricchio A, Hummel JD, *et al.* Comparison of stimulation sites within left ventricular veins on the acute hemodynamic effects of cardiac resynchronization therapy. *Heart Rhythm* 2005;2(4):376–381.

63 Ypenburg C, van Bommel RJ, Delgado V, *et al.* Optimal left ventricular lead position predicts reverse remodeling and survival after cardiac resynchronization therapy. *J Am Coll Cardiol* 2008;52(17):1402–1409.

64 Becker M, Kramann R, Franke A, *et al.* Impact of left ventricular lead position in cardiac resynchronization therapy on left ventricular remodelling. A circumferential strain analysis based on 2D echocardiography. *Eur Heart J* 2007;28(10):1211–1220.

65 Auricchio A, Stellbrink C, Block M, *et al.* Effect of pacing chamber and atrioventricular delay on acute systolic function of paced patients with congestive heart failure. The Pacing Therapies for Congestive Heart Failure Study Group. The Guidant Congestive Heart Failure Research Group. *Circulation* 1999;99(23):2993–3001.

66 Chung ES, Leon AR, Tavazzi L, *et al.* Results of the Predictors of Response to CRT (PROSPECT) trial. *Circulation* 2008;117(20):2608–2616.

67 Ruschitzka F, Abraham WT, Singh JP, *et al.* Cardiac-resynchronization therapy in heart failure with a narrow QRS complex. *N Engl J Med* 2013;369(15):1395–1405.

68 Becker M, Hoffmann R, Kuhl HP, *et al.* Analysis of myocardial deformation based on ultrasonic pixel tracking to determine transmurality in chronic myocardial infarction. *Eur Heart J* 2006;27(21):2560–2566.

69 Delgado V, van Bommel RJ, Bertini M, *et al.* Relative merits of left ventricular dyssynchrony, left ventricular lead position, and myocardial scar to predict long-term survival of ischemic heart failure patients undergoing cardiac resynchronization therapy. *Circulation* 2011;123(1):70–78.

70 Delgado-Montero A, Tayal B, Goda A, *et al.* Additive prognostic value of echocardiographic global longitudinal and global circumferential strain to electrocardiographic criteria in patients with heart failure undergoing cardiac resynchronization therapy. *Circ Cardiovasc Imaging* 2016;9(6):e004241.

71 Gasparini M, Regoli F, Galimberti P, Ceriotti C, Cappelleri A. Cardiac resynchronization therapy in heart failure patients with atrial fibrillation. *Europace* 2009;11(Suppl 5):v82–v86.

72 Kleemann T, Becker T, Strauss M, *et al.* Impact of left ventricular lead position on the incidence of ventricular arrhythmia and clinical outcome in patients with cardiac resynchronization therapy. *J Interv Card Electrophysiol* 2010;28(2):109–116.

73 Foley PW, Chalil S, Ratib K, *et al.* Fluoroscopic left ventricular lead position and the long-term clinical outcome of cardiac resynchronization therapy. *Pacing Clin Electrophysiol* 2011;34(7):785–797.

74 Saxon LA, Olshansky B, Volosin K, *et al.* Influence of left ventricular lead location on outcomes in the COMPANION study. *J Cardiovasc Electrophysiol* 2009;20(7):764–768.

75 Singh JP, Klein HU, Huang DT, *et al.* Left ventricular lead position and clinical outcome in the Multicenter Automatic Defibrillator Implantation Trial-Cardiac Resynchronization Therapy (MADIT-CRT) trial. *Circulation* 2011;123(11):1159–1166.

76 DeRose Jr JJ, Ashton Jr RC, Belsley S, *et al.* Robotically assisted left ventricular epicardial lead implantation for biventricular pacing. *J Am Coll Cardiol* 2003;41(8):1414–1419.

77 Dong K, Shen W-K, Powell BD, *et al.* Atrioventricular nodal ablation predicts survival benefit in patients with atrial fibrillation receiving cardiac resynchronization therapy. *Heart Rhythm* 2010;7(9):1240–1245.

78 Plummer CJ, Frank CM, Bari Z, *et al.* A novel algorithm increases the delivery of effective cardiac resynchronization therapy during atrial fibrillation: The CRTee randomized crossover trial. *Heart Rhythm* 2018;15(3):369–375.

79 Wilton SB, Leung AA, Ghali WA, Faris P, Exner DV. Outcomes of cardiac resynchronization therapy in patients with versus those without atrial fibrillation: a systematic review and meta-analysis. *Heart Rhythm* 2011;8(7):1088–1094.

80 Lakkireddy D, Di Biase L, Ryschon K, *et al.* Radiofrequency ablation of premature ventricular ectopy improves the efficacy of cardiac resynchronization therapy in nonresponders. *J Am Coll Cardiol* 2012;60(16):1531–1539.

81 Hauser RG, Hayes DL. Increasing hazard of Sprint Fidelis implantable cardioverter-defibrillator lead failure. *Heart Rhythm* 2009;6(5):605–610.

82 Mullens W, Grimm RA, Verga T, *et al.* Insights from a cardiac resynchronization optimization clinic as part of a heart failure disease management program. *J Am Coll Cardiol* 2009;53(9):765–773.

83 Khan FZ, Virdee MS, Palmer CR, *et al.* Targeted left ventricular lead placement to guide cardiac resynchronization therapy. The TARGET study: a randomized, controlled trial. *J Am Coll Cardiol* 2012;59(17):1509–1518.

CHAPTER 10

ICD follow-up and troubleshooting

Kevin P. Jackson

Duke University, School of Medicine, Durham, NC, USA

Introduction

The implantable cardioverter–defibrillator (ICD) is an effective therapy for reducing the risk of sudden death in survivors of cardiac arrest and in patients with significant left ventricular systolic dysfunction and heart failure. Expanding indications for ICD implantation across a broad spectrum of patients has led to a marked increase in the prevalence of these devices. Technological advances have resulted in increasingly complex devices with intricate algorithms that dictate the recognition of arrhythmias, delivery of therapy, and monitoring for device malfunction. While ICDs are also equipped with multifaceted pacing features, this chapter focuses on the follow-up and troubleshooting specific to defibrillator functions. In so doing, ICD follow-up recommendations are reviewed and troubleshooting tips offered with an emphasis on evidence-based guidelines when possible.

ICD follow-up

To ensure proper functioning and appropriate programming of ICDs, frequent monitoring is essential. With modern devices, this may be achieved through a combination of in-person visits and remote monitoring. Consensus guidelines recommend an initial in-person follow-up visit 2–12 weeks after ICD implantation. During this visit, the implant incision site is inspected for any signs of infection and sutures removed when applicable. Interrogation of the ICD is performed to assess device function and review diagnostics and program device parameters for optimal performance. Demonstration of audible and vibratory alerts should be performed. Thereafter, device evaluation should be performed every 3–6 months either via in-person visits or remote monitoring [1]. Factors which influence the decision between in-office and remote device evaluation include the presence of comorbidities which need close follow-up (e.g. heart failure or antiarrhythmic drug monitoring), anticipation of device reprogramming, geographical location, or patient preference. Even if remote monitoring is preferred, at least one annual visit should be in person. Routine follow-up typically consists of ensuring that the patient is clinically stable, that device performance is intact, that clinical data are retrieved and reviewed, and that bradycardia and tachycardia programming is verified and optimized. Guideline-recommended content for ICD follow-up is presented in Table 10.1.

Considering that ICD patients constitute a relatively sick population, at each in-person visit a directed history should inquire about syncope,

Cardiac Pacing and ICDs, Seventh Edition. Edited by Kenneth A. Ellenbogen and Karoly Kaszala.
© 2020 John Wiley & Sons Ltd. Published 2020 by John Wiley & Sons Ltd.

Table 10.1 Content of ICD follow-up (every 3–6 months)

- Battery voltage (and impedance)
- Capacitor charge time
- Sensing threshold(s) for all leads
- Pacing threshold(s) for all leads
- Impedance(s) for all leads including shocking coil(s)
- Percentage of pacing in each chamber
- Arrhythmias detected by device
- Therapies required for termination of SVT/VT/VF
- Review of main programmed parameters
- Review of any device triggered alerts
- Review of hemodynamic measurements (when available)

SVT, supraventricular tachycardia; VF, ventricular fibrillation; VT, ventricular tachycardia.

shocks, and heart failure symptoms. A brief examination should focus on the ICD wound and signs of heart failure. Pertinent medications, such as antiarrhythmic drugs and oral anticoagulants, should be reviewed. Amiodarone, for example, slows the ventricular tachycardia (VT) cycle length, and this should be factored into device programming. Physicians should also be aware of the potential for antiarrhythmic agents to alter the defibrillation threshold (DFT). Knowledge of the anticoagulation status is helpful in the event that atrial fibrillation (AF) is detected.

Remote monitoring

All modern defibrillators allow remote monitoring using a home transmitter, which interrogates the device either by a telemetry wand or automated wireless technology. Data are transmitted using a landline, cellular phone line, or wireless network to a secure server accessible on the web. A transmission schedule is typically programmed in the pacemaker/ICD clinic and unscheduled transmissions may be sent by the patient or in the event of triggered programmed alerts. Daily automated interrogations provide nearly continuous monitoring for out-of-range parameters, with the benefit of early notification of critical events.

In the ICD population, several large randomized controlled trials have demonstrated that replacing in-person evaluations with remote monitoring results in earlier detection of actionable events and reduces the number of healthcare visits without compromising patient safety [2]. In the Lumos-T Safely Reduces Routine Office Device Follow-up (TRUST) trial, remote monitoring reduced the number of scheduled and unscheduled hospital visits by nearly 50% [3]. In addition, time to detection of arrhythmic events was reduced to a median of 1 day in the remote monitoring arm, compared to more than 30 days in patients with scheduled quarterly conventional visits. Similarly, in the Clinical Evaluation of Remote Notification to Reduce Time to Clinical Decision (CONNECT) trial, remote monitoring with automatic clinician alerts significantly reduced the time to a clinical decision in response to events and was associated with a significant reduction in mean length of cardiovascular hospital stay [4]. Multiple studies have reported a high rate of patient satisfaction with remote monitoring, including the economic benefit of eliminating the cost of travel and loss of income due to time off work compared to in-person visits [5].

Automated remote monitoring allows early detection and prompt treatment of critical device malfunction, including early battery depletion and lead failure. Inappropriate shocks due to device malfunction, including lead fracture or oversensing of noise or T waves, are significantly decreased for patients enrolled in remote monitoring compared to routine in-person evaluation only. In addition, remote monitoring provides an efficient means of frequent follow-up when a component requires closer surveillance, such as device approaching elective replacement indicator (ERI), unstable lead parameters, or device or lead advisory. Most devices remotely execute the same tests performed in clinic, with modern ICDs conducting threshold tests for all leads, followed by automated adjustments to output parameters to maintain secure pacing margins.

The role of remote monitoring in disease management such as heart failure or AF is less clear. While remote monitoring can reliably detect episodes of asymptomatic AF in patients with pacemakers and ICDs, the benefit of initiating anticoagulation in response to these events is unproven [6]. Observational studies suggest that episodes of AF as brief as 6 min bear prognostic relevance with regard to stroke risk. Risk appears to be proportional to the CHADS2 score and arrhythmia duration, with higher risk for episodes of greater than 6 hours per day. However, there appears to be a temporal dissociation between the occurrence of stroke and AF episodes. In the ASSERT trial, only 8% of patients had a detected AF episode within 1 month of stroke occurrence, suggesting the decision to initiate or continue anticoagulation should not be based solely on the timing of events [7,8]. Ultimately, a combination of detected AF events with thromboembolic and bleeding risk score determination may better guide appropriate treatment in this population. In addition to considerations regarding stroke, observational data have also linked the detection of rapid AF (≥1 hour with average rates of ≥110 bpm) to inappropriate shocks [9]. It is thus reasonable to expect that adequate control of ventricular response rates during AF will reduce inappropriate shocks.

Heart failure diagnostics, specifically the use of serial transthoracic impedance measurements to predict heart failure decompensation, have similarly yielded mixed results. Combining multiple device-based measurements, such as resting or nocturnal heart rate, physical activity, occurrence of arrhythmias, and percentage pacing (right ventricular or biventricular), may improve the ability to identify low- or high-risk patients. The Implant-based Multiparameter Telemonitoring of Patients with Heart Failure trial demonstrated that daily remote monitoring with early management of decompensated heart failure resulted in fewer heart failure hospitalizations and lower mortality compared to standard care [10]. Management of this potentially large amount of data, including interpretation and therapy implementation, poses significant challenges, including communication of the findings with the patient and heart failure specialist.

Workflows around remote monitoring should be clearly defined, including timeliness of data review, responsibility for interpretation, and communication of results with patients and other healthcare providers. There may be a fear among some providers regarding the legal implications of delayed action or inaction to alert events, to the extent that remote monitoring is not routinely offered to patients. However, given the proven benefits of the technology, there is likely great risk in not informing patients of its availability. Patient education regarding limitations of the technology, including delays in alert transmissions and time schedules of data review, is critical. In addition, patients should be made aware that remote monitoring is not a substitute for emergency medical care.

Advisories

The most common ICD advisories concern early battery depletion, higher than expected lead failure rates, or device software malfunction. Pacemaker/ICD clinics are generally responsible for identifying and informing patients of a device advisory or recall. It is the responsibility of the manufacturer to keep physicians up to date. While the manufacturer may offer recommendations, the resulting action ultimately remains the decision of the physician. Remote monitoring is the modality of choice for close surveillance of patients with ICDs under advisory status, although more frequent in-person office visits may be necessary in some circumstances.

Lead integrity

The weakest link in an ICD is the high-voltage lead, such that the integrity of the conductor and shocking coils must be monitored closely. Intermittent noise often precedes observed changes in standard lead parameters (i.e. impedance, sensing, pacing threshold) [11]. Electrograms (EGMs) of noise reversion events and non-sustained VT should therefore be reviewed in detail. The make–break potential seen with ICD lead fracture can lead to inappropriate shocks (Figure 10.1) [12]. Alerts for out-of-range lead impedance values have been available for many years, although the sensitivity of this parameter alone for timely detection of lead fracture is low as the conductors contribute only a small fraction to nominal impedance measurements. In order to enhance sensitivity, algorithms have been developed which detect an abrupt change in lead impedance or the presence of non-physiological signals, such as very short V–V intervals (<130 ms) that are not common with a true arrhythmia. Short V–V intervals are not exclusively due to lead fracture, as other causes include T-wave oversensing, lead dislodgement, electromagnetic interference (EMI), and double counting of QRS complexes. Other noise-detecting algorithms compare the

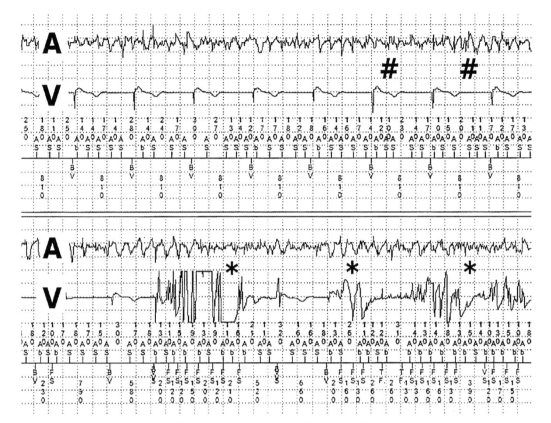

Figure 10.1 Make–break connections. Recording from a biventricular ICD with a fractured ICD lead. The patient presented with multiple ICD shocks. The tracing shows atrial fibrillation in the atrial channel and biventricular pacing in the middle panel. There are sudden non-physiological intervals (RR intervals <130 ms) with make or break-type electrogram abnormalities and saturation of the amplifier channel (*). This is consistent with lead integrity failure. Note the difference between a fibrillatory wave recording in the atrial channel as compared to the noise on the ventricular channel. While some short A–A intervals may be seen even during atrial (or VV in ventricular) fibrillation (#), the characteristics of the signals are markedly different. A, atrial tip–ring; V, ventricular tip–ring.

near-field and far-field right ventricular (RV) signals during high-rate episodes, and ICD therapy is withheld if the signals are discordant. Lead integrity algorithms, especially in the case of an ICD lead on recall status, combined with a timely intervention (e.g. within 24–72 hours) have been associated with a significant reduction in inappropriate shocks beyond standard remote monitoring alone [13].

Ventricular sensing
In contrast to the fixed sensing of a traditional pacemaker, ventricular sensing in an ICD is dynamic. It auto-adjusts to the R-wave amplitude and decays to reach the maximum programmed sensitivity, while avoiding T-wave sensing. Alternatively, the signal gain may be adjusted in a beat-to-beat fashion to adjust sensing of variable signal amplitudes. Longstanding experience suggests that an R-wave amplitude greater than 5 mV is usually adequate to ensure appropriate detection of ventricular fibrillation (VF). Ventricular oversensing in patients with ICDs may present with an audible patient alert, an alert on interrogation, or more severely as single or multiple inappropriate shocks [14]. Insights into the potential mechanism of oversensing may be gleaned from analyzing real-time and event log EGMs (i.e. non-sustained VT and VT) during device interrogation and analyzing the corresponding annotated event markers. Possible causes of ventricular oversensing are presented in Table 10.2. Physiological causes include T-wave oversensing, double count-

ing of R waves, sensing of diaphragmatic myopotentials (Figure 10.2), and oversensing P waves when leads are close to the tricuspid annulus. Non-physiological oversensing may be caused by lead fracture, header connection issues (make–break potential), or EMI. The latter is often present on both atrial and ventricular leads (Figure 10.3). Since integrated leads have larger "antennas," with sensing from tip to coil, historically they were associated with a higher incidence of oversensing, but this is less common in modern devices with better filtering [15]. Additionally, some devices allow bipolar leads to be programmed to sense integrated bipolar or true bipolar configuration. This allows additional versatility in programming options to manage small R waves or prominent T waves.

Table 10.2 Causes of ventricular oversensing

Physiological

- T-wave oversensing
- P-wave oversensing
- Double counting R waves
- Sensing of diaphragmatic myopotentials

Non-physiological

- Lead fracture
- Loose lead–header connection
- Electromagnetic interference

In the event that noise is recorded, the patient should be questioned about recent hospitalizations, since the hospital environment is the leading cause of EMI. Provocative maneuvers (e.g. arm lifting, deep breathing, pocket stimulation, and isometric exercises) should be performed in an attempt to reproduce detected noise, especially in the setting of a suggestive history. Interrogation may be followed by chest radiography to verify lead positioning and rule out a lead fracture or loose connection (e.g. pin not fully engaged in the generator header).

Solutions to oversensing depend on the cause. Reprogramming the ICD to a less sensitive setting can be an option in cases of near-field oversensing (R wave and T wave). This must be balanced against a potentially higher risk of undersensing true VT or VF. Another method of adjusting sensitivity is to modify the decay delay and threshold start. As illustrated in Figure 10.4, increasing the sensing threshold percentage and/or delaying the plateau interval may help to eliminate R-wave double counting or T-wave oversensing. Any time that sensing parameters are modified, the physician must judge whether or not a defibrillation test is warranted to verify VF detection. In cases where oversensing cannot be overcome by programming (e.g. small R wave, large T wave), reintervention should be considered.

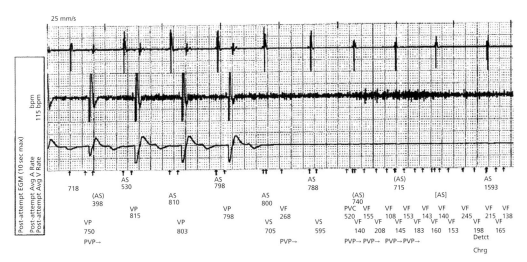

Figure 10.2 Sensing of diaphragmatic myopotentials. Tracing, from top to bottom, shows atrial electrogram, ventricular near-field, and ventricular far-field (shock) channels. A regular atrial (sinus) rhythm is present throughout. High-frequency diaphragmatic myopotentials are sensed as ventricular fibrillation (VF), leading to suppression of ventricular pacing, VF detection and charging of the defibrillator.

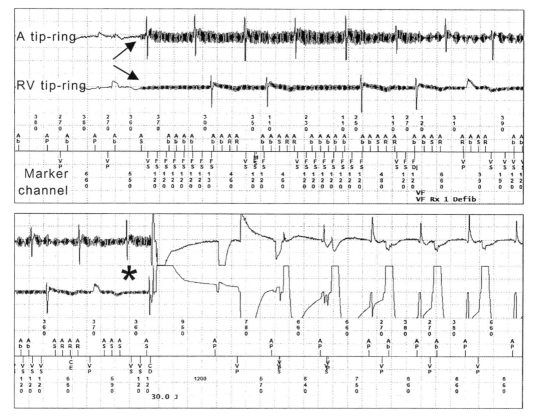

Figure 10.3 Electromagnetic interference (EMI) and ICD shock due to poorly grounded electrical equipment. The patient was working in an outside shed; he touched a wet surface and felt a tingle and soon afterwards received a shock. Device interrogation showed EMI with oversensing in both the atrial and the ventricular channels (Ab and FS events, respectively) and subsequent delivery of an ICD shock (*). The electrical signals were sudden onset, continuous, and high frequency. Typical 60-Hz signals are commonly seen when patients interact with poorly grounded electrical currents. Sudden termination of EMI is common following an ICD shock as patients usually stop the provoking activity immediately. A tip–ring, near-field atrial channel; RV tip–ring, near-field RV bipolar signal; AP, atrial-paced event; AS, atrial-sensed event; Ab, atrial event in the blanking period; CE, charge ended; CD, charge delivered; FS, ventricular-sensed event in VF rate zone; FD, VF detected; MS, mode switch episode; VS,ventricular-sensed event; VP, ventricular-paced event. Source: courtesy of Karoly Kaszala, MD.

Some devices incorporate algorithms not to eliminate but to identify oversensing, thereby averting inappropriate shocks. One T-wave over-sensing algorithm uses a differential sense EGM to magnify the ratio of R-wave to T-wave amplitude, enabling RT pattern recognition (Figure 10.5) [16]. Sensitivity for VF is maintained at 100% with this algorithm, with 96% specificity for detecting T-wave oversensing. A noise algorithm is meant to avoid shocks secondary to lead fractures. It functions on the premise that noise secondary to a conductor fracture will be detected by the near-field (tip-to-ring) EGM, but not the far-field (coil-to-can) EGM. The algorithm cross-checks the EGMs and withholds therapy if fast events are detected only by the near-field EGM. Patients with EMI that affects both near- and far-field EGMs will not be protected against inappropriate shocks.

Electromagnetic interference

In patients with ICDs, ventricular oversensing from EMI can lead to inappropriate ventricular arrhythmia detection and shock delivery (Figure 10.6). In pacemaker-dependent patients, EMI may lead to suppression of pacing with resultant dizziness or syncope. ICDs are well

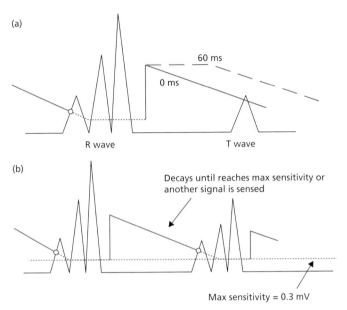

Figure 10.4 Decay delay and threshold start. Digitally rectified signals as used in detection algorithms. (a) Sensing begins at the open circle, initiating a sensed refractory period. The sensed refractory period is marked by the dashed line that crosses the R wave. In this example, 62.5% of the peak of the maximum amplitude signal recorded during this period is defined as the next "threshold start" value, indicated by the vertical line. As the sensed refractory period elapses, two examples of decay are provided, the first with no delay (solid blue line) and the second with a delay of 60 ms (dashed line). (b) Decay continues until maximum sensitivity is reached (dotted line at 0.3 mV) or another signal is sensed. Source: St. Jude Medical, Inc. Reproduced with permission of St. Jude Medical, Inc.

shielded from most sources of EMI due to bipolar sensing (versus integrated), electronic filtering, and noise reversion modes. Despite these improvements, EMI can still occur from both medical and non-medical sources. Medical sources include electrocautery, magnetic resonance imaging (MRI), radiation therapy, transcutaneous electrical nerve stimulation devices, and radiofrequency ablation [17]. Electrocautery delivers alternating current from a cauterizing device to a large return electrode on the skin (monopolar) or between two electrodes on the tip of the device (bipolar). Bipolar electrocautery generally does not interfere with ICD function and can be used without special precautions. Monopolar cautery, on the other hand, is a frequent cause of EMI in the operative setting and therefore requires special consideration. Use of electrocautery at distances more than 15 cm from the ICD generator is unlikely to result in inappropriate device interaction. For surgical procedures performed below the umbilicus, therefore, no device intervention (e.g. magnet application) is required [18]. For procedures above the umbilicus or where significant device interaction is anticipated, ICD arrhythmia detection can be suspended by placing a magnet over the pulse generator. In this situation, patients should have transcutaneous patches placed in case of need for emergent defibrillation. Reprogramming of the device is generally not required, except in cases where magnet placement or stability during surgery is expected to be challenging, or additional adjustments to pacing function (e.g. turning off rate-responsive pacing) are required. Preoperative management of ICDs in the setting of electrocautery is summarized in Table 10.3.

Interactions from medical sources of EMI aside from electrocautery are less common. All device manufacturers offer MRI-conditional devices as standard, since patients with pacemakers or ICDs will have a high likelihood of requiring MRI during their lifetime. Legacy devices, or devices with older components not classified as MRI-conditional, require special consideration. A large prospective database of

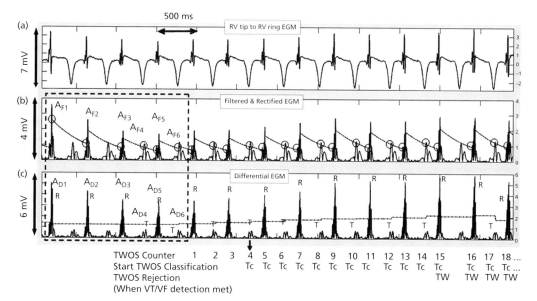

Figure 10.5 T-wave oversensing (TWOS) rejection algorithm. (a) Device stored right ventricular (RV) tip-to-RV ring electrogram (EGM) during spontaneous TWOS. (b) Filtered and rectified EGM (solid line) and auto-threshold (dashed line) with a sensitivity setting of 0.3 mV. The initial value of sensitivity is at 75% of sensed peak R or T wave (up to 10× the programmed sensitivity setting). Circles indicate the sense markers when sensing EGM exceeds the auto-threshold. (c) Differential EGM (solid line) based on filtered EGM. Specifically, Differential EGM(*i*) – Filtered EGM(*i*) – Filtered EGM(*i* – 1) at a sampling frequency of 1024 Hz. A_{Fi} and A_{Di} (*i* = 1–6) indicate the peak amplitudes for filtered and differential filtered signals, respectively. Comparing signal amplitude (differential versus filtered), T-wave amplitude is reduced more than the R-wave amplitude. The dashed line in (c) represents the threshold used to identify candidate R waves and T waves. In the six sensed event windows, the 3R3T or 4R2T pattern and other TWOS criteria will trigger the increment of TWOS counter. This event window moves beat by beat. TWOS is identified when four or more of the last 20 sensed events meet TWOS criteria (see "Tc" annotation). When ventricular tachycardia (VT)/ventricular fibrillation (VF) detection and TWOS detection criteria are both met, the "TW" marker is displayed, indicating VF or VT detection withholding due to TWOS rejection. The algorithm will not withhold VT/VF detection when the corrected RR interval as determined by the TWOS algorithm is less than max (SVT Limit, FDI; VT detection "off" or Monitor) or less than max (SVT Limit, TDI; VT detection "on"). SVT, supraventricular tachycardia; FDI, fibrillation detection interval; TDI, tachycardia detection interval. Source: Cao *et al.* [16]. Reproduced with permission of Elsevier.

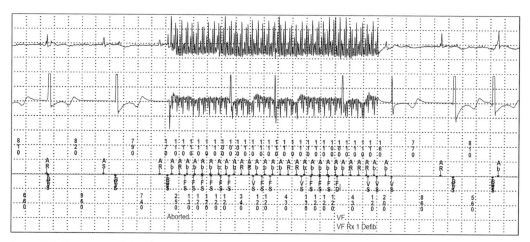

Figure 10.6 Electromagnetic interference due to electrocautery during surgery. Electrograms (EGMs) are displayed from episode stored on the ICD memory. High-frequency, non-physiological signals are seen on both the atrial and ventricular EGMs and recorded as ventricular fibrillation (VF) on the marker channel. Enough events are detected to satisfy VF detection (FD) and an ICD shock is delivered (not shown).

Table 10.3 Perioperative management of ICDs

General preoperative management
- Management in conjunction with the device clinic
- Device interrogation within prior 6 months to ensure proper function
- Clarify dependency status and magnet response (default is to inhibit detection, but programmable in some models)

General intraoperative management
- Patients with ICDs deactivated should be on a cardiac monitor with immediate availability of external defibrillation
- Use plethysmography or arterial pressure monitoring during procedure
- Limit electrocautery to short bursts (<5 s) in the absence of ICD reprogramming or magnet inhibition of therapies
- For monopolar electrocautery, place the return patch so as to keep the ICD system outside the current flow (thigh or ipsilateral limb)

Infraumbilical surgery
- Risk of interference minimal: either do nothing or place magnet over ICD generator

Supraumbilical surgery
- Inactivate ICD detection by placing magnet over ICD generator (preferred) or programming detection "off"
- In pacemaker-dependent ICD recipients: inactivate detection and pace in VOO/DOO mode (magnet has no effect on pacing)

Cardioversion/defibrillation with external pads
- Place pads in an anteroposterior position ≥8 cm away from the ICD generator

Postoperative management
- Identify the person responsible for reprogramming at the end of surgery
- If not reprogrammed, interrogate the ICD prior to discharge for cardiothoracic surgery or post cardioversion, or within a month for other situations, remote or in-person examination as per clinical situation

undergoing thoracic and non-thoracic MRI examinations with non-conditional devices reported no clinically significant long-term adverse effects [19]. Pacemaker-dependent patients should be programmed in an asynchronous pacing mode to avoid inappropriate inhibition of pacing resulting from detection of EMI, while an inhibited pacing mode is appropriate for patients without pacing dependence. Interaction of ICDs with other medical sources of EMI is rare. Transurethral prostate resection carries minimal risk of EMI in modern devices. Lithotripsy also incurs minimal risk, especially if it is directed more than 18 cm away from the device system. Risks of EMI associated with cataract and laser surgery are negligible.

Interactions with non-medical sources of EMI are rare. Airport metal detectors, laser therapy for cosmetic purposes, cellular phones, and all well-grounded appliances are unlikely to interfere with ICDs. *In-vitro* studies have prompted the recommendation to avoid keeping a cellular phone over the ICD pocket. Similarly, devices with small magnets, such as earphones, should not be kept near the ICD generator [20]. Interactions with anti-theft detectors are variable, with highest EMI risk associated with magneto-acoustic and electromagnetic devices. It is recommended that patients do not linger around such detectors. Arc welding and transcutaneous electrical nerve stimulation are generally not recommended due to the risks of ventricular oversensing.

Troubleshooting

Individual patients have unique risks of ICD malfunction or ICD therapy (appropriate or inappropriate). However, troubleshooting is guided by several general principles, including a careful clinical history surrounding the index event, physical examination, radiographic examination, and device interrogation (Figure 10.7). In addition, a clear understanding of device algorithms is essential when determining the reason a therapy was delivered or withheld. Delivery of inappropriate shocks or absence of appropriate shocks is most commonly due to improper programming or insufficient understanding of device algorithms.

Patient evaluation
After a single shock, it may be reasonable for an asymptomatic patient to non-urgently present to or notify a pacemaker/ICD clinic. However, in the presence of symptoms or multiple shocks, evaluation in the emergency department is warranted for rapid management. The clinical history surrounding the shocks should be elicited. Inappropriate shocks due to oversensing are suggested by a lack of

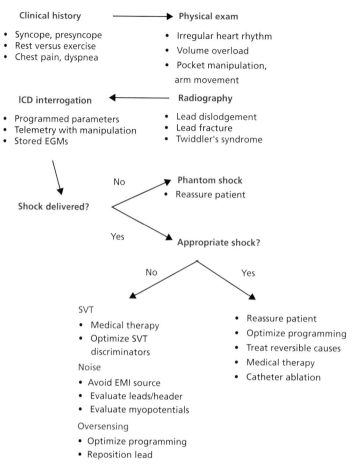

Figure 10.7 Flow diagram for evaluating ICD shocks. EGM, electrogram; EMI, electromagnetic interference; SVT, supraventricular tachycardia.

heralding symptoms (Figure 10.8). An ICD shock during exercise may be appropriate due to VT or inappropriate due to sinus tachycardia or rapidly conducted AF. ICD shocks associated with arm movement or body position suggest lead fracture, lead instability, or loose set-screw. Palpitations preceding ICD therapy may be due to either supraventricular tachycardia (SVT) or VT.

Physical examination helps provide further clues as to the cause of ICD therapy. Evidence of volume overload may suggest VT due to exacerbation of congestive heart failure. An irregular pulse suggests AF, which can be confirmed by electrocardiogram (ECG). When lead fracture is suspected, device pocket manipulation or arm movements with simultaneous device interrogation may elicit electrical noise artifact. Chest radiography can identify

improperly positioned pin connectors in the ICD header, a fractured lead, or a displaced ventricular lead (Figure 10.9).

Single shock

When a shock is delivered, one must determine whether it is appropriate (VT/VF) or inappropriate. Inappropriate shocks can be further classified as due to SVT, intracardiac oversensing (P, R, or T waves; Figure 10.8), or extracardiac oversensing (e.g. myopotentials, EMI, lead fracture). When reviewing EGMs, analyzing the rhythm using the same logic employed by ICD discriminators may help to determine whether a shock is appropriate. In single-chamber devices, an irregular rhythm is more likely to represent AF and gradual acceleration is more compatible with sinus tachycardia. The

(a)

ID#	Date/Time	Type	V. Cycle	Last Rx	Success	Duration
6	Aug 03 14:55:32	VF	210 ms	VF Rx 1	Yes	8 sec

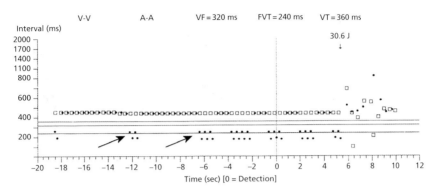

(b)

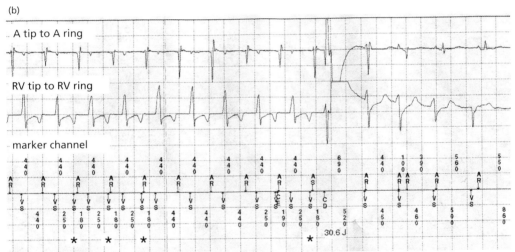

Figure 10.8 Inappropriate ICD shock due to T-wave oversensing. (a) Plot diagram in a dual-chamber device. Note the typical railroad-track appearance of intermittent T-wave oversensing events (arrows). (b) Electrograms retrieved from the device memory. T-wave oversensing is recognized by ventricular sense events corresponding to the T wave (*) and double counting. Due to baseline sinus tachycardia, these intermittent oversensing episodes resulted in an ICD shock. Source: courtesy of Karoly Kaszala, MD.

most challenging rhythm strips to classify are sudden-onset regular tachycardias that can be either SVT (e.g. AV nodal reentrant tachycardia, atrial tachycardia, atrial flutter) or VT. Arrhythmia termination by antitachycardia pacing (ATP) supports a diagnosis of VT, although the differential diagnosis may include atrioventricular (AV) reciprocating tachycardia or termination of an SVT by retrograde penetration of the AV node (Figure 10.10). Morphology can be useful when comparing the far-field channel from sinus rhythm with the one in arrhythmia. Morphology of beats that immediately

follow shocks should not be relied on for comparison because of possible EGM distortion. This does not apply to arrhythmias terminated by ATP.

In dual-chamber ICDs, addition of an atrial channel significantly increases physician accuracy for recognizing SVT, even if its value in reducing inappropriate shocks remains debated [21,22]. The simplest and most reliable method for differentiating VT from SVT is by identifying more ventricular than atrial events. This single criterion correctly classifies the vast majority of VTs. Transient ventriculoatrial (VA) block helps to identify VTs with 1 : 1 retrograde

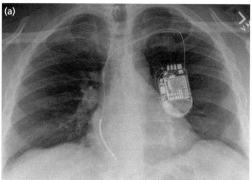

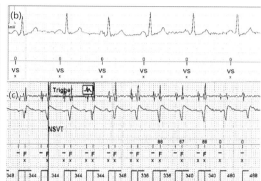

Figure 10.9 ICD lead dislodgement. (a) Chest X-ray demonstrating single-chamber ICD system with right ventricular lead displaced into the right atrium. (b) Simultaneous ECG and device marker channels demonstrating ventricular sensed (VS) events corresponding to P waves on ECG. (c) Non-sustained VT (NSVT) event due to double-counting (P waves and R waves). Due to intermittent undersensing of R waves, VF counters are reset and ICD therapy is not delivered.

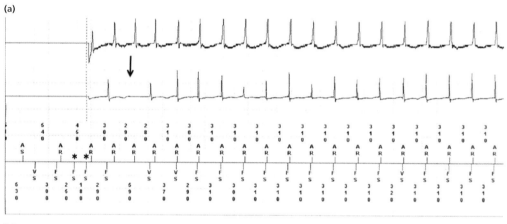

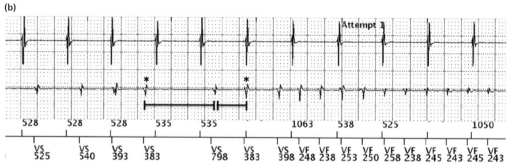

Figure 10.10 Two examples of tachycardia initiation by a premature ventricular contraction (PVC) in an ICD. (a) Consecutive PVCs (asterisks) result in initiation of supraventricular tachycardia with transient atrioventricular (AV) block (arrow) consistent with AV nodal reentrant tachycardia or atrial tachycardia. (b) PVCs result in long–short sequence initiating ventricular tachycardia with ventriculoatrial (VA) block. In both panels, top tracing is atrial electrogram, middle is ventricular electrogram, and bottom is marker channel.

conduction, which accounts for less than 10% of all VTs. Conversely, transient AV block (with V < A) favors a diagnosis of SVT. Additionally, it is useful to see how the arrhythmia was initiated. If initiated by a premature atrial contraction (PAC), SVT is likely; however, VT is more likely initiated with a premature ventricular contraction (PVC), although SVT may on occasion be initiated from a PVC as well (Figure 10.10).

Other situations may benefit from considering additional discriminators. In the presence of a double tachycardia, AV association may be useful in identifying atrial flutter, whereas a regular ventricular response during AF favors VT. When V = A, identifying slight variations in cycle length can further help to differentiate SVT from VT by determining the "driving chamber." A change in A–A interval that precedes a corresponding change in V–V interval supports a diagnosis of SVT, and vice versa for VT. For discriminators to function appropriately, reliable sensing is a prerequisite. Atrial undersensing can lead to an incorrect diagnosis of VT. Far-field R-wave sensing on the atrial channel may result in underdetection of VT if constant (A > V) or to an inappropriate diagnosis of VT if inconsistent.

Multiple shocks

Multiple shocks may be appropriate due to incessant or repetitive VT/VF or inappropriate due to SVT, oversensing or lead failure (Table 10.4). ICD shocks, whether appropriate or inappropriate, are associated with increased mortality [23]. Furthermore, they frequently cause significant psychological distress to the patient. The occurrence of multiple ICD shocks is a medical emergency and requires prompt evaluation and hospitalization for diagnostic work-up and patient management and support. Management of ICD shocks begins with determination of the underlying rhythm. If incessant or repetitive VT is the cause, treatment with intravenous beta-blockers or antiarrhythmic drugs (e.g. amiodarone) is usually effective [24]. If episodes

Table 10.4 Multiple ICD shocks

Cause	Management options
Incessant or repetitive VT/VF	• Judicious use of a magnet or inactivation of ICD therapy • Pharmacological therapy for VT (intravenous beta-blockers, amiodarone) • Replace electrolytes (K+, Mg2+) • Treat ischemia or other precipitating factors such as heart failure • Intra-aortic balloon pump or hemodynamic support for hypotension • Intubate and sedate patient • Sympathetic blockade with stellate ganglionic block in selected patients • Catheter ablation
Supraventricular tachycardia (SVT)	• Place magnet or inactivate ICD therapy • Pharmacological therapy for SVT (intravenous beta-blockers, calcium-channel blockers) • Program higher cutoff rates and/or discriminators if feasible • Catheter ablation
Lead failure	• Turn off detection and admit patient for lead replacement
Loose connection	• Reoperate
T-wave oversensing	• Reprogram if possible • Reposition lead • Force pacing if T-wave oversensing not present during pacing and patient not a candidate for lead repositioning
Diaphragmatic myopotential	• Change sensitivity and retest for sensing during VF • Reposition lead
P-wave oversensing	• May be difficult to program around since usually in integrated lead near tricuspid annulus or as a result of lead dislodgement • Reoperate
R-wave oversensing	• Decrease sensitivity and retest for sensing during VF • Adjust blanking period if programmable • Reposition lead
Electromagnetic interference (EMI)	• Identify source of EMI • Avoid source of EMI

VT, ventricular tachycardia; VF, ventricular fibrillation.

continue despite adequate drug therapy, sedation and intubation of the patient may relieve the sympathetic drive precipitating ventricular arrhythmias. Similarly, sympathetic blockade with injection of local anesthetic along the stellate ganglion has been shown to acutely reduce VT/VF episodes and may identify patients who will benefit from surgical cardiac sympathetic denervation [25,26]. Once the patient is stabilized, work-up and treatment of secondary causes of ventricular arrhythmia should be initiated. This may include correction of electrolyte abnormalities, treatment of heart failure, and evaluation and treatment of coronary ischemia. Monomorphic VT commonly occurs as a result of prior myocardial substrate and scar rather than acute ischemia. Coronary evaluation may be indicated for prognostic purposes but coronary intervention is unlikely to eliminate the source of the tachycardia. Ischemia typically causes polymorphic VT or VF and aggressive coronary evaluation is more appropriate in those cases in the right clinical context.

If ICD shocks are determined to be inappropriate due to abnormal but non-life-threatening arrhythmia (e.g. SVT, AF or atrial flutter) or to have occurred during sinus rhythm due to oversensing of T waves, EMI, or electrical noise artifact from a fractured lead conductor, the ICD should be immediately disabled via programming or placement of a magnet over the pulse generator. Accurate diagnosis of SVT (versus VT with 1 : 1 VA conduction, for instance) requires careful examination of the device EGMs, including tachycardia initiation (Figure 10.10a), changes in cycle length during tachycardia to identify the "driving" chamber, tachycardia termination or response to ATP (when present) as well as changes in far-field EGM morphology. In the setting of underlying AF, it is critical to distinguish between an inappropriate ICD shock due to rapid ventricular conduction versus an appropriate shock due to concomitant VT (Figure 10.11).

The characteristics of inappropriate shocks due to oversensing differ based on the cause (Figure 10.12). Improvements in device algorithms and programming have resulted in an overall decrease in the incidence of inappropriate therapy due to oversensing or lead fracture [27]. Non-physiological sensed signals due to lead fracture have several characteristics which allow accurate determination by device algorithms, namely (i) sensed intervals too short to occur due to successive ventricular depolarizations, (ii) non-continuous rapidly sensed signals, and (iii) absence of matching sensed signals on the far-field shock EGM (in bipolar leads). Of these, only the last is used by some devices to withhold ICD therapy, while the presence of non-continuous short V–V intervals is used to alert the physician of possible impending lead fracture but not to withhold therapy.

Unsuccessful shock

Failure to appropriately detect or treat a ventricular arrhythmia may be due to improper ICD function, ICD programming, or underlying cardiovascular substrate (Table 10.5). In the presence of an unsuccessful shock, all potential scenarios must be considered. The integrity of the ICD system should be verified, including the battery, leads, and high-voltage (HV) coils. SVT must be ruled out. The shocking vector is suboptimal for atrial arrhythmias such that it is not uncommon for shocks to fail to convert SVT (e.g. AF) in this setting. In interpreting a single isolated unsuccessful shock, one should bear in mind the probabilistic nature of defibrillation. However, in the presence of multiple unsuccessful maximum output shocks, the substrate should be reevaluated (e.g. ischemia/scar, progressive heart failure) and changes in drug therapy such as addition of amiodarone or sodium channel blockers should be considered. After an appropriate washout period, the DFT should be (re)assessed in the electrophysiology laboratory. In the event of a persistently high DFT, options include modifying the shock waveform (e.g. polarity, waveform duration, or tilt) and testing other shock vectors (including or excluding the superior vena cava coil or "can"). A suboptimal DFT can occur in the setting of an active "can" that has migrated inferiorly, thereby altering the shock vector. Additional options include lead repositioning, changing to a high-output generator, adding HV coils (e.g. superior vena cava, coronary sinus, azygous vein, subcutaneous array), or the use of drugs (e.g. dofetilide, sotalol) to help decrease the DFT.

Figure 10.11 (a) Rapid monomorphic ventricular tachycardia (VT) treated with antitachycardia pacing (ATP). The tachycardia is converted to a slightly slower VT with different morphology. Tracings top to bottom: NF EGM, NF EGM, FF EGM, Marker. (b) The continuation of the previous arrhythmia. Another round of ATP was delivered which resulted in termination of the VT. (c) Rapid monomorphic VT or ventricular flutter. Because of very rapid cycle length, ATP was not delivered because the tachycardia was faster than the minimum allowed VT cycle length. Primary defibrillation therapy was administered with termination of the arrhythmia. Tracings top to bottom: NF EGM, FF EGM, Marker. (d) Primary ventricular fibrillation successfully terminated by ICD shock. Tracings top to bottom: A EGM, NF EGM, Marker. (e) Onset of VT in a patient with chronic atrial fibrillation. Distinguishing features include an abrupt increase in ventricular rate with regularization of the cycle length. Additionally, a change in the far-field morphology on the shock EGM is evident (asterisk). Note that occasional undersensing of atrial fibrillation is present but does not affect the device's ability to appropriately classify the ventricular arrhythmia. A, atrial; NF, near field; FF, far field; EGM, electrogram.

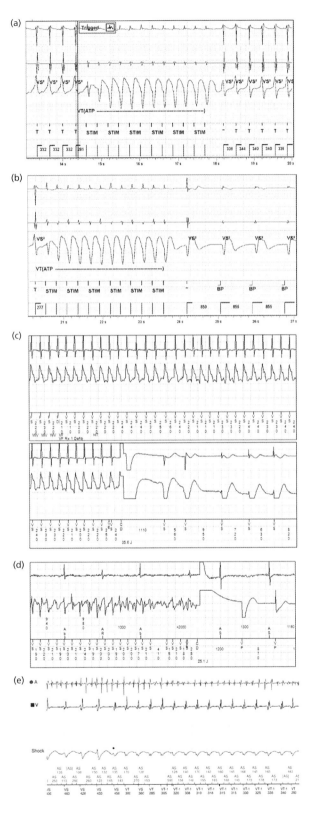

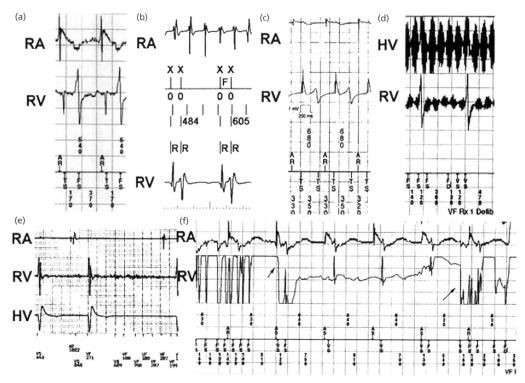

Figure 10.12 Types of oversensing resulting in inappropriate detection of ventricular tachycardia and fibrillation: (a–c) oversensing of physiological intracardiac signals; (d–f) oversensing of extracardiac signals. (a) P-wave oversensing in sinus rhythm from integrated bipolar lead with distal coil near the tricuspid valve. (b) R-wave double counting during conducted atrial fibrillation in a biventricular-sensing ICD. (c) T-wave oversensing in a patient with a low-amplitude R wave (note mV calibration marker). (d) Electromagnetic interference from a power drill has higher amplitude on a widely spaced high-voltage electrogram than on a closely spaced true bipolar sensing electrogram. (e) Diaphragmatic myopotential oversensing in a patient with an integrated bipolar lead at the right ventricular apex. Note that the noise level is constant, but oversensing does not occur until automatic gain control increases the gain sufficiently, about 600 ms after the sensed R waves. (f) Lead fracture noise results in intermittent saturation of amplifier range (arrow). RA, right atrium; RV, right ventricular sensing electrogram; HV, high-voltage electrogram. Source: Swerdlow and Friedman [28]. Reproduced with permission of John Wiley & Sons Ltd.

Failure to detect or treat sustained VT

In a functioning ICD system, the most common cause of absence of appropriate VT therapy is VT slower than the lower programmed rate cutoff [29]. This may occur in patients with high programmed cutoff rates or, more commonly, when VT is slowed by antiarrhythmic drug therapy. In patients with symptoms suggestive of an arrhythmic event with unremarkable device interrogation, a monitoring zone may detect slow VT. Lead sensing issues can compromise VT/VF detection. Undersensing can occur in the presence of small VF waves. In the presence of a second pacing device (e.g. epicardial pacemaker in a post-cardiac surgery patient), the ICD may interpret pacing stimuli as a normal rhythm leading to underdetection of VT/VF.

Less frequently, pacing or arrhythmia discrimination algorithms may result in VT underdetection. When SVT discriminators are programmed "on," criteria other than tachycardia rate must be satisfied to trigger therapies in the VT zone. Common discriminators, including sudden onset and rate stability, may falsely withhold therapy for VT with gradual acceleration into the VT zone or irregular cycle length. Underdetection of VT has also been reported

Table 10.5 Failure to detect or treat ventricular arrhythmia

Cause	Management options
ICD component failure	
• Lead dislodgement, fracture	• Revise lead
• Loose header screw	• Revise lead/system
• Battery depletion	• Replace ICD generator
• Energy shunting (abandoned electrode)	• Extract redundant hardware
Failure to detect	
• VT below detection rate	• Reprogram VT detection rate
• Undersensing	• Increase sensitivity, reposition lead
• Inappropriate classification as SVT	• Disable SVT discriminators
Failure to treat	
• Change in underlying myocardial substrate (ischemia, heart failure)	• Treat underlying ischemia, heart failure
• High defibrillation threshold	• Reposition RV lead; additional shock coil
• Electrical overstress (EOS)	• Replace ICD generator

VT, ventricular tachycardia; VF, ventricular fibrillation.

due to pacing algorithms such as rate smoothing, which reduces the maximum variation in cycle length by a programmable value. By minimizing short–long–short intervals, rate smoothing was developed to reduce the ventricular arrhythmia burden. Underdetection of VT may occur due to the ventricular blanking period that follows atrial pacing provoked by the algorithm. In addition, after each ventricular stimulus, the ventricular channel is blanked for a fixed interval. Although initially thought to be predominantly mediated by aggressive programming of rate smoothing (e.g. <12%), the potential for underdetection was later shown to be unpredictable. Thus, its routine use does not appear to be justified.

Finally, ventricular undersensing may rarely occur as a result of auto-adjusting sensitivity features and decay delay [30]. In certain sensing algorithms, the peak amplitude of a ventricular signal serves to establish the "threshold start" value, which is used to define sensitivity at the onset of the following cardiac cycle. This value remains fixed for a programmable amount of time, termed the "decay delay," after which it declines linearly. The higher the threshold start value and the longer the decay delay, the less sensitive the settings.

Patients with polymorphic VT, such as torsades de pointes, can have highly variable threshold start values that may undulate in an erratic or patterned fashion. Undersensing may occur when higher amplitude signals are followed by lower amplitude signals, particularly with longer decay delays (Figure 10.13).

Device proarrhythmia

Empirical programming of ATP for VT is an effective method for decreasing the frequency of ICD shocks. On rare occasions, however, ATP may accelerate or decelerate VT, or induce VT if inappropriately delivered. Shocks for VT or SVT, particularly low-energy shocks, can induce VF. When multiple consecutive events are recorded, an analysis of the first episode is critical, since subsequent ATP and shocks can cloud the initial event. Rarely, antibradycardia ventricular pacing can induce ventricular arrhythmias [31]. Typically, a pause followed by a back-up paced beat induces monomorphic or polymorphic VT. Algorithms aimed at minimizing pacing may occasionally result in lengthy pauses with ventricular proarrhythmic effects via short–long–short sequences (Figure 10.14). Proarrhythmia associated with biventricular pacing has also been described, likely due to preferential

(a)

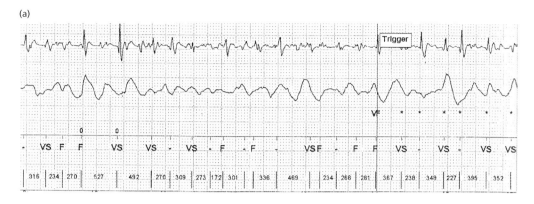

(b)

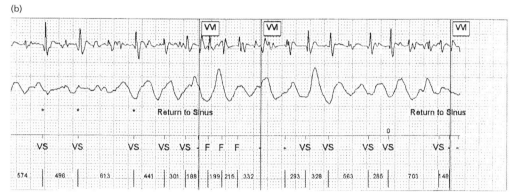

Figure 10.13 (a) Ventricular fibrillation (VF) triggered and (b) followed by return to sinus. Each panel, from top to bottom, shows intracardiac ventricular electrogram (EGM) recordings, far-field EGMs (ICD can-to-right ventricular coil), and telemetered marker channels. (a) Polymorphic ventricular tachycardia is noted with a variable amplitude and cycle length. The term "trigger" marks the recognition of VF. (b) Subsequently, due to ventricular undersensing, the ICD considers the arrhythmia to have reverted back to sinus rhythm. No shock is delivered. VS, ventricular-sensed event. Source: Michaud *et al.* [30]. Reproduced with permission of Elsevier.

conduction into slowly conducting myocardial channels in the scarred left ventricle initiating reentrant arrhythmia. Deactivation of the left ventricular lead may be required.

Subcutaneous ICD

The widely spaced electrodes on the subcutaneous ICD (S-ICD) have a sensing function that more closely resembles an external defibrillator than transvenous system. As the S-ICD does not provide bradycardia pacing, the device is not required to sense and classify each EGM. Rather, the device utilizes a sensing algorithm consisting of a detection phase, certification phase, and decision phase. In the US pivotal study, 99.8% of VT/VF episodes were appropriately detected [33]. Oversensing can occur, particularly when T-wave and R-wave

amplitudes are similar, and a screening process to evaluate for this possibility is mandatory prior to implant. If T-wave oversensing occurs after implant, causes such as subcutaneous air around the electrodes, metabolic derangements such as hyperkalemia, or migration of the lead or generator should be investigated (Figure 10.15). Reprogramming to an alternate sensing vector with larger R waves or a larger R-wave to T-wave ratio may eliminate the problem.

Conclusion

ICD programming options, governing algorithms, and potential therapies have evolved considerably over time, with important repercussions regarding follow-up and troubleshooting. Optimization of

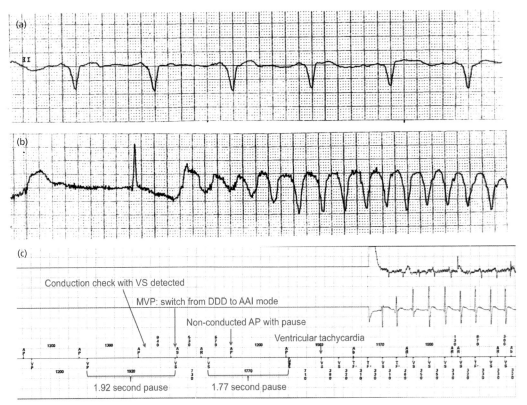

Figure 10.14 Electrical storm due to managed ventricular pacing. (a) Patient's underlying atrial and ventricular paced rhythm (lead II) at the lower programmed rate limit of 50 bpm. (b) A >1.9-s pause is terminated by a ventricular escape beat with a seemingly long QT interval (albeit recorded on only one lead), followed by the onset of ventricular tachycardia at approximately 170 bpm. (c) Tracing, from top to bottom, shows intracardiac atrial electrograms (EGMs), ventricular EGMs, and telemetered marker channels. The ICD initially functions in a DDD mode, with atrial (AP) and ventricular (VP) pacing. In accordance with the managed ventricular pacing (MVP) algorithm, verification for intrinsic atrioventricular conduction occurs after the third paced atrial beat. A 1.92-s pause is terminated by a ventricular escape beat (VS). Since a ventricular beat is detected between the two consecutive atrial events, the ICD reverts to an AAI pacing mode. The first atrial-paced beat is non-conducted, resulting in an additional 1.77-s ventricular pause, followed by the onset of ventricular tachycardia. Source: Mansour and Khairy [32]. Reproduced with permission of Elsevier.

device settings and effective troubleshooting require an appreciation for the various components of the ICD, their potential limitations and interactions, and the sophisticated rules and algorithms that determine signal recognition and interpretation and guide therapeutic responses. In order to fully understand ICD responses and troubleshoot accordingly, the clinician is challenged to keep pace with novel and emerging algorithms and options. While an in-depth understanding of ICD functions is critical, effective troubleshooting should extend beyond the ICD interrogation and incorporate all relevant external information, such as changes to pharmacological therapy, sources of device interference, triggers for events, and underlying substrates.

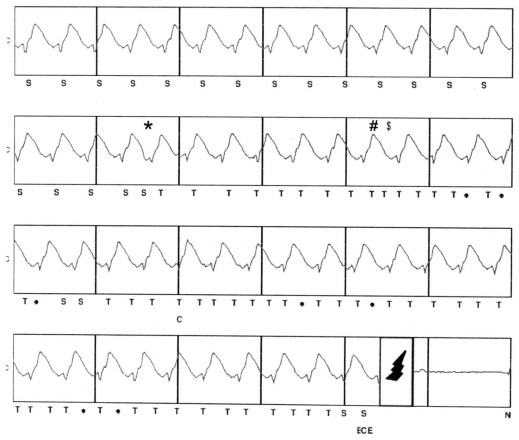

ECE

Figure 10.15 Inappropriate shock in S-ICD. The inappropriate therapy occurred in an end-stage renal failure patient without obvious electrolyte abnormality. Regular tachycardia is properly sensed (marked as "S" in the top tracing; note that the R wave is smaller than the T wave) until intermittent oversensing of P wave (examples marked by * and $) or T wave (example marked with #) occurs with double or triple counting and ICD shock at the end of the tracing. Note that for nearly all R waves there is more than one marker in the second half of the tracing. S, sensed event; T, tachycardia event. Source: courtesy of Karoly Kaszala, MD.

References

1 Wilkoff BL, Fauchier L, Stiles MK, *et al*. 2015 HRS/EHRA/APHRS/SOLAECE expert consensus statement on optimal implantable cardioverter–defibrillator programming and testing. *J Arrhythm* 2016;32(1):1–28.

2 Slotwiner D, Varma N, Akar JG, *et al*. HRS Expert Consensus Statement on remote interrogation and monitoring for cardiovascular implantable electronic devices. *Heart Rhythm* 2015;12(7):e69–e100.

3 Varma N, Epstein AE, Irimpen A, Schweikert R, Love C. Efficacy and safety of automatic remote monitoring for implantable cardioverter–defibrillator follow-up: the Lumos-T Safely Reduces Routine Office Device Follow-up (TRUST) trial. *Circulation* 2010;122(4):325–332.

4 Crossley GH, Boyle A, Vitense H, Chang Y, Mead RH. The CONNECT (Clinical Evaluation of Remote Notification to Reduce Time to Clinical Decision) trial: the value of wireless remote monitoring with automatic clinician alerts. *J Am Coll Cardiol* 2011;57(10):1181–1189.

5 Ricci RP, Vicentini A, D'Onofrio A, *et al*. Economic analysis of remote monitoring of cardiac implantable electronic devices: results of the Health Economics Evaluation Registry for Remote Follow-up (TARIFF) study. *Heart Rhythm* 2017;14(1):50–57.

6 Martin DT, Bersohn MM, Waldo AL, *et al*. Randomized trial of atrial arrhythmia monitoring to guide anticoagulation in patients with implanted defibrillator and cardiac resynchronization devices. *Eur Heart J* 2015;36(26):1660–1668.

7 Brambatti M, Connolly SJ, Gold MR, *et al.* Temporal relationship between subclinical atrial fibrillation and embolic events. *Circulation* 2014;129(21):2094–2099.

8 Hohnloser SH, Capucci A, Fain E, *et al.* ASymptomatic atrial fibrillation and Stroke Evaluation in pacemaker patients and the atrial fibrillation Reduction atrial pacing Trial (ASSERT). *Am Heart J* 2006;152(3):442–447.

9 Fischer A, Ousdigian KT, Johnson JW, Gillberg JM, Wilkoff BL. The impact of atrial fibrillation with rapid ventricular rates and device programming on shocks in 106,513 ICD and CRT-D patients. *Heart Rhythm* 2012;9(1):24–31.

10 Hindricks G, Taborsky M, Glikson M, *et al.* Implant-based multiparameter telemonitoring of patients with heart failure (IN-TIME): a randomised controlled trial. *Lancet* 2014;384(9943):583–590.

11 Swerdlow CD, Gunderson BD, Ousdigian KT, *et al.* Downloadable software algorithm reduces inappropriate shocks caused by implantable cardioverter–defibrillator lead fractures: a prospective study. *Circulation* 2010;122(15): 1449–1455.

12 Schoenfeld MH. Contemporary pacemaker and defibrillator device therapy: challenges confronting the general cardiologist. *Circulation* 2007;115(5):638–653.

13 Blanck Z, Axtell K, Brodhagen K, *et al.* Inappropriate shocks in patients with Fidelis® lead fractures: impact of remote monitoring and the lead integrity algorithm. *J Cardiovasc Electrophysiol* 2011;22(10):1107–1114.

14 Swerdlow CD, Asirvatham SJ, Ellenbogen KA, Friedman PA. Troubleshooting implanted cardioverter defibrillator sensing problems I. *Circ Arrhythm Electrophysiol* 2014;7(6):1237–1261.

15 Powell BD, Asirvatham SJ, Perschbacher DL, *et al.* Noise, artifact, and oversensing related inappropriate ICD shock evaluation: ALTITUDE noise study. *Pacing Clin Electrophysiol* 2012;35(7):863–869.

16 Cao J, Gillberg JM, Swerdlow CD. A fully automatic, implantable cardioverter–defibrillator algorithm to prevent inappropriate detection of ventricular tachycardia or fibrillation due to T-wave oversensing in spontaneous rhythm. *Heart Rhythm* 2012;9(4):522–530.

17 Misiri J, Kusumoto F, Goldschlager N. Electromagnetic interference and implanted cardiac devices: the medical environment (Part II). *Clin Cardiol* 2012;35(6):321–328.

18 Crossley GH, Poole JE, Rozner MA, *et al.* The Heart Rhythm Society (HRS)/American Society of Anesthesiologists (ASA) Expert Consensus Statement on the perioperative management of patients with implantable defibrillators, pacemakers and arrhythmia monitors: facilities and patient management. *Heart Rhythm* 2011;8(7):1114–1154.

19 Nazarian S, Hansford R, Rahsepar AA, *et al.* Safety of magnetic resonance imaging in patients with cardiac devices. *N Engl J Med* 2017;377(26):2555–2564.

20 Lee S, Fu K, Kohno T, Ransford B, Maisel WH. Clinically significant magnetic interference of implanted cardiac devices by portable headphones. *Heart Rhythm* 2009;6(10): 1432–1436.

21 Orlov MV, Houde-Walter HQ, Qu F, *et al.* Atrial electrograms improve the accuracy of tachycardia interpretation from ICD and pacemaker recordings: the RATE Registry. *Heart Rhythm* 2016;13(7):1475–1480.

22 Defaye P, Boveda S, Klug D, *et al.* Dual- vs. single-chamber defibrillators for primary prevention of sudden cardiac death: long-term follow-up of the Defibrillateur Automatique Implantable-Prevention Primaire registry. *Europace* 2017;19(9):1478–1484.

23 Poole JE, Johnson GW, Hellkamp AS, *et al.* Prognostic importance of defibrillator shocks in patients with heart failure. *N Engl J Med* 2008;359(10):1009–1017.

24 Chatzidou S, Kontogiannis C, Tsilimigras DI, *et al.* Propranolol versus metoprolol for treatment of electrical storm in patients with implantable cardioverter–defibrillator. *J Am Coll Cardiol* 2018;71(17):1897–1906.

25 Vaseghi M, Gima J, Kanaan C, *et al.* Cardiac sympathetic denervation in patients with refractory ventricular arrhythmias or electrical storm: intermediate and long-term follow-up. *Heart Rhythm* 2014;11(3):360–366.

26 Meng L, Tseng CH, Shivkumar K, Ajijola O. Efficacy of stellate ganglion blockade in managing electrical storm: a systematic review. *JACC Clin Electrophysiol* 2017;3(9): 942–949.

27 Auricchio A, Schloss EJ, Kurita T, *et al.* Low inappropriate shock rates in patients with single- and dual/triple-chamber implantable cardioverter–defibrillators using a novel suite of detection algorithms: PainFree SST trial primary results. *Heart Rhythm* 2015;12(5):926–936.

28 Swerdlow CD, Friedman PA. Advanced ICD troubleshooting: Part I. *Pacing Clin Electrophysiol* 2005;28(12): 1322–1346.

29 Thøgersen AM, Larsen JM, Johansen JB, Abedin M, Swerdlow CD. Failure to treat life-threatening ventricular tachyarrhythmias in contemporary implantable cardioverter–defibrillators: implications for strategic programming. *Circ Arrhythm Electrophysiol* 2017;10(9): e005305.

30 Michaud J, Horduna I, Dubuc M, Khairy P. ICD-unresponsive ventricular arrhythmias. *Heart Rhythm* 2009;6(12):1827–1829.

31 Theis C, Mollnau H, Sonnenschein S, *et al.* Reduction of ICD shock burden by eliminating back-up pacing induced ventricular tachyarrhythmias. *J Cardiovasc Electrophysiol* 2014;25(8):889–895.

32 Mansour F, Khairy P. Electrical storm due to managed ventricular pacing. *Heart Rhythm* 2012;9(5):842–843.

33 Weiss R, Knight BP, Gold MR, *et al.* Safety and efficacy of a totally subcutaneous implantable cardioverter defibrillator. *Circulation* 2013;128(9):944–953.

CHAPTER 11

Follow-up of the patient with a CIED

Arun R.M. Sridhar and Kristen K. Patton
University of Washington, Seattle, WA, USA

Introduction

Cardiovascular implantable electronic devices (CIEDs), which include cardiac pacemakers, transvenous and subcutaneous implantable cardioverter–defibrillators (ICDs), biventricular and His-pacing devices, require long-term follow-up and a thoughtful approach. The CIED patient differs from other procedural patients in that implantation of an indwelling device does not effect a cure for a disease, but creates the requirement for an enduring relationship with an overseeing clinician. This chapter outlines general principles of CIED follow-up over the course of the patient's life. Additionally, approaches to management of CIEDs in commonly encountered clinical situations, such as programming in the perioperative period, when using magnetic resonance imaging (MRI) and radiation therapy, and in other electromagnetic interference (EMI)-generating environments, are summarized. We review decision-making across the time course of device therapy, including reassessment of clinical need for device therapy at time of generator replacement, and management when the patient is nearing the end of life. For details of troubleshooting device malfunction and programming, see Chapters 7 and 10.

Acute CIED implant follow-up

Immediate post implantation

Following implantation of a new CIED system or after system revision of a transvenous lead, the patient is traditionally observed on a cardiac monitor overnight on an observational status. Increasing data support favorable safety of same-day discharge in many patients [1–3]. Adoption of this strategy has expanded due to the ability to perform next-day remote device interrogation Simple generator replacements are nearly always performed as a same-day discharge procedure (Table 11.1).

A 12-lead electrocardiogram (ECG), ideally with pacing, is obtained postoperatively. When ventricular pacing is not present, it can be useful to obtain an ECG with a magnet applied to the pacemaker generator site in order to capture the paced morphology (ICDs would inhibit therapy and would not pace with magnet application). This can be particularly helpful after a His-pacing lead implant in patients who are programmed to avoid ventricular pacing. A portable chest radiograph is usually obtained immediately following implantation to exclude a pneumothorax. Posteroanterior (PA) and lateral chest radiographs are usually obtained the following day to confirm satisfactory positioning

Cardiac Pacing and ICDs, Seventh Edition. Edited by Kenneth A. Ellenbogen and Karoly Kaszala.
© 2020 John Wiley & Sons Ltd. Published 2020 by John Wiley & Sons Ltd.

Table 11.1 Example same-day discharge (SDD) protocol for patients with cardiovascular implanted electronic device (CIED)

Inclusion criteria
- Patients having the following procedures may be considered for SDD:
  - Single, dual, leadless, or biventricular pacemaker
  - Single, dual, or biventricular defibrillator
  - S-ICD

Exclusion criteria
- Patient has a history of any of the following:
  - Cardiac arrest, sustained ventricular fibrillation or ventricular tachycardia
  - Pacemaker dependency
- Patient requires periprocedural bridging with heparin
- Patient lives >40 miles from a hospital or emergency department
- Patient is unable to monitor postoperative complications and/or follow standard wound care instructions. This includes circumstances that preclude next-day remote transmission (i.e. travel)
- Patient experiences an intraprocedural or postprocedural complication that increases risk of SDD
- Postprocedural device interrogation is not within expected parameters
- Physician discretion

Protocol
- Patients identified as potential SDD in clinic will be identified preoperatively
- Patients will receive a home monitor for device data transmission and be paired
- Patient is evaluated after implant for complications (surgical site inspection, telemetry, chest X-ray)
- Patients will be observed for 1–5 hours post procedure:
  - S-ICD or no leads placed: monitor for anesthesia recovery
  - Cephalic access: does not require 4 hour wait before PA/lateral chest X-ray
  - Axillary or subclavian access: PA and lateral chest X-ray 4 hours after access
- Patient teaching performed prior to discharge:
  - Review remote transmitter unit, what a transmission is and its importance, and what remote monitoring is not (not telemetry)
  - Sling and dressing removal instructions
  - Contact information (mobile phone number) for the patient to be reviewed/obtained from patient
- Discharge home with pain medications as needed

Postoperative day 1
- Remote transmission reviewed on website
- Results communicated to patient and attending physician

Follow-up
- Patients will undergo routine clinic follow-up (7–14 days) for an incision check and device interrogation

of the pacing and/or ICD lead(s) and generator and to serve as a baseline for subsequent comparisons. A CIED evaluation with assessment of the lead parameters and programming is performed the following day prior to discharge in order to assess stability and confirm appropriate programming.

Pre-discharge patient education

Education of the patient and/or caregiver is critical in the early postoperative period. Patients receive a tremendous amount of information regarding CIEDs, and often benefit from repetition and use of both verbal and written communication. Important topics include what to expect in the postoperative healing phase, warning signs of complications or device malfunction, expected follow-up protocols, the remote monitoring system, issues to be aware of when living with a CIED (e.g. what can produce EMI), traveling, what to expect for lead and generator longevity, and how to reach the clinic (Table 11.2).

The patient should be instructed on incision care as appropriate for the institution. Often, patients are asked to keep the surgical site dry for

Table 11.2 Spectrum of CIED patient knowledge areas

Knowledge topic	Patient illustration
Operative pocket complications	Normal healing and bruising, and warning signs (redness, swelling, drainage)
Postoperative lead complications (dislodgement, perforation, pneumothorax)	Symptoms: dyspnea, palpitations, syncope
Activity restrictions	Do not abduct arm >90° for first 4 weeks, or lift >4.5 kg on ipsilateral side
Remote follow-up	Keep transmitter plugged in, usually at bedside Mode of communication of transmissions Purpose, procedure (who to call) and effect of sending an unscheduled transmission Usual transmission schedule and what communication to expect from device clinic
Living with a CIED	Carry identification card What to do during travel Use of cellphone Driving Sources of EMI (? uncommon hobbies) and common household sources of unnecessary concern for EMI Education on ICD shock

1–2 days if skin glue is used or 5–7 days for sutures alone to minimize the chance of dehiscence. Patients should also be educated to recognize any signs of fever or infection, such as pain, redness, swelling, or drainage at the incision site, and must be informed of who to call if questions arise.

Patients are commonly instructed to refrain from vigorous activity involving the ipsilateral arm for a period of approximately 4 weeks to minimize the possibility of lead dislodgement and minimize undue stress on the incision. However, some data do indicate that shoulder immobilization can increase the risk of long-term pain and disability [4]. In small series, forgoing immobilization has not been shown to increase the risk of dislodgment, hematoma, or other postoperative complications [5,6].

Precautions to minimize interference from industrial and medical sources of electromagnetic energy should be discussed; equally important, the patient should be reassured regarding the safety in use of most common household appliances such as microwave ovens, cellular phones, electric vehicles, gardening equipment, and wireless communication devices. Driving restrictions should be based on the preprocedure diagnoses; from a CIED surgical standpoint, driving may be resumed after the patient is no longer taking pain medications [7].

Long-term CIED clinic follow-up

Organization of the CIED clinic

Most CIED clinics engage several types of clinicians, including physicians, physician assistants, nurse practitioners, nurses, and device technicians, and both the division of labor and workflow are highly variant. What has become increasingly important, as the number of patients followed in CIED clinics increases, is that procedures are set in place that allow appropriate long-term follow-up of patients and their device system, preferably as a dataset that is searchable in the advent of a device advisory or recall.

First postoperative visit

The first visit is routinely scheduled 1–4 weeks after implantation, and the focus is directed toward evaluation of the healing wound and health of the pocket. This is particularly important in patients with comorbidities that increase risk of impaired wound healing or infection. Worrisome medical conditions include diabetes, obstructive pulmonary disease, chronic renal insufficiency, heart failure, anticoagulation, and steroid use [8]. A relatively focused, yet comprehensive cardiovascular evaluation is merited, concentrating on excluding postoperative complications (pocket hematoma, infection, venous occlusion, lead dislodgement or perforation, etc.) and assessment of how the patient is functioning clinically, and if any changes in programming of the device are warranted (Table 11.3). The details of the examination will differ for conventional transvenous devices compared with leadless, subcutaneous defibrillator, or surgical epicardial devices.

Table 11.3 CIED clinic visit

Clinic visit component	Example
History	Overall status: energy level, exertional tolerance, fevers and other infectious symptoms, near-syncope, syncope, palpitations, dyspnea, arrhythmia, coronary and heart failure symptomatology Local symptoms: wound healing, amount of pain, vascular/thrombotic complications
Physical examintion	Assess vital signs Incision and pocket examination Examination for signs of heart failure Check access site if leadless pacemaker implant or after use of a temporary pacing wire
CIED evaluation	Interrogation of battery voltage, lead parameters, programming Assessment for arrhythmias Evaluate need to optimize programming parameters (rate response, maximum tracking rate, resynchronization or physiological pacing parameters, arrhythmia therapies)
Troubleshooting	Abnormalities of CIED function or of underlying medical condition
Communication	Documentation for clinical care and for tracking of device function over time

Second postoperative visit

A second follow-up clinic visit is arranged 6 weeks to 3 months post implant to reassess for complications, clinical benefit, appropriate programming and, importantly in systems that are not programmed to automatically assess pacing thresholds, to program pacing output downward from acute outputs to a twice-safety margin in order to conserve battery longevity. Most increases in pacing threshold necessitate evaluation with chest radiography, particularly when acute.

Annual or biannual visit

Annual follow-up visits should focus on evaluation of the patient's symptomatology and arrhythmia, heart failure, or device-related issue, device maintenance and optimization of programming. Because of the close follow-up afforded by remote monitoring, many patients are seen only yearly in device clinic. In-person visits offer distinct advantages, including the ability to perform a physical examination, assess physical signs not readily described by an untrained eye, perform specific maneuvers when assessing lead integrity and, lastly, develop and maintain an empathetic physician–patient relationship. However, office visits may be particularly burdensome for patients who are frail, have difficulties with mobility, or who live far from medical facilities. With increasing reliability and automaticity in modern CIEDs, and with the availability of reliable remote monitoring systems, less

frequent in-office checks have become more feasible and safe.

The standard assessment is similar to the previously described postoperative visits, although emphasis shifts to chronic management of arrhythmia-related issues and continuing assessment of the CIED system.

History and physical examination

Historical information sought is similar to that of prior visits (Table 11.2), with attention to how optimization of programming may serve to improve quality of life or lessen symptoms. New angina may develop following device implantation, and might require the lower rate and the rate response algorithm to be decreased pending evaluation. Sharp pleuritic chest pain can result from pericarditis. Dyspnea can result from pericardial effusion or from pulmonary thromboembolism. Either substernal chest pain or new dyspnea should raise concern for perforation and effusion. Exertional dyspnea or fatigue can occur due to lack of rate-adaptive pacing or inadequate rate response in a patient with chronotropic incompetence. On the other hand, an older patient might experience exertional angina or dyspnea due to an over-aggressive rate response. Upper rate behavior can account for exertional symptoms, for example a previously vigorous patient who receives a dual-chamber system for complete heart block may be exertionally limited with an upper tracking rate of only 120 bpm, especially if electrical Wenckebach or 2 : 1 heart block develops at the pacemaker's upper rate limit. Symptoms may also result from exercise-induced arrhythmias, pacemaker-mediated tachycardia, or other pacemaker programming features causing pacemaker syndrome.

Examination includes consideration of the chronic pocket to assess whether the device is normally mobile and not adhered to the skin and in danger of eroding, yet not too freely mobile and causing pain or risk of twisting in the pocket. Review of systems includes evaluation of symptoms and signs that might indicate need for changes in device programming (i.e. heart rate histogram and chronotropic incompetence, arrhythmia burden, maximization of battery longevity).

CIED pocket

The most common early pocket complication is hematoma (Figure 11.1), which occurs in 2–10% of initial implants, and is strongly associated with anticoagulant use [9–11]. Most hematomas can be managed conservatively by close attention and with consideration for withholding of anticoagulation [9]. Hematomas that are large enough to cause pressure on the skin, or that cause incision dehiscence or drainage, may need to be addressed invasively. Percutaneous aspiration of pocket swelling is not recommended, due to the risk of introducing skin bacterial flora into a potentially non-infected space. The development of hematoma is strongly associated with subsequent pocket infection. Unfortunately, data do not support a benefit to treating hematoma with antibiotics to prevent infection, although strategies aimed at reducing hematoma formation may decrease future infection risk [12]. Despite lack of supporting data, many experts advocate treating with prophylactic antibiotics until the hematoma has resolved. Conservative management is otherwise all that is usually required, with temporary cessation of anticoagulants, consideration of pressure dressing if hematoma is enlarging, and more frequent follow-up to look for signs of pressure on the pocket skin or incision dehiscence.

Pocket infections are rare in the initial postoperative period, and when present are usually due to *Staphylococcus aureus*, which is usually not subtle in presentation. Delayed infections are most often seen

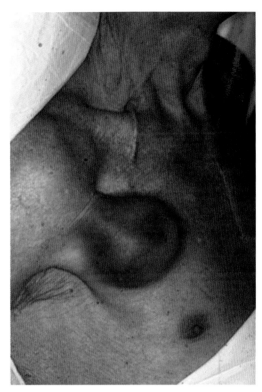

Figure 11.1 Large hematoma managed conservatively by withholding anticoagulation.

more than 6 months to even 2 years after generator replacement or revision [13,14]. It is not unusual for late pocket infections to be difficult to recognize or differentiate from insidious progression of pocket abnormalities, such as device migration, mild swelling, and skin adherence prior to erosion.

Patients may note caudal migration of the generator or superficiality of the pacemaker leads, but these phenomena are infrequent and of concern only rarely. In a healthy pocket, the generator is freely mobile beneath the skin. An immobile generator, especially when firmly adherent to the overlying skin, raises the possibility of occult infection or pre-erosion. Erosion of a generator or a lead is serious and may result in systemic infection.

CIED interrogation

A detailed review of device interrogation and programming is discussed in Chapters 6 and 8. The general approach includes a systematic evaluation of the CIED system, which comprises

Table 11.4 Approach to CIED interrogation

- Review of programmed parameters

- Display of real-time electrograms, marker channels, and ECG

- Evaluation of measured data and comparison with historical trends
  - Pacing thresholds
  - Lead impedance(s)
  - Lead sensing characteristics
  - Battery voltage and longevity

- Review of diagnostics
  - Heart rate histograms
  - Arrhythmia events
  - Pacemaker-mediated tachycardia (PMT) events: differentiate PMT, arrhythmia, or inadequate maximum tracking rate

- Special considerations
  - Minimizing right ventricular pacing with AV delay or algorithms
  - Adjusting rate response
  - Conserving battery longevity by adjusting pacing output or using autocapture
  - Assessing functionality of autocapture
  - Dynamic maneuvers for provocation of noise/oversensing

- Consideration of programming changes

review of programmed parameters, assessment of lead electrical parameters, evaluation of diagnostics, and consideration of programming changes (Table 11.4).

Battery follow-up

Various stages in the life of a pacemaker or ICD battery are recognized. A new battery is said to be at beginning of life (BOL) or beginning of service (BOS). With progressive battery depletion, most devices have a certain point designated the *elective replacement indicator* (ERI), *elective replacement time* (ERT), or *recommended replacement time* (RRT), when replacement is recommended within a short period (about 3 months). Beyond the ERI, devices reach *end of life* (EOL) or *end of service* (EOS), when immediate replacement of the generator is warranted since the functions become unpredictable. It is important to distinguish EOL from ERI. The former connotes gross device malfunction or lack of function; the latter strives to

indicate a time when generator replacement should be considered within a period of a few weeks to months. At or near EOL, transient high current drain from the battery may further reduce the output voltage. This may result in temporary or persistent loss of device function (Figure 11.2). Some devices identify an earlier point before ERI called *elective replacement near* (ERN), when close follow-up is recommended. ICD batteries (lithium–silver–vanadium oxide) have a *middle of life* (MOL) when they reach a plateau following the initial dip in voltage. Battery voltage drops gradually from an implant value of around 3.2 V to around 2.6 V, where it plateaus during the MOL of the device, and declines again as the device reaches ERI.

The behavior of devices approaching battery depletion is highly variable among different manufacturers and even among different models from the same manufacturer. Importantly, with some pacemakers (but not with most ICDs), the pacing rate in response to magnet application is altered at ERI and provides the primary means of discerning the triggering of ERI. Other device functions may be altered at ERI that are specific to the manufacturer and the device. With all manufacturers, rate response and certain diagnostic and storage features are disabled at ERI. With certain manufacturers, the mode of pacing at ERI is changed as well, i.e. DDD to VVI. These changes may produce symptoms of pacemaker syndrome in some patients; in such patients, it may be necessary to schedule generator replacement before ERI is triggered.

Lead performance trends

Historical information (including initial implant values) regarding lead impedance, electrogram (EGM) amplitude, and pacing threshold is recorded in most devices and is available for recall during interrogation (Figure 11.3). Lead conductor or insulation problems can be identified by the recording of non-physiologically short intervals between intracardiac events, which indicate lead noise. Algorithms incorporating several of these parameters may be useful in early identification of lead problems, for example the lead integrity alert from Medtronic has proven to be useful in early identification of Sprint Fidelis™ lead fractures (Figure 11.4) [15].

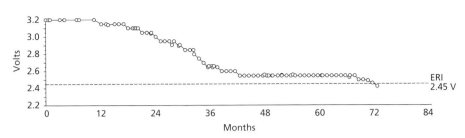

Figure 11.2 Graphic display of change in battery voltage over time of a St. Jude Medical ICD.

1: V Unipolar Tip 2.0 mm/mV
2: Markers

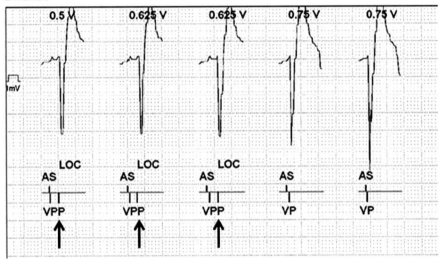

Test Results: Ventricular Capture

0.75 V @ 0.4 ms (Bi)   Dec 27, 2012
0.625 V@ 0.4 ms (Bi)   Jul 30, 2012

AutoCapture Trend

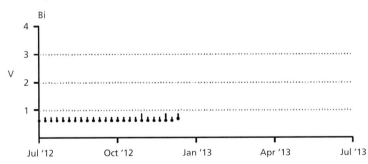

Figure 11.3 Right ventricular pacing auto-capture threshold test and historical trend. (a) There is loss of capture at 0.625 V at 0.5 ms, and appropriate capture at 0.75 V. With loss of capture, a back-up safety pulse (arrows) is delivered. (b) Display of pacing threshold over time.

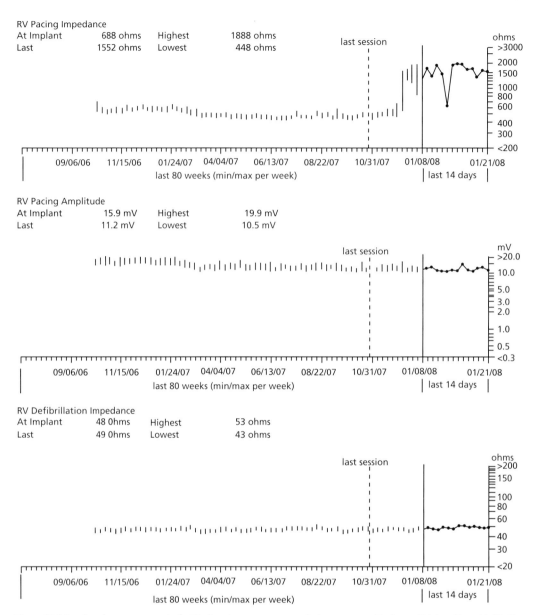

Figure 11.4 Lead performance report of a Medtronic Sprint Fidelis ICD lead from a patient implanted with a Medtronic ICD system showing trends in pacing imped- ance, electrogram amplitude, and high-voltage (defibrilla- tion) impedance. Lead fracture was diagnosed based on the sudden elevation in pacing impedance.

Programmability of polarity is often available in current pacemakers and, unfortunately, is not infrequently required. Problems with insulation defects in certain polyurethane leads subject to the "subclavian crush" syndrome, resulting in low impedance values, may be temporarily addressed by reprogramming from bipolar to unipolar mode. Some devices will automatically reprogram the lead con- figuration to unipolar polarity when bipolar imped- ances are abnormal. This maneuver will generally increase the lead impedance in these situations and prevent loss of capture and possible undersensing, but will not prevent oversensing from make–break electrical transients arising from contact between the two conductors. Ultimately, lead replacement is required in the pacemaker-dependent patient.

Occasionally, pacing or sensing thresholds will be significantly better in one polarity compared with the other. This may be helpful in the setting of marginal threshold values.

ICD shock

Patients require education about what to do in the case of an ICD shock, syncope, or tachycardia episodes. In general, patients who experience a single shock should be evaluated within 24–48 hours, as long as they are feeling well enough to wait. Initial evaluation in the otherwise well patient can be via remote interrogation, the clinic, or the emergency department. If a patient has received more than one shock, or if they are feeling unwell, they should be instructed to call the emrgency services for transport, or to come to the emergency room, since more than one shock may indicate either ventricular tachycardia storm or a lead malfunction.

Remote monitoring

CIEDs often are life-preserving or life-saving devices, and frequent monitoring of device function is extremely important. Remote monitoring has revolutionized the care of CIED patients by reducing the need for in-person visits, thus easing the burden for both the patient and the medical facility while not compromising on the quality of care [16].

There are different modalities of remote transmission (Figure 11.5). Transtelephonic monitoring is the oldest remote monitoring technology and has been in use since the 1970s. It requires the patient to make contact with two electrodes that record a single-lead ECG, which is then transmitted through a telephone connection to the device clinic. By studying the patient's ECG strips both during baseline and applied magnet rates, information can be deduced regarding device status, battery function, and problems with sensing and capture. This technology has limitations. Only real-time information is available, and no correlation can be made with past events or symptoms. Certain older device models only allow for this modality of ambulatory monitoring and not the newer forms of remote monitoring described here. Because of the widespread uptake of current remote-enabled CIEDs, the use of transtelephonic monitoring is rare and waning, in favor of current remote monitoring systems.

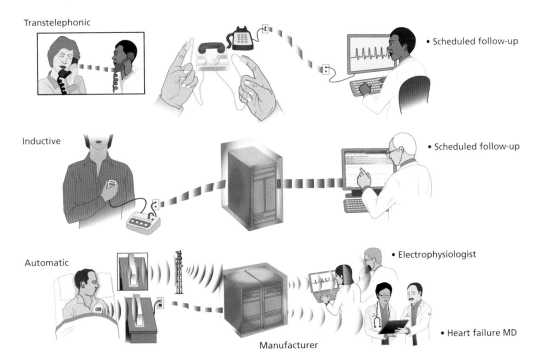

Figure 11.5 Technologies for remote monitoring.

Remote interrogation can be performed by inductive technologies or be automatic. Inductive technology requires the patient to hold a transceiver's inductive wand over the CIED generator to perform an interrogation. The drawbacks of an inductive system are reliance on the patient to establish contact with the transceiver and lack of CIED monitoring between scheduled interrogations. Automatic remote monitoring is wireless, does not require a wand or patient effort, and allows for nearly continuous monitoring of CIED system parameters and the occurrence of clinical arrhythmias. Most wireless remote monitoring systems rely on radiofrequency or Bluetooth contact for communication from the transceiver to the CIED system [16]. Usually the patient will have to be within about 4–5 m of the receiver, making placement of the device on the nightstand in a patient's bedroom ideal. Once set up, daily communication between the CIED and the transceiver ensues, without the need for any patient involvement. The transmitter delivers the data via a landline (increasingly uncommon) or cellular connection to a central repository, where the data are stored and processed. These data are then available for the device clinic or the physician for download and review. Most information obtained during an in-clinic visit check-up can now be obtained remotely (Table 11.5). Patients can also manually initiate a transmission by pushing a button on the transceiver. Automatic remote monitoring systems are set up to transmit information on a prespecified schedule, i.e. every 3–6 months. Certain "alert" situations, such as battery at ERI, lead impedances out of range, defibrillator shocks, or onset of atrial fibrillation, can be set as "alert criteria" to trigger immediate transmissions. Depending on the system being used, the device clinic, monitoring service, or clinician can be advised of these alert transmissions via page, fax, phone, or internet review. These systems still allow the patient to "trigger" a transmission if concerned about a symptom such as palpitations or syncope, a sensation of shock, or an audible alert.

Substantial data have indicated the benefit of both remote inductive follow-up and automatic remote monitoring in both pacemaker and defibrillator therapy, leading to the development of a Heart Rhythm Society (HRS) Expert Consensus Statement on this important topic [16]. Studies have shown that replacing in-clinic visits with remote monitoring or follow-up is safe and decreases the time to clinical response for actionable events [16–18]. A systematic review of remote monitoring of ICD therapy showed comparable mortality, with a reduction in all-cause mortality in the three trials that used daily remote monitoring [odds ratio (OR) 0.65, $P = 0.021$] [19]. Although the odds of receiving an ICD shock were similar in both populations, the risk of inappropriate shock was reduced in the home monitoring groups (OR 0.55, $P = 0.002$) [19,20]. Importantly, not only is remote monitoring associated with substantial clinical benefits, it is often preferred by patients, as it reduces associated costs such as time off work and necessity of travel to the clinic [16].

Frequency and mode of follow-up

The advantages of reliable and convenient remote monitoring has resulted in a paradigm shift in follow-up monitoring of CIEDs, from frequent in-office visits to frequent remote visits with periodic in-clinic care. This is reflected in the HRS expert consensus document, which is summarized in Table 11.6.

In-person follow-up is crucial in the immediate post-implantation period for CIEDs (before discharge, in 2–4 weeks, and in 4–12 weeks) to evaluate wound healing and recognize early complications. Subsequent follow-up can be predominantly clinic based (every 6–12 months for pacemakers, every 3–6 months for ICDs) or remote (every 3–6 months), with yearly clinic visits. Intensified follow-up (every 1–3 months) is recommended as the device nears battery depletion, depending on the platform and alert system.

Table 11.5 Available remote interrogation information

Battery status
Lead impedance
Lead sensing characteristics
Pacing threshold (if autocapture is programmed "on")
Activity sensor statistics
Percentage of pacing
Stored arrhythmic events

Table 11.6 Follow-up recommendations for CIEDs (pacemakers, ICDs, CRT devices)

	In person	Remote
Initial	Before discharge: same or next day	Next day if same-day discharge
	1–4 weeks	
Subsequent		
Pacemakers and CRT-P	6 weeks to 6 months	3–6 months
ICDs and CRT-D	1–3 months	1–3 months
Long term		
Clinically stable	Annual	3–6 months
Actionable event	Days to weeks as indicated	As indicated

CRT, cardiac resynchronization therapy.

For implantable loop recorders (ILRs), in-person or remote follow-up every 1–6 months is recommended. Patients with a CIED component on advisory may require more frequent in-clinic or remote evaluation. Deviations from the recommended schedule may also be needed for changes in the patient's clinical condition. Patients experiencing symptoms potentially related to CIED malfunction or arrhythmia are encouraged to transmit their rhythm when they are symptomatic, independent of these scheduling guidelines.

Advisories

Special considerations apply to patients who are identified as having devices that are listed in an advisory for a risk of malfunction (software or hardware). The nature of the abnormality, the clinical profile of the patient, and the probability of occurrence of the abnormality should serve as the basis for forming management recommendations. While the Food and Drug Administration (FDA) and device companies along with independent physician experts usually make overall recommendations, the final treatment decision should fall on the treating physician after the risks and benefits of all treatment options are carefully reviewed and explained to the patient. The device clinic is also responsible for timely identification and notification of those patients who may be affected by the advisory. Evaluation of the risk is commonly derived from return product analysis, a process that is seriously underutilized. It remains the responsibility of the implanting or treating physician to assure timely notification of any adverse events to the company and also to the FDA via the Medwatch reporting system in order to accurately capture possible systematic problems.

Special situations encountered by the CIED patient

Electromagnetic interference

EMI is the interruption of normal operation of an electronic device due to an electromagnetic field in the radiofrequency spectrum that is generated by another device. Common sources of EMI are found in the medical, industrial, public, and home environments. Electromagnetic fields are classified by frequency and wavelength, and have variable effects on devices [21]. Static magnetic fields, found in permanent magnets (i.e. MRI) or batteries, can trigger the magnet mode of a device, which can cause asynchronous pacing in a pacemaker or disable tachyarrhythmia therapies in a defibrillator. Low-frequency electromagnetic fields (LF-EMF) are the most commonly encountered type of EMI and can be difficult to filter due to overlap with local intracardiac EGM signals. Oversensing is common with all sources of EMI (Figure 11.6).

In a CIED being utilized for the pacing function, the most important clinical issue is that oversensing of EMI can lead to inhibition of pacing, which can result in asystole in the pacemaker- dependent patient. Most devices have noise response (noise reversion) algorithms, which can be triggered when EMI is sensed, leading to asynchronous pacing. Asynchronous pacing may trigger an arrhythmia

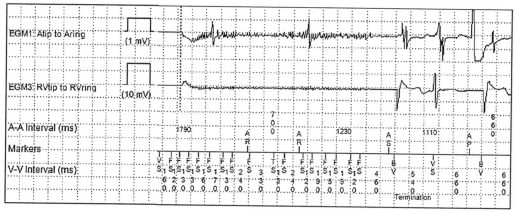

Figure 11.6 An episode of oversensing of electromagnetic interference (EMI) retrieved during device follow-up. Transient electrical noise artifact is seen on both the atrial and ventricular channels.

due to ventricular pacing in the vulnerable period, although in practice this risk is quite low. Oversensing of EMI can also result in inappropriate tracking, mode switch, or safety pacing. Oversensing of EMI by an ICD may result in inappropriate therapies, including antitachycardia pacing and shocks. Inappropriate therapies can cause significant discomfort to the patient, and carry the additional risk of triggering a true arrhythmia due to ventricular pacing and shock in the vulnerable period. In addition to oversensing, EMI can trigger the magnet mode or the power-on reset mode, and can rarely cause device malfunction. Various effects of EMI on CIEDs are summarized in Table 11.7.

General management strategies

General management strategies for EMI (Table 11.7) primarily focus on reducing the likelihood of exposure to EMI (avoiding known EMI sources if possible, keeping the source of EMI as far away as possible, and reducing the time of exposure) or minimizing the consequences of EMI [22]. The latter is targeted against oversensing of EMI, and may be accomplished by application of a magnet over the CIED or by reprogramming. In general, magnet application results in asynchronous pacing (DOO or VOO) in a pacemaker or disabling of tachycardia detection in an ICD. Reprogramming of the device to an asynchronous pacing mode and/or disabling of tachycardia detection can be done instead of using a magnet. Either strategy is appropriate in a patient with a pacemaker or in a patient with an ICD who is not pacing dependent. However, reprogramming to an asynchronous pacing mode along with disabling of tachycardia therapies is essential in a pacemaker-dependent patient who has an ICD. It is important to note that either magnet application or reprogramming only minimizes the effects of oversensing of EMI, and other effects of EMI can still occur. Strategies to minimize some of these source-specific effects are briefly discussed in the following sections.

Non-medical sources of EMI

Common household appliances, such as microwave ovens, toasters, and televisions, do not usually interact with CIEDs. Reports of EMI from household sources often relate to improper grounding or technical defects of the source device [21]. When using electrical tools, such as drills and chainsaws, it is prudent to maintain a safe distance (15 cm or more) between the motor and the CIED. It is important to ensure that all electrical equipment is properly grounded. Arc welders can interact with CIEDs and special precautions are necessary. Most CIED manufacturers have specific recommendations regarding these circumstances. Although it is commonly recommended to avoid magnetic mattresses or chairs, and devices that deliver electrical current through the body such as body fat estimators (bioelectrical impedance analyzers), some evidence suggests that these interactions may be safe [23].

It is increasingly recognized that cellphones may pose less risk of EMI than previously noted [24,25].

Table 11.7 Electromagnetic interference and CIEDs

Effects and consequences	
Oversensing	Pacing inhibition
	Inappropriate tracking (atrial channel)
	Inappropriate mode switch (atrial channel)
	Safety pacing (ventricular channel)
	Asynchronous pacing (noise response/noise reversion)
	Inappropriate therapies (ICD and S-ICD)
Magnet mode (response)	Asynchronous pacing (pacemakers)
	Inhibition of tachycardia functions (ICD and S-ICD)
Power-on (electrical) reset	Change in bradycardia parameters (pacemakers and ICDs)
	Change or loss of tachycardia functions (ICDs)
Device malfunction	Unpredictable failure of device function
Lead–tissue interface damage	Elevated pacing thresholds
	Induction of arrhythmias
Other	
Activation of rate response	Rapid pacing
Direct myocardial capture	Inappropriate pacing
Spurious programming	
General management strategies	
Reduce exposure	Avoid known sources if possible
	Keep source as far away as possible
	Minimize time of exposure
Minimize consequences (of oversensing)	Magnet application
	Reprogramming

Interference was more common in older devices without feed-through filters [26], and current CIEDs are less susceptible to interference [21,27]. Since most interactions occur at distances of less than 10 cm, a reasonable recommendation would be to avoid placing cellphones in the breast pocket over the device [21]. Some advocate holding the phone over the ear contralateral to the device while using it. Particular care should be exercised with high-powered fixed cellular devices such as those in cars and boats.

Digital music players can cause interference with programmer telemetry but are unlikely to affect CIED function. Portable headphones use a magnetic substance that can cause EMI and interfere with device function. All reported interactions occurred when the headphones were within 3 cm of the device, so the headphones should be kept a safe distance from the device [28].

Anti-theft (electronic article surveillance, EAS) devices are becoming ubiquitous in retail centers. Several different technologies are used to detect metal alloy-containing tags on merchandise. These have been observed to potentially interact with implanted devices, resulting in inappropriate device triggering or, in the case of implanted defibrillators, inappropriate discharge. Device reset with reversion from dual-chamber pacing to single-chamber ventricular pacing with resultant pacemaker syndrome has been observed. These interactions appear to be clinically infrequent, particularly with diminishing use of acoustomagnetic technology. Since interactions are more likely with prolonged close exposure, patients should be told to walk through the store threshold without either lingering or leaning directly against the gates [29].

Walk-through or hand-held metal detectors are used at airports and other places requiring high security. The detector alarm will usually be triggered by the CIED, but device function is unlikely to be affected because of the transient nature of exposure to EMI. Patients may pass through security metal detectors without lingering. Patients with implanted devices should notify security staff of the presence of the device. The metal-detecting wand may be passed over the device quickly in a single stroke. Repeated back-and-forth motions over the device are to be avoided. Tasers are sometimes used by law-enforcement agencies. These weapons use electrical current that can interfere with pacemaker or ICD function. Slot machines have been reported to cause EMI resulting in ICD shocks.

Some common non-medical sources of EMI and recommendations for patients with CIEDs are summarized in Table 11.8.

Medical sources of EMI

Interactions between CIEDs and various medical sources of EMI have been well described in the literature. The 2011 joint HRS/American Society of Anesthesiologists (ASA) consensus has an excellent summary of these studies [22].

Electrocautery

Electrocautery is often required intraoperatively and is the most common source of EMI in the medical environment. The monopolar configuration is commonly used and involves delivery of current between the cauterizing device and a return electrode placed on the skin. The bipolar configuration, which is less commonly used, involves delivery of energy between two electrodes at the tip of the device. Monopolar cautery can affect CIED function, whereas bipolar cautery does not cause any significant interaction.

Similar to any other source of EMI, electrocautery can cause oversensing that may result in inhibition of pacing output or inappropriate ICD therapies. In addition, it can cause irreversible damage to the generator or resetting of the device to a back-up mode. Procedures performed below the umbilicus are less likely to cause interference

Table 11.8 Selected non-medical sources of electromagnetic interference and recommendations for the CIED patient

Non-medical sources	Specific precautions
Household appliances (microwave, TV, toasters, electric can openers, food processors) Remote control devices Electric blankets Digital music players (iPods) Electric cars	No specific precautions required (minimal to no interactions)
Cellphones	Do not place in breast pocket ipsilateral to CIED Hold over contralateral ear Keep fixed high-output phones (car and boat) at least 15 cm away from device
Portable headphones	Keep at least 3 cm away from device
Electric tools	Proper grounding At least 15 cm distance between motor and device
Welding	Wear non-conductive gloves Keep welding cables away from device At least 1 m between welding arc and device Follow manufacturer recommendations for amperage
Anti-theft devices (EAS systems)	Walk through without lingering or leaning directly on the device
Airport metal detectors	Inform security personnel of device Walk through quickly (may trigger alarm) Hand-held wand may be passed quickly over the device
Devices that pass electrical current through the body (e.g. body fat estimators, TENS units) Magnetic mattresses or chairs	Avoid using without further testing

with a CIED located in the usual position in the upper chest if the return electrode is placed on the lower body. Interference should be anticipated with procedures above the umbilicus, and magnet application or reprogramming should be considered, especially if the patient is pacemaker dependent and/or has an ICD.

It is important to maximize the distance between the site of cautery and the CIED. It is best to avoid cautery entirely near the pulse generator, if possible. Bipolar cautery should be considered if required near the CIED. For monopolar cautery, the grounding pad should be placed as far as possible from the CIED and in a location where the vector from the cautery tip to the pad moves directly away from the pulse generator. Short bursts of cautery and the least required power settings are recommended. Surface ECG monitoring becomes unreliable when cautery is used, and an alternative mode of rhythm monitoring, such as arterial pressure or plethysmography, is essential. The device should be interrogated after the procedure if cautery is used near the device site.

Defibrillation/cardioversion

Transient undersensing and both acute and chronic rises in pacing threshold have been observed with defibrillation and cardioversion [30]. Some of this may relate to transmission of current down the lead(s) causing injury at the tissue–electrode interface, resulting in the potential for exit block. The majority of problems seen after electrical cardioversion are encountered with unipolar pacemakers implanted in the right pectoral fossa. To minimize these types of phenomena, cardioversion or defibrillation should be performed via an anteroposterior rather than anteroapical patch or paddle placement. Minimizing the defibrillating energy by using more efficient biphasic defibrillators is desirable. In addition, pacing and sensing thresholds should be checked following external defibrillation, either in person or remotely. Finally, equipment for temporary pacing should be close at hand, especially for a pacemaker-dependent patient.

Both electrocautery and defibrillation can produce irreversible damage to the generator. This is more likely in older devices that lack protective mechanisms such as Zener diodes, which shunt energy away from the delicate device circuitry.

They may also result in resetting of the generator to a back-up mode.

Endoscopy

Certain endoscopic procedures require the use of cautery, including treatment of bleeding ulcers and the removal of colonic polyps. Although there is a paucity of reports in the literature regarding interactions during these procedures, a cautious approach still seems rational. With endoscopic procedures where cautery will be used, placing a magnet over the generator in pacemaker-dependent patients and using a magnet or temporarily turning off tachycardia detection in patients with an ICD are reasonable approaches. Capsule endoscopy is an increasingly used novel system for visualizing the small intestine. The labeling on this device reports that it is contraindicated in patients with ICDs, although the contraindication was based more on theoretical concerns rather than hard data. Several publications have reported absolutely no effect of the capsule on pacemaker function. The largest report involved 100 pacemaker patients tested with an external device simulating the capsule transmissions and moved over the generator and along the chest wall. The distances between device and simulator were closer than those that would occur *in vivo*. There were no dangerous interactions. In four patients, the device briefly switched to a noise reversion, asynchronous pacing mode [31]. In rare instances, the output of the cardiac device can interfere with video acquisition from the capsule, i.e. with an abdominal pacemaker generator.

Left ventricular assist devices

Left ventricular assist devices (LVADs) may be used as a bridge to transplant or as destination therapy in patients with end-stage heart failure. Following LVAD placement, certain changes may be observed in lead function, including a decrease in sensed ventricular EGM amplitude, rise in capture threshold, and decrease in lead impedance. EMI between an LVAD and CIED resulting in oversensing is rare, but has been reported. A unique interaction occurs between the HeartMate™ II LVAD and St. Jude Medical ICDs, resulting in loss of telemetry [32]. This occurs because the LVAD pulse width modulator operates at approximately the same frequency as used for telemetry by the St. Jude Medical programmer. Metal shielding may be necessary to restore communication between the programmer and the ICD. Replacement with a device that communicates on a different frequency may be required.

Lithotripsy

Lithotripsy has the potential to cause pacing inhibition, triggered pacing at the upper rate limit, and activation of rate modulation [33]. The pacemaker circuitry, particularly piezoelectric crystals, may be damaged if they are located within several centimeters of the lithotripter focal point. Great care should be taken with abdominal implants. Lithotripsy synchronized to the R wave is less frequently used nowadays, particularly as it can add to the length of the procedure. This mode should be strongly considered in those with significant ventricular irritability, as the synchronized pulses are less likely to result in ventricular arrhythmias. If the lithotripter is used in a synchronized mode, care should be taken to ensure that the pulses are synchronized to the R wave and not the P wave or atrial spike, which can result in oversensing and ventricular pacing inhibition. In general, rate modulation should be disabled and consideration given

to programming to an asynchronous mode, particularly with pacemaker-dependent patients.

Transcutaneous electrical nerve stimulation

Transcutaneous electrical nerve stimulation (TENS) units do not readily interfere with modern bipolar pacemakers. In pacemaker-dependent patients, particularly those with unipolar leads, the ECG tracing should be monitored during treatment or reprogrammed to an asynchronous mode. TENS units have clearly resulted in inappropriate defibrillator shocks (Figure 11.7) [34]. Patients with ICDs who absolutely require TENS should have the marker channel observed with the device in a "monitor-only" mode with the first treatment to rule out any interference.

Radiofrequency catheter ablation

Radiofrequency ablation is undertaken in the electrophysiology laboratory for various atrial and ventricular tachyarrhythmias. Potential interactions include asynchronous pacing due to noise reversion, pacing inhibition, inappropriate ICD therapies, and device reset to the back-up mode. Rarely, threshold rises may be observed. Pacing inhibition is particularly relevant in the patient undergoing

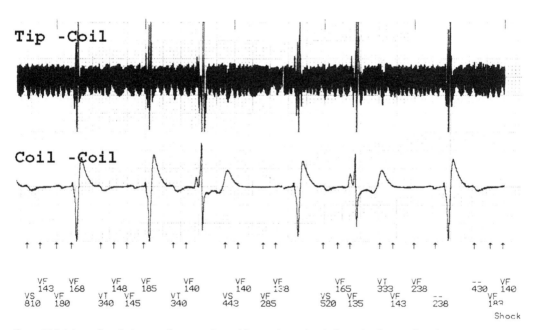

Figure 11.7 Intracardiac electrogram from a patient with a single-lead ICD undergoing transcutaneous electrical nerve stimulation. In the hope of achieving better pain relief, the patient independently turned up the output to maximum. This resulted in inappropriate detection of ventricular fibrillation and high-output shock delivery.

atrioventricular (AV) node ablation, which results in complete heart block and pacemaker dependency. Reprogramming the device to an asynchronous mode will prevent this interaction but loss of capture may occur if the right ventricular lead is at the His position. Tachycardia detection should be disabled in ICDs.

Other therapies

Electroconvulsive therapy (ECT) is safe in the pacemaker patient, although rare case reports of adverse effects on CIEDs exist in the literature, and underlie a recommendation to interrogate the CIED within a month of therapy [22]. Neurostimulators (deep-brain stimulators and spinal cord stimulators) may be used concomitantly in patients with pacemakers or ICDs, but testing for interactions is recommended [22]. Medical diathermy should be avoided in patients with pacemakers or ICDs.

Magnetic resonance imaging in the patient with a CIED

MRI presents a potentially harmful environment for cardiac devices. All components of MRI – the static magnetic field, gradient magnetic field, and pulsed radiofrequency field – can potentially interfere with device function.

- The static magnetic field can cause reed switch closure, resulting in magnet mode, and can cause unpredictable magnetic sensor activation.
- The gradient magnetic field and rapid radiofrequency pulses can result in oversensing of EMI, which can cause pacing inhibition, noise response, inappropriate tracking, or inappropriate ICD shocks.
- Heating can occur at the electrode–myocardial interface as a result of the radiofrequency field, resulting in thermal injury, increase in pacing thresholds, or myocardial perforation. This heating may theoretically be more pronounced with abandoned leads than with leads connected to a pulse generator.
- Rapid pacing corresponding to the pulse frequency can occur due to the effects on the output circuits.

Extensive research over the past several decades has resulted in the engineering redesign to modify the CIED system to allow for MRI-conditional labeling. In addition, considerable research has documented the methodology to allow for safe MRI of non-conditional CIED systems. These data and techniques are well detailed in the HRS Expert Consensus Statement on MRI and radiation exposure in patients with CIEDs [35].

MRI-conditional devices

Pacing and ICD systems specially designed for the MRI environment (MRI-conditional systems) incorporate several features: replacing the reed switch by a Hall sensor, changing the lead input-filtering capacitance to minimize energy induced on leads, adding internal power supply circuit protection, reducing ferromagnetic components, and developing lead geometry changes to reduce lead heating. MRI-conditional CIEDs also have a special software mode that must be activated by programming prior to entering the MRI environment. These modes temporarily disable therapy and feature high-voltage pacing output in asynchronous modes for pacemaker-dependent patients. Having MRI-conditional labeling therefore still requires programming changes and evaluation of lead parameters in order to protect the patient and the CIED system. This means that it is unsafe to send the patient into the MRI environment without appropriate programming, monitoring, and reprogramming after MRI (Table 11.9) [35].

Other considerations for safe imaging include (i) normal lead and battery parameters; (ii) no fractured, abandoned, or epicardial leads; (iii) 1.5 T MRI is preferred; (iv) gradient slew rate set to less than 200 T/m per second; (v) emergency equipment with external defibrillator and device programmer present during MRI; (vi) continuous patient monitoring with ECG and pulse oximetry during the imaging session; and (vii) specific absorption rate (SAR) and scan time limited.

It is important to understand that labeling of a CIED system as MRI-conditional requires that the leads and the generator have been investigated as a unit; therefore, if an individual patient's system has "MRI-conditional" leads from one manufacturer and a "MRI-conditional" generator from a different manufacturer, the system is a "non-MRI conditional" one.

Non-MRI-conditional devices

It has been estimated that 50–75% of patients with implanted devices will have MRI recommended over the lifetime of the device, and therefore

Table 11.9 Suggested considerations for institutional protocol for MRI in patients with a CIED

Radiology
- For all MRI requests, the presence of CIED and/or leads is noted
- Consider requiring chest X-ray image in system
- Evaluation of diagnostic need and potential alternatives

Cardiology
- Evaluation of CIED implanted system
  - MRI conditionality
  - Exclusion of abandoned, fractured, or epicardial leads
- CIED current status evaluation
  - Battery status, lead parameters, programming
  - Pacemaker dependence
  - ICDs: recent therapies that may warrant closer monitoring
  - Consider if MRI procedure requires patient consent

Scanning
- Schedule scan with device company representative or cardiology representative for programming as required by institutional protocol
- Pre-scan programming
  - MRI mode in MR-conditional systems
  - VOO/DOO high-voltage output in pacemaker-dependent patients
  - ICD detections "off"
- Continuous monitoring during scan
  - Pulse oximetry and ECG
- In pacemaker-dependent patients, understand need for closer monitoring
  - Appropriate personnel during scan in patients with non-MRI-conditional systems and pacemaker dependence
  - Abort scan if bradycardia in dependent patient
- Post-scan interrogation and reprogramming

Follow-up
- Continue usual remote and clinic device follow-up
- Include patients in quality assurance dataset

millions of patients with non-MRI-conditional systems will be candidates for MRI [36]. Fortunately, abundant data have demonstrated that patients with non-conditional CIED systems can safely undergo clinically required scanning, and specified how best to care for these patients [35]. These data led to a class IIa (moderate/"it is reasonable") recommendation for patients with non-MRI-conditional systems to undergo scanning if MRI was considered the best test for the patient, there was an absence of

contraindications, and there was an institutional protocol and responsible physician [35].

Specific adjustments for the patient with a non-conditional CIED system in the MRI environment include (i) programming to asynchronous pacing mode in pacemaker-dependent patients or to a non-sensing or non-tracking mode in patients who require rare pacing support; (ii) disabling tachycardia therapy in ICD patients; and (iii) disabling rate-response algorithms. Careful monitoring of the patient, including continuous verbal communication, ECG, and pulse oximetry, is essential, as is the presence of emergency resuscitation equipment and staff or designee to program the device, monitor as needed clinically, and resuscitate if needed.

For any patient with a CIED who will undergo MRI, there remain unknowns with respect to static magnetic field strengths in excess of 1.5 T, safety in patients with abandoned, fractured, or epicardial leads, or with high SARs, and how to maximize image quality of thoracic and cardiac studies.

Radiation therapy

Ionizing radiation has been used for over a century to treat malignancy. Photon-based radiation is the most commonly used modality, although in some circumstances electrons, protons, neutrons, and carbon ions are used [35]. A linear accelerator (LINAC) is used to create a beam of energy aimed at the target and multiple beams are used for convergence, which allows sparing of adjacent tissue. There are risks to the CIED system from therapeutic radiation, including random component failure due to interactions with high-energy neutrons produced by the LINAC, (possibly) transient oversensing, and cumulative dose delivered to the generator. The use of complementary metal oxide semiconductors (CMOS) in current devices makes them vulnerable to reset errors. Most malfunctions are recoverable reset errors that affect memory or programming; device failure is rare [35]. In previous decades, there was substantial concern regarding the total dose to the generator, due to older *in-vitro* and *in-vivo* studies; however, this paradigm has changed due to recent work. Three relatively large studies published in 2015, with substantially larger numbers of patients than prior studies, confirmed that the strongest association with device malfunction was not the total dose to the device, but use of a photon beam energy in excess of 10 MV [37–39]. These stochastic effects are due to inadvertent production of neutrons that occurs in association with higher beam energies [40,41].

These data underlie current management recommendations detailed in the 2017 HRS Expert Consensus on MRI and radiation exposure in patients with CIEDs [35] (Table 11.10).

Despite the updated guidelines in this expert consensus document, all major manufacturers recommend against radiation therapy if the CIED is within the radiation field. However, radiation therapy to the chest (e.g. for breast or lung cancer) may be unavoidable in certain patients with pacemakers and ICDs. In rare instances, a newly placed contralateral system or generator repositioning using lead extenders should be considered if the device blocks the intended target.

Table 11.10 Recommendations for management of patients with a CIED undergoing radiation therapy (RT)

CIED evaluation prior to initiation of RT	• Pacemaker or ICD • Location of device (left or right pectoral, left axillary S-ICD, leadless pacemaker) • Pacing dependence • Programming (lower and upper rates)
Beam energy	• Non-neutron producing if possible (<10 MV)
CIED follow-up	• Consider weekly interrogations in patients undergoing neutron-producing RT (may be unnecessary if remote monitored) • Consider weekly evaluation in pacemaker-dependent patients (may be unnecessary if remotely monitored) • Evaluation for all patients at conclusion of RT (may be unnecessary if remotely monitored)
During RT	• Visual and voice contact recommended
Generator relocation	• Only recommended if location interferes with adequate tumor treatment • Not recommended for maximum cumulative doses <5 Gy

Perioperative (periprocedural) management

The device physician is often asked to evaluate a CIED patient before surgery or other procedure. The main concern in this situation is EMI from various sources: many procedures involve use of electrocautery or cardioversion/defibrillation; other sources of EMI are specific to the procedure being performed. The periprocedural management of the CIED patient is to recognize and manage various sources of EMI pertinent to the procedure; these have already been discussed in detail. A recent expert consensus statement provides general guidelines for perioperative management of patients with CIEDs [22].

Most patients will not require a *de-novo* preoperative evaluation. Review of records should be sufficient to provide recommendations as long as the device has been interrogated recently (within the past 12 months for pacemakers and within the last 6 months for ICD and CRT devices). Patient factors (pacemaker dependency, programmed parameters), procedural factors (type of surgery, whether cautery will be used), and device factors (battery life, chronicity of leads, magnet response) should all be taken into consideration. Recommendations for use of a magnet during surgery or for device reprogramming should be individualized. It is essential to have equipment for cardioversion/defibrillation and external pacing readily available; placement of pads for this purpose should be considered in most patients in whom tachycardia therapies are disabled. Given the potential interaction of electrocautery and other sources of EMI with ECG monitoring, an alternative method of rhythm monitoring (plethysmography or invasive arterial pressure) should be considered.

After the procedure, the device must be reprogrammed prior to discharge or transfer from telemetry if the device was reprogrammed prior to the procedure, following major vascular or cardiothoracic surgeries, or if significant events including cardiac arrest occurred intraoperatively. In some situations with moderate exposure to EMI (monopolar cautery, ECT, lithotripsy), device follow-up within a month is recommended, or remote interrogation may be used. In other situations, routine follow-up should be sufficient.

Table 11.11 Selected medical sources of electromagnetic interference (EMI) and recommendations for the CIED patient

Source	Specific effects/comments	Recommendations
Electrocautery	Most common medical cause of EMI Device reset or malfunction can occur	Reprogramming or magnet application for procedures above the umbilicus Place grounding pad away from device Use short bursts of cautery Limit power settings Use bipolar cautery if close to device Monitor pulse with arterial line or oximetry
Cardioversion and defibrillation	Undersensing and elevated thresholds Device reset or malfunction can occur	Use anteroposterior pads, away from device Use biphasic shocks 5-min interval between successive shocks
Cardiac radiofrequency ablation	Random component failure and premature battery depletion	Reprogramming or magnet application
Left ventricular assist device (LVAD)	Interaction between LVAD and some St. Jude Medical/Abbott, Sorin/LivaNova, Biotronik ICDs	Metal shielding Generator replacement
Lithotripsy		Reprogram device (asynchronous mode, disable ICD therapies, disable rate response) Synchronize pulses to R wave Avoid submersion of generator
Transcutaneous electrical nerve stimulation (TENS)		Test ICDs in monitor mode with first session Turn off impedance-based sensor
Deep-brain stimulators and spinal cord stimulators		Test for interactions with CIED
Electroconvulsive therapy (ECT)		Disable ICD therapies
Medical diathermy		Contraindicated
Bipolar cautery Diagnostic radiation (X-ray, CT) Capsule endoscopy Nerve conduction studies (EMG) Dental equipment Wireless technology (RFID, wireless telemetry, flow pumps)	No significant interference	

EMG, electromyogram; RFID, radiofrequency identification.

Table 11.11 summarizes common medical sources of EMI and the recommendations for patients with CIEDs to minimize interference from these sources.

Improving the experience of patients with CIEDs

Caring for a patient with a CIED allows for the development of some of the more rewarding relationships in medicine. These longstanding connections can foster a deep understanding of a patient, and provide insight into their individual set of values, preferences, and support system. The natural habitat of an electrophysiology service, one that is based in a team approach to clinical care with various clinical members, can be effective in providing critical access, information and education, and coordination of care. CIEDs and the circumstances that lead to implantation can be complex; the amount of information available about devices is sometimes overwhelming and, depending on the source, can be inaccurate. Opportunities to educate patients about their device and cultivate a trusted bond are plentiful and worthwhile.

Shared decision-making and preference-sensitive decisions

In February 2018, the Centers for Medicare and Medicaid Services released a decision memo for ICDs which established a requirement for a formal shared decision-making encounter using an evidence-based decision tool prior to most primary prevention ICD implantations. The core principle motivating this concept – ensuring good understanding of the patient's values and medical preferences – should be extended to clinical decisions throughout the lifetime of the patient and their device. This applies to clinical situations as variant as arm movement restrictions, which range from none to chronic in different practices, to whether pocket pain is sufficiently bothersome to a patient to warrant the risks of intervention. Other common examples of occasions when patient preference is key to decision-making include whether to replace an ICD generator at ERI voltage in a patient with extensive comorbidities [42] or with a recovered ejection fraction, whether to downgrade to a pacemaker and forgo ICD therapies in a patient with response to biventricular pacing therapy or who is quite old or frail, and whether to follow, abandon, or extract a malfunctioning lead [43]. As in all areas of medicine, a good outcome is defined by what is valued and meaningful to the individual.

Patients nearing end of life or requesting withdrawal of CIED therapy

With aging and disease progression, the benefit of ICD therapy wanes [44]. Despite the reduction in mortality benefit of ICD therapy in patients with multiple comorbidities, data from the National ICD Registry indicates that over 40% of new ICDs are implanted in patients older than 70 years, and over 10% in patients older than age 80 [45]. Regrettably, a study of Medicare beneficiaries revealed that over 10% of primary prevention ICD recipients had dementia, and the corresponding 1-year mortality rate in this group was 27% [46]. Over 50% of Medicare aged patients who receive an ICD are referred to hospice or die within 5 years of implantation [47]. Some studies have revealed an astonishingly high rate of 20–30% of patients receiving ICD shocks in the last weeks to hours of life [48,49]. There is a critical need for clinicians caring for these patients to understand the palliative care requirements of this vulnerable population and to engage in forthright conversations about mode of death and patient preferences regarding shock therapies. The HRS Expert Consensus on the management of CIEDs in patients nearing end of life provides an excellent review of the ethical and legal underpinnings of this issue, and suggests conversational prompts to aid in exploring these issues [50]. Patient decisions may be nuanced; for example, many patients wish to leave shock therapies programmed on while forgoing cardiopulmonary resuscitation, especially if their current quality of life is reasonable [51]. What is not acceptable is the low frequency of clinicians engaging in conversations about the options of disabling therapies.

While there is general agreement about management of ICD therapies at end of life, deactivation of pacemaker therapy can be more challenging [50]. Although both legal and ethical precedents are clear that disabling pacemaker therapy in a patient with decision-making capacity (or when directed by a surrogate) is not equivalent to patient-assisted suicide or euthanasia but is withdrawing a burdensome therapy and allowing a disease process to continue [50], some clinicians are unwilling. In this case, the responsibility of the clinician is to refer to an alternative clinician who is willing to support the patient's goals of care. It is worth noting that in some cases the requesting patient/family may not understand the function of a pacemaker, and a conversation about the effects of disabling pacing therapies may allow reconciliation of views. For example, in the case of a patient who is actively dying, family members may need reassurance that the pacer is unable to create a heartbeat in a patient at the end of life. Likewise, understanding that pacing therapy may be allowing a better quality of life in someone who is not actively dying, but who relies on cardiac resynchronization, intermittent pacing for pauses that may prevent falls, or chronotropic competence and symptoms, may be useful.

We are privileged in cardiac electrophysiology to work in a specialty that allows for care across the lifespan of a patient. Communication regarding CIED therapy and the nuances of deactivation is a quintessential aspect of CIED care that starts before implantation and continues over the life of the patient.

Acknowledgments

We are indebted to the previous authors of this revised chapter, Drs. Harish Doppalapudi, Mark L. Blitzer, and Mark H. Schoenfeld.

References

1 Atherton G, McAloon CJ, Chohan B, et al. Safety and cost-effectiveness of same-day cardiac resynchronization therapy and implantable cardioverter defibrillator implantation. Am J Cardiol 2016;117(9):1488–1493.

2 Darda S, Khouri Y, Gorges R, et al. Feasibility and safety of same-day discharge after implantable cardioverter defibrillator placement for primary prevention. Pacing Clin Electrophysiol 2013;36(7):885–891.

3 Hess PL, Greiner MA, Al-Khatib SM, et al. Same-day discharge and risks of mortality and readmission after elective ICD placement for primary prevention. J Am Coll Cardiol 2015;65(9):955–957.

4 Findikoglu G, Yildiz BS, Sanlialp M, et al. Limitation of motion and shoulder disabilities in patients with cardiac implantable electronic devices. Int J Rehabil Res 2015; 38(4):287–293.

5 Naffe A, Iype M, Easo M, et al. Appropriateness of sling immobilization to prevent lead displacement after pacemaker/implantable cardioverter-defibrillator implantation. Proceedings Baylor University Medical Center 2009; 22(1):3–6.

6 Miracapillo G, Costoli A, Addonisio L, et al. Early mobilization after pacemaker implantation. J Cardiovasc Med 2006;7(3):197–202.

7 Watanabe E, Abe H, Watanabe S. Driving restrictions in patients with implantable cardioverter defibrillators and pacemakers. J Arrhythm 2017;33(6):594–601.

8 Polyzos KA, Konstantelias AA, Falagas ME. Risk factors for cardiac implantable electronic device infection: a systematic review and meta-analysis. Europace 2015;17(5): 767–777.

9 Wiegand UKH, LeJeune D, Boguschewski F, et al. Pocket hematoma after pacemaker or implantable cardioverter defibrillator surgery: influence of patient morbidity, operation strategy, and perioperative antiplatelet/anticoagulation therapy. Chest 2004;126(4):1177–1186.

10 Kutinsky IB, Jarandilla R, Jewett M, Haines DE. Risk of hematoma complications after device implant in the clopidogrel era. Circ Arrhythm Electrophysiol 2010;3(4): 312–318.

11 Masiero S, Connolly SJ, Birnie D, et al. Wound haematoma following defibrillator implantation: incidence and predictors in the Shockless Implant Evaluation (SIMPLE) trial. Europace 2016;19(6):1002–1006.

12 Essebag V, Verma A, Healey JS, et al. Clinically significant pocket hematoma increases long-term risk of device infection: Bruise Control Infection Study. J Am Coll Cardiol 2016;67(11):1300–1308.

13 Hussein AA, Baghdy Y, Wazni OM, et al. Microbiology of cardiac implantable electronic device infections. JACC Clin Electrophysiol 2016;2(4):498–505.

14 Poole JE, Gleva MJ, Mela T, et al. Complication rates associated with pacemaker or implantable cardioverter-defibrillator generator replacements and upgrade procedures: results from the REPLACE Registry. Circulation 2010;122(16):1553–1561.

15 Tzogias L, Bellavia D, Sharma S, Donohue TJ, Schoenfeld MH. Natural history of the Sprint Fidelis lead: survival analysis from a large single-center study. J Interv Card Electrophysiol 2012;34(1):37–44.

16 Slotwiner D, Varma N, Akar JG, et al. HRS Expert Consensus Statement on remote interrogation and monitoring for cardiovascular implantable electronic devices. Heart Rhythm 2015;12(7):e69–e100.

17 Crossley GH, Chen J, Choucair W, et al. Clinical benefits of remote versus transtelephonic monitoring of implanted pacemakers. J Am Coll Cardiol 2009;54(22):2012–2019.

18 Varma N, Epstein AE, Irimpen A, Schweikert R, Love C. Efficacy and safety of automatic remote monitoring for implantable cardioverter-defibrillator follow-up. Circulation 2010;122(4):325–332.

19 Parthiban N, Esterman A, Mahajan R, et al. Remote monitoring of implantable cardioverter-defibrillators: a systematic review and meta-analysis of clinical outcomes. J Am Coll Cardiol 2015;65(24):2591–2600.

20 Guédon-Moreau L, Kouakam C, Klug D, et al. Decreased delivery of inappropriate shocks achieved by remote monitoring of ICD: a substudy of the ECOST Trial. J Cardiovasc Electrophysiol 2014;25(7):763–770.

21 Napp A, Stunder D, Maytin M, et al. Are patients with cardiac implants protected against electromagnetic interference in daily life and occupational environment? Eur Heart J 2015;36(28):1798–1804.

22 Crossley GH, Poole JE, Rozner MA, et al. The Heart Rhythm Society (HRS)/American Society of Anesthesiologists (ASA) Expert Consensus Statement on the perioperative management of patients with implantable defibrillators, pacemakers and arrhythmia monitors: facilities and patient management. Heart Rhythm 2011;8(7):1114–1154.

23 Chabin X, Taghli-Lamallem O, Mulliez A, et al. Bioimpedance analysis is safe in patients with implanted cardiac electronic devices. Clin Nutr 2019;38(2):806–811.

24 Hekmat K, Salemink B, Lauterbach G, et al. Interference by cellular phones with permanent implanted pacemakers: an update. Europace 2004;6(4):363–369.

25 Burri H, Mondouagne Engkolo LP, Dayal N, *et al.* Low risk of electromagnetic interference between smartphones and contemporary implantable cardioverter defibrillators. *Europace* 2016;18(5):726–731.

26 Hayes DL, Wang PJ, Reynolds DW, *et al.* Interference with cardiac pacemakers by cellular telephones. *N Engl J Med* 1997;336(21):1473–1479.

27 Ismail MM, Badreldin AMA, Heldwein M, Hekmat K. Third-generation mobile phones (UMTS) do not interfere with permanent implanted pacemakers. *Pacing Clin Electrophysiol* 2010;33(7):860–864.

28 Wolber T, Ryf S, Binggeli C, *et al.* Potential interference of small neodymium magnets with cardiac pacemakers and implantable cardioverter-defibrillators. *Heart Rhythm* 2007;4(1):1–4.

29 McIvor ME, Reddinger J, Floden E, Sheppard RC. Study of Pacemaker and Implantable Cardioverter Defibrillator Triggering by Electronic Article Surveillance Devices (SPICED TEAS). *Pacing Clin Electrophysiol* 1998;21(10): 1847–1861.

30 Levine PA, Barold SS, Fletcher RD, Talbot P. Adverse acute and chronic effects of electrical defibrillation and cardioversion on implanted unipolar cardiac pacing systems. *J Am Coll Cardiol* 1983;1(6):1413–1422.

31 Dubner S, Dubner Y, Gallino S, *et al.* Electromagnetic interference with implantable cardiac pacemakers by video capsule. *Gastrointest Endosc* 2005;61(2):250–254.

32 Mehta R, Doshi AA, Hasan AK, *et al.* Device interactions in patients with advanced cardiomyopathy. *J Am Coll Cardiol* 2008;51(16):1613–1614.

33 Cooper D, Wilkoff B, Masterson M, *et al.* Effects of extracorporeal shock wave lithotripsy on cardiac pacemakers and its safety in patients with implanted cardiac pacemakers. *Pacing Clin Electrophysiol* 1988;11(11 Pt 1):1607–1616.

34 Philbin DM, Marieb MA, Aithal KH, Schoenfeld MH. Inappropriate shocks delivered by an ICD as a result of sensed potentials from a transcutaneous electronic nerve stimulation unit. *Pacing Clin Electrophysiol* 1998; 21(10):2010–2011.

35 Indik JH, Gimbel JR, Abe H, *et al.* 2017 HRS Expert Consensus Statement on magnetic resonance imaging and radiation exposure in patients with cardiovascular implantable electronic devices. *Heart Rhythm* 2017;14(7):e97–e153.

36 Kalin R, Stanton MS. Current clinical issues for MRI scanning of pacemaker and defibrillator patients. *Pacing Clin Electrophysiol* 2005;28(4):326–328.

37 Brambatti M, Mathew R, Strang B, *et al.* Management of patients with implantable cardioverter-defibrillators and pacemakers who require radiation therapy. *Heart Rhythm* 2015;12(10):2148–2154.

38 Grant JD, Jensen GL, Tang C, *et al.* Radiotherapy-induced malfunction in contemporary cardiovascular implantable electronic devices: clinical incidence and predictors. *JAMA Oncol* 2015;1(5):624–632.

39 Zaremba T, Jakobsen AR, Søgaard M, *et al.* Risk of device malfunction in cancer patients with implantable cardiac device undergoing radiotherapy: a population-based cohort study. *Pacing Clin Electrophysiol* 2015;38(3): 343–356.

40 Zaremba T, Jakobsen AR, Thøgersen AM, Oddershede L, Riahi S. The effect of radiotherapy beam energy on modern cardiac devices: an in vitro study. *Europace* 2014; 16(4):612–616.

41 Zecchin M, Morea G, Severgnini M, *et al.* Malfunction of cardiac devices after radiotherapy without direct exposure to ionizing radiation: mechanisms and experimental data. *Europace* 2016;18(2):288–293.

42 Beattie JM, Kirkpatrick JN, Patton KK, Eiser AR. Hardwired for life? Implantable defibrillator dilemmas in older patients. *Am J Med* 2018;131(10):1143–1145.

43 Kusumoto FM, Schoenfeld MH, Wilkoff BL, *et al.* 2017 HRS Expert Consensus Statement on cardiovascular implantable electronic device lead management and extraction. *Heart Rhythm* 2017;14(12):e503–e551.

44 Levy WC, Hellkamp AS, Mark DB, *et al.* Improving the use of primary prevention implantable cardioverter-defibrillator therapy with validated patient-centric risk estimates. *JACC Clin Electrophysiol* 2018;4(8):1089–1102.

45 Wright GA, Klein GJ, Gula LJ. Ethical and legal perspective of implantable cardioverter defibrillator deactivation or implantable cardioverter defibrillator generator replacement in the elderly. *Curr Opin Cardiol* 2013;28(1):43–49.

46 Green AR, Leff B, Wang Y, *et al.* Geriatric conditions in patients undergoing defibrillator implantation for prevention of sudden cardiac death: prevalence and impact on mortality. *Circ Cardiovasc Qual Outcomes* 2016; 9(1):23–30.

47 Kramer DB, Reynolds MR, Normand S-L, *et al.* Hospice use following implantable cardioverter-defibrillator implantation in older patients: results from the National Cardiovascular Data Registry. *Circulation* 2016;133(21): 2030–2037.

48 Goldstein NE, Lampert R, Bradley E, Lynn J, Krumholz HM. Management of implantable cardioverter defibrillators in end-of-life care. *Ann Intern Med* 2004;141(11): 835–838.

49 Kinch Westerdahl A, Sjöblom J, Mattiasson A-C, Rosenqvist M, Frykman V. Implantable cardioverter-defibrillator therapy before death. *Circulation* 2014; 129(4):422–429.

50 Lampert R, Hayes DL, Annas GJ, *et al.* HRS Expert Consensus Statement on the management of cardiovascular implantable electronic devices (CIEDs) in patients nearing end of life or requesting withdrawal of therapy. *Heart Rhythm* 2010;7(7):1008–1026.

51 Kobza R, Erne P. End-of-life decisions in ICD patients with malignant tumors. *Pacing Clin Electrophysiol* 2007;30(7):845–849.

Index

Page locators in **bold** indicate tables. Page locators in *italics* indicate figures. This index uses letter-by-letter alphabetization.

Cardiac Pacing and ICDs, Seventh Edition. Edited by Kenneth A. Ellenbogen and Karoly Kaszala.
© 2020 John Wiley & Sons Ltd. Published 2020 by John Wiley & Sons Ltd.